D1643971

Pain Procedures
in Clinical Practice
Second Edition

Edited by
Ted A. Lennard, MD
Clinical Assistant Professor
Department of Physical Medicine and Rehabilitation
University of Arkansas for Medical Sciences
Little Rock, Arkansas
Private Practice
Springfield, Missouri

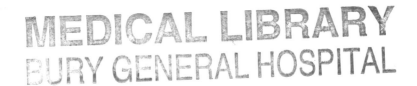
HANLEY & BELFUS, INC. / Philadelphia

Publisher   HANLEY & BELFUS, INC.
Medical Publishers
210 S. 13th Street
Philadelphia, PA 19107
(215) 546-4995
FAX (215) 790-9330
www.hanleyandbelfus.com

Library of Congress Cataloging-in-Publication Data

Pain procedures in clinical practice / edited by Ted A. Lennard. — 2nd ed.
     p. ; cm.
     Includes bibliographical references and index.
     ISBN 1-56053-367-6 (alk. paper)
       1. Medicine, Physical. 2. Medical rehabilitation. I. Lennard, Ted A., 1961–
     [DNLM: 1. Physical Medicine—methods. 2. Rehabilitation. WB 460 P577 2000]
   RM700 .P46 2000
   617'.03—dc21

                                             99-042857

PAIN PROCEDURES IN CLINICAL PRACTICE, 2nd edition   ISBN 2-56053-367-6

Last digit is the print number: 9   8   7   6   5   4   3   2   1

Contents

IV. SOFT TISSUE AND PERIPHERAL JOINT PROCEDURES

V. SPINE PROCEDURES

Contributors

Russell R. Bond, D.O.
Southwest Physical Medicine and Rehabilitation, Springfield, Missouri

Kenneth P. Botwin, M.D.
Fellowship Director, Florida Spine Institute, Clearwater, Florida; Sun Coast Hospital, Largo, Florida

D. Wayne Brooks, M.D.
Northwest Rehabilitation Hospital, Fayetteville, Arkansas

Martin K. Childers, D.O.
Assistant Professor, Department of Physical Medicine and Rehabilitation, University of Missouri, Columbia, School of Medicine; Faculty Member, Rusk/HealthSouth Rehabilitation Center; Courtesy Faculty, University of Missouri Hospital and Clinics, Columbia, Missouri

Susan M. Donnelly, J.D.
Attorney, Murphy & Riley, P.C., Boston, Massachusetts

Susan J. Dreyer, M.D.
Assistant Professor, Departments of Orthopaedic Surgery and Physical Medicine and Rehabilitation, Emory University School of Medicine; Emory Spine Center, Atlanta, Georgia

Paul Dreyfuss, M.D.
Clinical Associate Professor, Department of Rehabilitation Medicine, University of Texas Health Science Center at San Antonio, San Antonio, Texas; East Texas Medical Center, Tyler, Texas

Frank J. E. Falco, M.D., FAAPMR, FAAEM, FAAPM
Department of Physical Medicine and Rehabilitation, Temple University School of Medicine, Philadelphia, Pennsylvania; Mid-Atlantic Pain Institute, Wilmington, Delaware

Andrew A. Fischer, M.D., Ph.D.
Associate Clinical Professor, Department of Rehabilitation Medicine, Mount Sinai Medical School, City University of New York, New York, New York; St. Francis Medical Center, Roslyn, New York

Joseph D. Fortin, D.O.
Clinical Assistant Professor, Department of Physical Medicine and Rehabilitation, Indiana University School of Medicine; Medical Director, Spine Technology and Rehabilitation, Fort Wayne, Indiana

Steve R. Geiringer, M.D.
Professor, Department of Physical Medicine and Rehabilitation, Wayne State University School of Medicine, Detroit, Michigan

Herman C. Gore, M.D.
Co-Director, The Pain Center, Department of Anesthesia, Gaston Memorial Hospital, Gastonia, North Carolina

Richard P. Gray, M.D.
Department of Physical Medicine and Rehabilitation, University of Arkansas for Medical Sciences; Staff Physician, Central Arkansas Veterans Affairs Health Care System, Little Rock, Arkansas

Robert D. Gruber, D.O.
Medical Director, Florida Spine Institute; Morton Plant/Meese Hospital, Clearwater, Florida; Sun Coast Hospital; Largo Medical Center; HealthSouth Hospital, Largo, Florida

Phala A. Helm, M.D.
Professor, Department of Physical Medicine and Rehabilitation, University of Texas Southwestern Medical Center at Dallas; Parkland Hospital; Zale Lipsky Hospital, Dallas, Texas

Joseph M. Helms, M.D.
Chairman, Physician Acupuncture Education, Office of Continuing Medical Education, University of California, Los Angeles, UCLA School of Medicine, Los Angeles, California; Director, Helms Medical Institute, Berkeley, California

Stanley A. Herring, M.D.
Clinical Professor, Departments of Rehabilitation Medicine and Orthopaedics, University of Washington School of Medicine; Puget Sound Sports and Spine Physicians, Seattle, Washington

Marta Imamura, M.D., Ph.D.
Attending, Division of Physical Medicine and
Rehabilitation, Institute of Orthopedics and
Traumatology, University of Sao Paulo, Sao Paulo,
Brazil

Michael Kaplan, M.D.
Department of Physical Medicine and
Rehabilitation, Gem City Bone and Joint, P.C.;
Gem City Bone and Joint Ambulatory Center;
Ivinson Memorial Hospital, Laramie,
Wyoming

Ted A. Lennard, M.D.
Clinical Assistant Professor, Department of Physical
Medicine and Rehabilitation, University of Arkansas
for Medical Sciences, Little Rock, Arkansas; Private
Practice, Springfield, Missouri

Dennis M. Lox, M.D.
All Florida Orthopaedic Associates, St. Petersburg,
Florida

Dennis J. Matthews, M.D.
Associate Professor and Chairman, Department of
Rehabilitation Medicine, University of Colorado
School of Medicine; Children's Hospital, Denver,
Colorado

Charles C. Mauldin, M.D.
Springfield Physical Medicine and Rehabilitation,
P.C., Springfield, Missouri

Marcie A. Merson, M.D.
Fellow, Georgia Pain Physicians, P.C., Marietta,
Georgia

David L. Nash, M.D.
Assistant Professor, Department of Physical Medicine
and Rehabilitation, Mayo Medical School; St. Mary's
Hospital, Rochester, Minnesota

David F. Neale, M.D.
Assistant Professor, Department of Physical
Medicine and Rehabilitation, University
of Arkansas for Medical Sciences, Little Rock,
Arkansas; Physical Medicine and Rehabilitation
Service, Central Arkansas Veterans Affairs Health
Care System, North Little Rock, Arkansas

Ricardo A. Nieves, M.D.
Spine Technology and Rehabilitation, Fort Wayne,
Indiana

John P. Obermiller, M.D.
Assistant Clinical Professor, Department of Physical
Medicine and Rehabilitation, University of Texas
Health Science Center at San Antonio, San Antonio,
Texas

Nicholas K. Olsen, D.O.
Rehabilitation Associates of Colorado, P.C.;
North Suburban Medical Center, Thornton,
Colorado; Swedish Medical Center, Englewood,
Colorado; Porter Medical Center, Denver,
Colorado

Kevin Pauza, M.D.
East Texas Medical Center, Neurological Institute,
Tyler, Texas

Inder Perkash, M.D., FRCS, FACS
Professor, Departments of Urology and Functional
Restoration, and Paralyzed Veterans of America
Professor of Spinal Cord Injury Medicine, Stanford
University School of Medicine; Stanford University
Medical Center; Chief, Spinal Cord Injury Service,
Veterans Affairs Palo Alto Health Care System, Palo
Alto, California

Elmer G. Pinzon, M.D., M.P.H.
Interventional Staff Physiatrist, Charlotte Spine
Center, Charlotte Orthopedic Specialists; Staff
Physiatrist, Presbyterian-Orthopaedic Hospital;
Presbyterian Hospital; Carolinas Medical Center;
University Hospital; Mercy Hospital, Charlotte,
North Carolina

Joel M. Press, M.D.
Assistant Professor, Department of Physical Medicine
and Rehabilitation, Northwestern University Medical
School; Rehabilitation Institute of Chicago, Chicago,
Illinois

K. Dean Reeves, M.D.
Section Chief, Department of Physical Medicine and
Rehabilitation, Bethany Medical Center; Providence
Medical Center, Kansas City, Kansas; Shawnee
Mission Medical Center, Shawnee Mission, Kansas;
Mid-America Rehabilitation Hospital, Overland
Park, Kansas

Christopher J. Rogers, M.D.
Assistant Clinical Professor, Department of
Orthopaedics, University of California, San Diego,
School of Medicine; Thornton Hospital, San Diego,
California

Robert G. Schwartz, M.D.
Piedmont Physical Medicine and Rehabilitation, P.A.,
Greenville, South Carolina

Nalini Sehgal, M.D.
Spine Technology and Rehabilitation, Fort Wayne,
Indiana

Chunilal P. Shah, M.D.
Florida Spine Institute, Clearwater, Florida

Daniel Y. Shin, M.D.
Associate Clinical Professor, Department of
Orthopedics, University of Southern California
School of Medicine, Los Angeles, California;
Director, Rehab West Medical Group, and Medical
Director, Acute Physical Rehabilitation Center,
Downey Community Hospitals Foundation;
Director, Neuromuscular Diagnostics Laboratory,
Rancho Los Amigos Medical Center, Downey,
California

Julie K. Silver, M.D.
Instructor, Department of Physical Medicine and
Rehabilitation, Harvard Medical School, Boston,
Massachusetts; Medical Director, Spaulding
Framingham Outpatient Center, Framingham,
Massachusetts

David G. Simons, M.D.
Clinical Professor, Department of Rehabilitation
Medicine, Emory University School of Medicine;
Veterans Affairs Medical Center, Atlanta, Georgia

Randall Smith, M.D.
Clinical Assistant Professor, Department of Physical
Medicine and Rehabilitation, University of Missouri,
Columbia, School of Medicine; Medical Director of
Physical Medicine and Rehabilitation, Harry S.
Truman Veterans Hospital, Columbia,
Missouri

Thomas Sowell, M.S.
Instructor, Department of Physical Medicine and
Rehabilitation, University of Arkansas for Medical
Sciences; Speech Pathologist, Central Arkansas
Veterans Affairs Health Care System, Little Rock,
Arkansas

Vikki A. Stefans, M.D.
Associate Professor, Departments of Pediatrics and
Physical Medicine and Rehabilitation, University of
Arkansas for Medical Sciences; Arkansas Children's
Hospital, Little Rock, Arkansas

**Robert E. Windsor, M.D., FAAPMR, FAAEM,
FAAPM**
Assistant Clinical Professor, Department of Physical
Medicine and Rehabilitation, Emory University
School of Medicine; West Paces Ferry Hospital,
Atlanta, Georgia; President, Georgia Pain Physicians,
P.C., Marietta, Forest Park, and Calhoun, Georgia

Jeffrey L. Woodward, M.D., M.S.
Springfield Physical Medicine and Rehabilitation,
P.C., Springfield, Missouri

Jeffrey L. Young, M.D.
Department of Physical Medicine and Rehabilitation,
Northwestern University Medical School; Director,
Spine and Sports Fellowship, Rehabilitation Institute
of Chicago, Chicago, Illinois

Preface

The second edition of *Pain Procedures in Clinical Practice*, formerly *Physiatric Procedures in Clinical Practice*, is larger and more comprehensive than the original version published in 1995. Some chapters have been consolidated while others have been expanded and include additional or new authors. New chapters contain more in-depth discussions of drugs, radiation safety, complications, medicolegal issues, botulinum toxin injections, and radiofrequency procedures. Injection procedures are described in greater detail in the section on myofascial pain and trigger point injections. The spine injection chapters have been expanded and feature new radiographic photos. The peripheral nerve injection section has been expanded to include gross specimen comparisons. As in the first edition, the authors are well-known in their respective fields and represent both clinical and academic physicians throughout the United States.

One of the largest considerations for a second edition was changing the name of the book. The new name, *Pain Procedures in Clinical Practice*, clearly reflects the content of the book. It also appeals to a wider range of medical specialties with expertise in pain management. The first edition dealt almost entirely with pain procedures with a few chapters on functional and rehabilitation procedures. These chapters—serial casting, urologic testing, removable rigid dressings, videofluoroscopy, and skin procedures—were purposefully maintained in the second edition because many of the patients that rehabilitation and pain physicians treat deal with these issues.

Interest in pain procedures by physicians has increased significantly since this reference was originally published. Reimbursement issues, new procedural techniques, training courses, and residency program curricula are ever developing. These rapid changes have forced pain physicians to continually update their skills. This edition attempts to combine many of these new developments into an easy-to-read volume that will assist the physician with many of these changes.

Once again, a large supporting cast made this second edition possible. I owe a huge amount of gratitude to the numerous photographers, artists, consultants, and x-ray technicians for their contributions. A big thanks goes out to each author for his or her efforts on each chapter. The authors' willingness to share their expertise is greatly appreciated. Read and enjoy!

Ted A. Lennard, M.D.

1

Commonly Used Medications in Pain Procedures

Susan J. Dreyer, M.D.

Local anesthetics, corticosteroids, and contrast agents are administered in many pain procedures. Sometimes neurolytic agents and medications to treat adverse reactions are required. Every interventional physician must know the pharmacology, pharmacokinetics, and potential adverse reactions of the drugs he or she administers. Furthermore, the physician needs to be familiar with medications used to treat potential procedure complications. This chapter examines medications commonly used during pain procedures.

LOCAL ANESTHETICS

Local anesthetics are widely used and generally safe when administered properly. They are therapeutically used in most injections to provide local anesthesia or analgesia of a painful structure. The ability of local anesthetics to relieve pain also can be used diagnostically to help confirm a pain generator. Common applications include skin and soft-tissue anesthesia for other procedures; intra-articular injections; injection for bursitis, tenosynovitis, entrapment neuropathies, and painful ganglia; spinal injections; and nerve blocks.

Local anesthetics are subdivided into esters and amides, referring to the bond that links the hydrophilic and lipophilic rings. The amide class is less allergenic and more commonly used in local, intra-articular and spinal injections. The most widely used agents in clinical practice are the amide local anesthetics lidocaine (Xylocaine) and bupivacaine (Marcaine).

Amide local anesthetics are hydrolyzed by the liver microsomal enzymes to inactive products. Thus, patients with hepatic failure or reduced hepatic flow are more sensitive to such agents. For this reason, patients taking beta blockers or who have congestive heart failure have a lower maximum dosage because

of their reduced hepatic flow and decreased elimination rates of the amide local anesthetics.

In contrast, the ester anesthetics are rapidly hydrolyzed by plasma cholinesterase into para-aminobenzoic acid (PABA) and other metabolites that are excreted unchanged in the urine. PABA is a known allergen in certain individuals. However, the rapid metabolism of ester local anesthetics lowers their potential for toxicity. Procaine is an aminoester commonly but not exclusively used in differential spinal blocks. 2-Chloroprocaine can be used for infiltration, epidural, or peripheral nerve block and also is an ester.

Mechanism of Action

Local anesthetics exert their effect by reversibly inhibiting neural impulse transmission. The local anesthetic molecules diffuse across neural membranes to block sodium channels and inhibit the influx of sodium ions; therefore, proximity of the local anesthetic to the nerve to be blocked is required. Only a short segment of the nerve (5–10 mm) needs to be affected to cease neural firing. Epidural analgesia from local anesthetic is believed by some to occur because of uptake across the dura, a backdoor approach to spinal block.

The ability of a local anesthetic to diffuse through tissues and then block sodium channels relies on the ability of these molecules to dissociate at physiologic pH of 7.4. The pK_as for local anesthetics are greater than the pH found in tissue. As a result, local anesthetics in vivo exist primarily as cations, the form of the molecule that blocks the sodium channel. The base form of the local anesthetic allows it to penetrate the hydrophobic tissues and arrive at the axoplasm.

In addition to host factors, neural blockade by local anesthetics is affected by the volume and concentration of local anesthetic injected, the absence or presence of vasoconstrictor additives, the site of injection, the addition of bicarbonate, and temperature of the local anesthetic. Increasing the total milligrams of a local anesthetic dose shortens the onset and increases the duration of the local anesthetic.[54] Epinephrine, norepinephrine, and phenylephrine are sometimes added to local anesthetics to reverse the intrinsic vasodilatation effects of many of the local anesthetics and thereby reduce their systemic absorption. This increases the amount of local anesthetic available to block the nerve, and more anesthetic means a quicker onset and longer duration. Application of the local anesthetic close to the nerve improves its ability to diffuse across the axon and block sodium channels. Highly vascular sites such as the intercostal nerve and caudal epidural space tend to result in slightly shorter duration of action. The addition of bicarbonate or CO_2 (700 mmHg) to local anesthetics hastens their onset. Bicarbonate raises the pH and the amount of uncharged local anesthetic for diffusion through the nerve membrane. CO_2 will diffuse across the axonal membrane and lower the intracellular pH and makes more of the charged form of the local anesthetic available intracellularly to block the sodium channels. Temperature elevations decrease the pK_a of the local anesthetic and speed onset of action.

Individual Agents

Local anesthetics are administered in the intradermal, subcutaneous, intra-articular, intramuscular, perineural, and epidural spaces during pain procedures. Injections into vascular regions, such as the oral mucosa and epidural space, may result in rapid absorption and higher systemic concentrations. Local anesthetics administered into or near the epidural space should be preservative-free. Methylparaben is a common preservative in multidose vials and also is a common allergen.[47]

Lidocaine

Lidocaine is the most versatile and widely used of the local anesthetics. It has a short onset of action (0.5–15 min) and short duration of action, typically 0.5–3 hours. The difference between the effective dose and the toxic dose is wide, resulting in a high therapeutic index compared to other common local anesthetics. Maximum doses are variably reported in the range of 400–500 mg of lidocaine given epidurally or 300 mg for infiltration. Typical concentrations are 0.5–2%. Final concentration is often diluted by the addition of a corticosteroid.[54]

Concentration percentages easily convert to milligrams. For example, a 1% solution of lidocaine has 1 gm of lidocaine in 100 ml of fluid, which is equivalent to 1000 mg/100 ml or 10 mg/ml. Volume of lidocaine injected varies greatly with location and practitioner. Using the aforementioned guidelines, total injection of 1% lidocaine should remain below 30 ml (30 ml × 10 mg/ml = 300 mg).

Bupivacaine

Bupivacaine (Marcaine) is another widely used local anesthetic. Its duration of action (2–5 hr) is longer than lidocaine's as is its onset of action (5–20 min). Bupivacaine is commonly used in concentrations of 0.125–0.75%. Final concentrations are often diluted by 30–50% by the addition of a corticosteroid. The higher concentrations generally have a faster onset of action. Bupivacaine has a higher cardiotoxicity than lidocaine, especially if an injection is inadvertently given intravenously . The toxic dose of bupivacaine is only 80 mg (16 ml of a 0.5% solution) when given intravascularly, but may rise up to 225 mg with an extravascular injection.[54]

Toxicity

Action of local anesthetics is affected by numerous factors reviewed above. Location of injection plays a primary role in determining the onset, duration, and toxic dose of these agents (Table 1-1). Vasoconstrictors such as epinephrine reduce local bleeding and thereby prolong the onset and duration, but generally are not used in physiatric practice.

Excess amounts of local anesthetics may cause central nervous system (CNS) effects, including confusion, convulsions, respiratory arrest, seizures, and even death. The risk for complications increases if the local anesthetics are given intravascularly. Other potential adverse reactions to local anesthetics include cardiodepression, anaphylaxis, and malignant hyperthermia. Patients with decreased renal function, hepatic function, or plasma esterases eliminate local anesthetics more slowly and, therefore, have an increased risk of toxicity. Toxic blood levels of lidocaine are approximately 5–10 μg, but adverse effects may be seen at lower blood levels.

Patients should be monitored for signs of toxicity, which include restlessness, anxiety, incoherent speech, light-headedness, numbness and tingling of the mouth and lips, blurred vision, tremors, twitching, depression, or drowsiness. Injections into the head and neck area require the utmost care.[8] Even small doses of local anesthetic may produce adverse

TABLE 1-1. Classification and Uses of Local Anesthetics

	Clinical Uses	Usual Concentration (%)	Usual Onset	Usual Duration (hours)	Maximum* Single Dose (mg)	Unique Characteristics
Aminoesters						
2-Chloroprocaine	Infiltration	1	Fast	0.5–1.0	1000 + EPI	Lowest systemic toxicity
	PNB	2	Fast	0.5–1.0	1000 + EPI	Intrathecal route may be
	Epidural	2–3	Fast	0.5–1.5	1000 + EPI	neurotoxic
Procaine	Infiltration	1	Fast	0.5–1.0	1000	Used for differential
	PNB	1–2	Slow	0.5–1.0	1000	spinal
	Spinal	10	Moderate	0.5–1.0	200	
Tetracaine	Topical	2	Slow	0.5–1.0	80	
	Spinal	0.5	Fast	2–4	20	
Aminoamides						
Lidocaine	Topical	4	Fast	0.5–1.0	500 + EPI	
	Infiltration	0.5–1.0	Fast	1–2	500 + EPI	
	IV regional	0.25–0.5		1–3	500	
	PNB	1.0–1.5	Fast	1–2	500 + EPI	
	Epidural	1–2	Fast	0.5–1.5	500 + EPI	
	Spinal	5	Fast		100	
Prilocaine	IV regional	0.25–0.5	Fast	1.5–3.0	600	Least toxic amide
	PNB	1.5–2.0	Fast	1.0–2.5	600	Methemoglobinemia
	Epidural	1–3			600	possible when > 600 mg
Mepivacaine	PNB	1.0–1.5	Fast	2–3	500 + EPI	Duration of plain solutions
	Epidural	1–2	Fast	1.0–2.5	500 + EPI	longer than lidocaine with EPI, useful when EPI contraindicated
Bupivacaine	PNB	0.25–0.5	Slow	4–12	200 + EPI	Exaggerated cardiotoxicity
	Epidural	0.25–0.75	Moderate	2–4	200 + EPI	with accidental IV injection
	Spinal	0.5–0.75	Fast	2–4	20	Low doses produce sensory > motor blockade
Etidocaine	PNB	0.5–1.0	Fast	3–12	300 + EPI	Motor > sensory blockade
	Epidural	1.0–1.5	Fast	2–4	300 + EPI	

PNB = peripheral nerve block; EPI = epinephrine.
* Maximum single dosage is affected by many factors; this figure is only a guide.
Modified from Barash PG, Cullen BF, Stoelting RK: Handbook of Clinical Anesthesia, 2nd ed. Philadelphia, J.B. Lippincott, 1993, pp 206–207.

reactions similar to systemic toxicity seen with unintentional intravascular injections of larger doses. Deaths have been reported.[35]

Resuscitative equipment and drugs should be immediately available when local anesthetics are used. Management of local anesthetic overdose begins with prevention by monitoring total dose administered, frequently aspirating for vascular uptake, and using contrast to avoid vascular uptake when appropriate. Recognition of symptoms of toxicity and support of oxygenation with supplemental oxygen are keys to initial management. The airway must be maintained and respiratory support provided as needed. Hypotension is the most common circulatory effect and should be treated with intravenous fluids and a vasopressor such as ephedrine in appropriate candidates. Convulsions that persist despite respiratory support often are treated with a benzodiazepine (e.g., diazepam). If cardiac arrest occurs, standard cardiopulmonary resuscitation measures should be instituted.

CORTICOSTEROIDS

Corticosteroids are administered for their potent anti-inflammatory properties. These injections that relieve pain and inflammation temporarily work well, but questions remain regarding their role in the management of many chronic musculoskeletal conditions. Corticosteroids may result in significant side effects. The potential for adverse effects range from a relatively innocuous facial flushing effect to joint-destroying avascular necrosis and must be weighed against potential benefits. Locally injected corticosteroids are sometimes partially absorbed systemically and can produce transient systemic effects.

Corticosteroids may be helpful in a variety of conditions, including rheumatoid arthritis, bursitis, tenosynovitis, entrapment neuropathies, crystal-induced arthropathies in patients who cannot tolerate systemic treatment well, radiculopathies, and, at times, osteoarthritis. Corticosteroids never should be injected directly into a tendon or nerve, subcutaneous fat, or an infected joint, bursa, or tendon.

Mechanism of Action

All corticosteroids have glucocorticoid, anti-inflammatory, and mineralocorticoid activity. Agents with significant glucocorticoid and minimal mineralocorticoid activity include betamethasone (Celestone), dexamethasone (Decadron), methylprednisolone acetate (Depo-Medrol), and triamcinolone hexacetonide (Aristospan). Corticosteroids can be mixed in the same syringe with local anesthetics. Commonly two parts of anesthetic are mixed with one part steroid.

Corticosteroids produce both anti-inflammatory and immunosuppressive effects in humans. The primary mechanism of action may be their ability to inhibit the release of cytokines by immune cells.[9] The effects of corticosteroids are species-specific. Lymphocytes in humans are much less sensitive to the effects of corticosteroids than lymphocytes in common laboratory animals, including the mouse, rat, and rabbit. In humans, corticosteroids reduce the accumulation of lymphocytes at inflammatory sites by a migratory effect.[37] In contrast to this lymphopenia is the neutrophilia seen by demargination of neutrocytes from the endothelium and an accelerated rate of release from the bone marrow.[14] For this reason a temporary rise in white blood cell count is commonly observed after a corticosteroid dose and in isolation does not indicate a postinjection infection.

The anti-inflammatory effects of corticosteroid also occur at the microvascular level. They block the passage of immune complexes across the basement membrane, suppress superoxide radicals and reduce capillary permeability and blood flow.[46] Corticosteroids inhibit prostaglandin synthesis,[44] decrease collagenase formation, and inhibit granulation tissue formation.

The immunosuppressant effects of corticosteroids generally impact T-cells. Such effects are not the desired effect of corticosteroid used in physiatric procedures and are not observed following epidural injections.[45] A review of these immunosuppressant effects can be found elsewhere in the literature.[3,10,15,45]

Individual Agents

Commonly used corticosteroid preparations include betamethasone, methylprednisolone, triamcinolone, dexamethasone, prednisolone, and hydrocortisone. Of these, betamethasone and dexamethasone have the strongest glucocorticoid or anti-inflammatory effects. Corticosteroid effects can be highly variable among individuals, and it is not possible to definitively state a safe dosage of corticosteroid. The following should serve only as a guide and must be tailored to each individual.

Betamethasone

An equal mixture of two betamethasone salts (Celestone Soluspan) allows for both immediate and delayed corticosteroid responses. Betamethasone sodium phosphate acts within hours, whereas betamethasone acetate is a suspension that is slowly absorbed over approximately two weeks. Betamethasone (Celestone Soluspan) is approved for intraarticular or soft-tissue injection to provide

TABLE 1–2. Comparison of Commonly Used Glucocorticoid Steroids

Agent	Anti-inflammatory Potency*	Salt Retention Property	Plasma Half-Life (min)	Duration†	Equivalent Oral Dose (mg)
Hydrocortisone (Cortisol)	1	2+	90	S	20
Cortisone	0.8	2+	30	S	25
Prednisone	4–5	1+	60	I	5
Prednisolone	4–5	1+	200	I	5
Methylprednisolone (Medrol, Depo-Medrol)	5	0	180	I	4
Triamcinolone (Aristocort, Kenalog)	5	0	300	I	4
Betamethasone (Celestone)	25–35	0	100–300	L	0.6
Dexamethasone (Decadron)	25–30	30	100–300	L	0.75

* Relative to hydrocortisone
† S = Short, I = Intermediate, L = Long

From Lennard TA: Fundamentals of procedural care. In Lennard TA (ed): Physiatric Procedures in Clinical Practice. Philadelphia, Hanley & Belfus, 1995, p 6.

short-term adjuvant therapy in osteoarthritis, tenosynovitis, gouty arthritis, bursitis, epicondylitis, and rheumatoid arthritis.[33] It also is commonly utilized in epidural injections. Typical intra-articular doses vary with joint size and range from 0.25 to 2 ml (1.5–12 mg). Typically, epidural injections range from 1 to 3 ml (6–18 mg). Betamethasone should not be mixed with local anesthetics that contain preservatives such as methylparaben because these may cause flocculation of the steroid.

Dexamethasone

Dexamethasone acetate (Decadron-LA) has a rapid onset and long duration of action. It usually is given in doses of 8–16 mg intramuscularly or 4–16 mg for intra-articular or soft-tissue injections. The most common preparations have 8 mg of dexamethasone acetate per milliliter; 0.5–2 ml quantities are the most common. Most preparations contain sodium bisulfite that can trigger allergic reactions in susceptible individuals. Dexamethasone sodium phosphate (Decadron Phosphate) is a rapid-onset, short-duration formulation of dexamethasone available in a variety of strengths ranging from 4 mg/ml to 24 mg/ml. Large joints often are injected with 2–4 mg, small joints 0.8–1 mg, bursae 2–3 mg, tendon sheaths 0.4–1 mg, and soft-tissue infiltration 2–6 mg.[33] Sulfites are common in the preparations of this salt. Dexamethasone is approved for the treatment of osteoarthritis, bursitis, tendonitis, rheumatoid arthritis flares, epicondylitis, tenosynovitis, and gout arthritis.[33]

Methylprednisolone

Methylprednisolone acetate (Depo-Medrol) has ⅕ to ⅙ the glucocorticoid potency of betamethasone but similar anti-inflammatory effects to prednisolone. It has an intermediate duration of action. Like the other corticosteroids, it is approved for intra-articular and soft-tissue injections for short-term adjuvant therapy of osteoarthritis, bursitis, tenosynovitis, gouty arthritis, epicondylitis, and rheumatoid arthritis.[33] Depo-Medrol also has been used for epidural administration. Preparations of methylprednisolone acetate include polyethylene glycol as a suspending agent. Concerns arose as to whether the polyethylene glycol can cause arachnoiditis with (inadvertent) intrathecal injections.[34] Animal studies have not demonstrated any adverse effects on neural tissues from the application of glucocorticoid.[12] Methylprednisolone is now available without polyethylene glycol. Typical doses range from 4 to 80 mg. Small joints are typically

injected with 4–10 mg, medium joints 10–40 mg, large joints 20–80 mg, and bursae and peritendon 4–30 mg.[33]

Triamcinolone

Triamcinolone is available as three different salts: triamcinolone diacetate (Aristocort Forte), triamcinolone hexacetonide (Aristospan), and triamcinolone acetonide (Kenalog). Duration of action is shortest with the diacetate and longest with the acetonide formulations. Triamcinolone has similar glucocorticoid activity to methylprednisolone with a long half-life. Approved uses are the same as the above agents and include use in epidural injections. Unfortunately, it has a higher incidence of adverse reactions, including fat atrophy and hypopigmentation.[33]

Adverse Reactions

Corticosteroid use should be carefully considered and if possible avoided in patients who are at increased risk for adverse reactions, including those with active ulcer disease, ulcerative colitis with impending perforation or abscess, poorly controlled hypertension, congestive heart failure, renal disease, psychiatric illness or a history of steroid psychosis, or a history of severe or multiple allergies. Intra-articular injections have been associated with osteonecrosis, infection, tendon rupture, postinjection flare, hypersensitivities, and systemic reactions.[33] Intraspinal injections have been associated with adhesive arachnoiditis, meningitis, and conus medullaris syndrome.[34]

Adverse reactions to injected corticosteroids include a transient flare of pain for 24–48 hours in up to 10% of patients. Diabetics and individuals with a predisposition to diabetes may become hyperglycemic; appropriate monitoring and corrective measures should be instituted. Adrenal cortical insufficiency generally is not seen associated with intermittent injections of corticosteroids but remains a serious adverse reaction that may be precipitated by indiscriminate and frequent high-dose corticosteroid injections. Allergic reactions to systemic glucocorticoids have been reported, and if slow-release formulations are used, the allergic response may not occur until one week after the injection. Some systemic response may occur even with local injections of corticosteroids.

Less serious side effects of corticosteroids include facial flushing, injection site hypopigmentation, subcutaneous fat atrophy, increased appetite, peripheral edema or fluid retention, dyspepsia, malaise, and insomnia.[33] Prolonged or repeated doses can result in cushingoid changes.

Drug Interactions

A number of drug–drug interactions for corticosteroids have been reported. Some of the more common ones encountered in physiatric practice are mentioned here. Estrogens and oral contraceptives may potentiate the effect of the corticosteroid. Macrolide antibiotics (e.g., erythromycin, azithromycin) may greatly increase the effect of methylprednisolone by decreasing its clearance. In contrast, the hydantoins (e.g., phenytoin), rifampin, phenobarbital, and carbamazepine may increase corticosteroid clearance and decrease the anti-inflammatory therapeutic effect. Theophylline and oral anticoagulants can interact variably with corticosteroids.[33]

NEUROLYTIC AGENTS

Neurolytic drugs such as phenol are utilized in clinical practice primarily to treat spasticity. Neurolytic agents also have been used for treating chronic pain, including intractable cancer pain and facet denervation procedures. The use of neurolytic agents for facet joint neurotomies is being replaced by radiofrequency lesioning.[13,29] Neurolytic agents are nonspecific in destroying all nerve fiber types. Phenol, ethyl alcohol, propylene glycol, chlorocresol, glycerol, cold saline, hypertonic solutions, and hypotonic solutions have been used as neurolytics. Of these, phenol is the most studied and widely used neurolytic.

Phenol

Phenol is the most widely instilled agent to treat severe spasticity. It can be injected around a motor nerve to selectively reduce hypertonicity.[26,55] Intrathecal injections of phenol have been used to treat spasticity of spinal cord origin and intractable pain disorders. Sympathectomies for peripheral vascular disease also have been accomplished by injection of phenol along the paravertebral and perivascular sympathetic fibers.[21,42]

Mechanism of Action

Phenol (carbolic acid) denatures protein and thereby causes denervation. Histologic sections show nonselective nerve destruction, muscle atrophy, and necrosis at the site of phenol injections.[16,19,31] Higher concentrations of phenol are associated with greater tissue destruction. An optimal concentration has not been determined, and a long-term difference between injection of 2% and 3% solution has not been noted.[31] Denervation potentials are seen as early as three weeks following phenol blocks.[2] A clinical response of decreased pain or spasticity lasts between two months and two years irrespective of underlying disorder.[19,31] Endoneural fibrosis is seen following phenol injections and is believed to impede reinnervation of the muscle by slow wallerian regeneration.

Dosage

Phenol is placed in an aqueous solution, glycerin, or lipids for administration. Commercially available phenol is an 89% solution and must be diluted to the desired concentration, typically 2–3%. Commonly it is mixed with an equal part of gylcerin and then diluted with normal saline to 2–5%. The maximum daily injectable dose is 1 gm. Toxic effects are uncommon in doses ≤ 100 mg. Phenol is eliminated through the liver; use in patients with significant liver disease should be avoided.

Adverse Reactions

Local reactions to phenol injection include delayed soreness from the associated necrosis and inflammation.[16] This discomfort can be relieved with ice packs and analgesics and typically resolves within 24 hours. If the needle is withdrawn without flushing it with saline, phenol may come in contact with the skin and cause erythema, sloughing, and skin necrosis. Protective eyewear can minimize the chance of eye irritation and conjunctivitis from any phenol splashing into the patient's or physician's eyes.

Paresthesias or dysesthesias from mixed somatic nerve blocks probably are due to an incomplete block. Paresthesias/dysesthesias occur in up to one quarter of nerve blocks and resolve within 3 months. Repeat blocks often alleviate these symptoms, which indicates that the dysesthesias may stem more from an incomplete block than from phenol-induced dysesthesias.

Systemic reactions to phenol usually result from inadvertent intravascular or central blockade.[1,20,51,52] Adverse systemic reactions most commonly affect the cardiovascular and central nervous systems.[51] Cardiac dysrhythmias, hypotension, venous thrombosis, spinal cord infarcts, cortical infarcts, meningitis, and arachnoiditis have been reported.[30,32,51]

CONTRAST AGENTS

Contrast agents are administered to help visualize the location of the needle tip, confirm the flow of injectant, or visualize the involved structure (e.g., joint, bladder, bursa). Inadvertent vascular uptake in spite of negative aspiration is not uncommon. The toxicity of local anesthetics and corticosteroids increases with intravascular injection, and contrast-enhanced fluoroscopic guidance helps minimize such toxicities. All contrast agents are iodinated compounds that allow opacification of structures for visualization. Contrast media are divided into ionic and nonionic agents. The nonionic contrast agents have low osmolality and may decrease the potential for adverse reactions. Although these nonionic agents decrease minor reactions such as nausea and urticaria, they have not been shown to decrease the incidence of more severe reactions.[21,50] They do not eliminate the possibility of severe or fatal anaphylactic reactions. Potential for adverse reactions can be minimized by limiting the quantity of the contrast media injected and adequately screening patients.

Patients with a history of prior contrast reaction, significant allergies, impaired cardiac function/limited cardiac reserve, blood-brain barrier breakdown, and severe anxiety are at increased risk for generalized reactions, including urticaria, nausea, vomiting, and anaphylaxis. Patients with impaired renal function and paraproteinemias are at increased risk for renal failure with the administration of contrast agents. Renal complications can be minimized by limiting the volume of contrast agent, ensuring adequate hydration before, during, and after the procedure, and using the low-osmolality agents for patients > 70 years with a creatinine ≥ 2 mg/dl.

Ideally, spinal procedures, including epidural steroid injections, facet joint injections, sympathetic blocks, discography, spinal nerve blocks, and sacroiliac joint injections, are all performed with the aid of fluoroscopy and contrast enhancement.[43,53] Nonionic contrast agents are used for these injections because the potential for subarachnoid spread exists with any of these procedures. The two most common nonionic agents are iopamidol (Isovue) and iohexol (Omnipaque). Both agents are nonionic, readily available as an injectable liquid, water-soluble, and quickly cleared. The first of the nonionic contrast agents, metrizamide (Amipaque), is a powder that must be reconstituted. Metrizamide also is associated with a higher incidence of seizures than either iohexol or iopamidol and rarely is used now for physiatric procedures. Generally, 0.2–2 ml of nonionic contrast is sufficient for the experienced injectionist to confirm location and spread of the contrast. Ninety percent of these agents are eliminated through the kidneys within 24 hours. Side effects are uncommon but include nausea, headaches, and CNS disturbances.[36]

Ionic contrast agents such as diatrizoate (Renografin) and iothalamate (Conray) may be used for other contrast-enhanced injections, including arthrograms, cystometrograms, and bursa injections. These agents are well tolerated when total volume of contrast is limited to ≤ 15 ml.

Premedication for Allergic Reactions

The risk of anaphylactoid reactions is 1–2% when radiopaque agents are used. This risk increases to 17–35% when repeat exposure to radiopaque agents occurs in individuals with known sensitivities.[4,22,36,48] If premedication with diphenhydramine (Benadryl) and methylprednisolone is given, the risk of anaphylactoid reactions is reduced to approximately 3.1%.[36] The current recommended prophylactic protocol is 32 mg of oral methylprednisolone 12 and 2 hours prior to contrast use.[27] Concurrent use of specific H_1 and H_2 blockers also is recommended.[11,18]

Treatment of Adverse Reactions to Medication

Medication adverse reactions may be minimized by careful patient selection and vigilance during the procedure. However, it is impossible to completely eliminate the possibility of allergic or other reactions, so the practitioner must be prepared to deal with these emergency situations. Immediate access to and familiarity with emergency medications and protocols is critical.

Minor medication reactions can be treated with observation to ensure symptoms do not worsen, and moderate reactions can be treated in the procedure area and do not require hospitalization. Reactions include symptomatic urticaria, bronchospasm, and vasovagal reactions. Symptomatic urticaria can be treated with 25–50 mg of diphenhydramine intramuscularly. Bronchospasm should be treated with supplemental oxygen by nasal cannula and O_2 saturation monitoring, intravenous access, and electrocardiogram monitoring. If needed, a beta agonist inhaler can be administered as long as bronchospasm has not worsened to laryngotracheal edema. Epinephrine 1:1000 sometimes is required in doses of 0.1–1 ml subcutaneously. In refractory bronchospasm and more severe reactions of laryngotracheal edema or symptomatic facial edema, intravascular epinephrine 1:10,000 is given in doses of 1–3 ml.

Vasovagal reactions are heralded by symptomatic bradycardia and hypotension. Simple measures of reassurance, leg elevation, and intravenous fluids may alleviate such reactions if promptly initiated. Vital signs must be monitored, and supplemental oxygen should be initiated promptly if oxygen saturation begins to drop. For more severe vasovagal reactions, drops in blood pressure and pulse can be treated with atropine, 0.3–0.5 mg IV given incrementally up to 2 mg. Vasovagal reactions with hypotension and bradycardia must be distinguished from anaphylactoid or cardiac reaction when the hypotension is associated with tachycardia.

Toxic convulsions may be treated with oxygen, airway management, and diazepam, 1–10 mg intravenously in 1-mg increments. Hospitalization and appropriate consultation are recommended. Cardiopulmonary arrest should be treated following standard advanced cardiac life support protocols: assess vital signs, secure airway and oxygenation, begin resuscitation, ensure intravenous access, and follow the appropriate treatment algorithm. After successful recuscitative attempts, the patient should be hospitalized for observation and any necessary treatment.

Physicians use a core group of medications for their procedures. It is imperative that the injectionist has a solid understanding of these agents to maximize benefit and minimize risk. Integration of injection procedures in appropriately selected patients increases the physician's effectiveness.

REFERENCES

1. Benzon HT: Convulsions secondary to intravascular phenol: A hazard of celiac plexus block. Anesth Analg 58:150-151, 1979.
2. Brattstrom M, Moritz U, Svantesson G: Electromyographic studies of peripheral nerve block with phenol. Scand J Rehabil Med 2:17–22, 1970.
3. Brown PB: The use of steroidal agents in the oral route. In Wilkens RF, Dali SL (eds): Therapeutic Controversies in the Rheumatic Diseases. Orlando, FL, Grune & Stratton, 1987, p 71.
4. Caro JJ, Trindade E, McGregor M: The risks of death and of severe nonfatal reactions with high vs. low-osmolality contrast media: A meta-analysis. Am J Roentgenol 156:825–832, 1991.
5. Claman HN: Corticosteroids and lymphoid cells. N Engl J Med 287:388–397, 1972.
6. Copp EP, Harris R, Keenan J: Peripheral nerve block and motor point block with phenol in the mangement of spasticity. Proc R Soc Med 63:17–18, 1970.
7. Copp EP, Keenan J: Phenol nerve and motor point block in spasticity. Rheum Phys Med 11:287–292, 1972.
8. Covino BG: Clinical pharmacology of local anesthetic agents. In Cousins MJ, Bridenbaugh PO (eds): Neural Blockade in Clinical Anesthesia and Pain Management. Philadelphia, J.B. Lippincott, 1996, pp 111–144.
9. Crabtree GR, Gillis S, Smith KA, Munck A: Glucocorticoids and immune responses. Arthritis Rheum 22:1246–1256, 1979.
10. Cupps RR, Fauci AS: Corticosteroid-mediated immunoregulation in man. [Review]. Immunol Rev 65:133–155, 1982.
11. Cusmano J: Premedication regimen eases contrast reaction. Diagn Imaging 181–182;185–186, 1992.
12. Delaney T, Rowlingson RC, Carron H: Epidural steroid effects on nerve and meninges. Anesth Analg 59:610– 614, 1980.
13. Dreyfuss P, Halbrook B, Pauza K, et al: Lumbar Percutaneous RF Medial Branch Neurotomy for Chronic Zygapophysial Joint Pain—A Pilot Study. Denver, International Spinal Injection Society, 1997.
14. Fauci AS: Immunosuppressive and anti-inflammatory effects of glucocorticoids. In Baxter JO, Rousseau CG (eds): Glucocorticoid Hormone Action. New York, Springer-Verlag, 1979.
15. Fauci AS, Dale DC, Balow JE: Glucocorticosteroid therapy: Mechanism of action and clinical considerations. Ann Intern Med 84:304–315, 1976.
16. Garland DE, Lucie RS, Waters RI: Current uses of open phenol nerve block for adult acquired spasticity. Clin Orthop Rel Res 165:217–222, 1982.
17. Goebert HW, Jallo SJ, Gardner WJ, Wasmuth CE: Painful radiculopathy treated with epidural injections of procaine and hydrocortisone acetate: Results in 113 patients. Anesth Analg 140:130–134, 1961.
18. Greenberger PA, Patterson R: The prevention of immediate generalized repeated reactions to radiocontrast media in high-risk patients. J Allergy Clin Immunol 87:867–872, 1991.
19. Halpern D: Histologic studies in animals after intramuscular neurolysis with phenol. Arch Phys Med Rehabil 58:438–443, 1977.
20. Holland AJC, Yousseff M: A complicaton of subarachnoid phenol blockade. Anesthesia 34:260–262, 1979.
21. Hughes-Davies DI, Rechman LR: Clinical lumbar sympathectomy. Anesthesia 31:1068, 1970.
22. Katayama H, Yamaguchi K, Kozuka T, et al: Adverse reactions to ionic and nonionic contrast media: A report from the Japanese Committee on the Safety of Contrast Media. Radiology 175:621–628, 1990.
23. Katz JK, Knott LW, Feldman MD: Peripheral nerve injections with phenol in the management of spastic patients. Arch Phys Med Rehabil 48:97–99, 1967.
24. Khalili AA: Physiatric management of spasticity by phenol nerve and motor point block. In Ruskin AP (ed): Current Therapy in Physiatry. Philadelphia, W.B. Saunders, 1984, pp 464–474.
25. Khalili AA, Betts HB: Peripheral nerve block with phenol in the management of spasticity. JAMA 200:1155–1157, 1967.
26. Khalili AA, Harmel MH, Forster S, et al: Management of spasticity by selective peripheral nerve block with dilute phenol solutions in clinical rehabilitation. Arch Phys Med Rehabil 45:513–519, 1964.
27. Lasser EC, Berry CC, Talner LB, et al: Pretreatment with corticosteroids to alleviate reactions to intravenous contrast material. N Engl J Med 317:845–849, 1987.
28. Lawrence V, Matthai W, Hartmaier S: Comparative safety of high-osmolality and low-osmolality radiographic contrast agents. Report of a multidisciplinary working group. Invest Radiol 27:2–18, 1992.

29. Lord SM, Barnsley L, Wallis BJ, et al: Percutaneous radio-frequency neurotomy for chronic cervical zygapophyseal-joint pain. N Engl J Med 335:1721–1726, 1996.
30. Macek C: Venous thrombosis results from some phenol injections. JAMA 249:1807, 1983.
31. Mooney V, Frykman G, McLamb J: Current status of intra-neural phenol injections. Clin Orthop 63:122–131, 1969.
32. Morrison JW, Matthews D, Washington R, et al: Phenol motor point blocks in children: Plasman concentrations and cardiac dysrhythmias. Anesthesiology 75:359–362, 1992.
33. Olin BR: Hormones: Adrenal corticosteroids. In Olin BR (ed): Facts and Comparisons. St. Louis, Wolters Kluwer, 1993, pp 465–486.
34. Nelson DA: Intraspinal therapy using methylprednisolone acetate. Spine 18:278–286, 1993.
35. Olin BR: Miscellaneous products: Local anesthetics, injectable. In Olin BR (ed): Facts and Comparisons. St. Louis, Wolters Kluwer, 1993, pp 2654–2665.
36. Olin BR: Miscellaneous products: Radiopaque agents. In Olin BR (ed): Facts and Comparisons. St. Louis, Wolters Kluwer, 1993, pp 2824–2831.
37. Peters WP, Holland JF, Senn H, et al: Corticosteroid administration and localized leukocyte mobilization in man. N Engl J Med 286:342–345,1972.
38. Petrillo C, Chu D, Davis S: Phenol block of the tibial nerve in the hemiplegic patient. Orthopedics 3:871–874, 1980.
39. Petrillo C, Knoploch S: Phenol block of the tibial nerve for spasticity: A long-term followup study. Int Disabil Studies 10:97–100, 1988.
40. Preuss L: Allergic reactions to systemic glucocorticoids: A review. Am Allergy 55:772–775, 1985.
41. Reevew DK, Baker A: A mixed somatic peripheral phenol nerve block for painful or intractable spasticity: A review of 30 years of use. Am J Pain Manage 2:205–210, 1992.
42. Reid W, Watt JK, Gray TG: Phenol injections of the sympathetic chain. Br J Surg 57:45–50, 1970.
43. Renfrew DL: Correct placement of epidural steroid injections: Fluoroscopic guidance and contrast administration. AJNR 12:1003–1007, 1991.
44. Robinson DR: Prostaglandins and the mechanism of action of anti-inflammatory drugs. [Review]. Am J Med 75:26–31, 1983.
45. Robinson JP, Brown PB: Medications in low back pain. Phys Med Rehabil Clin North Am 2:97–126, 1991.
46. Schayer RS: Synthesis of histamine, microcirculatory regulation and the mechanisms of action of the adrenal glucocorticoid hormones. Prog Allergy 7:187, 1963.
47. Schorr WF: Paraben allergy. JAMA 204:107–110, 1968.
48. Shehadi WH: Contrast media adverse reactions: Occurrence, recurrence and distribution patterns. Radiology 143:11–17, 1982.
49. Spira R: Management of spasticity in cerebral palsied children by peripheral nerve block with phenol. Develop Med Child Neurol 13:164–173, 1971.
50. Steinberg EP, Moore RD, Powe NR, et al: Safety and cost effectiveness of high-osmolality as compared with low-osmolality contrast material in patients undergoing cardiac angiography. [comments]. N Engl J Med 326:425–430, 1992.
51. Swerdlow M: Complications of neurolytic neural blockade. In Cousins MJ, Bridenbaugh PO (eds): Neural Blockade in Clinical Anesthesia and Management of Pain. Philadelphia, J.B. Lippincott, 1988, pp 719–735.
52. Totoki T, Kato T, Nomoto Y, et al: Anterior spinal artery syndrome: A complication of cervical intrathecal phenol injections. Pain 6:99–104, 1979.
53. White AH, Derby R, Wynne G: Epidural injections for diagnosis and treatment of low-back pain. Spine 5:78–86, 1980.
54. Williams MJ: Pharmacology for regional anesthetic techniques. In Hahn MB, McQuillan PM, Sheplock GJ (eds): Regional Anesthesia: An Atlas of Anatomy and Techniques. St. Louis, Mosby, 1996, pp 3–17.
55. Wood KM: The use of phenol as a neurolytic agent: A review. Pain 5:205–229, 1978.

2

Complications of Common Selective Spinal Injections: Prevention and Management

Robert E. Windsor, M.D., Elmer G. Pinzon, M.D., M.P.H., and Herman C. Gore, M.D.

Selective spinal injections are being performed with increasing frequency in the management of acute and chronic pain syndromes.[1,2,3] Because these procedures require a needle to be placed in or around the spine, there is always a risk of complications. As a result, prevention and the early recognition and management of complications are paramount to appropriate patient care. This chapter discusses physician training, patient preparation, patient monitoring, and specific complications and their treatment.

PHYSICIAN TRAINING

The level of physician training required to perform selective spinal injections safely is a topic of debate; standards vary from one region of the United States to another and one specialty to another. Some physicians perform selective spinal injections without appropriate training thereby placing their patients at undue risk. Although uncomplicated lumbar procedures in an otherwise healthy population do not require the degree of training and expertise that high-risk procedures performed in a medically unstable population do, certain standards still must be met. The American Academy of Physical Medicine and Rehabilitation (AAPM&R) and the Physiatric Association of Spine, Sports, and Occupational Rehabilitation (PASSOR) have adopted guidelines that recommend a minimal level of documented didactic and clinical training that should be provided in a reasonable training program.[4] Training should include spinal injections, how to recognize, evaluate, and treat related complications, and advanced cardiac life support (ACLS) certification. The fellowship director or residency chairman must be comfortable with a physician's abilities before recommending privileging for spinal interventions. Selective spinal injection courses, although valuable, do not provide a sufficient amount or breadth of training for the novice injectionist to safely perform spinal injections in practice.

PATIENT PREPARATION

Patient preparation includes patient education, informed consent, NPO status, IV access, ascertaining that no procedural contraindications exist, patient positioning, sterile preparation and draping, supplemental IV fluids and oxygen, and appropriate recovery after the procedure. Depending on the procedure and the patient's status, prophylactic antibiotics also may be indicated.

Patients should be given a thorough description of the procedure, including potential risks, benefits, alternatives, and likely outcome. Informed consent should include signature by the patient, the doctor, and a witness. Before the procedure, the patient should take no solid foods for 12 hours and no fluids for 8 hours preoperatively to ensure that all gastric contents are distal to the ligament of Treitz.[5] A large-bore IV (ideally ≥ 20 gauge) should be started in a large proximal upper extremity or neck vein to allow immediate IV access in an emergent setting. Smaller gauge or peripherally placed IV catheters do not allow adequate access to the central venous supply for resuscitative purposes after peripheral vasoconstriction occurs. Procedural contraindications or relative contraindications that may not have been present or recognized during the last physician office visit should be reviewed, such as chest pain, shortness of breath, fever, systemic infection, uncontrolled hypertension, or other medical problems. Preprocedure laboratory work is necessary if the procedure involves placement of a needle or other instrument through the skin and into a disc or implantation of a device. Preprocedure laboratory work also should be done if the patient is recovering from a known systemic infection (e.g., pneumonia or urinary tract infection). If the patient is infirm (e.g., chronic obstructive pulmonary disease [COPD], heart disease), clearance from the patient's primary care physician or specialist must be obtained. Depending on the patient's problem, preprocedure laboratory work may include a complete blood count with differential, liver function tests, urinalysis, chest x-ray, electrocardiogram, blood culture and sensitivity, urine culture and sensitivity, and sedimentation rate.

The patient should be comfortably positioned on the procedure table so that the treating physician is allowed unencumbered access to the body region under treatment. The patient's position should be comfortable enough for him or her to lie still for the duration of the procedure. Care must be taken to make certain that no region of neural compression or stretch exists, especially if sedating medication will be used. Areas particularly vulnerable to neural compression or stretch include the ulnar nerve at the elbow and the brachial plexus.[6] If necessary, use an arm board, tape, strapping, or padding to make the patient more comfortable, to help him or her hold the appropriate position, and to keep his or her hands from inadvertently extending beyond the sterile field.

Sterile preparation minimally includes scrubbing the region of the body to be treated and the surrounding areas with a povidone-iodine preparation and allowing it to dry. If the patient has an iodine allergy, chlorhexidine gluconate and/or isopropyl alcohol may be used. For discography or any type of implant, the authors do a triple scrub that lasts at least 5 minutes and that includes isopropyl alcohol, chlorhexidine gluconate, and povidone-iodine. The povidone-iodine is allowed to dry. We also use pre- and postprocedure antibiotics for these procedures.

The degree of sterile draping required depends on the procedure. Draping the immediate area to be penetrated with sterile towels is adequate for a lumbar epidural. In the case of a spinal implant, percutaneous discectomy, or other more invasive spinal procedure, full-body draping with a fenestrated drape, iodine-impregnated adhesive biodrapes, sterile towels, and half sheets should be used as needed in order to ensure a sterile field.

Supplemental fluids are important during most procedures whether it is a high-risk procedure or not. Patients who have been NPO for 3 hours, particularly those who have been scheduled for morning procedures who have been NPO since the night before, may be volume-depleted and more prone to vasovagal reactions. Supplemental fluids before, during, and after the procedure help prevent such reactions. In addition, it is helpful to have fluids readily available during the procedure in the event that the patient becomes hypotensive or to help flush medications through the line. Supplemental fluids should be used cautiously if the patient is volume-sensitive as in congestive heart failure or renal pathology.

Supplemental oxygen use is determined by the situation. If IV sedation is administered, supplemental oxygen should be used as needed to help maintain the patient's oxygen saturation above 92%. If the patient has COPD or other pulmonary pathology, supplemental oxygen should be used sparingly, because too much oxygen may further suppress his or her respiratory drive. In addition, if the patient has chronic pulmonary disease, the treating physician must confirm that he or she can tolerate the position required by the procedure. If necessary, consult his or her pulmonologist or internist.

PATIENT MONITORING

At a minimum, patient monitoring should include blood pressure and heart rate monitoring. Cardiac monitoring and pulse oximetry also should be done if the patient is infirm, if a high-risk procedure is being performed, or if IV sedation is being used. Baseline vital signs are obtained before the procedure for purposes of comparison during and after the procedure. Preprocedure hypertension should be approached with caution. A patient with cerebrovascular disease may require a higher-than-normal blood pressure to maintain cerebral perfusion; thus, adjusting the blood pressure may incite a stroke. If lowering the blood pressure is deemed medically safe and appropriate, gentle IV sedation is sufficient. Sublingual calcium channel blockers should be avoided. In addition, if IV sedation is planned, blood pressure reduction with other medications should not be carried out before sedation, because this drug combination may lower the blood pressure to dangerous levels.

Any patient with a significant cardiovascular history or for whom procedural risks are planned that may place him or her at risk for cardiovascular complications should undergo cardiac monitoring. In general, it should be performed in any patient with a known history of myocardial infarction or angina; a significantly invasive procedure (e.g., spinal implant); an intraspinal cervical or thoracic procedure; a procedure that may place a significant volume of local anesthetic or narcotic in the spinal canal or systemic circulation; or a procedure that requires a significant amount of IV sedation. A rhythm strip should be run before, during, and after the procedure and placed on the patient's chart.

PATIENT RECOVERY

Patient recovery following the procedure is critically important and often is ignored. Most procedure-related complications occur during the postprocedural period. Such complications include hypotension, vasovagal reactions, sensorimotor blockade, excessive somnolence, respiratory suppression, and cardiovascular complications.

Therefore, a medically reasonable recovery protocol is needed to ultimately allow the patient to recover in a monitored situation until he or she is alert, oriented, tolerating fluids, and ambulating as well as expected. The following represents an abbreviated version of the author's protocol for routine spinal injection procedures with minimal or no sedation:

The patient is allowed to remain in the procedure room in the recumbent position for 5–10 minutes under the watchful eye of a nurse while two additional sets of vital signs are taken. If the patient is feeling well, he or she is slowly moved to a sitting position and transferred to a wheelchair or assisted with ambulation to the recovery area. In the recovery area the patient is observed with intermittent vital sign monitoring for at least 20 minutes or until the above outlined criteria have been met. If the patient received IV sedation during the procedure, someone else must drive him or her home.

If the specific intervention is more significant than a simple spinal injection (e.g., spinal implant, percutaneous discectomy), the recovery period may last up to 8 hours. If the patient does not meet the discharge criteria listed above, he or she is held overnight if necessary. After discharge criteria have been met, the patient is discharged with appropriate safety and follow-up instructions.

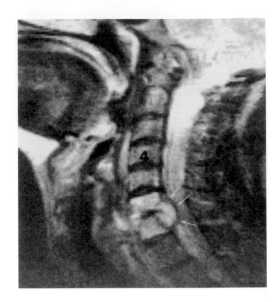

FIGURE 2-1. Lumbar epidural abscess (MRI). T2-weighted image demonstrates an epidural abscess (*white arrows*) severely compressing the thecal sac at C6 and C7 levels.

GENERAL COMPLICATIONS OF SPINAL INJECTIONS

Infection

Infections occur in 1–2% of spinal injections and range from minor to severe conditions such as meningitis,[7,8] epidural abscess,[9,10,11] and osteomyelitis[12,13] (Figs. 2-1 and 2-2). Severe infections are rare and occur between 1 in 1,000 and 1 in 10,000 spinal injections. Severe infections may have far-reaching sequelae, such as sepsis, spinal cord injury, or spread to other sites of the body via Batson's plexus or direct contiguous spread. Poor sterile technique is the most common cause of infection. *Staphylococcus aureus* is the most common infectious organism and is contracted from skin structures. Infection from gram-negative aerobes and anaerobes may occur from inadvertent intestinal penetration. Usually, discitis from lumbar discography involves a gram-negative aerobe, is self-limited, and resolves with early recognition and administration of appropriate antibiotics. Cervical discitis, however, often is life-threatening due to the aggressive gram-negative anaerobes that colonize the esophagus. If the infection is a mild cutaneous one and the patient is immunocompetent, it probably will resolve with local disinfection. The physician should make specific hygiene recommendations and follow the infection expectantly. If it appears to be pursuing a

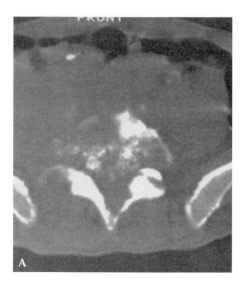 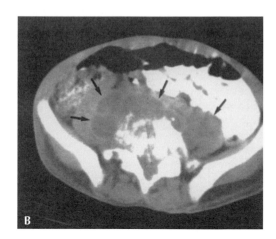

FIGURE 2-2.   Vertebral osteomyelitis and paraspinal abscess (CT). *A,* Note the paraspinal soft tissue mass in front of the destructive process of the L5 vertebra. *B,* Soft tissue windows following intravenous contrast enhancement show a large, multilocular abscess in the soft tissues enhanced (*black arrows*).

more aggressive course but does not appear to involve spinal structures, appropriate oral antibiotics on an outpatient basis and frequent follow-up may suffice. If the infection appears to be progressing to spinal structures or spaces or if the patient is infirm or otherwise predisposed to infection, inpatient evaluation and care with appropriate IV antibiotics usually are appropriate. If epidural abscess occurs, emergent surgical drainage must be considered to avoid neural damage or other complications.[14]

Early detection and treatment of epidural or intrathecal infection is necessary in order to avoid morbidity and mortality. Usually it presents with severe back or neck pain, fever, and chills with a leukocytosis developing on the third day following the injection.[11] Patients with diabetes or other immunocompromising conditions are more susceptible to infection and should be followed closely following spinal injections. After infection is suspected or confirmed in such patients, they must be evaluated and treated aggressively. Preexisting systemic infection is a relative contraindication to spinal injection. If spinal injection is critical to the overall care of the patient with preexisting systemic infection, the risks and benefits must be carefully weighed. In addition, prophylactic antibiotics for 72 hours before the injection should be considered. It is important to know the standard of care for preventing or treating spinal injection–related infections and to routinely review current microorganism susceptibilities.

Cardiovascular Complications

Bleeding is a risk inherent to all injection and surgical procedures. The potential for bleeding during spinal injection is increased by liver disease, the use of Coumadin or other anticoagulants, certain inherited anemias such as G6PD deficiency or sickle cell anemia, coagulopathy from any cause, and venous puncture. On average, the epidural vasculature is injured in 0.5–1% of spinal injections and is more common with placement of the needle in the lateral portion of the spinal canal than the midline.[15] Significant epidural bleeding may cause the development of an epidural hematoma. Clinically significant epidural hematomas are rare and have a reported incidence of less than 1 in 4,000[16,17] to 1 in 10,000 lumbar epidural cortisone injections, but they may lead to irreversible neurologic compromise if not surgically decompressed within 24 hours.[15,16,17,18,19,20,21] Retroperitoneal hematomas may occur following spinal injection if the large vessels are inadvertently penetrated. These hematomas usually are self-limited but may cause acute hypovolemia or anemia.

In addition to bleeding, a variety of dysrhythmias for which treatment should be initiated immediately may occur. The entire team of primary care physicians (PCPs) must be able to function synergistically when treating a dysrhythmia. ACLS code scenarios should be run in the procedure facility no less frequently than quarterly, all PCPs should know how to alert other staff and extended PCPs immediately, and everyone should know his or her individual roles. In addition, all PCPs must know where emergency care equipment is located and how to use it as their roles require. Treatment of individual dysrhythmias is beyond the scope of this chapter; the reader is directed to the emergency cardiac care algorithms included in Appendix 1 and to other sources for more detailed information.[22,23]

Neurologic Complications

Neurologic complications are rare. The most common causes of neural injury during spinal injection are direct trauma to the spinal cord or nerve roots from a needle, compression from an epidural hematoma, or involvement by infectious exudate. Other causes include injection-induced stroke, sedation-induced or cardiac-induced hypotension, the dislodgement of plaque from intra-arterial injection, and anoxia from respiratory arrest or laryngeal obstruction. The proximity of the vertebral artery during cervical transforaminal or facet joint injections requires specific knowledge of the three-dimensional anatomy of the cervical spine as well as specific training and expertise in cervical spinal injection procedures in order to consistently protect such structures. Injection into the vertebral artery may cause a posterior circulation stroke, hematoma formation and occlusion of the vessel, or the injection of air. Seizure also may occur if local anesthetic is injected into the vessel. Studies demonstrate that fluoroscopically guided spinal injections are less apt to cause inadvertent neural injury or injection into a vascular structure.[24] A pertinent neurologic review of symptoms and physical exam should be performed immediately if a neurologic complication is suspected.

Respiratory Complications

Respiratory arrest occurs when a patient becomes apneic for more than one minute due to lack of central respiratory drive or paralysis of the muscles of inspiration.[25] Respiratory arrest may occur from a variety of causes, including oversedation, central nervous system trauma, and the intrathecal or epidural injection of a sufficient amount of local anesthetic to cause spinal anesthesia. Treatment includes the immediate recognition of the condition and emergent support of vital signs. If the cause is self-limited, the treatment may require respiration support and other vital signs as needed until spontaneous and adequate respiration resumes. If possible,

the cause should be easily reversed (e.g., when too much opioid or sedative has been given). In such a situation it is important to consider the half-life of the reversing agent as compared to the half-life of the narcotic or sedative being reversed. If the narcotic or sedative's half-life is longer than that of the reversing agent, respiratory compromise may resume after the reversing agent has been metabolized.

The true incidence of respiratory depression due to spinal opioid administration is unknown. Agents that may cause respiratory depression include sedatives, parenteral or spinal opioids, and local anesthetics. One of the main advantages of spinal versus parenteral opioid administration is the lack of respiratory depression with the former.[26] Note that respiratory rate alone is inadequate to establish the presence or lack of respiratory depression: measurement of blood gases remains the gold standard.[25]

Other respiratory complications due to spinal injections include pneumothorax and injury to the recurrent laryngeal nerve. A pneumothorax may occur during a lower cervical procedure, such as a discogram or selective nerve root block, or a thoracic procedure, such as an intercostal nerve block. As a general rule, a pneumothorax may not occur if a needle penetrates the pleural cavity or lung parenchyma unless it is placed through a bleb, if the needle is ≥ 18-gauge, or if a solution has been injected. When a pneumothorax does occur, usually it is self-limited and causes only minor lung collapses (10%).[27] Treatment includes close observation with supportive care in a hospital setting and serial chest x-rays. A chest tube should be placed if the pneumothorax advances significantly over 25% or if the patient develops shortness of breath or other signs of respiratory distress.

Injury to the recurrent laryngeal nerve may cause unilateral vocal cord paralysis, reduction in the ability to protect the airway, and hoarseness. This injury usually is self-limited and resolves on its own but may be clinically significant while the patient is recovering from sedation or if there is preexisting underlying pathology that causes marginal airway protection (e.g., stroke, laryngeal cancer).

Urologic Complications

The application of local anesthetics and/or opioids to the lumbar and sacral nerve roots results in higher incidence of urinary retention.[28] This side effect of lumbar epidural nerve block is seen more commonly in elderly males, multiparous females, and patients who have undergone inguinal and perineal surgery. Overflow incontinence may occur if such a patient is unable to void or if bladder catheterization is not used. It is advisable that all patients undergoing lumbar epidural nerve blocks should demonstrate the ability to void the bladder prior to discharge from the pain center.

Dural Puncture

In the hands of an experienced interventional spine specialist, inadvertent dural puncture during lumbar epidural injections should occur in < 0.5% of cases (or 1 in 200 epidural injections).[29] Dural puncture occurs when the dura mater is violated by the epidural needle and a sufficient amount of cerebrospinal fluid leaks out from the thecal sac to cause a positional headache.[30,31,32,33] The rare occurrence of postdural puncture (spinal tap) headache is an unpleasant side effect but is generally relatively benign and will pass without permanent harm or morbidity to the patient. Rarely, with dehydration and severe nausea and vomiting, uncal herniation may occur with associated brain-stem involvement and, potentially, death.[34] If a needle is placed subdurally and epidural doses of local anesthetics are administered, the signs and symptoms are similar to subarachnoid injection.[35] The subdural or subarachnoid injection of large doses of local anesthetics may cause total spinal anesthesia, loss of consciousness, hypotension, cardiovascular arrest, apnea, and death. This condition requires immediate resuscitative measures and support of all vital signs until the condition resolves. Intubation usually is required to adequately control the airway and ventilate the patient.

Fluoroscopic Exposure

Epidural injections performed without fluoroscopy are not always placed into the epidural space or at the desired vertebral interspace, and sometimes the medication does not target the intended organ due to anatomic abnormality.[36–43] For this reason, most spine management specialists recommend fluoroscopic direction and the use of nonionic or low ionic contrast agents for epidural injections, which helps confirm accurate needle placement and the delivery of the injected solution to the appropriate target organ. The risk of fluoroscopic exposure to the patient is minimal for one or several isolated procedures, because each procedure should require minimal (< 20 seconds) fluoroscopic exposure time.

Fluoroscopic exposure to the physician, attending nurse, x-ray technician, and anyone else consistently in the procedure room should be viewed as cumulative. In limiting PCPs from exposure, it is important to note that radiation dissipates at the inverse of the square of the distance from the tube. As a result, if the PCP is able to stand 6 feet or more from the fluoroscopic tube, the risk of excessive exposure is minimal. As the radiation source, the fluoroscopy anode also should be kept under the procedure table. In this way, the patient absorbs the bulk of the directed radiation, and the vast majority of the small amount of radiation spilled into the room, known as "scatter radiation," has a significantly reduced ability to penetrate tissues than directed radiation. In addition, PCPs should wear protective garments. The physician should wear a lead apron, thyroid shield, radiation-attenuating gloves, and perhaps lead-lined glasses. The nurse and x-ray technician should wear wrap-around lead aprons (because their backs are frequently turned to the radiation source) and a thyroid shield. All PCPs should wear radiation badges under their thyroid shield and apron, and the physician should consider wearing a ring badge if his or her hand is routinely in the field during active fluoroscopy. Finally, the fluoroscopy unit must be routinely maintained and inspected to confirm its proper function and safety. With the proper use of fluoroscopy and radiation safety, the use of fluoroscopy to direct and confirm proper needle placement should maximize the benefit while limiting potential risks to the patient or PCPs (see chapter 3 for more information on fluoroscopy).

Adverse Drug Reactions

Adverse drug reactions rarely are seen with medications used during spinal injections. The treating physician should be aware of drug toxicity, side effects, allergic reactions, and concentration and dosing of all medications used. Lidocaine and bupivacaine are the most common local anesthetics used during spinal injections; it is important to be aware of their CNS and cardiovascular toxicity and side effects. Strict cardiovascular and neurologic monitoring is required before, during, and after the procedure. Although most anaphylactic reactions most often occur within 2 hours after the epidural injection, they have been known to occur up to 6 hours later.[44]

Local anesthetics primarily function by reversibly blocking the sodium channels in nerve and muscle membranes that have a direct effect on sympathetic nerves when injected into the subarachnoid space and the cardiac tissue when injected intravascularly. If the sympathetic system is sufficiently blocked, hypotension may result; if cardiac muscle is sufficiently blocked, decreased contractility may result. When injected intravenously, lidocaine is fast-in and fast-out, reaching steady-state in 1–2 beats. Bupivacaine is fast-in and slow-out, and its blocking action increases as the heart works harder. These direct effects may cause cardiac arrest. Cervical and thoracic level blocks have an increased risk for complications due to the regional neural supply cardiac and respiratory control.

Central nervous system toxicity by 1% lidocaine has an onset at plasma concentrations of 5–10 μg/ml, which is slightly more than 400 mg (or 40 ml) of total intravenous bolus. Bupivacaine is about four times more toxic than lidocaine with a toxic bolus of 100 mg (or 10 ml).[45] Patients with CNS toxicity usually present with complaints of circumoral numbness, disorientation, light-headedness, nystagmus, tinnitus, and muscle twitching in the face or distal extremities. Peak plasma concentrations occur 10–20 minutes after injection; thus, patient monitoring for at least 30 minutes following an epidural injection with a significant bolus of lidocaine or bupivacaine is mandatory.

Methylprednisolone, triamcinolone, and betamethasone are the most commonly used corticosteroid preparations. Side effects are uncommon but include headaches, dizziness, insomnia, facial erythema, rash and pruritis, low-grade fever (< 100°F), hyperglycemia, transient hypotension and hypertension, increased back or limb pain, fluid retention, mood swings, euphoria, menstrual irregularities, headaches, and gastritis. Other rare side effects include elevation of cerebrospinal fluid protein levels, septic or aseptic meningitis, worsening of symptoms of multiple sclerosis, sclerosing spinal pachymeningitis, exacerbation of latent infection, near-fatal septic meningitis (intrathecal injection), hypercorticism, and congestive heart failure (see chapter 1 for more details on commonly used drugs and potential reactions).

Anaphylactic and Allergic Reactions

Anaphylactoid reaction (without histologic immune response) or anaphylaxis (with histologic immune response) most often occurs within 2 hours after the epidural injection and have been known to develop up to 6 hours later.[44] They usually cause fatalities by respiratory-related complications involving mechanical airway obstruction. Close patient

monitoring after the procedure is recommended for approximately 30 minutes, and informing the patient of possible risks may expedite early identification of complications.

Bleeding

Epidural hematoma formation following injection is extremely rare. Bleeding usually occurs because of damage to the veins in the highly vascular epidural space. Medications that interfere with the clotting mechanism include heparin, Coumadin, aspirin, and most nonsteroidal anti-inflammatory drugs (NSAIDs). Patients usually present with severe neck or back pain associated with any significant neurologic complaint right after the procedure. An immediate physical exam followed by a CT or MRI scan is essential for patients thought to have an epidural hematoma, because early surgical intervention can limit or even prevent permanent neurologic damage (Fig. 2-3).

SPECIFIC COMPLICATIONS OF SELECTIVE SPINAL INJECTIONS

Lumbar Epidural Injections

The lumbar epidural space is highly vascular. Inadvertent intravenous placement of the epidural needle occurs in approximately 0.5–1% of patients

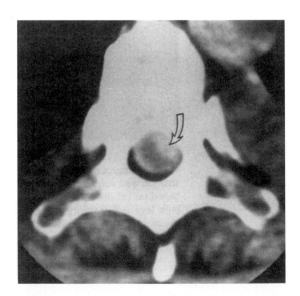

FIGURE 2-3. Acute epidural hematoma and subarachnoid hemorrhage (CT). Thoracic spine view shows a lenticular, high-density epidural hematoma (*open arrow*) causing spinal cord compression. Acute hemorrhage is noted in the subarachnoid space.

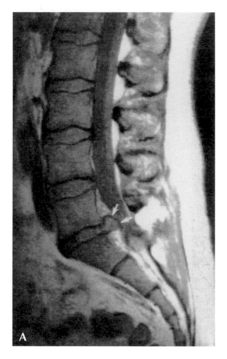
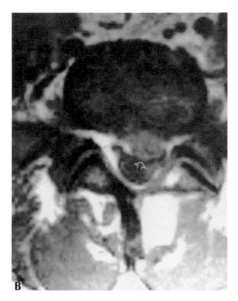

FIGURE 2-4.   Herniated nucleus pulposus (MRI). *A*, T1-weighted sagittal image shows impingement of the thecal sac by the herniated nuclear material (*white arrows*). *B*, Axial sagittal gradient echo image reveals that the herniation has shifted to the left (*black arrows*).

undergoing lumbar epidural anesthesia.[29] This rare complication primarily is seen with distended epidural veins that occur during pregnancy and in patients with a large abdominal tumor mass. If the misplacement goes unrecognized, injection of a large volume of local anesthetic directly into an epidural vein may result in significant local anesthetic toxicity.[46] Careful, four-quadrant aspiration (aspiration in all four quadrants by rotating the needle) prior to injection of drugs into the epidural space is mandatory in identifying the vascular placement of the needle when performing a "blind" (non–fluoroscopically guided) epidural injection.

Neurologic complications of lumbar nerve block are uncommon if proper technique is used. Usually these complications are associated with a preexisting neurologic lesion or with surgical or obstetric trauma rather than with the lumbar block itself.[28] Direct trauma to the spinal cord or nerve roots is usually accompanied by pain. Any significant pain that occurs during placement of the epidural needle or catheter or during injection should warn the injectionist to pause and confirm needle placement before proceeding.[29] The use of deep intravenous sedation or general anesthesia prior to initiation of epidural nerve block may reduce the patient's ability to provide accurate verbal feedback if needle misplacement occurs. As a result, conscious sedation or general anesthesia before epidural nerve block should be used with caution.[47]

If the patient's lower extremity neurologic status deteriorates rapidly or if a cauda equina syndrome is suspected within 24–48 hours after an epidural procedure, an expanding epidural hematoma should be suspected.[48] An immediate and complete clinical evaluation is mandatory in this situation. If the diagnosis is still entertained following the clinical evaluation, a lumbar CT scan or MRI should be obtained (Figs. 2-4, 2-5, and 2-6). If the diagnosis is confirmed, an emergent surgical consult to consider decompression should be arranged.

Caudal Epidural Injections

Incorrect needle placement during caudal epidural injection occurs 25–40% of the time.[49,50] The needle may be placed outside the sacral canal, resulting in the injection of air or fluid into the subcutaneous tissues, periosteum, sacrococcygeal ligament, sacral marrow cavity, and pelvic cavity, possibly entering both the rectum or vaginal vault. The application of local anesthetic and opioids to the sacral nerve roots results in an increased incidence of urinary retention, noted especially in elderly

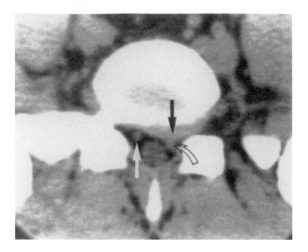

FIGURE 2-5. Posterolateral disc herniation (CT). Focal protrusion of the disc on the left (*black arrow*), leading to posterior displacement of the left S1 nerve root (*open arrow*) and effacement of the anterior epidural fat. This contrasts with the epidural fat on the right and the normal location of the right S1 nerve root (*white arrow*).

males and multiparous females and after inguinal and perineal surgery. The use of smaller doses of local anesthetic helps avoid such complications without adversely affecting the efficacy of caudal

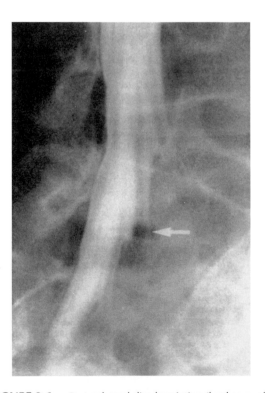

FIGURE 2-6. Posterolateral disc herniation (lumbar myelogram view). Oblique view performed with water-soluble contrast reveals the abrupt termination and widening of the S1 nerve root sleeve (*white arrow*).

epidural steroid injections when treating painful conditions. Because of the proximity of the sacral hiatus to the perineum, the incidence of epidural abscess and meningitis is increased compared to the translaminar or transforaminal injection route. When placing the epidural needle, remember that the thecal sac usually ends at the S2 bony level but may end as low as S4; thus, the needle should be placed no higher than absolutely necessary to assure epidural injection. If the needle penetrates the thecal sac, this may cause a positional headache and lower the body's protection against meningitis, because the thecal sac will have been violated. In addition, if the needle malposition is not detected before injection, an intrathecal injection may occur and potentially cause a spinal block and its associated sequelae.

Cervical Epidural Injections

Because of the potential for hematogenous spread via Batson's plexus, local infection and sepsis are absolute contraindications to the cervical approach to the epidural space. Anticoagulation and coagulopathy represent absolute contraindications to cervical epidural nerve block because of the risk of epidural hematoma.

The fact that the spinal cord is present within the spinal canal increases the risk for spinal cord injury with the cervical epidural injection technique as compared to lower or mid-lumbar injections. Central canal stenosis from bony eburnation, central disc herniation, or congenital shortening of the pedicles represents an *absolute* contraindication to performing a translaminar epidural injection at that level (Figs. 2-7 and 2-8).[51,52]

Thoracic Epidural Injections

Thoracic epidural techniques are similar to lumbar injections, but the presence of the narrow epidural space and close proximity to the spinal cord in the thoracic vertebral canal makes spinal cord trauma more likely with the latter. The incidence of spinal cord damage is unknown; however, the incidence of infection is increased in the thoracic spine compared to the lumbar spine.[53] The presence of the lungs on either side of the spine makes a pneumothorax a potential complication that usually is not a consideration with either a cervical or lumbar injection. The injection of local anesthetic in the mid-thoracic epidural space may inhibit the cardiac accelerator zone and cause hypotension and bradycardia and their potential sequelae. In addition, a thoracic motor block from either the epidural or intrathecal injection of local anesthetic can cause up to a 50% reduction in tidal volume, making adequate ventilation of a patient with pulmonary disease difficult.

Selective Nerve Root Blockade

Selective nerve root blockade has been used interchangeably as a spinal nerve block, selective epidural, or anterior ramus block. In this brief section each type is separately discussed.

An anterior ramus block is an extra spinal injection of the anterior ramus. This occurs 1–2 cm outside of the neural foramen, so local anesthetic does not reach the spinal canal or spinal nerve. The main complication of this blockade is direct trauma to the anterior ramus from the needle or the disruption of the neural vasculature, causing an intraparenchymal hematoma or neural infarct.

A spinal nerve block occurs when the needle tip is placed within the neural foramen and local anesthetic only affects the spinal nerve and does not migrate inside the spinal canal. The main risk of this injection technique is trauma to the spinal nerve or dorsal root ganglion. If the needle penetrates the dural sleeve, an intrathecal injection and its associated risks and complications may occur.

A selective epidural occurs when fluid is injected into the epidural space via a neural foramen. To accomplish this, the needle also is placed within the neural foramen, and therefore trauma to the spinal nerve or dorsal root ganglion is possible. Injection with all of its associated risks and complications into the dural sleeve also is possible.

Discography

The most common severe complication after discography is infection of the disc, which is commonly referred to as *discitis*. Discitis should occur no more frequently than 1 in 500 to 1 in 750 discs injected.[54,55] The most common organisms infecting the lumbar disc are *Staphylococcus aureus* and *Staphylococcus epidermidis*.[54,56] Occasionally a colonic organism involves the lumbar discs as a result of penetrating the colon with the discography needle. Because of the limited blood supply to the disc, such infections may prove difficult to eradicate. Discitis usually presents as an increase in spine pain 5–14 days following discography. Acutely, no change in the patient's neurologic status should be evident. An

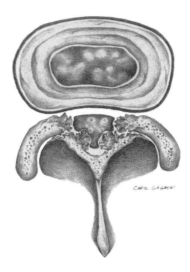

FIGURE 2-7. Degenerative central spinal stenosis (schematic view). Lumbar vertebra at the disc level is noted in the axial view. The osteophytes derived from the articular processes can lead to thecal sac compression.

elevated sedimentation rate will be seen within the first week to 10 days.[57,58,59] Magnetic resonance imaging is now considered the gold standard in the detection of discitis, which was found to be superior to bone scan with 92% sensitivity, 97% specificity, and a 95% overall accuracy (Fig. 2-9).[60,61,62]

The incidence of thoracic discitis following a thoracic discogram is unknown, but the organisms infecting those discs after discography should be similar to those involving the lumbar discs. Similarly, the incidence of pneumothorax and large vessel damage following thoracic discography also is unknown. In one series of 230 outpatient thoracic

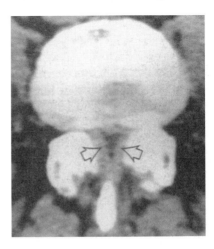

FIGURE 2-8. Central spinal stenosis (CT). Marked hypertrophy of the ligamentum flavum (*open arrows*) is noted to directly cause thecal sac compression; mild annular bulging and facet joint arthropathy also are seen.

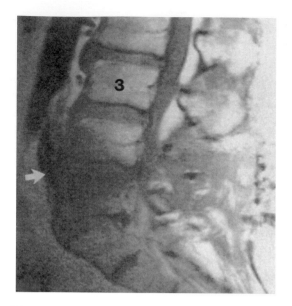

FIGURE 2-9. Lumbar disc space infection (MRI). T1-weighted image shows areas of low signal of L4 and L5. The anterior paraspinal mass is noted (*white arrow*).

discograms, Schell reported a zero incidence of pneumothorax.[63] However, the complication does still occur, and thus the procedure should not be attempted without substantial experience and training.

Cervical discitis generally is profound and life-threatening. The esophagus has gram-negative and anaerobic bacteria as components of its normal flora; placing the discography needle through it and into the disc may seed the disc with bacteria that may initiate a profound infection. In the mid and lower cervical spine, the esophagus lies on the left side of the larynx. The carotid sheath lies on the anterolateral surface of the cervical spinal column. Therefore, a cervical discogram should be performed using a right paralaryngeal approach. In performing this approach, the esophagus should be pushed to the left and the carotid sheath to the right to minimize the risk of trauma to these structures. If the needle does penetrate the carotid sheath, direct injury to the vagus nerve or carotid artery can occur.

In addition to infectious complications, pneumothorax may occur after cervical and thoracic discography but rarely should occur if appropriate technique is used. Most pneumothoraces following cervical or thoracic discography are small (10–15% of lung volume) and often can be treated conservatively. However, all pneumothoraces must be taken seriously and watched overnight with serial chest x-rays and close monitoring of vital signs and blood gases. If the pneumothorax advances, a chest tube must be placed.

Direct trauma to the nerve roots and the spinal cord can occur if the needle is allowed to traverse the entire disc or is placed too laterally. These complications rarely should occur if appropriate technique and precautions are used. Such needle-induced trauma to the cervical spinal cord can result in syrinx formation with attendant progressive neurologic deficit, including quadriplegia.

Intercostal Nerve Blocks

Given the proximity of the pleural space, pneumothorax after intercostal nerve blocks is a distinct possibility. The incidence of the complication is less than 1% (0.082%)[64] but occurs with greater frequency in patients with COPD. Because of the proximity to the intercostal nerve and artery, when analgesia is produced from the intercostal block, the compensatory vasoconstriction eases and the patient may become hypotensive. In a similar manner, intercostal blocks can lead to respiratory failure when pain relief from the block unmasks the ventilatory depression of previously administered but ineffective parenteral narcotics.[65]

Facet Joint Nerve Blocks

The most often cited problem is a transient exacerbation in pain (about 2% incidence) lasting as long as 6 weeks to 8 months in some cases.[66] Spinal anesthesia may occur after facet joint injection if the needle is positioned within the thecal sac or if there is an abnormal communication between the facet joint capsule and the thecal sac. Chemical meningitis after lumbar facet block has been reported.[66,67,68] Both of these complications are thought to have occurred after inadvertent dural puncture. Facet capsule rupture also occurs, especially if more than 2.0 ml of injectate is used for intra-articular injections.

During performance of cervical facet blockade, the potential risk of entry into the intervertebral foramen, spinal canal, and vertebral artery is present. Such complications occur more frequently with a lateral intra-articular technique than with blockade of the medial branches innervating the cervical facets, because the former technique requires deeper penetration of the needle into the joint and toward the spinal structures. Local anesthetic may leak out of the joint into these areas and cause motor and sensory blockade with its attendant risks and complications.

Third occipital nerve blocks can cause transient ataxia and unsteadiness due to partial blockade of the upper cervical proprioceptive afferents and the righting response.[69,70] In one study of cervical facet joint radiofrequency denervation, 13% of the patients complained of postprocedure pain that resolved in 2–6 weeks, and 4% complained of occipital hypesthesia (probably due to a lesion of the third occipital nerve) that resolved in 3 months.[70] No persistent motor or sensory deficits occurred.

Sympathetic Nerve Blocks

In the cervicothoracic (stellate ganglion) block, acute, potentially life-threatening complications may occur, including seizures, spinal block, hypotension, or pneumothorax.[71–75] Additional complications include block or injury to the recurrent laryngeal nerve, phrenic nerve, sympathetic trunk, apex of the lung, or brachial plexus.

In the lumbar sympathetic block, potential complications include intravascular injections, intradural injections with spinal anesthesia or postural headaches, hypotension, lumbar plexus block, renal puncture, or genitofemoral neuralgia.[72,76,77] Other risks include injury to the spleen, intestines, and liver and injection of large volumes of local anesthetic into the aorta or inferior vena cava.

REFERENCES

1. Falco FJ: Lumbar spine injection procedures in the management of low back pain. Occup Med 13:121–149, 1998.
2. Moskovich R: Epidural injections for the treatment of low back pain. Bull Hosp Jt Dis 55:178–184, 1996.
3. Kinard RE: Diagnostic spinal injection procedures. Neurosurg Clin North Am 7:151–165, 1996.
4. PASSOR: PASSOR Fellowship Guidelines. Endorsed by the AAPM&R Board of Governors; April, 1998.
5. Demling R: Preoperative care in current surgical diagnosis and treatment. Curr Surg Diag Treatment 2:11, 1991.
6. Sunderland S: Nerves and Nerve Injuries, 2nd ed. Edinburgh, Churchill Livingstone, 1978.
7. Dougherty JH Jr, Fraser RA: Complications following intraspinal injections of steroids: Reports of two cases. J Neurosurg 48:1023–1025, 1978.
8. Gutknecht DR: Chemical meningitis following injections of epidural steroids [letter]. Am J Med 82:570, 1987.
9. Shealy CN: Dangers of spinal injections without proper diagnosis. JAMA 197:1104–1106, 1966.
10. Goucke CR, Graziotti P: Extradural abscess following local anesthetic and steroid injection for chronic low back pain. Br J Anaesth 65:427–429, 1990.
11. Chan ST, Leung S: Spinal epidural abscess following steroid injection for sciatica. Case report. Spine 14:106–108, 1989.
12. Tham EJ, Stoodley MA, Macintyre PE, Jones NR: Back pain following postoperative epidural analgesia: An indicator of possible infection. Anaesth Intensive Care 25:297–301, 1997.
13. Cooper AB, Sharpe MD: Bacterial meningitis and cauda equina syndrome after epidural steroid injections. Can J Anaesth 43:471–474, 1996.
14. Baker AS, Ojemann RG, Swartz MN, Richardson EP: Spinal epidural abscess. N Engl J Med 293:463–468, 1975.
15. Bonica JJ: Diagnostic and therapeutic blocks. A reappraisal based on 15 years experience. Anesth Analg Curr Res 37:58, 1958.
16. Odom J, Sih I: Epidural analgesia and anticoagulant therapy: Experience with one thousand cases of continuous epidurals. Anesthesia 38:550–551, 1983.
17. Rao T, El-Etr A: Anticoagulation following placement of epidural and subarachnoid catheters. Anesthesiology 55:618–620, 1981.
18. Delaney T, Towlingson JC, Cannon H, Butler A: Epidural steroid effects on nerves and meninges. Anaesth Analg Curr Res 59:610–614, 1980.
19. Knight C, Burnell J: Systemic side effects of extradural steroids. Anaesthesia 35:593–594, 1980.
20. Goebert H, et al: Sciatica: Treatment with injections of procaine and hydrocortisone acetate. Results in 113 patients. Anesth Analg 40:130–134, 1960.
21. Knutsen O, Ygge H: Prolonged extradural anesthesia with bupivacaine at lumbago and sciatica. Acta Orthop Scand 42:338–352, 1971.
22. American Heart Association: Textbook of Advanced Cardiac Life Support, 3rd ed. Dallas, AHA, 1993.
23. American Heart Association: Guidelines for Cardiopulmonary Resuscitation and Emergency Cardiac Care. JAMA 268:2171–2302, 1992.
24. El-Khoury GY, Renfrew DL: Percutaneous procedures for the diagnosis and treatment for lower back pain: Discography, facet-joint injection, and epidural injection. AJR 157:685–691, 1991.
25. Rawal N, Wattwil M: Respiratory depression following epidural morphine: An experimental and clinical study. Anesth Analg 63:8–14, 1984.
26. Rawal N, Arner S: Present state of extradural and intrathecal opioid analgesia in Sweden: A nationwide follow-up survey. Br J Anaesth 59:791–799, 1987.
27. Bridenbaugh PO, DuPen SL, Moore DC, et al: Post-operative intercostal nerve block analgesia versus narcotic analgesia. Anesth Analg 52:81–85, 1973.
28. Armitage EN: Lumbar and thoracic epidural. In Wildsmith JAW, Armitage EN (eds): Principles and Practice of Regional Anesthesia. New York, Churchill Livingstone, 1987, p 109.
29. Bromage PR: Complications and contraindications. In Bromage PR (ed): Epidural Analgesia. Philadelphia, W.B. Saunders, 1978, pp 654–711.
30. Benzon H: Epidural steroid injections for low back pain and lumbosacral radiculopathy. Pain 24:277–295, 1986.
31. Swerdlow M, Sayle-Creer W: A study of extradural medication in the relief of the lumbosciatic syndrome. Anaesthesia 25:341–345, 1970.
32. Warr A, Wilkinson JA, Burn JM, Langdon L: Chronic lumbosciatic syndrome treated by epidural injection and manipulation. Practitioner 209:53–59, 1972.
33. Kepes E, Duncalf D: Treatment of low back ache with spinal injections of local anesthetics, spinal and systemic steroids: A review. Pain 22:33–47, 1985.
34. Deisenhammer E: Clinical and experimental studies on headaches after myelography. Neuroradiology 9:99–102, 1985.
35. Waldman SD: Subdural injection as a cause of unexplained neurological symptoms. Reg Anesth 17:55, 1992.
36. El-Khoury GY, Ehara S, Weinstein JN, et al: Epidural injections: A procedure ideally performed under fluoroscopic control. Radiology 168:554–557, 1988.
37. Mehta M, Salmon N: Extradural block. Confirmation of the injection site by x-ray monitoring. Anesth 40:1009–1012, 1985.

38. Dreyfuss P: Epidural steroid injections: A procedure ideally performed with fluoroscopic control and contrast media. ISIS Newsletter 1(5): 1993.
39. Stewart HD, Quinnell RC, Dann N: Epidurography in the management of sciatica. Br J Rheumatol 26:424–429, 1987.
40. Forrest JB: The response to epidural steroid injections in chronic dorsal root pain. Can Anaesth Soc J 27:40–46, 1980.
41. White AH: Injection techniques for the diagnosis and treatment of low back pain. Spine 5:78–82, 1980.
42. Renfrew DL, Moore TE, Kathol MH, et al: Correct placement of epidural steroid injections: Fluoroscopic guidance and contrast administration. AJNR 12:1003–1007, 1991.
43. White AH: Injection techniques for the diagnosis and treatment of low back pain. Orthop Clin North Am 14:553–567, 1983.
44. Simon DL, Kunz RD, German JD, Zivodovich V: Allergic or pseudoallergic reaction following epidural steroid deposition and skin testing. Reg Anesth 14:253–255, 1989.
45. Covino BG: Clinical pharmacology of local anesthetic agents. In Cousins MJ, Bridenbaugh PO (eds): Neural Blockade in Clinical Anesthesia and Management of Pain, 2nd ed. Philadelphia, J.B. Lippincott, 1988, pp 111–144.
46. Braid DP, et al: The systemic absorption of local analgesic drugs. Br J Anaesth 37:394, 1965.
47. Cousins MJ, et al: Epidural neural blockade. In Cousins MJ, Bridenbaugh PO (eds): Neural Blockade in Clinical Anesthesia and Management of Pain, 2nd ed. Philadelphia, J.B. Lippincott, 1988, pp 340–341.
48. Cousins MJ: Hematoma following epidural block. Anesthesiology 37:263, 1972.
49. Waldman SD, Winnie AD: Caudal epidural nerve block. In Interventional Pain Management. Philadelphia, W.B. Saunders, 1996, pp 381–382.
50. Derby R, et al: Precision percutaneous blocking procedures for localizing spinal pain. Part 2. The lumbar neuroaxial compartment. Pain Digest 3:175–178, 1993.
51. Lerner SM, Gutterman P, Jenkins F: Epidural hematoma and paraplegia after numerous lumbar punctures. Anesthesia 39:550–553, 1973.
52. Waldman SD: Cervical epidural steroid blocks—a prospective study of complications occurring during 790 consecutive nerve blocks. Reg Anesth 11:149–152, 1989.
53. Redekop GJ, Del Maestro RF: Diagnosis and management of spinal epidural abscess. Can J Neurol Sci 19:180–187, 1992.
54. Fraser RD, Osti OL, Vernon-Roberts B: Discitis after discography. J Bone Joint Surg 69B:26–35, 1987.
55. Crock H: Practice of Spinal Surgery. New York, Springer-Verlag, 1983.
56. Guyer RD, Collier R, Stith WJ, et al: Discitis after discography. Spine 13:1352–1354, 1988.
57. Fernand R, Lee CK: Post-laminectomy disc space infection. A review of the literature and a report of three cases. Clin Orthop 209:215–218, 1986.
58. Lindholm TS, Pylkkanen P: Discitis following removal of intervertebral discs. Spine 7:618–622, 1982.
59. Thibodeau AA: Closed space infection following the removal of lumbar intervertebral discs. J Bone Joint Surg 50A:400–410, 1968.
60. Arrington JA, Murtagh FR, Silbiger ML, et al: MRI of postdiscogram discitis and osteomyelitis in the lumbar spine: Case report. J Fla Med Assoc 73:192–194, 1986.
61. Modic MT, Feiglin DH, Hinton CE, et al: Vertebral osteomyelitis: Assessment using MR. Radiology 157:157–166, 1985.
62. Szypryt EP, Hardy JG, Hinton CE, et al: A comparison between MRI and scintigraphic bone imaging in the diagnosis of disc space infection in an animal model. Spine 13:1042–1048, 1988.
63. Moore DC, et al: Pneumothorax: Its incidence following intercostal nerve block. JAMA 174:842, 1960.
64. Cory PC, Mulroy MF: Postoperative respiratory failure following intercostal block. Anesthesiology 54:418, 1981.
65. Bous RA: Facet joint injections. In Stanton-Hicks M, Bous R (eds): Chronic Low Back Pain. New York, Raven Press, 1982, pp 199–211.
66. Thomson SJ, Lomax DM, Collett BJ: Chemical meningism after lumbar facet joint nerve block with local anesthetic and steroids. Anesthesia 46:563–564, 1993.
67. Berrigan T: Chemical meningism after lumbar facet joint block. Anesthesia 47:905–906, 1992.
68. Pawl RP: Headache, cervical spondylosis, and anterior cervical fusion. Surg Ann 9:391, 1971.
69. Bogduk N, Mansland A: The cervical zygopophyseal joints as a source of neck pain. Spine 13:610–617, 1988.
70. Carron H, Litwiller R: Stellate ganglion block. Anesth Analg 54:567, 1975.
71. Lofstrom J, et al: Sympathetic neural blockade of upper and lower extremity. In Cousins MJ, Bridenbaugh PO (eds): Neural Blockade in Clinical Anesthesia and Management of Pain, 2nd ed. Philadelphia, J.B. Lippincott, 1988, p 461.
72. Malmqvist EL, Bengtsson M, Sorensen J: Efficacy of stellate ganglion block: A clinical study with bupivacaine. Reg Anesth 17:340–347, 1992.
73. Sachs BL, Zindrick MR, Beasley RD: Reflex sympathetic dystrophy after operative procedures on the lumbar spine. J Bone Joint Surg 75A:721–725, 1993.
74. Wallace MS, Millholland AV: Contralateral spread of local anesthetic with stellate ganglion block. Reg Anesth 18:55–59, 1993.
75. Schmidt S, Gibbons JJ: Postdural puncture headache after fluoroscopically-guided lumbar paravertebral sympathetic block. Anesthesiology 78:198, 1993.
76. Sprague R, Ramamurthy S: Identification of the anterior psoas sheath as a landmark for lumbar sympathetic block. Reg Anesth 15:253–255, 1990.
77. Waldman SD, Winnie AP: Interventional Pain Management. Philadelphia, W.B. Saunders, 1996.
78. Kricun R, Kricun ME: Computed Tomography of the Spine: Diagnostic Exercises. Gaithersburg, MD, Aspen, 1987.
79. Daffner RH: Clinical Radiology: The Essentials. Baltimore, Williams & Wilkins, 1993.

Appendix I

American Heart Association's ACLS Protocols, Version 2.0. ACLS Pocket References. Arlen Advertising, 1993.

Appendix II
Treatment of Acute Reactions

Urticaria
Discontinue injection
Benadryl or Vistaril, PO/IM/IV, 25–50 mg
Cimetidine PO/IV, 300 mg, or ranitidine PO/IV, 50 mg
If severely disseminated, give Epinephrine SC (1:1000), 0.1–0.3 ml

Facial and Laryngeal Edema
Epinephrine SC (1:1000), 0.1–0.2 ml, or if hypotensive give 1:10,000, slowly IV, 0.1 ml
Oxygen via mask/endotracheal tube, 6–10 L/min*
If resuscitation needed, initiate ACLS protocol and call EMS

Bronchospasm
Oxygen via mask, 6–10 L/min*
Monitor vital signs (BP, pulse oxygen, and EKG)
Beta agonist inhalers (e.g., albuterol)
Epinephrine SC (1:1000), 0.1–0.2 ml, or if hypotensive give 1:10,000, slowly IV, 0.1 ml
If oxygen saturations persist at < 88%, initiate ACLS protocol and call EMS

Hypotension with Tachycardia
Reverse Trendelenburg position
Monitor vital signs (BP, pulse oxygen, and EKG)
Oxygen via mask, 6–10 L/min*
Rapid IV administration of large volumes of isotonic Ringer's lactate or normal saline solution
If poorly responsive: epinephrine SC (1:10,000), 1.0 ml, slowly IV

Hypotension with Bradycardia—Vagal Reaction
Reverse Trendelenburg position
Monitor vital signs (BP, pulse oxygen, and EKG)
Oxygen via mask, 6–10 L/min*
Secure IV access and initiate rapid IV administration of large volumes of isotonic Ringer's lactate
  or normal saline solution
If poorly responsive: atropine, 0.6–1.0 mg, slowly IV
Repeat atropine to reach total dose of 0.04 mg/kg (2–3 mg) in adult

Hypertension—Severe
Monitor vital signs (BP, pulse oxygen, and EKG)
Nitroglycerin, 0.4 mg, SL, or Nitrol topical ointment, 1–2 inch
If persistent, transfer for further evaluation to an ER or ICU setting
For pheochromocytoma: give phentolamine, 5 mg (adults), 1 mg (children)

Seizures or Convulsions
Monitor vital signs (BP, pulse oxygen, and EKG)
Oxygen via mask, 6–10 L/min*
Maintain IV access
Protect patient from physical injury during seizure
Insert bite block
If seizure lasts longer than 2 minutes, secure airway and oxygenate
Obtain neurologic consult
Give diazepam (Valium), 5 mg IV, or midazolam (Versed), 2.5 mg IV
If longer effect needed, consider phenytoin (Dilantin) infusion, 15–18 mg/kg at rate of 50 mg/min
Consider ACLS protocol, if intubation is needed

Pulmonary Edema
Elevate the torso; rotating tourniquets (venous compression)
Oxygen via mask, 6–10 L/min*
Diuretics: furosemide (Lasix), 40 mg IV, slow push
Consider morphine
Transfer to an ICU or ER setting, for further management

Prophylaxis for Adverse Intravascular Iodinated Contrast Media Reactions
Avoid unnecessary exposure to contrast medium
Substitute nonionic for ionic contrast medium
In adults, give prednisone, 50 mg PO, 12 hrs then 2 hrs prior to procedure
Give diphenhydramine (Benadryl), 50 mg PO, 1 hour prior to procedure
For pheochromocytoma: give phenoxybenzamine, 10–20 mg, 3–4 times/day PO for 7–10 days; or 24 hours prior to the procedure, give phenoxybenzamine 0.5 mg/kg in 250 ml of D5W slowly IV, over 2 hours

Dysrhythmias
Refer to ACLS protocol

* Always administer supplemental oxygen with caution in a patient with chronic pulmonary disease.

3

Radiation Safety for the Physician

Robert D. Gruber, D.O., Kenneth P. Botwin, M.D., and Chunilal P. Shah, M.D.

Currently, fluoroscopic guidance is used routinely for many interventional pain management procedures in order to obtain more precise localization of anatomic target areas. Fluoroscopy is used in many procedures, including swallowing studies, urologic evaluations, peripheral joint injections, and, perhaps most commonly, interventional spine procedures. The ability to perform many spinal injections, including transforaminal epidurals, facet joint injections, medial branch blocks, sympathetic blocks, discograms, and sacroiliac joint injections, is entirely dependent on fluoroscopic imaging. This chapter reviews the basic concepts of radiation safety and their practical application in the fluoroscopy suite to minimize exposure risks for the patient and spinal interventionalist.

RADIATION CONCEPTS

Radiologic nomenclature describes the quantity of radiation in terms of *exposure*, *dose*, *dose equivalent*, and *activity*. Conventional terms are used in the United States, and an international system of units defined in 1960 by the General Conference of Weights and Measurements is primarily used in Europe. Each system has its unique terms[16] (Table 3-1).

Terminology

Like matter, energy can be transformed from one type to another. When ice (solid) melts and turns to H_2O (liquid) and then evaporates (gas), a transformation of matter has occurred. Similarly, x-rays transform electrical energy (electricity) into electromagnetic energy (x-rays), which then transforms into chemical energy (radiographic film). Electromagnetic energy emitted into and transferred through matter is called **radiation**. The spectrum of electromagnetic radiation extends over twenty-five orders of magnitude and includes not only x-rays, but also the wavelengths responsible for visible light, magnetic resonance imaging (MRI), microwaves, radio, television, and cellular phone transmission (Fig. 3-1). **Irradiation** occurs when matter is exposed to radiation and absorbs all or part of it.

Ionizing Radiation

The two basic types of electromagnetic radiation are ionizing and nonionizing. A unique characteristic of **ionizing radiation** is the ability to alter the molecular structure of materials by removing bound orbital electrons from its atom to create an electrically charged positive ion. The ejected electron and the resulting positively charged atom are called an **ion pair**. Ionizing radiation gradually uses its energy as it collides with the atoms of the material through which it travels. This transfer of energy and the resulting electrically charged ions can induce molecular changes and potentially lead to somatic and genetic damage.

X-Rays and Gamma Rays

Ionizing radiation includes **x-rays** and **gamma rays**, which are emitted from x-ray machines, nuclear reactors, and radioactive materials. Gamma rays and x-rays are identical in their physical properties and biologic effects; the only difference is that gamma rays are natural products of radioactive atoms, whereas x-rays are produced in machines. In the production of x-rays, a high dose of voltage, measured in kilovolts (kVp), and a sufficient dose of electrical current, measured in milliamperes (mA), are required.

X-ray is a form of electromagnetic energy of very short wavelength (0.5–0.06 angstrom [Å]), which allows it to readily penetrate matter. When an object or body is exposed to ionizing radiation, the total amount of exposure is a unit of measurement called the **roentgen** (R). The definition

TABLE 3-1.   Radiation Quantities and Units

Quantity	Conventional Unit	SI Unit	Conversion
Exposure	Roentgen (R)	Coulomb/kg of air (C/kg)	1 C/kg = 3876 R 1 R = 258 µC/kg 1 R = 2.58×10^{-4} C/kg
Dose	Rad (100 ergs/g)	Gray (Gy) (joule/kg)	1 Gy = 100 rad 0.01 Gy = 1 cGy = 1 rad 0.001 Gy = 1 mGy = 100 mrad
Dose equivalent	Rem (rad × Q)	Sievert (Sv) (Gy × Q)	1 Sv = 100 rem 0.01 Sv = 1 cSv = 1 rem 0.001 Sv = 1 mSv = 100 mrem
Activity	Curie (Ci)	Bequerel (Bq)	1 mCi = 37 MBq

Adapted from Wycoff HO: The international system of units. Radiology 128:833–835, 1978.

describes the electrical charge per unit mass of air (1 R = 2.58×10^{-4} coulombs/kg of air). The output of x-ray machines usually is specified in roentgen (R) or milliroentgens (mR). Ionizing radiation exposed to a body interacts with the atoms of the material it comes in contact with in the form of transfer of energy. This dose of transferred energy is called absorption, and the quantity of absorbed energy in humans is referred to as the **radiation absorbed dose** (rad). By definition, 1 rad = 100 ergs/g where the erg (joule) is a unit of energy and the gram is a unit of mass. The **gray** (Gy) is a commonly used international unit of measurement to describe absorbed dosages and can be calculated by multiplying the rad by 0.01. Biologic effects usually are related to the rad, which is the unit most often used to describe the quantity of radiation received by a patient. The **rad equivalent man** (rem) is the unit of occupational

radiation exposure and is used to monitor personnel exposure devices such as film badges.

RADIOLOGIC PROCEDURES

Fluoroscopy

In general, there are two types of x-ray procedures: radiography and fluoroscopy. Conventional fluoroscopic procedures, such as myelography, barium enemas, upper gastrointestinal series, and swallowing studies, usually are conducted on a fluoroscopic table. The conventional fluoroscope consists of an x-ray tube located above a fixed examining table. The physician is provided with dynamic images that are portrayed on a fluoroscopic screen and the ability to hold and store ("freeze frame") an image in memory for review or to print as a radiograph

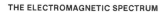
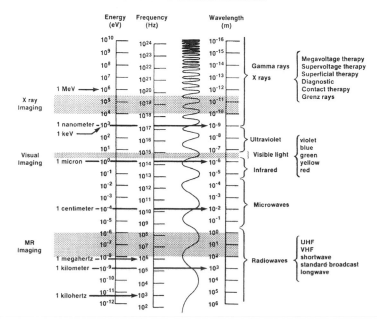

THE ELECTROMAGNETIC SPECTRUM

FIGURE 3-1.   The electromagnetic spectrum extends over more than twenty-five orders of magnitude. This chart shows the values of energy, frequency, and wavelength and identifies some common values and regions of the spectrum. (From Bushong S: Radiologic Science for Technologists: Physics, Biology, and Protection, 4th ed. St. Louis, Mosby, 1988, with permission.)

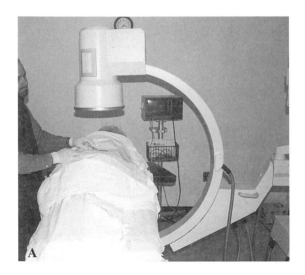
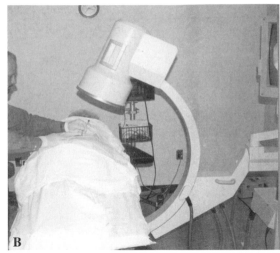
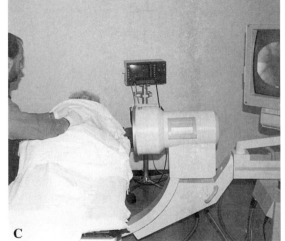

FIGURE 3-2. The C-arm rotated to the anteroposterior projection (A), oblique projection (B), and lateral projection (C).

("spot view") for future reference. Conventional fluoroscopy is considered suboptimal for spinal interventional procedures because of the inability to manipulate the x-ray tube around the patient, and it has been virtually replaced by C-arm fluoroscopes with image **intensification** for use in spinal injection procedures. The C-arm permits the physician to rotate and angle the x-ray tube around the patient while the patient rests on a radiolucent support table (Fig. 3-2). Image intensification is achieved through the addition of an image-intensifier tube located opposite the x-ray tube. The intensifier receives remnant x-ray beams that have passed through the patient and converts them into light energy, thereby increasing the brightness of the displayed image and making it easier to interpret. In the current image-intensified fluoroscopy, the x-ray tube delivers currents between 1 and 8 mA. Federal regulations limit the maximum output for C-arm fluoroscopes to 10 R/min at 12 inches from the image intensifier.

FACTORS AFFECTING RADIATION EXPOSURE

Exposure to ionizing radiation is an unavoidable event while performing fluoroscopic procedures. If one cannot avoid the radiation, then one must minimize its absorption by biologic tissues. The primary source of radiation to the physician during such procedures is from **scatter** reflected back from the patient. Of lesser concern is the small amount of **radiation leakage** from the equipment housing.

The cardinal principles of radiation protection are: (1) maximize *distance* from the radiation source; (2) use *shielding* materials; and (3) minimize *exposure* time. These principles are derived from protective measures that were adopted by individuals who worked on the atomic bomb in the Manhattan Project; such measures also may be instituted in the fluoroscopic suite. In addition, the concept of

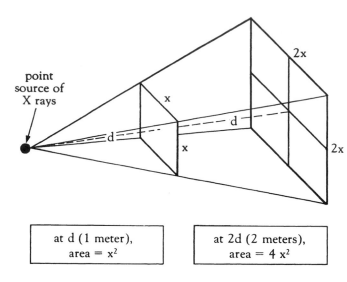

point source of X rays

FIGURE 3-3. When the distance from a point source of radiation is doubled, the radiation covers an area four times larger than the original area. However, the intensity at the new distance is only one fourth of the original intensity. (From Statkiewicz MA, Ritenour ER: Radiation Protection for Student Radiographers. St. Louis, Mosby, 1983, with permission.)

| at d (1 meter), area = x^2 | at 2d (2 meters), area = $4 x^2$ |

ALARA should be applied in all situations of radiation exposure to keep radiation *as low as reasonably achievable* within the limits of effectiveness.

Distance

Distance is the most effective means of minimizing exposure to a given source of ionizing radiation. According to the inverse square law, the intensity of the radiation is inversely proportional to the square of the distance. That is, when a given amount of radiation travels twice the distance, the covered area becomes four times as large and the intensity of exposure reduces to one-fourth (Fig. 3-3). Therefore, at four times the distance from the source, exposure is reduced to one-sixteenth the intensity.

A rough estimate of the physician's exposure at a distance of 1 meter from the x-ray tube is 1/1000th of the patient's exposure. It is therefore recommended that the technician and physician remain as far away from the examining table as practical during fluoroscopic procedures. The position of the physician's body, especially the hands, should be closely monitored and his or her position should be kept at a maximum distance from the fluoroscope at all times.[2] For example, it is advisable that the physician deliberately step away from the patient before acquiring each image and also use extension tubing during contrast injection to maximize the physician's distance from the beam.

Shielding

Shielding factors include filtration, beam collimation, intensifying screens, protective apparel (e.g., leaded aprons, eyewear, and gloves), and protective barriers (e.g., leaded glass panels or drapes). Appropriate shielding of critical tissues (i.e., gonads, thyroid, lungs, breast, eyes, and bone marrow) from ionizing radiation is critical to the safe use of fluoroscopic equipment.[7] In **filtration**, metal filters (usually aluminum) are inserted into the x-ray tube housing so that low energy x-rays emitted by the tube are absorbed before they reach the patient or medical staff. **Beam collimation** constricts the useful x-ray beam to the part of the body under examination, thereby sparing adjacent tissue from unnecessary exposure. It also serves to reduce scatter radiation and thus enhances imaging contrast. **Protective apparel**, such as a leaded apron ≥ 0.5 mm Pb, is mandatory to reduce exposure to the physician and technologist.[7] Such shielding decreases radiation exposure by 90% to critical body areas.[6] Lead-impregnated leather or vinyl aprons and gloves may be ordered in different thicknesses ranging from 0.55 mm Pb protection, which protects at 80 kVp, to 0.58 mm Pb, which protects at 120 kVp.[14] The use of a leaded thyroid shield also is recommended because of the superficial location and sensitivity of the thyroid gland and to protect a limited amount of cervical bone marrow. Protective, flexible lead-lined gloves also may reduce exposure without sacrificing dexterity; however, their use is no substitute for vigilant avoidance of direct x-ray beam exposure.[15] Leaded glasses or goggles will effectively eliminate approximately 90% of scatter radiation from frontal and side eye exposure. The leaded acrylic shields are made of clear lead equivalent to 0.3 mm Pb at 7-mm thickness. The lenses are leaded glass with a minimum thickness of 2.5 mm, which creates a lead shielding with over 97% attenuation up to 120 kV.[13] Clear, leaded glass x-ray

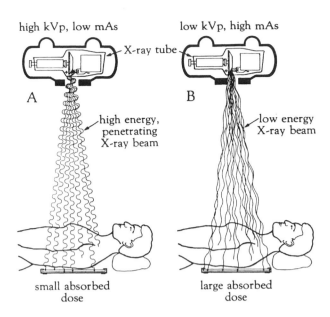

FIGURE 3-4. The use of higher kilovoltage (kVp) and lower milliamperage (mAs) reduces patient dose. *A,* The use of high kVp and low mAs results in a high-energy, penetrating x-ray beam and a small patient (absorbed) dose. *B,* The use of low kVp and high mAs results in a low-energy x-ray beam most of which is easily absorbed by the patient. (From Statkiewicz MA, Ritenour ER: Radiation Protection for Student Radiographers. St. Louis, Mosby, 1983, with permission.)

protective barriers are available in several styles and shapes. They may be height-adjustable or full-height, floor-rolling radiation barriers or suspendable on an overhead track. They weigh between 100 and 400 lbs with lead thicknesses of 0.5–1.0 mm. When it is necessary to remain near the x-ray beam during a procedure, additional shielding should be used.

Exposure Time

To minimize exposure time to ionizing radiation, the clinician and radiologic technician need to work together as a team. The technologist assists by optimally orienting the C-arm around the patient before beginning any kind of interventional procedure. The technologist also should ensure that the orientation of the C-arm is such that the x-ray tube is positioned directly under the patient to minimize scatter to that which is attenuated through the patient. The operator should minimize exposure time through the judicious use of the "beam on" controls (i.e., a foot or hand switch). If the technologist is responsible for the controls, then communication with the physician is critical to avoid unintended exposure. Training and experience of all personnel in the intricacies of complex procedures help to reduce unnecessary exposure. Fluoroscopic equipment may have features such as high- and low-dose modes, pulsed fluoroscopy, hold-and-store image capability, and beam collimation, all of which can minimize exposure time. A high kilovolt–low milliamperage approach to imaging will minimize the absorption of x-ray by the

patient and improve the contrast of the visualized image (Fig. 3-4). Freeze-frame capabilities minimize repeated exposures and should be used to review the last image in preparation for needle adjustments during the procedure.

RADIATION RISKS TO THE PATIENT DURING FLUOROSCOPIC PROCEDURES

Ionizing radiation occurs naturally in the environment: the general population usually is exposed to an individual effective dose equivalent of 360 millirem (mrem) of radioactivity per year. This exposure comes from numerous sources, the most significant of which is naturally occurring radon[9] (Table 3-2).

Assessment of Risk

Risk assessment for patients subject to diagnostic and therapeutic radiographs is an inexact science, and the body of knowledge is constantly evolving. Current estimation of risk from radiographic exposure to a specific body part is based on the biologic effects of whole-body exposure (e.g., a survivor of an atomic bomb attack) converted by weight factors specific for individual organs and tissues. This concept was adopted by the International Commission on Radiological Protection in 1977 and was modified in 1991.[4] Termed the *effective dose equivalent,* the calculation has been adopted by most authoritative bodies that determine radiation risk and recommend protective measures.

TABLE 3-2.   Average Annual Effective Dose Equivalent of Ionizing Radiations to a Member of the U.S. Population

Source	Dose Equivalent[a]		Effective Dose Equivalent	
	mSv	**mrem**	**mSv**	**%**
Natural				
Radon[b]	24	2,400	2.0	55
Cosmic	0.27	27	0.27	8.0
Terrestrial	0.28	28	0.28	8.0
Internal	0.39	39	0.39	11
Total natural	—	—	3.0	82
Artificial				
Medical				
X-ray diagnosis	0.39	39	0.39	11
Nuclear medicine	0.14	14	0.14	4.0
Consumer products	0.10	10	0.10	3.0
Other				
Occupational	0.009	0.9	< 0.01	< 0.3
Nuclear fuel cycle	< 0.01	< 1.0	< 0.01	< 0.03
Fallout	< 0.01	< 1.0	< 0.01	< 0.03
Miscellaneous[c]	< 0.01	< 1.0	< 0.01	< 0.03
Total artificial	—	—	0.63	18
Total natural and artificial	—	—	3.6	100

[a] To soft tissues.
[b] Dose equivalent to bronchi from radon daughter products. The assumed weighting factor for the effective dose equivalent relative to whole-body exposure is 0.08.
[c] Department of Energy facilities, smelters, transportation, etc.
From National Council on Radiation Protection and Measurements (NCRP): Ionizing Radiation Exposures of the Population of the United States. Report No. 87b. Washington, DC, NCRP, 1987, with permission.

Extent of Exposure

Radiation exposure to the patient during fluoroscopic procedures can exceed those associated with routine radiographs. The amount of radiation absorbed by an individual patient depends on a number of unalterable factors relating to his or her habitus, including the type, density, and location of tissue involved. For instance, bone absorbs more ionizing radiation than soft tissues. An obese person will absorb more radiation than a slender one. Because of the frequency of exposure, skin at the entry site is the area most susceptible to radiation-induced injury. Different tissues have varying degrees of sensitivity to ionizing radiation[4] (Table 3-3).

For instance, transient skin erythema can result from as little as 200 rad, and at 300 rad temporary hair loss may occur. The threshold for permanent injury is 700 rad, and doses > 1800 rad can cause dermal necrosis. The skin dose is typically used to interpret a patient's radiation exposure to diagnostic x-rays. In the absence of a dosimeter, the skin dose may be calculated using a variety of complicated techniques. In fluoroscopy, the patient's exposure is more difficult to estimate because of the movement and variation in size of the radiation field. In the absence of absolute measurements, it usually is sufficient to estimate the fluoroscopic skin dose at 2 rad/mA-min. In order to determine the approximate exposure, first it is necessary to know the exposure time and milliamperage. For example, if a

TABLE 3-3.   Specific Organ Cancer Risks of Radiation (Per 10,000 per Sv or Per 1,000,000 per Rem)

Organ or Cancer	Probability of Radiation-Induced Cancer
Breast	50–200
Thyroid	50–150
Lung	50
Leukemia	15–25
Stomach	10–20
Brain	5–20
Colon	10–15
Liver	10–15
Lymphoma	4–12
Uterus	7–10
Salivary glands	5–10
Ovary	8
Bladder	4–7
Bone	2–5
Esophagus	2–5
Pancreas	2–5
Paranasal sinuses	2–5

From International Commission on Radiological Protection: Recommendations of the International Commission on Radiation Protection 26. Ann Int Commission Radiat Prot 1:1–53, 1977, with permission.

TABLE 3-4.   Radiation Exposure Comparison

Procedure/Activity	Exposure	Body Part
Natural background	100–200 mrem/yr	Total body
Lumbar epidural with fluoroscopy—patient	2.5 rem/30 sec	Lumbar region
Lumbar epidural with fluoroscopy—physician	2.5 mrem*/30 sec	Total body
Swallowing videofluoroscopy (patient)	3 mrem/min†	Face/neck
Posteroanterior chest x-ray	10–30 mrem	Chest
CT scan of head	3–5 rem	Head

* Exposure estimated without shielded protection and at a distance of approximately 1 meter.
† Data collected by Charles Beasley, Radiation Safety Officer, St. John's Regional Hospital, Springfield, MO, based on operation
   at 85 kVp/0.2 mA.

fluoroscopically guided transforaminal epidural corticosteroid injection requires 30 seconds to perform and the average milliamperage is 8 mA, exposure is estimated as follows: 2 rad/mA-min (8 mA)(0.5 min) = 8 rad.

The primary controllable factor contributing to patient exposure is the length of the procedure. Depending on the complexity of the procedure, exposure times can last a few moments to an hour or more. Fluoroscopes usually produce between 1 and 5 R/min of ionizing radiation. The typical rem exposure to patients during common diagnostic and treatment procedures is shown in Table 3-4.

Calculating the health risks from radiation is a relatively inexact science, but the risk from low-level exposure is clearly small. With the exception of the effects on a developing fetus from exposure through the mother's abdomen, no direct evidence of human harm from low doses of radiation exists.[3]

RADIATION RISKS TO THE PHYSICIAN AND ASSISTING PERSONNEL

The maximum safe allowable exposure limits have been established by the National Council on Radiation Protection and Measurement as a *maximum permissible dose* (MPD).[11] The general radiation whole-body exposure guidelines allow no more than 5 rem/year (Table 3-5).

Guidelines for Exposure

Several studies have evaluated radiation exposure to clinicians during fluoroscopically assisted orthopedic procedures. One study demonstrated that unprotected individuals working ≤ 24 inches from a fluoroscopic beam received significant amounts of radiation, whereas those working ≥ 36 inches from the beam received an extremely low amount of radiation.[1] Risk of radiation exposure to orthopedic surgeons also has been studied. One prospective

study showed that radiation doses over a 6-month period were well below the maximum dose limits for ionizing radiation as recommended by the European Economic Communities (EURATOM) directives.[12] Using a phantom patient, this experiment revealed that exposure to ionizing radiation during the insertion of a dynamic hip screw was minimal. Caution during fluoroscopy was recommended nevertheless. The cutaneous effects of long-term skin exposure in a physician are clearly visible (Fig. 3-5).

Protective Measures

In order to monitor the amount of radiation the technologist and physicians are exposed to, a film dosimetry system should be used to provide accurate personal dosimetry and comprehensive diagnostic evaluation. The Gardray® film consists of a slim, light, clip-on badge that can easily be worn on either the torso (body badge) or extremities (finger/ring badge). The film is placed in a holder that incorporates 6 absorbers to optimize the determination of the type and level of exposure. Metal absorbers are U-shaped to permit the film to be filtered for radiation exposure not only from the

TABLE 3-5.   National Council on Radiation Protection and Measurements Recommendations for Occupational Radiation Exposure

1. Effective dose limits		
Annual	50 mSv	(5 rem)
Cumulative	10 mSv	(1 rem) x age
2. Annual dose limits for tissues and organs		
Lens of the eye	150 mSv	(15 rem)
Skin, hands, and feet	500 mSv	(50 rem)
3. Embryo/fetus		
Total dose equivalent	5 mSv	(0.5 rem)
Monthly dose equivalent	0.5 mSv	(0.05 rem)

mSv = millisievert
Adapted from National Council on Radiation Protection and Measurements (NCRP): Ionizing Radiation Exposures of the Population of the United States. Report No. 116. Washington, DC, NCRP, 1993, with permission.

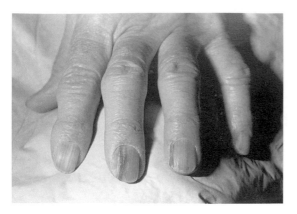

FIGURE 3-5. Fingers of an 83-year-old general practitioner who set fractures under fluoroscopy for 35 years. Note the changes in the nails. A basal cell carcinoma was earlier resected from a proximal phalynx. (From Lennard TA: Fundamentals of procedural care. In Lennard TA (ed): Physiatric Procedures in Clinical Practice. Philadelphia, Hanley & Belfus, 1995, pp 1–13, with permission.)

front but also from the bottom and behind. The finger/ring badge should be worn with the film facing the inside part of the hand nearest the radiation source. The body badge is worn in the same position closest to the radiation source each day. A badge also may be placed on protective eyewear to determine exposure to the lenses of the eye. The badges and rings are sent in monthly for processing to monitor the type and amount of radiation exposure (as measured in mrem) received by each participant. Results are reported as monthly and 12-month accumulated dosages. Exposure is divided into three dose-equivalent columns for shallow, deep, and eye lens exposures. The shallow dose equivalent applies to the external exposure of the skin or extremity and is taken as the dose equivalent at a tissue depth of 0.007 cm averaged over an area of 1 cm squared[5]; the deep dose equivalent applies to external whole-body exposure and is the dose equivalent at a tissue depth of 1 cm; and the eye dose equivalent applies to the external exposure of the lens of the eye and is taken as the dose equivalent at a tissue depth of 0.3 cm. Cataract development may occur with cumulative eye lens exposure of ≥ 400 rad.[8]

CONCLUSION

Through compliance with an occupational dosimetry program, the application of cautious work habits, and attention to the three essentials of radiation safety—distance, time, and shielding—the physician can minimize exposure and maximize long-term safety in the fluoroscopy suite.

Acknowledgment

The authors would like to acknowledge Carol Barragen for secretarial assistance and Rita Cotraccia, RRT, and Nicole Belsanti, RRT, for supporting literature.

REFERENCES

1. Barendsen GW: Parameters of linear-quadratic radiation dose-effect relationships: Dependence on LET and mechanisms of reproductive cell death. Int J Radiat Biol 71:649–655, 1997.
2. Boone JM, Levin DC: Radiation exposure to angiographers under different fluoroscopic imaging conditions. Radiology 180:861–865, 1991.
3. Gray JE: Safety risk of diagnosis radiology exposures. In American College of Radiology Commission on Physics and Radiation Safety (ed): Radiation Risks: A Primer. Reston, VA, American College of Radiology, 1996, pp 15–18.
4. International Commission on Radiological Protection: Recommendation of the International Commission on Radiation Protection 26. Ann Int Commission Radiat Prot 1:1–53, 1977.
5. Landauer, Inc., 2 Science Road, Glenwood, IL 60425-1586.
6. Larimore E (Radiation Consultants): [Personal communication to TA Lennard], 1994. Reported in Lennard TA: Fundamentals of procedural care. In Lennard TA (ed): Physiatric Procedures in Clinical Practice. Philadelphia, Hanley & Belfus, 1995, pp 1–13.
7. Marx VM: Interventional procedures: Risks to patients and personnel. In American College of Radiology Commission on Physics and Radiation Safety: Radiation Risks: A Primer. Reston, VA, American College of Radiology, 1996, pp 22–25.
8. Marx MV, Niklason L, Manger EA: Occupational radiation exposure to the interventional radiologist: A prospective study. J Vasc Interv Radiol 3:597–606, 1992.
9. National Council on Radiation Protection and Measurements (NCRP): Ionizing Radiation Exposures of the Population of the United States. Report No. 93. Washington, DC, NCRP, 1987.
10. National Council on Radiation Protection and Measurements (NCRP): Ionizing Radiation Exposures of the Population of the United States. Report No. 115. Washington, DC, NCRP, 1993, UN publication E.94.IX.2, UN Publication E.94.IX.11.
11. National Council on Radiation Protection and Measurements (NCRP): Ionizing Radiation Exposures of the Population of the United States. Report No. 116. Washington, DC, NCRP, 1993.
12. O'Rourke PJ, Crerand S, Harrington P, et al: Risks of radiation exposure to orthopedic surgeons. J R Coll Surg Edinb 1:40–43, 1996.
13. ProTech Leaded Eyewear, Palm Beach Gardens, FL.
14. ProTech Radiation Apparel and Accessories, Palm Beach Gardens, FL.
15. Vehmas T: Finger doses during interventional radiology: The value of flexible protective gloves. Fortschr Roentgenstr 154:555–559, 1991.
16. Wycoff HO: The international system of units. Radiology 128:833–835, 1978.

4

Basic Principles of Neural Blockade

Ted A. Lennard, M.D.

Percutaneous nerve blocks can be used in a variety of clinical circumstances (Table 4-1). They are easy to perform when one understands the regional anatomy, block technique, indications, and pharmacology of the medication injected. These blocks can provide anesthesia for procedures, as well as rapid diagnostic, prognostic, and therapeutic information when applied in the appropriate clinical setting. The result, either temporary or permanent, promotes a higher level of function when used within the framework of a well-designed rehabilitation program.

NEUROVASCULAR BUNDLE ANATOMY

The neurovascular bundle consists of peripheral nerve fibers wrapped in connective tissue intermingled by a capillary plexus (Fig. 4-1). Three types of connective tissue are present within the peripheral nerve: endoneurium, perineurium, and epineurium. The endoneurium is a delicate, supporting structure located adjacent to individual axons within a fascicle. Individual fasicles are bound by the perineurium, a layer felt to monitor intrafascicular fluid diffusion.[14,20] These fascicles are bound in groups by the outermost layer, the epineurium (Fig. 4-2). This layer contains the vasa nevorum, which divides into arterioles that penetrate the perineurium (Fig. 4-3). Ultimately a network of capillaries reach each fascicle to supply individual axons.

The neurovascular bundle usually lies well protected between muscle or bone. At its most proximal location—the spinal root level—the neurovascular bundle contains motor, sensory, and autonomic fibers. These roots divide into dorsal and ventral rami, the latter of which reconnect to form a plexus of nerves. Ultimately, terminal nerve branches of isolated fiber types—sensory or motor branches—are formed.

NEURAL BLOCK TECHNIQUE: GENERAL CONSIDERATIONS

Several techniques can be used to block a peripheral nerve. Each technique requires a thorough knowledge of both surface and gross anatomy as well as good manual dexterity. When selective motor nerves are blocked, an understanding of kinesiology is helpful.

The two common approaches used to block nerves are the paresthesia technique (PT) and nonparesthesia technique (NPT). PT attempts to purposefully provoke paresthesias of the nerve before injection. These paresthesias indicate that the needle is in contact with the nerve and serve as a warning of potential nerve injury. This technique assumes that the patient's sensory pathways are intact and that the patient is able to cooperate fully with the injection. The second approach, NPT, avoids this deliberate probing for paresthesias and relies on anatomic landmarks, but may require greater volumes of medication to achieve the desired block. With NPT the needle tip may not approximate the nerve as closely as PT. As expected, PT is associated with a greater incidence of nerve injury[13,15,18] and should be avoided if possible.

As an alternative technique, a nerve stimulator (Fig. 4-4) can be used to locate and block peripheral nerves. These stimulators are available commercially, although office electrodiagnostic equipment often will suffice. An electrical impulse generated by the stimulator and controlled by a rheostat is transmitted through a needle. The entire shaft of this needle is coated with Teflon except the bevel. The Teflon prevents spread of stimulus into surrounding tissue and directs electrical current to the needle tip. As the needle approaches the nerve, either a motor, sensory, or mixed response can be elicited depending on the fiber types contained

TABLE 4-1. Indications for Percutaneous Nerve Blocks

With local anesthetics
1. Provides anesthesia for procedures
2. Differentiates pain problems and helps better understand nociceptive pathways
3. Serves as a treatment for inflammatory compression neuropathies in combination with corticosteroids
4. Provides treatment for sympathetic mediated pain syndromes
5. Differentiates spasticity from joint contractures
6. Helps predict the effect of a neurolytic procedure
7. Allows selective recording in nerve conduction studies[8]
8. Promotes functional activities in an occupational or physical therapy program
9. Assists in serial or inhibitory casting

With normal saline
10. Provides placebo response

With neurolytic agents (chemical neurolysis)
11. Facilitates functional goals in the spastic patient: positioning, ambulation, bracing, transfers
12. Improves caregiver tasks (such as hygiene) in the spastic patient: perineal, axillary, elbow, or hand regions
13. Improves self-image of the spastic patient by reducing joint deformities and improving cosmesis
14. May improve residual voluntary muscle control by eliminating unwanted hypertonia in the spastic patient
15. Reduces pain caused by hypertonia
16. Provides treatment for specific, intractable pain disorders
17. Prevents nerve compression injuries in hyperflexed joints, i.e., median nerve at the wrist from wrist flexor spasticity
18. Prevents skin breakdown by promoting proper seating and positioning

within the nerve. The neural response should increase as the needle tip approaches the nerve. It is desirable to obtain a strong neural response with a low stimulus output, thereby assuring accurate needle placement. This technique is preferred when injecting neurolytic agents for the treatment of spasticity.

One can quickly identify selective motor responses, such as musculocutaneous nerve stimulation causing elbow flexion, and quickly determine the effect of chemical neurolysis after injection.

Regardless of the technique used, the needle tip should remain in the epineural space when solution is injected (Fig. 4-5). Solution should not be injected into the nerve because intraneural injections have a high association with fascicular damage.[6,7] If paresthesias are elicited, the needle should be repositioned before solution is injected. Forceful injection is not recommended, because it may be a sign of injecting into a fixed space such as tendon or adjacent to bone. Intravascular injection can usually be avoided by aspirating for blood in several planes prior to injecting. Slow administration of the drug is advisable to allow detection of early side effects from vascular injection.

Repeat anesthetic injections close to the same nerve within a single office visit should be avoided. Because warning paresthesias may not be present, occult iatrogenic nerve injury may occur.

NERVE INJURIES

Three major factors contribute to nerve injury from injections: trauma, toxicity, and ischemia. Many nerve injection injuries are due to a combination of these factors.[15]

Trauma to the nerve during injection occurs with overly vigorous probing during insertion of the needle. This can directly injure the nerve fascicles. Selander et al. demonstrated a lower risk of nerve fascicle injury using short beveled needles. They

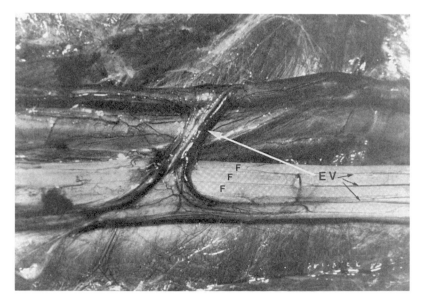

FIGURE 4-1. Under magnification, the neurovascular bundle with extrinsic blood vessels and a segmental supplying artery are apparent (*EV*). The linear extrinsic vessels parallel grooves created by adjacent fascicles (*F*). (From Beek AV, Kleinert HE: Peripheral nerve injuries and repair. In Rand R (ed): Microneurosurgery, 3rd ed. St. Louis, Mosby, 1985, p 742, with permission.)

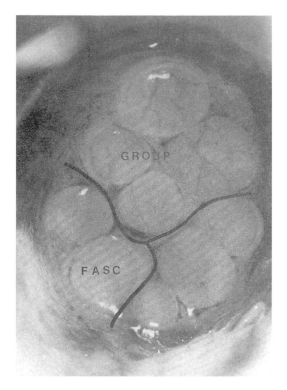

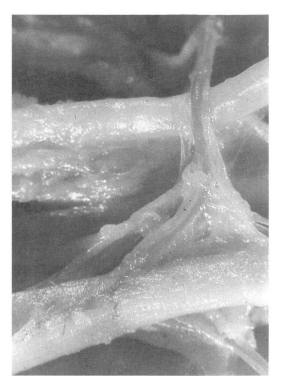

FIGURE 4-2.   Under magnification, a cross-section of the median nerve demonstrates individual and groups of fascicles (FASC). Note the connective tissue between each fascicle and surrounding the entire nerve. (From Beek AV, Kleinert HE: Peripheral nerve injuries and repair. In Rand R (ed): Microneurosurgery, 3rd ed. St. Louis, Mosby, 1985, p 742, with permission.)

FIGURE 4-3.   Neurovascular bundle demonstrating the entrance of the arterial supply into the epineurium with surrounding connective tissue. (From Zancolli EA, Cozzi EP: Nerves of the upper limb. In Zancolli EA, Cozzi EP (eds): Atlas of Surgical Anatomy of the Hand. New York, Churchill Livingstone, 1992, p 685, with permission.)

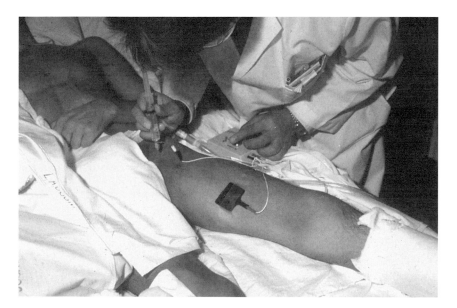

FIGURE 4-4.   As the physician holds the syringe in his right hand, the rheostat is adjusted on the block stimulator with the left hand. The syringe is attached to a Teflon-coated hypodermic needle, which is attached to the stimulator. Note the surface ground pad on the patient's inner thigh.

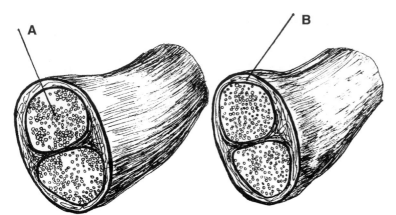

FIGURE 4-5.   Needle placement in the intrafascicular space (*A*) compared to the extrafascicular space (*B*). (Adapted from Gentili F, Hudson A, Kline D, et al: Peripheral nerve injection injury: An experimental injury. Neurosurgery 4:244, 1979, © Congress of Neurological Surgeons.)

also demonstrated that nerve fascicles rolled or slid with needle contact.[15]

Intraneural injections of solution not only directly injure both myelinated and unmyelinated nerve fibers but also cause a breakdown in blood-nerve barrier function.[6,7] The spread of anesthesia with intraneural injections has been demonstrated and, when near the spine, may cause unexpected spinal anesthesia.[19] Neural compression or stretching also may result from large volumes of solution injected into a fixed space, thereby traumatizing the nerve.

Neurotoxicity can be caused by direct injection of drugs into nervous tissue. Intrafascicular injections of anesthetics cause profound nerve damage. The degree of damage depends on the type and amount of drug injected.[6,7] Ester anesthetics generally demonstrate greater toxicity than amides when injected into the intrafascicular space.[5,12] Extrafascicular injections of anesthetics in routine concentrations rarely cause significant histologic nerve damage or disruption of the blood-nerve barrier but can alter the permeability of the perineurium, leading to endoneurial edema.[5,12] The epineurium provides some neuroprotective function during injection, thereby reducing toxicity from medication.

Additives, such as epinephrine, increase the toxicity of the anesthetics when injected intrafascicularly.[3,16] Consequently, if extended duration of anesthesia is desired from a nerve block, a long-acting anesthetic or continuous infusion technique is preferable to the addition of epinephrine.[18]

Mackinnon et al. found that corticosteroid injections into the epineural tissue did not cause nerve damage.[10] When injected into the intrafascicular space, corticosteroids exerted a direct neurotoxic effect with disruption of the blood-nerve barrier, similar to anesthetics. Severe nerve fiber damage was noted with hydrocortisone (Solu-Cortef) and triamcinolone hexacetonide (Aristospan), moderate damage with triamcinolone acetonide (Kenalog) and methylprednisolone (Depo-Medrol), and the least damage with dexamethasone (Decadron) (Fig. 4-6).

Ischemia may result not only from application of a tourniquet or improper positioning of the patient, but also by the nerve block itself if the injection is given into the intrafascicular space. The ischemia results from increased intraneural compartment pressure by the injectate volume, which reduces neural perfusion. This intraneural pressure has been shown experimentally to remain above the blood perfusion pressure for 15 minutes without damage.[19]

GENERAL PRINCIPLES OF NEURAL BLOCKADE

Drugs in isolation or in combinations can be injected to block nerves. The most common mixtures include anesthetic agents in combination with corticosteroids. When chemical neurolysis is desired, neurolytic drugs are injected. Under the correct clinical circumstance, these neurolytic agents can be successfully used to treat hypertonicity and chronic intractable pain disorders. The following section will briefly discuss the principles behind anesthetic motor and sensory blocks and neurolytic blocks for spasticity and pain.

Anesthetic Blocks

As a result of an anesthetic's reversible properties, nerve blocks can be performed to intentionally paralyze or deactivate specific muscles and/or selectively disrupt sensory pathways. This effect has numerous clinical applications, especially when prior

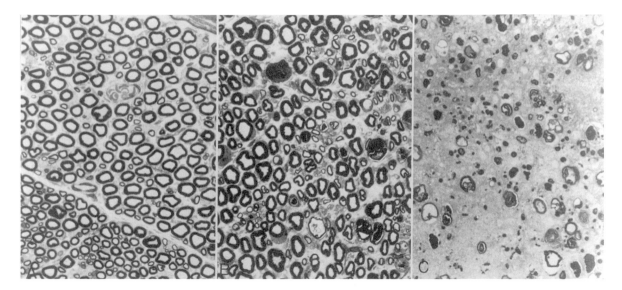

FIGURE 4-6. *Left,* Cross-section of a normal myelinated nerve fiber population within a sciatic nerve (×585). *Center,* Cross-section 12 days afer intrafascicular injection of dexamethasone (Decadron), demonstrating relatively normal appearance with minimal evidence of nerve injury (×585). *Right,* Cross-section 12 days after intrafascicular injection of triamcinolone hexacetonide (Aristospan), demonstrating severe widespread axonal and myelin degeneration (×585). (From Mackinnon SE, Hudson AR, Gentili F, et al: Peripheral nerve injection injury with steroid agents. Plast Reconstr Surg 69:482–489, 1982, with permission.)

treatment has failed or a diagnosis is unclear. With the exception of anesthesia for surgical procedures, blocks should seldom be the initial treatment of a disorder and always be integrated into a well-planned rehabilitation program.

Motor Blocks

Isolated blocks purely to motor nerves or to motor components of mixed nerves are useful to relax specific muscles. Motor blocks also may be useful in differentiating joint contracture from spasticity. For example, if a patient presents with an elbow flexion deformity, a musculocutaneous anesthetic nerve block can be performed. After injection, the patient's elbow is passively extended and any change in range of motion is evaluated. If only minimal improvement in passive elbow extension occurs, one would suspect contracture formation or bony ankylosis as the etiology. However, if full extension is achieved, the elbow flexion deformity is more likely to be related to spasticity. A neurolytic block may then be pursued. The information gained from the previous anesthetic block assists the clinician in predicting the outcome from subsequent chemical neurolysis. In addition, anesthetic peripheral nerve blocks can facilitate serial casting by relaxing spastic muscles. The effect allows placement of casts on extremity joints in the desired joint position.

Sensory Blocks

Anesthetic peripheral nerve blocks are most commonly used to facilitate surgical procedures by blocking sensory pathways. In an office practice setting, anesthetic blocks can be used to assist in the diagnosis of difficult pain problems. When sensory components to nerves are interrupted, expected dermatomal sensory changes can be evaluated and compared with actual "blocked" changes, thereby diagnosing nociceptive pain pathways undetected with conventional testing. For example, a radial sensory neuropathy masked by de Quervain's tenosynovitis may be diagnosed after a radial sensory nerve block. This and other compressive neuropathies, such as carpal tunnel syndrome, may later require corticosteroid injections.

Patients who malinger or magnify symptoms also may be evaluated using blocks. Response to injections with various concentrations of anesthetic versus placebo can be analyzed and, thus, the patient's reliability determined.

Another way to use sensory blocks is to "reset" the pain generators, especially in cases of sympathetic mediated pain disorders with serial injections.[1] Once a response to painful stimuli is attenuated, the patient can participate in a therapy program that emphasizes functional tasks, joint range of motion, stretching, and skin desensitization. The goal is to gradually eliminate the painful stimulus over time.

Neurolytic Blocks

Spasticity

Hypertonicity due to upper motor neuron dysfunction may be caused by lesions at many levels within the brain and spinal cord. Among patients with traumatic brain injury (TBI), the most severe hypertonicity is found in those with diffuse axonal injury (DAI) or hypoxic-ischemic injury (HII) following cardiopulmonary arrest. Rigidity, spasticity, and dystonia all contribute to joint abnormalities and restricted function. Hypertonicity is usually greatest within the first 6 months of injury. Because this is the period of spontaneous neurologic recovery, one should avoid any permanent surgical procedure intended to control hypertonicity. Without any treatment, disabling musculotendinous contracture and abnormal, dyssynergic patterns of movement occur, further complicating the patient's recovery and outcome. Peripheral nerve blockade may be useful during this interval to assist in the treatment of spasticity.

A large number of patients with TBI and spinal cord injury require localized nerve blocks designed to depress the final common pathway during reorganization and recovery of the central nervous system. If nerve blocks are performed early in the course of rehabilitation, therapy may be facilitated. Noninvasive treatment of spasticity should be maximized before proceeding with percutaneous neurolytic blocks. This includes medications, stretching, serial casting, icing, electrical stimulation, and positioning. Any cerebral or spinal cord anomalies, such as hydrocephalus and syringomyelia, should be corrected surgically. Any noxious stimuli, such as urinary tract infection and skin lesion, should be eliminated when possible. Drug-induced movement disorders should be evaluated and, when possible, the offending drug discontinued.

The prognosis for motor return and stage of recovery should be established. The physician must determine if the hypertonicity is generalized or focal. Generalized hypertonicity is usually not responsive to nerve blocks, and, unless hygiene is the primary concern, blocks should not be performed. Focal hypertonicity, however, does not respond well to nerve blocks. Consistent patterns of hypertonicity need to be established, and treatment should initially be directed toward proximal tone. Any block should affect the most proximal nerve capable of denervating the maximum number of spastic myotomes. All residual voluntary motor function of the affected limb is to be preserved.

Phenol generally results in alleviation of spasticity with little decrease of voluntary contraction.[11]

Pain Management

The most common use of neurolytic agents for pain management is to treat intractable cancer pain in patients with a limited life span. This can be done with intrathecal or peripheral nerve injections. Advancements in radiofrequency procedures are rapidly replacing injectable neurolytics for pain management. An in-depth discussion of this topic is beyond the scope of this chapter.

CONCLUSION

Any peripheral nerve can be blocked if a physician is familiar with the regional anatomy, indications, and technique. Judicious use of these procedures requires a thorough understanding of the appropriate indications for blockade and the medications to be used. With this understanding, outcomes are maximized while the potential for complications is reduced.

REFERENCES

1. Brown DL: Somatic or sympathetic block for reflex sympathetic dystrophy. Which is indicated? Hand Clin 13:485–497, 1997.
2. Choi YK, Liu J: The use of 5% lidocaine for prolonged analgesia in chronic pain patients. A new technique. Reg Anesth 23:96–100, 1998.
3. Covino BG: Potential neurotoxicity of local anesthetic agents [editorial]. Can Anaesth Soc J 30:111–116, 1983.
4. Fouch RA, Abram SE, Hogan QH: Neural blockade for upper extremity pain: The painful hand. Hand Clin 12:791–800, 1996.
5. Gentili F, Hudson A, Hunter D, et al: Nerve injection injury with local anesthetic agents: A light and electron microscopic, fluorescent microscopic and horseradish peroxidase study. Neurosurgery 6:263–272, 1984.
6. Gentili F, Hudson A, Kline D, et al: Peripheral nerve injection injury: An experimental study. Neurosurgery 4:244–253, 1979.
7. Hudson AR: Nerve injection injuries. Clin Plast Surg 11:27–30, 1984.
8. Kimura J: Electrodiagnosis in Diseases of Nerve and Muscle: Principles and Practice, 2nd ed. Philadelphia, F.A. Davis, 1989.
9. Kirvela O, Nieminen S: Treatment of painful neuromas with neurolytic blockade. Pain 41:161–165, 1990.
10. Mackinnon SE, Hudson AR, Gentili F, et al: Peripheral nerve injection injury with steroid agents. Plast Reconstr Surg 69:482–489, 1982.
11. Moritz U: Phenol block of peripheral nerves. Scand J Rehabil Med 5:160–163, 1973.
12. Myers R, Kalichman M, Reisner L, et al: Neurotoxicity of local anesthetics: Altered perineuial permeability, edema, and nerve fiber injury. Anesthesiology 64:29–35, 1986.
13. Plevak DJ, Linstromberg JW, Danielson DR: Paresthesia vs nonparesthesia: The axillary block. ASA Abstracts, Anesthesiology 59, 1983.
14. Ross MH, Reith EJ: Perineurium: Evidence for contractile elements. Science 165:604–606, 1969.

15. Selander D: Paresthesias or no paresthesias? Nerve complications after neural blockades. Acta Anaesthesiol Belg 39:173–174, 1988.
16. Selander D, Brattsand R, Lundborg G, et al: Local anesthetics: Importance of mode of application, concentration and adrenaline for the appearance of nerve lesions. Acta Anesthesiol Scand 23:127–136, 1979.
17. Selander D, Dhuner K, Lundborg G: Peripheral nerve injury due to injection needles used for regional anesthesia. Acta Anaesthesiol Scand 21:182–188, 1977.
18. Selander D, Edshage S, Wolff T: Paresthesiae or no paresthesiae? Acta Anaesthesiol Scand 23:27–33, 1979.
19. Selander D, Sjostrand J: Longitudinal spread of intraneurally injected local anesthetics. Acta Anaesthesiol Scand 22:622–634, 1978.
20. Thomas PK, Olsson Y: Microscopic anatomy and function of connective tissue components of peripheral nerve. In Dyck PJ, Thomas PK, Lambert EH, Bunge R (eds): Peripheral Neuropathy, vol 1. Philadelphia, W.B. Saunders, 1984, pp 97–120.

5

Medicolegal Issues

Julie K. Silver, M.D., and Susan M. Donnelly, J.D.

Physicians who routinely perform pain procedures need to understand certain elements of informed consent in order to minimize their risk of medicolegal entanglements. Often physicians have little or no training in obtaining informed consent. Even when they do obtain training, the instruction may be incomplete or incorrect. Understanding and documenting the consent process before the procedure is as important as the procedure itself.

UNDERSTANDING INFORMED CONSENT

The law implicitly recognizes that a person has a strong interest in being free from nonconsensual invasion of bodily integrity.[1] In short, the law recognizes the individual's interest in preserving the "inviolability of the person,"[1] an interest protected within the context of medical malpractice with the doctrine of informed consent. It has long been accepted that a patient must agree to any procedures or treatment. However, earlier it was accepted that the physician could steer the patient in the direction that he or she wanted. This has changed: it is now recognized that "[I]t is the prerogative of the patient, not the physician, to determine the direction in which his . . . interests lie."[1] Consequently, a body of law that dictates the manner in which the patient's consent or refusal needs to be obtained has developed. Some consider the right to informed consent to be the most important aspect of patients' rights.[3]

In order for patients to intelligently exercise control of their bodies and attendant medical care, they must be provided with appropriate and complete medical information upon which to base their decision. The dilemma facing medical practitioners is the determination of when such informed consent needs to be obtained and the manner in which to obtain it. This requires a knowledge of the type and extent of information to be given to an individual patient and the manner in which it is to be imparted.

Although the vast majority of claims of medical malpractice focus upon errors in diagnosis and improper treatment and performance of procedures, a recent analysis found that allegations of failure to inform and breach of warranty were present in 6% of cases.[4]

THE LEGAL FRAMEWORK FOR INFORMED CONSENT

Complete informed consent should be obtained for all therapeutic and diagnostic procedures. Any course of treatment that carries with it the risk of permanent injury requires a full disclosure before consent. Full informed consent should precede medical treatment even for procedures with a risk of temporary injury only. Indeed, it is recognized that only under emergency conditions or situations in which there are no therapeutic options that informed consent may be omitted. There is no excuse to fail to obtain informed consent for an elective procedure.

Moreover, the physician performing the procedure is the appropriate person to meet with the patient. Of course, other health care providers are of great assistance to reaffirm the consent, answer additional questions a patient may have, and continue a dialogue.

To enable a patient to make an informed decision, "the physician owes to his patient the duty to disclose in a reasonable manner all significant medical information that the physician possesses or reasonably should possess that is material to an intelligent decision by the patient whether to undergo a proposed procedure."[1] The specific law varies somewhat from jurisdiction to jurisdiction. Use of this language facilitates discussion of the two perspectives involved in the decision-making process: the physician and the patient.

ROLE OF THE PHYSICIAN

The major role of the physician in the process of obtaining informed consent is that of an expert. Through education and experience, he or she is able to recognize the risks and benefits of the proposed treatment. Because the patient has limited knowledge of the medical and technical aspects of the procedure, the physician should begin the discussion with a reasonable explanation of the medical diagnosis—an obvious but often overlooked point. Thereafter, significant information includes the nature and probability of risks involved in the procedure, expected benefits, the irreversibility of the procedure, the available alternatives to the proposed procedure, and the likely result of no treatment.[1] Whether a physician has provided appropriate information to a patient generally will be measured by what is customarily done or by the standard of what the average physician should tell a patient about a given procedure. It often is essentially the same information that the physician has imparted to countless previous patients. In general, the duty to disclose does not require the physician to disclose all possible and/or remote risks, nor does it require the physician to discuss with a patient the information that he believes the patient already has, such as the risk of infection or other inherent risks of a procedure.[1]

ROLE OF THE PATIENT

Although explanations to patients may be nearly identical for a given procedure, the law often also requires that the conversation be tailored to the particular patient. It is incumbent upon the physician to have an appreciation of what information is important to a particular patient. The patient has the right to know all information that he or she considers material to his or her decision. *Materiality* is defined as the significance a specific patient attaches to the disclosed risks in deciding whether to undergo the proposed procedure.[5] Materiality of information about a side effect or consequence is a function not only of the severity of that consequence, but also of the likelihood that it will occur.[5] Remote risks whose likelihood of occurrence is not more than negligible need not warrant discussion. In summary, provide the patient with a realistic appreciation of his or her medical condition and an appropriate explanation of the treatments available.

Never forget that however unwise his or her sense of values may be in the eyes of the medical profession, every patient has the right to forego treatment or even cure if it entails personally intolerable consequences or risks.[5]

AVOIDING LEGAL ENTANGLEMENTS

Lack of informed consent may develop into a lawsuit only when a physician fails to disclose a risk that subsequently becomes an injury. Otherwise, as one court stated, "an omission (of material information), however unpardonable, is legally without consequence."[2] Practically, the patient must demonstrate that, had the proper information been disclosed, he or she would not have consented to the course of therapy. To control the subjectivity of this application, some jurisdictions require the patient to prove that if the risk had been disclosed neither this patient, nor a reasonable person in this patient's situation, would have consented.[1]

REQUIREMENTS OF DOCUMENTATION

A signed form entitled "consent to treatment" is required for all procedures; note, however, that the form only proves consent, not that it was informed.[8] The exchange of information that precedes the signed consent is crucial to the process. Good chart documentation (including signed consent forms, which are often and appropriately recommended by attorneys and risk managers) does not insulate a physician from a lawsuit but does make the defense of one considerably less difficult. Malpractice claims often are made years after the treatment was rendered, by which time any specific discussion with the patient in question has long since faded from memory. A standard consent form does nothing to jog the memory of the physician or the patient about the discussion; thus, it is highly important to tailor the discussion (and the subsequent documentation) for each patient, regardless of the procedure. Gone are the days when the phrase "reviewed the risks and benefits and the patient consents" was sufficient. On the standard consent form there usually is an area in which additional information may be added—savvy doctors will make pertinent notes in this body before every procedure (see Fig. 5-1). For example, if trigger point injections are to be given in the piriformis muscle, note that injury to the sciatic nerve is possible. If the injections are to be done in the region of the middle trapezius, noting that potential complications include a pneumothorax is more appropriate. Any notations on the consent form may be bolstered by further documentation in the medical record regarding the details of the discussion. In certain circumstances, it may be advisable to provide the patient with a written summary of the discussion to take home and review before the procedure.

It is also advisable to document concerns that the patient expressed and how these concerns were addressed. Finally, note all persons present for the discussion, including other health care providers or individuals who accompanied the patient. If possible, have one of the additional medical persons present for the discussion also sign the consent form. This person can subsequently be available to the patient for further information, and, should there be an adverse outcome, this person can attest to the completeness of the consent discussion.

THE ROLE OF THE DOCTOR-PATIENT RELATIONSHIP

In studies that have explored the relationship between physicians' claims experience and the quality of care they provide, a common theme is that the differences between sued and never-sued physicians are not necessarily explained by their quality of care or their chart documentation. "[I]f quality of care, medical negligence and chart documentation are not the critical factors leading to litigation, what factors are critical? Patient dissatisfaction is critical."[9] Although the law dictates what needs to be said to a patient, experience dictates that the manner in which it is said and the amount of time it takes to say it are equally important in providing good quality care

PROCEDURE/TREATMENT CONSENT FORM

DATE: 7/23/99 UNIT NO.: ________

PATIENT: John Smith

PROCEDURE/TREATMENT: trigger point injections

I have explained to the patient the nature of his/her condition, the nature of the procedure/treatment and the benefits to be reasonably expected compared with alternative approaches.

I have discussed the likelihood of major risks or complications of this procedure/treatment including (if applicable) but not limited to loss of limb function, brain damage, paralysis, hemorrhage, infection, drug reactions, blood clots and loss of life. I have indicated that with any treatment/procedure there is always the possibility of an unexpected complication. I have also indicated the risks of not having the procedure/treatment.

List additional comments, if any, specific to the procedure/treatment. Identify other persons present during explanation. Note what, if any, information is being provided in writing (description, protocols, et cetera).

allergic reaction to the medication
injury to a blood vessel or nerve
punctured lung requiring hospitalization

Note - Mr. Smith's wife was present during consent discussion.

The patient consents to the procedure/treatment.

Joyce P. Jones M.D.

Dr. Joyce Jones has explained the above to me and I consent to the procedure/treatment.

x John Smith Date: 7/23/99

Signature of patient or (Guardian, or Agent, or, legal next-of-kin for a minor).
If signature cannot be obtained, indicate reason in comments section above.

x Barbara Smith

Barbara Smith (wife)

Revised/Approved: Medical Staff 11/89; 6/17/92; 5/95

FIGURE 5-1. Sample consent form.

and in avoiding a malpractice allegation. Effective communication between the patient and the physician not only enhances treatment outcomes but also enhances patient satisfaction. This combination tips the balance away from litigation, even in the face of unfavorable procedure outcomes.

A recent study found that routine visits with physicians with no malpractice claims were longer than routine visits with physicians who had experienced malpractice claims.[9] This same study found that the malpractice claims were more strongly correlated with the process and tone of a discussion than the content of that discussion.

WHEN MEDICAL NEGLIGENCE IS AN ISSUE

Full and complete informed consent is never a substitute for competent medical care. Claims arising exclusively under the doctrine of informed consent assume that the treatment was rendered appropriately and that a known and accepted risk occurred in the absence of negligence. When the procedure was not performed appropriately, there is a basis for the additional (and more common) claim for medical negligence.

By virtue of the doctor-patient relationship, a physician must exercise the degree of knowledge and skill of the average qualified physician practicing the specialty.[10] Any breach of this standard that results in injury to a patient may be actionable as a medical malpractice claim.

Proof of compliance with the standard of practice usually will come through a review by an expert witness, who will offer opinions based upon his or her education, training, and experience in the specialty, and, in particular, in the procedure at issue. In addition, an expert opinion must be based upon the facts of the case.

The medical records best demonstrate facts. It is essential to accurately and completely describe every procedure. The procedure note should contain the indications for the procedure, the details of its performance, and the patient's reaction or initial outcome. For example, the diagnosis for a trigger point injection may be fibromyalgia, and the indications may be to alleviate pain and muscle spasm.

Symptoms and their duration and prior treatment intervention also should be documented. The following sample documentation may be useful: "Under sterile conditions using a 1-inch, 27-gauge sterile disposable needle and a solution of 2 cc 1% Xylocaine and 10 cc 0.25% Sensorcaine, a total of 6 trigger point injections were done in the bilateral upper trapezii. A 2-cc aliquot of the mixture was used at each site. Patient tolerated the procedure well and reported immediate relief of pain in the cervical region." Finally, follow-up plans should be clearly documented. Once again, providing the patient with a copy of the plan may be appropriate.

After analysis of the records, an expert may evaluate the physician's proficiency with the procedure. "When a new procedure is instituted into clinical practice, proctorship and supervision by a more experienced colleague or other specialist with appropriate documentation may help establish a basis for indicating that the physician has attained the requisite degree of knowledge and skill for the procedure."[11]

In conclusion, informed consent involves explaining the diagnosis to the patient in language that he or she understands, possible treatment options, and the risks and benefits of the proposed treatment (procedure). Moreover, thoroughly documenting informed consent in an individualized manner is imperative.

REFERENCES

1. *Harnish v Children's Hospital Medical Center*, 387 Mass. 152, 439 N.E.2d, 240 (1982).
2. *Cobbs v Grant*, 8 Cal. 3d 229, 104 Cal. Rptr. 505, 502 P. 2d 1 (1972).
3. Annas G: A National Bill of Rights. N Engl J Med 338:695–699, 1998.
4. Physician Insurers Association of America: Cumulative Data Sharing Reports, 1997.
5. *Precourt v Frederick*, 395 Mass. 689, 481 N.E.2d 1144 (1985).
6. *Wilkinson v Vesey*, 110 R.I. 606, 295 A.2d 676 (1972).
7. *Canterbury v Spence*, 464 F. 2d 772 (D.C. Cir) cert. denied, 409 U.S. 1064, 93 S.Ct. 560, 34 L.Ed 2d 518 (1972).
8. Urbanski PK: Getting the "go ahead": Helping patients understand informed consent. Lifelines: 45–48, 1997.
9. Levinson W, Roter DL, Mullooly JP, et al: Physician-patient communication: The relationship with malpractice claims among primary care physicians and surgeons. JAMA 277: 553–559, 1997.
10. *Brune v Belinkoff*, 354 Mass. 102, 235 N.E.2d 793 (1968).
11. Brenner RJ: Interventional procedures of the breast: Medicolegal considerations. Radiology 195:611–615, 1995.

6

Wound Management

David F. Neale, M.D., and Phala A. Helm, M.D.

PERSPECTIVE AND HISTORY

Wound management has by tradition and rich historical precedent been the purview of the surgeon and, in antiquity, the battlefield surgeon. The fundamental principles of wound care that evolved through the centuries by clinical observation and trial and error were the "dividend of the tragedy of war."[28] Unfortunately, they were often discovered only to be forgotten, rediscovered, and relearned by succeeding generations of war surgeons.

The enduring wound treatment methods generally support the biologic dictum that "the good physician is truly 'nature's servant.'"[28] As the Swiss physician Paracelsus (1493–1541) stated: "The surgeon should know that not he but Nature is the healer."[26] Ambrose Paré (?1510–1590), the great military barber-surgeon, revolutionized the treatment of wounds in the 16th century by abandoning the use of cautery (with "scalding oyle") in favor of simple dressings[36] that protected rather than perturbed the wound. He humbly stated in his famous aphorism:

> Je le pensay, Dieu le guarit![28] (I dress him, God heals him!)

Good physicians are still "nature's servant" insofar as their modern wound management is an extension of the lessons and methods of predecessors who have as the central goal the optimization of the milieu in which protected natural healing can take place. In this regard we find ourselves on a continuum with the best efforts of the battlefield surgeons. The enduring Halstedian principles of atraumatic tissue handling, careful hemostasis, and appropriate irrigation of the wound enhance healing and prevent infection.[15]

Future scientific inquiry and practice will no doubt hone the ability to improve the milieu of the wound by identifying for correction the many impediments to healing and the few overlooked enhancements to healing. One such enhancement discovered (or perhaps rediscovered) in 1962 was the benefit of a moist wound environment. This was noted in Winter's work with experimental wounds treated with occlusive dressings versus air drying.[39,40] He proved that drying of the wound surface with scab formation impeded healing. Thus began the "dressings revolution" that continues today.

ULCER DEBRIDEMENT

An appreciation of local anatomy, the depth of necrosis, the presence or absence of infection, and the patient's level of nutrition and immune competence are all critical to outcome. In general, if the skin wound is large, if it exceeds full-thickness dermal destruction with necrosis of subcutaneous or deeper tissues (stage 3 or greater pressure ulcer), if it is associated with vascular insufficiency or bony deformity, or if a flap or graft is likely to be needed, it is in the patient's and physician's best interest to obtain appropriate, early surgical consultation for initial debridement.

Wound management implies a process. The first step in that process is protection from the localized pressure that causes the ulceration and further tissue damage.[9] Correction, where possible, of deficiency factors that influence wound healing must accompany the process. Systemic factors such as malnutrition, vitamin deficiency, anemia, hypoxemia, decreased circulating volume, and vascular insufficiency must be addressed.[2,9]

The second step is debridement. Debridement is "the removal of foreign material and devitalized or contaminated tissue from or adjacent to a traumatic or infected lesion until surrounding healthy tissue is exposed."[6] Sharp debridement of an ulcer may be *selective* in that only devitalized tissue is excised, or it may be *nonselective*, as in the case of total surgical excision of both devitalized and adjacent viable tissue prior to closure or grafting.[41] Selective debridement is well within the purview of the physician or his or her trained designee. It is particularly effective in the treatment of infected ulcers, because only nonviable, necrotic tissue is removed, thereby decreasing the bacterial contamination while hastening the removal of physical blocks to healing. When done sequentially on consecutive days, the ulcer can be rendered "clean" in a short time unless tissue damage is ongoing (e.g., as a result of pressure) or systemic host deficiency factors have not been corrected.

Undebrided devitalized tissue enhances infection by acting as a culture medium for bacterial growth. In addition, devitalized tissue inhibits leukocyte phagocytosis of bacteria and their subsequent destruction.[11] The bacteria present are protected from systemic or topically applied antimicrobials by avascular necrotic tissue. This allows infection to persist and may encourage the development of resistance to such antimicrobials.

The physical effect of devitalized material includes mechanical obstruction to wound contraction and a surface barrier to eventual reepithelialization from the wound perimeter. Epithelial cells require a moist environment in which to migrate. The presence of a dry eschar or necrotic debris forces these cells to burrow beneath such material, significantly delaying the healing process. Wound contraction by myelofibroblastic activity in and around the healing ulcer serves to shorten the healing process by reducing the size of the defect. This contraction is prevented by a hard eschar.[41]

Partial surgical debridement is usually painless and associated with minimal if any blood loss when performed properly and carefully. As with any psychomotor task, skill and confidence are acquired with practice and experience. A useful practice task described by Davis[5] closely simulates actual wound and burn debridement if necrotic tissue is of a less adherent type. This simulation involves peeling a navel orange of all skin down to its thin pulp membrane without the leakage of any juice (Fig. 6-1).

Debridement Procedure: Decubitus Ulcer

The procedure of debridement is easily divided into three parts: preparation, debridement, and dressing.

Preparation

1. Time. For the initial debridement, morning allows better coordination of nursing issues and

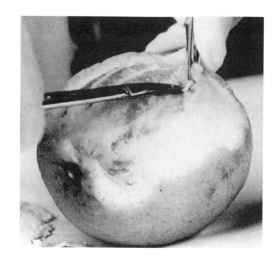

FIGURE 6-1. Peeled navel orange used for debridement simulation and practice. Goal: a clean, unbroken membrane. (From Razor BR, Martin LK: Validating sharp wound debridement. J ET Nurs 18:107, 1991, with permission.)

support systems as well as the convenience of an afternoon wound check.

2. Obtain the patient's informed consent for initial debridement to remove dead and/or infected tissues from the wound. Determine any allergies.

3. Supplies (see Table 6-1). These and other instruments are often in a minor surgery tray. A minor debridement tray can be arranged through the hospital's central sterile supply to provide only what is desired. Other disposable supplies should be ordered in the chart if not routinely available. They include povidone-iodine solution, normal saline irrigation solution, local anesthetic of choice (the author prefers 1% or 2% lidocaine without epinephrine), sterile gloves, glasses or goggles (optional), gown, silver nitrate sticks, Gelfoam (optional), and dressing supplies.

4. Arrange for an assistant familiar with sterile technique to retrieve additional supplies.

5. Position patient comfortably on an adjustable-height bed or plinth.

TABLE 6-1.   Instruments for Sharp Wound Debridement

Gloves
Adson forceps with teeth
No. 3 scalpel handle with no. 10 and no. 15 blades
Two mosquito clamps
Silver nitrate sticks
Absorbable gelatin film (Surgical or Gelfoam)
Gauze sponges
Curved iris scissors
Normal saline solution
Sterile towels

From Razor BR, Martin LK: Validating sharp wound debridement. J ET Nurs 18:107, 1991, with permission.

6. Cleanse the wound area and surrounding area with povidone-iodine solution and gauze sponges. Work from center outward in spirals, discarding sponges between spirals.

7. An adjustable local light source is recommended. If a gooseneck exam light is to be used, the bulb should be positioned no closer than 18 inches to the patient's skin.

8. Set up a sterile impermeable barrier on mobile bedside table, and set up a sterile field with instruments, supplies, and a basin of normal saline.

9. Drape the ulcer site with sterile towels, leaving the ulcer exposed. Simple cloth surgical towels work best, although paper, adhesive-stripped, windowed drapes are available.

10. Wipe povidone-iodine solution from exposed ulcer and skin with a saline-moistened gauze sponge or alcohol swabs.

11. If the site is inflamed and tender and not of neuropathic etiology, it may be necessary to infiltrate a local anesthetic in the skin edge of the dermatome proximal to the ulcer at this point. Lidocaine 2% without epinephrine injected subdermally via a 25-gauge, 1½-inch needle will give 2–4 hours of anesthetic time.

Debridement

12. Using toothed Adson forceps, pick up the edge of the eschar and develop a plane using the curved iris scissors by spreading the points and snipping. Traction on the freed eschar or any other tissue freed from the wound should always be perpendicular to the plane of the wound. This affords not only the best visibility of the wound, but the best chance of staying within the chosen tissue plane without inadvertently cutting into a deeper plane. In this manner the devitalized tissue of the ulcer can be removed in sequential layers. Adipose subcutaneous tissue, when necrotic, is gray in color with little, if any, tensile strength and must be picked from the wound. Curved mosquito hemostats are useful in this procedure.

Hemostasis

13. Occasionally (more often when using a scalpel) viable tissue will be entered and capillary or small vessel bleeding will occur. Usually this can be controlled with gentle pressure and a moist saline sponge, which has the added benefit of wicking away the blood before it stains nearby tissues pink. This unwanted staining of otherwise obviously necrotic tissue is the reason one should start debridement at the lowest point and work up whenever

possible. In this way any bleeding flows away from the work area. If small vessel bleeding or capillary ooze persists, a silver nitrate stick lightly touched to the area is usually sufficient. Persistent venous bleeders respond to Gelfoam and pressure for 5 minutes. A defiant arteriolar bleeder occasionally will require suture ligature.

14. Keep the wound moist. Do not allow it to dry out. A moist saline gauze should cover as much of the debrided ulcer bed and viable tissue as possible. This protects the tissue and, on removal, helps locate any unnoticed bleeding.

15. Remember, this is a process of debridement, not an event. If the clinician or the patient gets tired, it is best to stop and resume the process at a later time.

Dressing

16. Dressings and dressing orders should aid in the debridement effort. Coarse mesh gauze—wet-to-moist with normal saline—loosely packed into every corner of the ulcer deficit and covered with a sterile absorbent dressing should be changed every 8 hours.

17. Lastly, a procedure note should reflect what was done. For example: "Partial surgical debridement of necrotic eschar and tissue from (type of wound and location)." The note should record the position of the patient, the prep solution and sterile drapes, any local anesthetic and amount used, the condition of the ulcer before and after debridement, any bleeding encountered and how it was controlled, the estimated tissue layer depth of necrosis identified, estimated stage of necrosis, and any complications.

Delayed Debridement

Partial surgical debridement often can be delayed advantageously in the case of an intact dry eschar over a decubitus lesion so long as there are no signs or symptoms of infection. The skin eschar here should eventually be removed but acts a a temporary biologic dressing while pressure relief and host deficiency factors are addressed. Within 3–5 days the inflammatory phase of wound healing may become evident at the wound as leukocytes and macrophages collect in the viable interface. Often the eschar edges will "lift" from the surrounding well-vascularized, viable tissue as this wound-healing inflammation progresses. The lift gives a palpable mobile sensation and denotes an opportune time to initiate sharp partial surgical debridement prior to actual separation or the development of infection at the eschar borders. It should be noted that the differentiation of a stage 3 ulcer, which involves only subcutaneous fat, from a stage 4 ulcer extending into muscle or bone is difficult to assess beneath intact eschar. Generally, a knowledge of local anatomy, the history and condition of the patient, and the size of the surface involvement are the only clues. The area at the surface usually underrepresents the area of necrosis at maximum depth and, therefore, the total volume of necrosis. If a deep stage 3 or stage 4 ulcer is clinically suspected, consultation for initial debridement in a formal surgical setting is indicated.

Debridement Exceptions

Specialized tissues that perform important physical functions such as nerves, tendons, and fascia may be left undebrided. Although they are devitalized, such fibrous tissues often can be rendered surgically clean by local debridement and irrigation. With the granulation process, they act as transplant grafts of correct length and ideal location that are recellularized (Fig. 6-4A).[27]

Another exception is black eschar attached to underlying bone, such as a posterior heel or sacral decubitus. As long as bacterial growth beneath it is minimized, it serves as a temporary biologic dressing.[41]

Underlying Osteomyelitis

Longstanding or chronically draining decubitus ulcers frequently overlie osteomyelitis. Plain radiographs are frequently diagnostic. If normal, they serve as a baseline for later comparison because radiographic changes often lag up to 4 weeks behind acute bone infection.[37] The triple phase technetium 99m bone scan, when negative, rules out bone involvement at the 90% sensitivity level.[37] When positive, infectious etiologies can be differentiated at the 80–90% sensitivity level from noninfectious inflammatory processes by the addition of an indium 111 or a technetium 99m (Ceretec) labeled leukocyte scan. The spatial resolution of the latter can be enhanced by single photon emission computed tomography (SPECT) reconstruction to aid in the detection and localization of infected tissues.

When osteomyelitis is absent but overlying tissue condition warrants debridement, all viable tissues or a thin layer of necrotic tissue and periosteum should be left in place over intact cortical bone. In the interest of preventing bacterial invasion, this remaining thin necrotic tissue over bone can be kept moist while its bacterial contamination is reduced by local treatment with topical antimicrobials such as silver sulfadiazine.

Ulcer Dressings

In the remainder of the ulcer, daily sequential partial surgical debridement and mechanical wet-to-dry saline dressing debridement of the surrounding necrosis will reduce the bacterial growth and encourage the formation of granulation tissue.[3] Normal saline wet-to-dry dressings with coarse mesh gauze will debride nonselectively both residual necrotic debris and some surface granulation tissue while retarding epithelialization. It is, however, the dressing of choice for initial management of necrotic wounds. The frequently used solutions of 1% povidone-iodine, 0.25% acetic acid, 3% hydrogen peroxide, and 0.5% sodium hypochlorite (Dakin's) have useful antimicrobial activity in heavily infected ulcers but should be discontinued in favor of saline as soon as possible because of their proven cytotoxic effects on fibroblasts.[20]

After the bulk of necrotic tissue and debris have been removed by sequential, partial surgical debridements and wet-to-dry dressing, underlying granulation tissue should be visible in parts or all of the wound. The establishment of this granulation bed and its confluent spread in the wound is the goal of all subsequent efforts until healing occurs. Healing may be achieved by secondary intention: that is, by filling in of the defect by granulation tissue (so-called proud flesh), contraction of the defect by myofibroblasts and reepithelialization from the periphery, or by a formal surgical intervention such as secondary closure or a grafting procedure. The spreading granulation tissue enhances autolytic debridement of the remaining necrotic debris by bringing to the wound polymorphonuclear leukocytes and macrophages. The breakdown of fibrin, protein, mucopolysaccharides, glycoproteins, glycolipids, DNA, and RNA is performed by the enzymes of these cells, which add their activity to that of bacterial enzymes present in the ulcer fluid.[41]

Autolytic debridement requires a moist environment in which to occur. The thin-film, polymeric dressings are useful in noninfected superficial wounds to retain moisture and autolytic activity while allowing visualization of the wound. In deeper wounds, the moisture-retentive and absorptive properties of hydrocolloid dressings aid debridement by increasing tissue fluid flow across the wound, and, in the case of DuoDERM (ConvaTec, Princeton, NJ), providing fibrinolytic activity.[23] Both the thin, oxygen-permeable, polymeric films and the hydrocolloids change the wound environment beneficially by lowering the pH of the wound fluid (more so with hydrocolloids) and by reducing the partial pressure of oxygen (PO_2). Low oxygen tension has been shown to enhance fibroblast growth and macrophage production of angiogenesis factors in vitro and is now believed to enhance the healing process in clean wounds.[34] Although small amounts of necrotic tissue are still present, occlusive dressings should be changed once or twice a day to allow additional selective debridement and to monitor the wound for signs of infection. Such wounds are always colonized, but infection, as evidenced by the signs of tissue invasion (pain, erythema of peripheral skin, induration, tenderness, change in volume and character of wound exudate, or fever), should prompt the temporary suspension of occlusive, moisture-retentive dressings. Appropriate bacteriologic studies, antibiotic coverage, and a return to wet-to-dry or wet-to-moist dressing suffice until the infection is controlled. Selective debridement

should continue as tenderness permits because this removes necrotic nutrients from the wound and hastens resumption of moisture-retentive dressings.

DIABETIC FOOT CARE

Levin and others[7,10,19] have advocated the management of the diabetic foot by a clinic-based, multidisciplinary team that is dedicated to limb preservation and salvage. In centers where multidisciplinary teams exist, the rate of amputations in diabetic patients has decreased by 50–85%.[7,14] Unfortunately, such centers have been slow to develop.[12] Although all disciplines of the team do not have to be physically present, the availability of immediate, in-clinic consultation facilitates cross-education of the team, prevents fragmentation of care, and improves salvage rates for patients at risk for limb loss.

Outpatient management of the diabetic foot entails patient education;[1] physical examination for deformity, intrinsic foot and distal limb strength, level of protective sensation,[16,33] skin temperature, condition, and hair pattern; vascular assessment by pulses and Doppler ultrasound;[35,42] wound management and closure of neuropathic ulcers; and assessment and provision of protective footwear. Also, nail and callus trimming is essential in the diabetic patient. In many instances, patients cannot and should not attempt these procedures because of impaired vision, sensation, and dexterity.

Nail Reduction

The diabetic patient's toenails, if normal, should be trimmed straight across to avoid ingrowth at the distal margins. Often the toenails grow slowly because of impaired circulation and become thickened by fungal infections (onychomycosis).[17] If neglected, such nails may curve plantarly over fungal debris and form so-called ram's horn nails that are prone to avulsion or subungual bleeding and infection. Lateral curving may threaten adjacent toes with ulceration.[25]

Normal nails and thickened nails that have been softened by hydrotherapy can be safely reduced with plier type toenail nippers without risk of shatter or splitting (Fig. 6-2A).

Thickened hypertrophic nails are best reduced and smoothed with a high-speed, rotary tool (Dremel) fitted with a small emery disk (Fig. 6-2B). In this way, the nail and its subungual debris can be carefully shaped and reduced as well as smoothed to prevent shoe trauma or snagging on clothing and bedding.

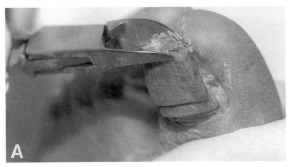
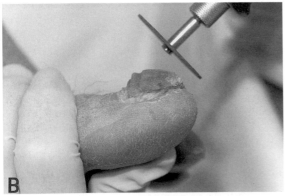

FIGURE 6-2. *A,* Normal to moderately thickened nails can be cut correctly with toenail nippers. *B,* Hypertrophic and "ram's horn" nails are best reduced and smoothed with a high-speed emery disk. Goggles and mask are recommended.

Callus Trimming

The sentinel sign of the diabetic foot at risk for neuropathic ulceration is the plantar callus. Loss of protective sensation allows repetitive high-pressure stress during ambulation without the normal shift of weight to protect the skin from damage.[4] Structural deformities such as hammer toes, bunions, and Charcot joints predispose the foot to develop areas of high pressure. The dermis responds initially with hyperkeratosis at the site of pressure. The callus thus formed becomes a "rock in the shoe." If the callus is kept trimmed, plantar pressures are reduced.[43] Continued hyperkeratosis and the subsequent increased local concentration of pressure leads to dermal necrosis and the tell-tale darkening of the callus by blood known as a preulcer (Fig. 6-3A).

Prophylactic trimming of the nonulcerated callus is easily accomplished with either a #10 scalpel or a single-edged razor blade. Care must be taken not to enter the vascular dermis but to remove only enough epidermal callus by serial tangential cuts to restore a supple surface.

Foot Grades

A classification of diabetic foot lesions has been described by Wagner based on clinical progression.[35] It is useful in determining treatment for six grades of foot lesions.

Grade 0: Intact skin. Bony deformity and/or keratotic skin thickenings may be present.

Grade 1: Superficial ulcer. Full-thickness skin or nail loss.

Grade 2: Deep ulcer. Penetrates subcutaneous fat down to tendon, ligament, joint capsule, or bone.

Grade 3: Ulcer with deep infection of tendon sheath, joint, bone, or abscess of deep tissues.

Grade 4: Gangrene of a portion of the foot requiring local amputation or possibly Syme's amputation.

Grade 5: Gangrene of foot sufficient to prevent surgical salvage. Amputation below knee or higher required.

Care for Neuropathic Grades 1 and 2 Ulcers

If a preulcer callus is removed, the bed of a true neuropathic ulcer is usually exposed (Fig. 6-3B). This bed, although necrotic, is usually clean and will heal if protected from further pressure. The ulcer must be probed to determine any undermining or sinus tracts. The ulcer must then be pared of its overlying and/or surrounding callus and debrided of its necrotic tissues.

A general principle for this debridement in Wagner grade 1 and 2 neuropathic ulcers is that the ulcer should be as wide as it is deep. This allows adequate drainage and prevents premature, superficial healing.[4] Sequential paring of the "ring callus" that often develops around healing ulcers reduces pressure and

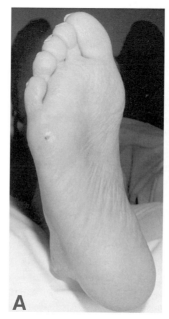 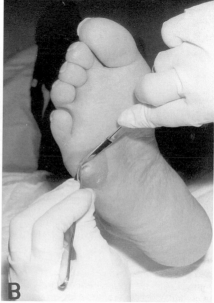

FIGURE 6-3. *A,* "Preulcer": telltale darkening beneath plantar callus at lateral metatarsal head. *B,* Unroofing callus exposes clean, neuropathic ulcer bed. Probing revealed no undermined edge or sinus tract.

shear at the ulcer rim and allows wound contracture to hasten closure.

Clean or granulating neuropathic superficial (Wagner grade 1) and deep (Wagner grade 2) ulcers without infection can usually be successfully treated with total contact walking casts on an outpatient basis. High rates of healing (72–90%) in 6 weeks or less have been reported.[4,13,24] Deep ulcers with tendon or joint sepsis, deep abscess, or osteomyelitis (Wagner grade 3) require hospitalization with antibiotics and appropriate surgical treatment. Once successfully treated and effectively rendered grade 1 or 2, the ulcer and surgical wound can be treated with total contact casts to aid healing (Fig. 6-4).[24]

Localized gangrene of the toes, forefoot, or heel (Wagner grade 4) requires hospitalization with local amputation and often vascular reconstruction. Gangrene of the entire foot (Wagner grade 5) requires major amputation above the ankle.[35]

Infected Grades 1 and 2 Ulcers

Frequently the patient presents with an open, infected superficial or deep (grade 1 or 2) neuropathic

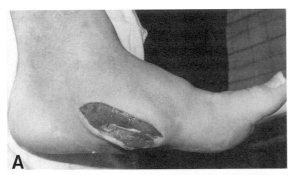

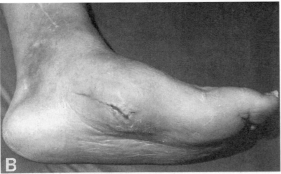

FIGURE 6-4. *A*, Attenuated plantar fascia exposed and left intact after incision and drainage of abscess at site of grade 3 chronic medial ulcer in Charcot deformed foot. Osteomyelitis was ruled out. Granulation is enveloping fascia. *B*, Irrigation and debridement and culture-specific antibiotics, followed by hydrotherapy, sequential local debridement, and serial total contact casting resulted in progressive closure.

ulcer. If the clinical examination reveals cellulitis, admission for elevation, intravenous antibiotics, and a search for deep, limb-threatening infection or osteomyelitis is indicated. In the absence of cellulitis, when probing reveals a sinus tract into joint, abscess, or bone, or when x-ray reveals joint or bone involvement, the lesion is grade 3, and admission is also indicated.

Locally infected Wagner grade 1 and 2 lesions without cellulitis can be managed in the outpatient setting. These ulcers should be cleansed in hydrotherapy to reduce soluble debris and bacterial load and begun on sequential partial surgical debridement to reduce adherent, necrotic tissue. Initial dressings of normal saline or dilute 10:1 saline–povidone-iodine wet-to-dry coarse mesh gauze changed three times daily will aid debridement.

Depending on the clinical setting, empirical antibiotics are often required. Adequate cultures to retrieve both aerobic and anaerobic organisms should be attempted before antibiotic treatment. Surface swab cultures are notoriously inaccurate,[32,38] and tissue aspirates may miss the pathogen[21]; however, deep biopsy cultures are not always indicated or available in grade 1 and 2 lesions. A curettage specimen culture obtained from the ulcer base and edges has been shown to correlate better with deep tissue biopsy and to be more sensitive for anaerobes and gram-negative bacilli.[21,31] The technique of collection involves surface decontamination of superficial colonizers with saline-soaked gauze, povidone-iodine or isopropyl alcohol pads, irrigation, and collection of tissue scrapings from the ulcer base and edges.

Acute and superfically infected ulcers tend to contain one or two aerobic, gram-positive cocci (frequently staphylococci or streptococci) species per infection and respond to either oral cephalexin or clindamycin. Detection of aerobic gram-negative bacilli (frequently *Proteus*, *Klebsiella-Enterobacter*, or *Pseudomonas* species and *Escherichia coli*) require a change to broader coverage such as trimethoprim-sulfamethoxazole, amoxicillin-clavulanate, or ciprofloxacin. Detection of obligate anaerobes, foul odor, or polymicrobial cultures suggest addition of metronidazole and consideration of inpatient management for deeper infection.

An adequate discussion of the microbiology and antimicrobial therapy of diabetic limb infections is beyond the scope of this chapter. The reader is referred to a review article on this subject by Lipsky et al.[22]

The patient should elevate the limb at home at bed rest to reduce edema while the infection comes under control. Wet-to-moist saline dressings changed three times a day, preferably by a family member, and diligent non–weight bearing via crutches, walker, or a wheelchair are essential. The wound is checked and debrided as necessary, initially every 2 or 3 days until it is clean and local signs of infection are resolving. Antibiotics are usually needed for 1 or 2 weeks.[21] However, continued swelling, excessive drainage, pain, or deterioration of the wound should prompt review of the antibiotic coverage and additional studies to rule out osteomyelitis or abscess.

When the ulcer is clean and edema resolved (often at the first or second follow-up visit), ambulatory care via total contact casting can be initiated. If the patient is not a candidate for casting due to conditions such as ataxia, blindness, fragile skin, morbid obesity, or claustrophobia, then non–weight-bearing mobility, dressing changes, and local wound care with foot protection in a molded Plastizote shoe or "healing sandal" are continued until healing occurs.

Total Contact Casting Technique

High rates of healing have been achieved by casting Wagner grade 1 and 2 neuropathic ulcers. This is probably due to the ability of the total contact cast to redistribute high pressures over the entire surface of the insensate foot while significantly reducing and controlling edema in the foot. This aids tissue fluid exchange and tends to localize infection. The plaster cast permits drainage to be absorbed from the wound while maintaining a moisture-retentive environment around the healing site. Lastly, it protects the foot from trauma, limits noncompliance, and allows weight bearing. Once healed, the patient is fitted with a custom-molded, rockered sandal for partial weight bearing until the skin toughens over the ulcer site. Alternatively, the patient may be placed directly into definitive extra-depth shoes with total contact molded insoles so long as he or she is limited to 1–2 hours of weight bearing a day initially for the first week with frequent foot checks the second week.

The classic technique of prone total contact cast application has been described by Coleman, Brand, and Birke of the National Hansen's Disease Center, Carville, Louisiana.[4] A slight variation in the technique is presented here, which allows immediate weight bearing, custom rocker molding, and level leg length. The addition of Webril cast padding allows safer removal of this fiberglass-reinforced cast with the cast saw.

Supplies

1. Fine mesh gauze or Xeroform gauze
2. Thin 2″ × 2″ or 4″ × 4″ gauze dressing
3. 1″ paper tape
4. 1 oz package (gas) sterilized lamb's wool or low density ½″ adhesive-backed foam (Sci-Foam by Next Generation, Rancho, CA)
5. 3″ stockinette sewn or folded over at toe and rolled into "donut"
6. Orthopedic felt ⅛″–¼″ thick (option: adhesive-backed) cut and beveled into 2½″-diameter maleolar pads and a 2″-wide tibial crest to dorsal arch pad
7. Two 3″ rolls of Webril cotton cast padding
8. Rockerbottom cast shoe
9. Plaster cast materials: three 3″ rolls, fast setting; three 4″ rolls, fast setting, two 5″ × 30″, five-thickness splints
10. Fiberglass casting tape: one 3″ roll; one 4″ roll
11. Bucket of cold water
12. Vinyl or latex gloves

Total Contact Cast Procedure

Preparation

1. Apply in the early morning following overnight elevation to ensure as little edema as possible in the foot and leg. Some centers use Ace wrapping or pneumatic pumping to reduce edema prior to casting.
2. Prepare the wound with diluted povidone-iodine solution and rinse.
3. Remove all necrotic ulcer tissue and surrounding callus. Excessive granulation tissue can be reduced with a silver nitrate swab and rinsed with saline.

Application

Step 1. The patient is positioned prone with the knee flexed 90° and the ankle at neutral. Pillows beneath the shoulders and hips improve comfort. Obese or breathless patients may be casted in the sitting position.

Step 2. The dressing of choice is applied and secured with paper tape at edges (Fig. 6-5).

Step 3. Lamb's wool is placed over the dressing, between the toes, and around the toes and secured with paper tape. This prevents maceration of toes and wound by wicking moisture away and into the cast. Alternate toe protection can be substituted here with low-density ½″ adhesive-backed foam (Sci-Foam) folded over the stockinette cut to form a

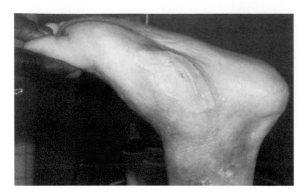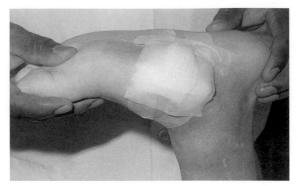

FIGURE 6-5

toe cap. Interdigital wicks of lamb's wool or thin cotton wisps are still required (Fig. 6-6).

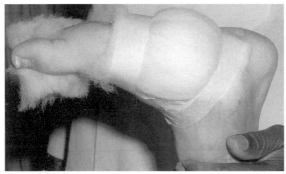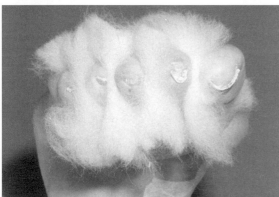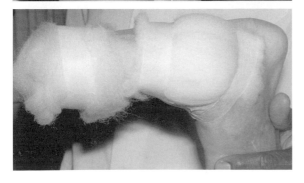

FIGURE 6-6

Step 4. A snug-fitting stockinette sewn or folded at the toe is rolled over the foot and leg to the tibial tubercle (Fig. 6-7).

Step 5. Beveled pads of orthopedic felt are taped over the maleoli, tibial crest, and dorsum of instep (Fig. 6-8).

Step 6. A single layer of overlapping 3″ Webril cotton cast padding is applied snugly from toe cap to just below the tibial tubercle (Fig. 6-9).

Step 7. An inner shell of plaster is applied using a 3″ roll for foot and ankle and a 4″ roll for ankle and leg (Fig. 6-10).

Step 8. In quick succession five-ply 5″ × 30″ plaster splints are applied from the calf around the toe cap and mediolaterally across the ankle stirrup and molded to the inner shell while ankle position is held. Cast is allowed to set (Fig. 6-11).

Step 9. Rocker bottom, sole height, and ankle position correction is adjusted with fan-folded layers of 3″ plaster roll (Fig. 6-12).

Step 10. Reinforcing layers of fiberglass cast tape are applied in sitting position (Fig. 6-13).

Step 11. A cast shoe is applied and the patient allowed to bear weight (Fig. 6-14).

Step 12. The patient is given written instructions for cast care and to return for signs of cast loosening, softening, or excessive drainage or symptoms of pain, fever, or lymphadenopathy.

Step 13. The first cast is changed after 2 or 3 days due to rapid loss of edema. Subsequent casts are changed at 1- to 3-week intervals, depending on ulcer condition and experience.

Skills Acquisition and Resources

The development of debridement, casting, and wound management skills can best be achieved by practice under experienced individuals. Most wound care specialists and multidisciplinary diabetic foot

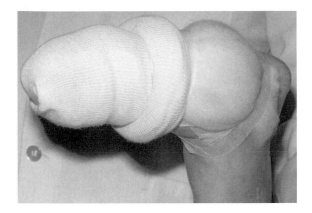

FIGURE 6-7

clinics welcome interest in their work and are eager to pass on their expertise to interested clinicians, nurses, and therapists. An excellent three-day course on comprehensive management of insensitive feet is given biannually by the U.S. Public Health Service's Gillis W. Long Hansen's Disease Center, Carville, Louisiana. Resources and information regarding continuing medical education courses are available through the American Diabetes Association. Additionally, several texts give excellent instruction and guidance on the entire

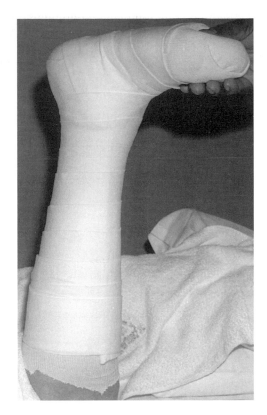

FIGURE 6-9

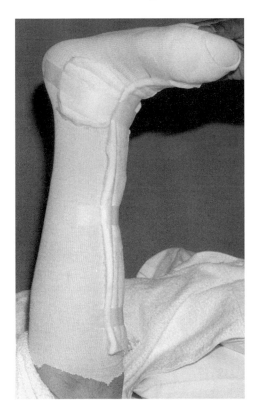

FIGURE 6-8

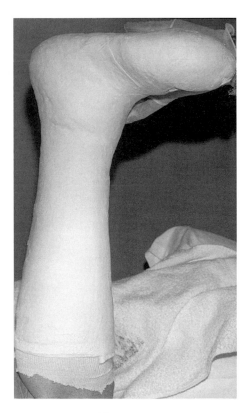

FIGURE 6-10

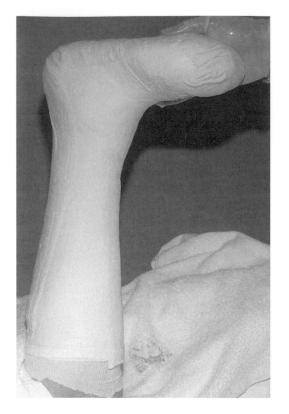 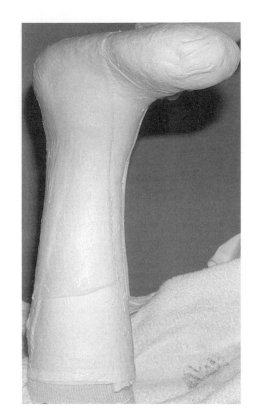

FIGURE 6-11

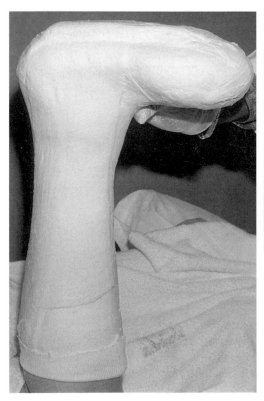 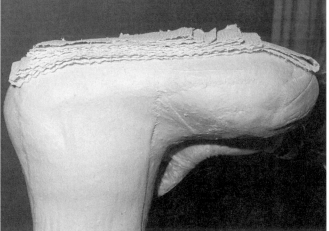

FIGURE 6-12

breadth and the intricacies of successful care of the diabetic foot.[8,18,30]

REFERENCES

1. Assal JP, Muhlhauser I, Pernet A, Gfeller R, et al: Patient education as the basis for diabetic foot care in clinical practice. Diabetologia 28:602–613, 1985.
2. Carrico TJ, Mehrhof AI Jr, Cohen IK: Biology of wound healing. Surg Clin North Am 64:721–733, 1984.
3. Coche W Jr, White RR IV, Lynch DJ, et al: Wound Care. New York, Churchill Livingstone, 1986.
4. Coleman WC, Brand PW, Birke JA: The total contact cast. A therapy for plantar ulceration on insensitive feet. J Am Podiatr Med Assoc 74:548–552, 1984.
5. Davis JT: Enhancing wound debridement skills through simulated practice. Phys Ther 66:1723–1724, 1986.
6. Dorland's Illustrated Medical Dictionary, 28th ed. Philadelphia, W.B. Saunders, 1994.
7. Edmonds ME, Blundell MP, Morris ME, et al: Improved survival of the diabetic foot: The role of a specialised foot clinic. Q J Med 601:763–771, 1986.
8. Frykberg RG (ed): The High Risk Foot in Diabetes Mellitus. New York, Churchill Livingstone, 1991.
9. Goode PS, Allman RM: The prevention and management of pressure ulcers. Med Clin North Am 73:1511–1524, 1989.
10. Grunfeld C: Diabetic foot ulcers: Etiology, treatment, and prevention. Arch Intern Med 37:123, 1991.
11. Haury B, Rodeheaver G, Vensko J, et al: Debridement: An essential component of traumatic wound care. Am J Surg 135:238–242, 1978.
12. Helm PA, Kowalski MD: Rehabilitation. In Levin ME, O'Neal LW, Bowker JH (eds): The Diabetic Foot, 5th ed. St. Louis, Mosby, 1993.
13. Helm PA, Walker SC, Pullium G: Total contact casting in diabetic patients with neuropathic foot ulcerations. Arch Phys Med Rehabil 65:691–693, 1984.
14. Hobgood E: Conservative therapy of foot abnormalities, infections, and vascular insufficiency. In Davidson JK (ed): Clinical Diabetes Mellitus. New York, Thieme, 1986.
15. Hochberg J, Murray GF: Principles of operative surgery. In Sabiston D (ed): Textbook of Surgery, 14th ed. Philadelphia, W.B. Saunders, 1991.
16. Holewskki JJ, Moss KM, Stess RM, et al: Prevalence of foot pathology and lower extremity complications in a diabetic outpatient clinic. J Rehabil Res Dev 26:35–44, 1989.
17. Jacobs RL, Karmody AM: Office care and the insensitive foot. Foot Ankle 2:230–237, 1982.
18. Levin ME, O'Neal LW, Bowker JH (eds): The Diabetic Foot, 5th ed. St. Louis, Mosby, 1993.
19. Levin ME: Pathogenesis and management of diabetic foot lesions. In Levin ME, O'Neal LW, Bowker JH (eds): The Diabetic Foot, 5th ed. St. Louis, Mosby, 1993.
20. Lineaweaver W, Howard R, Soucy D, et al: Topical antimicrobial toxicity. Arch Surg 120:267–270, 1985.
21. Lipsky BA, Pecoraro RE, Larson SA, et al: Outpatient management of uncomplicated lower-extremity infections in diabetic patients. Arch Intern Med 150:790–797, 1990.
22. Lipsky BA, Pecoraro RE, Wheat LJ: The diabetic foot: Soft tissue and bone infection. Infect Dis Clin North Am 4:409–432, 1990.
23. Lydon MJ, Hutchinson JJ, Rippon M, et al: Dissolution of wound coagulum and promotion of granulation tissue under DuoDERM. Wounds 1:95–106, 1989.
24. Myerson M, Papa J, Katulle E, et al: The total-contact cast for management of neuropathic plantar ulceration of the foot. J Bone Joint Surg 74A:261–269, 1992.
25. O'Neal LW: Surgical pathology of the foot and clinicopathologic correlations. In Levin ME, O'Neal LW, Bowker JH (eds): The Diabetic Foot, 5th ed. St. Louis, Mosby, 1993.
26. Paracelsus: Gross Chirurgie, 1536.
27. Peacock EE Jr: Wound Repair, 3rd ed. Philadelphia, W.B. Saunders, 1984.
28. Peterson CG: Perspectives in Surgery. Philadelphia, Lea & Febiger, 1972.
29. Razor BR, Martin LK: Validating sharp wound debridement. J ET Nurs 18:105–110, 1991.
30. Sammarco GJ (ed): The Foot in Diabetes. Philadelphia, Lea & Febiger, 1991.
31. Sapico FL, Witte JL, Canawati HN, et al: The infected foot of the diabetic patient: Quantitative microbiology and analysis of clinical features. Rev Infect Dis 6:S171–S176, 1984.
32. Sharp CS, Bessman AN, Wagner FW Jr, et al: Microbiology of superficial and deep tissue in infected diabetic gangrene. Surg Gynecol Obstet 149:217–219, 1979.
33. Sosenko JM, Kato M, Soto R, et al: Comparison of quantitative sensory-threshold measures for their association with ulceration in diabetic patients. Diabetes Care 13:1057–1061, 1990.
34. Varghese MC, Balin AK, Carter DM, et al: Local environment of chronic wounds under synthetic dressings. Arch Dermatol 122:52–57, 1986.
35. Wagner WF Jr: The treatment of the diabetic foot. Compr Ther 10:29–38, 1984.
36. Walton J, Beeson PB, Scott RB (eds): Oxford Companion to Medicine, vol. II. Birmingham, AL, Gryphon Editions, 1988.
37. Wegener WA, Alavi A: Diagnostic imaging of musculoskeletal infection. Orthop Clin North Am 22:401–418, 1991.
38. Wheat LJ, Allen SD, Henry M, et al: Diabetic foot infections: Bacteriologic analysis. Arch Intern Med 146:1935–1940, 1986.
39. Winter GD: Formation of the scab and the rate of epithelialization of superficial wounds in the skin of the young domestic pig. Nature 193:293–294, 1962.
40. Winter GD, Scales JT: Effects of air drying and dressings on the surface of a wound. Nature 197:91–92, 1963.
41. Witkowski JA, Parish LC: Debridement of cutaneous ulcers: Medical and surgical aspects. Clin Dermatol 9:585–591, 1992.
42. Yao ST, Hobbs JT, Irvine WT: Ankle systolic pressure measurements in arterial disease affecting the lower extremities. Br J Surg 56:676–679, 1969.
43. Young MJ, Cavanaugh PR, Thomas G, et al: The effect of callus removal on dynamic plantar foot pressures in diabetic patients. Diabetic Med 9:55–57, 1992.

7

Pediatric and Adult Swallowing Videofluoroscopy

Vikki Stefans, M.D., Richard P. Gray, M.D., and Thomas Sowell

Acceptance of the need for instrumental assessment of swallowing and greater general awareness and understanding of the principles of swallowing assessment are increasing, and an expanded repertoire of assessment techniques has become available to treat swallowing disorders. These instrumental techniques now include not only videofluoroscopic swallowing studies (VFSS; also known as modified barium swallow, oral pharyngeal video), but also pharyngeal-esophageal manometry and flexible endoscopic esophageal study (FEES) and other forms of videoendoscopy. Cervical auscultation and pharyngeal ultrasound may enhance specific aspects of the bedside evaluation as well. Radionuclide salivagram also may be added to this group of studies as a method to determine the efficacy of automatic swallowing of secretions at all times rather than only at mealtimes, particularly for individuals experiencing more severe respiratory complications.

Many patients with physically disabling conditions have associated swallowing disorders, and instrumental swallowing assessment is a recognized tool in all phases of management. The American Speech-Language-Hearing Association (ASHA) has recently approved guidelines for swallowing and swallowing disorders that specify these procedures to be within the scope of the speech and language pathologist and outline purposes, indications, and nonindications for instrumental study.[3] Study is not indicated if dysphagia is not confirmed on clinical history and evaluation, if a patient is too medically unstable for the study of choice, or if the swallow reflex is clinically absent. In addition, the Agency for Health Care Policy and Research recommends the following:

> Swallowing problems (dysphagia) are common after stroke and may cause aspiration. The patient's ability to swallow should be assessed before oral intake is begun, and techniques to facilitate swallowing should be implemented in affected patients. A feeding gastrostomy or nasogastric tube may be required if the patient does not regain the ability to swallow safely.... Assessment includes careful pharyngeal and laryngeal nerve examinations and testing of facial muscles, tongue function, and the cough response.... Videofluoroscopy using a modified barium swallow method can be used to evaluate swallowing time, pharyngeal motility, and the mechanism of aspiration.[1]

At least 12–13% of all patients with stroke experience dysphagia, although this decreases to 4% over the subsequent several months of recovery. Continued assessment and adjustment of recommendations is needed. For certain types of stroke, the incidence and likelihood is substantially higher, and in groups of people with stroke referred for inpatient rehabilitation, incidence figures double or triple in some studies. A VFSS has been used in these studies to help determine both the presence of aspiration and the likelihood of recovery, with either full oral feeding or normalized diet.[29]

Other conditions and categories of disability also are strongly associated with dysphagia, including pediatric conditions such as cerebral palsy and spina bifida with hydrocephalus and symptomatic Arnold-Chiari malformation and conditions in persons of all ages with neuromuscular disorders. The interaction of respiratory insufficiency and provision of respiratory supports with oral feeding is an increasingly common issue for patients with neuromuscular disorders. Studies continue to indicate that VFSS has a high sensitivity for dysphagia and for aspiration and should still be favored over endoscopic methods when the patient can tolerate transport to the fluoroscopy suite and be well positioned. One study of patients with motor neuron disease found that:

> Videofluoroscopy was the most sensitive technique in identifying oropharyngeal alterations of swallowing. Impairment of the oral phase, abnormal pharyngoesophageal motility, and incomplete relaxation of the

upper esophageal sphincter were the changes most sensitive in detecting dysphagia. Videofluoroscopy was also capable of detecting preclinical abnormalities in non-dysphagic patients who later developed dysphagia.[6]

Another study, with a variety of diagnoses involved, found that "impaired pharyngeal propulsion" was detectable nearly 90% of the time and aspiration was detectable 70% of the time compared to VFSS, with sensitivity increased further by correlation with manometry.[34] In this study's institution, the cost profile was also apparently much more favorable for endoscopy, and the advantage of using normal rather than barium-laced foods was cited.[34] Bach notes that fiber-optic evaluation can also assess airway opening and closing, closing in early swallowing, general vocal cord mobility, direct injury or infection of pharyngeal or laryngeal structures, and pooling of food or secretions; using methylene blue or blue food coloring can render the study more sensitive to aspiration.[4] Structural abnormalities such as small clefts will be more visible to direct methods as well, particularly in children with congenital anomalies. Nevertheless, the VFSS is still important to assess the phases of swallowing.[12]

Integration of information about the swallow itself with information about nutritional status and the functioning of the rest of the gastrointestinal (GI) tract, including attention to gastroesophageal reflux, cricopharyngeal spasm, and peptic ulcer disease, is the function of the physician leading the rehabilitation team. This team, as always, must include the physician(s), the patient and family, and the swallowing therapist(s), radiologist, and nutritionist. The most common medical specialists involved include neurologists, otolaryngologists, gastroenterologists, oncologists, pulmonologists, and physiatrists. Speech therapists and occupational therapists may serve as primary dysphagia therapists or may address different aspects of swallowing and functional eating activities. Physical therapists are sometimes involved directly but more commonly will aid in positioning for both studies and ongoing feeding activities. Patients and families today are often aware of the ramifications of swallowing problems and various management options. They are highly likely to have encountered partial information from the Internet or other health resources, sometimes finding very balanced views and a variety of perspectives but sometimes forming strong opinions and predeterminations about what will constitute acceptable management and quality of life for them or their loved ones. Including the patient and family in

decision making and education and showing respect for their concerns and desires remain paramount. However, parents often fail to perceive the severity of chronic malnutrition. Sometimes parents report being counseled to avoid excess weight gain even for a small, thin child or that weight maintenance was a satisfactory goal only during the growing years; this is usually done to spare parents difficulty in passive transfers and lifting.[8] Health benefits may not be apparent until after an intervention based on swallowing assessment has been performed. Up to 80% of children with some congenital conditions may aspirate silently, manifesting only as poor nutrition and apparent susceptibility to respiratory infection and general fatigue or decreased energy.[8] Not uncommonly, young children and even adolescents and young adults will have reported no eating difficulty but will present with evidence of serious nutritional or pulmonary problems, sometimes triggered by an illness, surgery, or minor injury leading to decompensation of a chronically precarious situation.

PHASES OF SWALLOWING

An understanding of the anatomy and physiology of swallowing is essential for all professionals involved in the evaluation and management of dysphagia (Fig. 7-1). Many excellent sources are available on this subject.[11,14,15,17,26,27] The swallowing phases include four phases:

1. The **oral preparatory phase** (Fig. 7-2): intake, mastication, and bolus formation.

2. The **oral or voluntary swallowing phase** (Fig. 7-3): control and movement of the bolus into a position to trigger the swallow.

3. The **pharyngeal or reflex swallowing phase** (Figs. 7-4 to 7-7): initiated normally with passage of the bolus at the faucial arch.

4. The **esophageal phase** (Fig. 7-8): passage of the bolus beyond the cricopharyngeus muscle.

The first phase is relatively, although not completely, accessible to evaluation through bedside examination. All phases except the esophageal phase may be influenced by therapeutic or compensatory swallowing techniques.

INDICATIONS FOR VIDEOFLUOROSCOPY

Indications for videofluoroscopy still include conditions that place patients at high risk for dysphagia as well as those with any complaints or signs referable to swallowing disorders such as decreased

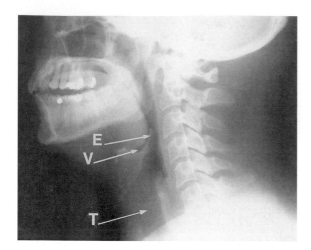

FIGURE 7-1. Lateral x-ray of the cervical spine demonstrating the epiglottis *(E)*, vallecula *(V)*, and trachea *(T)*.

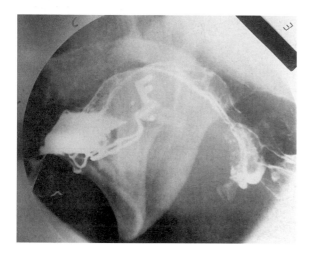

FIGURE 7-2. Bolus formation during the oral preparatory phase.

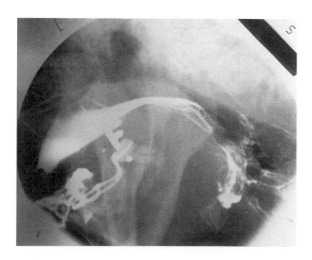

FIGURE 7-3. Advancement of the bolus from the oral swallowing phase.

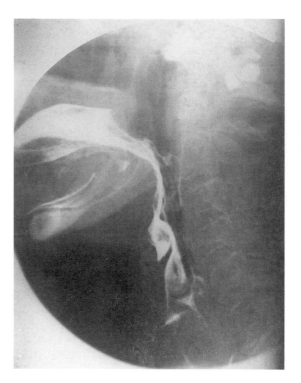

FIGURE 7-4. Movement of the bolus from the oral swallowing phase into the pharyngeal phase.

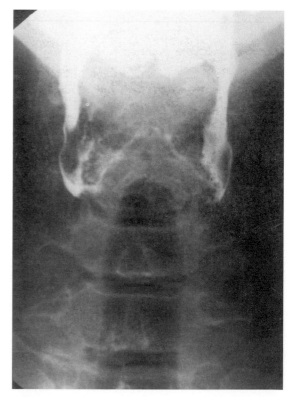

FIGURE 7-5. Posteroanterior radiograph demonstrating movement of the bolus from the oral swallowing phase into the pharyngeal phase.

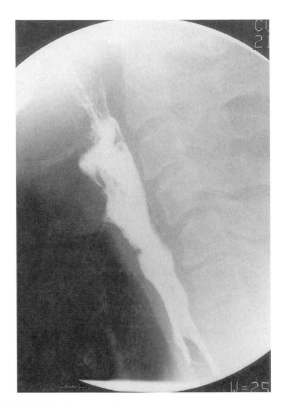

FIGURE 7-6. Lateral view demonstrating the pharyngeal phase of swallowing.

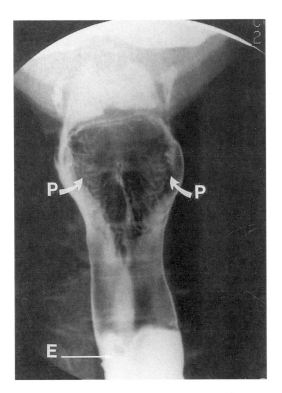

FIGURE 7-7. Posteroanterior radiograph demonstrating the pharyngeal phase of swallowing. Note the asymmetrical filling within the piriform sinuses *(P)* and esophagus *(E)*.

nutritional status (especially if they "eat like a horse" but still fail to gain or maintain weight and have no other symptoms of malabsorption), overt choking, coughing, tearing, gagging, oral hypersensitivity, explained or unexplained severity of respiratory problems, frequent infections, and reactive airway disease. The procedure may detect conditions that are not obvious at all during the best clinical or "bedside" evaluation (Fig. 7-9), because about 40% of patients at risk for dysphagia have silent aspiration, a percentage that has held up through many additional studies over the years. It appears that cervical auscultation may reduce but not eliminate the occurrence of clinically undetectable aspiration during swallowing.[41] Medical conditions known to be specifically associated with dysphagia are listed in Table 7-1. A more comprehensive list, along with a thorough review of diagnostic and therapeutic options for evaluation and management of dysphagia, is available from the American Gastroenterological Society on the World Wide Web at http://www.gastrojournal.org/cgi/content/full/116/2/455#T1.[2] The rationale for the detection of aspiration (though it is still not clear exactly how much aspiration is tolerable over what period of time) is the fairly consistent association with increased morbidity and

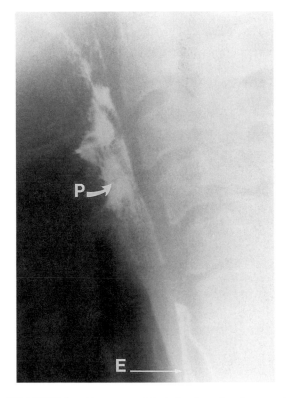

FIGURE 7-8. Movement of the bolus from the pharyngeal *(P)* phase into the esophageal *(E)* phase of swallowing.

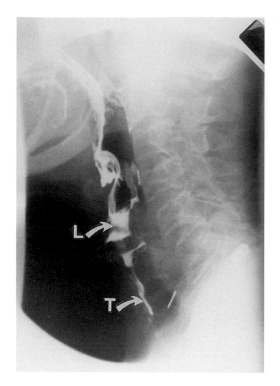

FIGURE 7-9. Lateral radiograph demonstrating laryngeal penetration *(L)* and tracheal aspiration *(T)*.

precise nature of oral phase problems, optimal food consistencies, positioning, and other compensatory techniques based on the details of oropharyngeal functioning. VFSS also is not the sole test for evaluating all causes of dysphagia; for example, it cannot determine the strength or pressure generation of pharyngeal contraction but can be coupled with manometry for that purpose. It may need to be followed by more distal barium studies or endoscopy to look for gastroesophageal causes of dysphagia, either functional or structural. Additionally, dysphagia is not the sole component of a comprehensive evaluation of feeding and nutritional status:

> Adequate nutrition and hydration can be compromised by altered consciousness, dysphagia, sensory or perceptual deficits, reduced mobility, or depression, which can cause decreased interest in eating. Poor hydration or metabolic imbalance, in turn, contributes to the development of infections, pressure sores, confusion, and poor physical endurance. Assessment includes monitoring intake, body weight, urinary and fecal outputs, caloric counts, levels of serum proteins, electrolytes, and blood counts.[1]

Given this background and information about its role, it is clear that VFSS is a major, but not exclusive, tool to be used in the context of comprehensive medical and rehabilitation team management for patients with feeding, swallowing, and nutrition issues. This chapter covers the performance and interpretation of this study and the specific techniques and protocols that have evolved and gradually become more standardized over time.

EVALUATION OF SWALLOWING

Three steps are necessary when evaluating swallowing function.

excess mortality attributable to chest infections, particularly for young people receiving tube feedings and for nursing home patients with stroke.[37] There are some controversies over aspiration detection, such as nonoral feeding itself being associated with higher mortality; however, these effects were not present in persons with tracheostomy or greater severity of disability, and the incidence of reflux possibly aggravated by tube placement without fundoplication was not accounted for in these studies.[40] Of course, VFSS is not useful solely for detecting aspiration; it also can determine the

TABLE 7-1. Medical Conditions Associated with Dysphagia

Central Nervous System–Static	Neuromuscular Disease
Cerebral palsy	Duchenne muscular dystrophy (late)[19]
Cerebrovascular accident	Myasthenia gravis
Traumatic brain injury	Myotonic dystrophy
Cervical spinal cord injury*	Polymyositis/dermatomyositis
Central Nervous System–Progressive	**Anatomic or Gastrointestinal**
Amyotrophic lateral sclerosis	Oral and oropharyngeal cancer†
CNS tumor	Laryngeal cancer†
Dysautonomia	Cleft palate
Dystonia	Tracheoesophageal fistula
Leukodystrophy	Esophageal stricture, tumor, web, or dysmotility
Multiple sclerosis	Cervical spondylosis
Parkinson's disease	Cricopharyngeal spasm
Other degenerative CNS disorders	Gastroesophageal reflux or ulcer disease

* May be mechanical, as for cervical spondylosis.
† May be related to either surgical therapy or radiotherapy.

1. **Preevaluation.** Usually a swallowing therapist performs a preevaluation that includes a medical history with emphasis on oropharyngeal function. The development of a hypothesis about the patient's swallowing disorder and its realistic management options, rationale, and any modification to the routine study are developed.[27,35,36,43] If indications for a study appear valid, a plan for the swallowing videofluoroscopy (SVF) can be made. There may be occasions when it is not appropriate or necessary to proceed. For example, the patient may not be in optimal medical condition or cannot be properly positioned to participate in the study.

2. **Swallowing study.** It is important to maintain a structured and sequenced videofluoroscopy procedure that can be kept standardized when needed, especially for research purposes, or allow flexibility for specific individual needs.

3. **Team decision making.** A philosophy and procedure for team notification and decision making on the basis of videofluoroscopic results should be outlined, including indications for planning follow-up studies.

PROTOCOLS

Most investigators agree that SVF should follow a protocol using specific consistencies and bolus sizes. For adults, liquid bolus sizes range from one third of a teaspoon (Logemann) to one half teaspoon (Robbins) and up to 30 ml (6 teaspoons) described by Rosenbeck.[31] Logemann's protocols use thin and thick liquids, paste, and solid. Robbins uses only liquid of thin-water consistency, semisolid, and solid, with three swallows. Foods that require chewing usually are not given unless indicated from the results of an oral motor evaluation and medical history. Less than one quarter of a Lorna Doone cookie coated with barium paste is sufficient and will tend to soften and crumble into a paste if held in the oropharynx rather than swallowed. Amounts and types of food selected can be advanced judiciously on subsequent trials during the study.

The rationale for the variety of consistencies is their different characteristics and risks with different types of swallowing pathophysiology. Liquids require little mastication and will pass easily through partially obstructed areas. However, they are more difficult to control and usually present greater anterior bolus loss with poor oral control and greater aspiration risks with impaired neurologic control of the pharyngeal phase. Semisolids or solids may be better controlled but are more likely to stagnate proximal to an anatomic obstruction or in pharyngeal recesses and to obstruct the airway if aspirated.

EQUIPMENT

Equipment required for videofluoroscopy includes 3- or 5-ml syringes, which are used to deliver the measured first bolus to the anterior or anterolateral oral cavity; injections into the posterior oropharynx are contraindicated. Also necessary are containers and utensils for mixing foods with barium to achieve desired consistencies; normal, "sippee," and cutaway cups; baby bottles with enlarged nipple holes or a device to make small crosscut incisions to enlarge holes as needed for thicker liquids; and some normal and rubber-tipped feeding spoons. Plastic spoons are contraindicated for patients who may exhibit a tonic bite reflex. Patients who can feed themselves may be encouraged to do so and should bring their own familiar or adaptive eating utensils if possible.

Food consistencies can be simulated with barium in many ways. The usual liquid barium is slightly thicker than most thin liquids but can be diluted with one or two parts of water, formula, clear juice, or Kool-Aid. It can be thickened with ice cream, rice cereal, or puree, such as baby food. Cold foods such as ice cream may help to stimulate the swallow reflex. Barium powder can be added to pureed foods or ice cream. Barium "cream" or paste can be mixed with less than an equal part liquid for a paste or semisolid consistency. Solids can be coated with or soaked in barium. Lorna Doone cookies are a traditional choice, but foods of the patient's choice may be used as long as they do not pose a major choking hazard. For instance, avoid popcorn or uncut hot dogs in children younger than 4 years. A small wire whip or electric mixer is helpful when preparing for the study. Newer, flavored types of barium products are not as chalky or ill-tasting as the older ones that many adults recall, and individual tolerance for these unusual preparations of foodstuffs may vary. Vanilla barium paste with chocolate ice cream seems palatable to most adults.

TECHNIQUE

The following are sample protocols for SVF in adults and children.

Test materials: thin liquid, thick liquid, paste, solid.

1. The patient is positioned to allow visualization of the oropharynx from a lateral approach under fluoroscopy.

2. The patient's swallow is observed with the following:

- one teaspoon of thin liquid barium
- one teaspoon of thick liquid barium
- one teaspoon of applesauce with barium paste

3. The feeder holds one corner of a cookie coated with barium paste and tells the patient to "bite the corner of this cookie and chew as you normally would until you feel you are ready to swallow."

4. Optional procedures such as the administration of 10- and 33-ml boluses of thin and thick liquid by cup and/or straw are undertaken if more information is desired.

5. Positions may be changed to allow an anteroposterior view. This view is used to assess symmetry of pharyngeal structures during the swallow and to evaluate function of the vocal cords.

6. If the anteroposterior view is used:

- The patient is instructed to tilt the head back or hold the chin up slightly. This position brings the mandible and other structures away from the pharynx and larynx for better visualization.
- The patient is told to say "ah" and prolong it at least twice.
- The patient is given one teaspoon of thick liquid barium.

7. If the patient is unable to protect the airway, additional positioning may be attempted or food consistencies changed, or the study may be terminated, especially if most of a bolus is aspirated. Criteria for terminating a study include the following:

- failure to initiate a swallow
- absence of a cough in response to significant (not just trace) aspiration
- significant amounts of material fill the pharyngeal space and do not pass into the esophagus with multiple dry swallows

Information obtained and conveyed to the treatment team should include the following:

1. Site of difficulty, either oral, pharyngeal, or both.

2. Aspiration, either nasopharyngeal, laryngeal, or both. For laryngeal aspiration, include timing (before, during, or after the swallow) and cause and/or source, i.e., during the swallow due to reduced laryngeal closure, or after the swallow due to reduced pharyngeal peristalsis, reduced laryngeal closure, or material moving back into the pharynx from a Zenker diverticulum.

3. Recommendations and documentation of counseling given to the patient and family.

Ideally, after the study, the whole team should come to a consensus and develop a single report.[18,33]

In practice, there may be separate reports from just the swallowing therapist and radiologist.

A careful history should be obtained regarding the administration of liquid medications, especially by syringe. A swallowing study with a barium tablet can clarify whether esophageal spasm or functional stricture creates a risk for localized medication-induced esophagitis.[33] Sedatives such as muscle relaxants and anticonvulsants also may have direct or indirect effects on swallowing coordination beyond simple central nervous system depression. Anticholinergic drugs such as antidepressants and bladder medications may impair esophageal motility. Optimizing treatment of Parkinson's disease or myasthenia gravis can improve swallowing if it improves other aspects of motor function and fatigue.

Based on the complete assessment of swallowing, various passive and active compensatory techniques are available to the swallowing therapist, and the reader is referred to existing texts and manuals for further details on their techniques and indications.[17,26–28,33] Passive techniques include positioning; methods of presentation such as straw, spoon, or a special cup designed to slow the rate of intake; consistencies chosen for ongoing use; supervision or assistance to control the rate or mode of intake; and thermal stimulation to facilitate the swallowing reflex. Active strategies include repeated swallows, swallow with effort, supraglottic swallow, and the Mendelsohn maneuver. The latter requires adequate cognition and cooperation by the patient. Oral exercises and swallowing training may improve performance or compensate effectively in the long term.[9,21,30]

Repeat studies are based on the rate of improvement or disease progression. Patients receiving active therapy may wait until the therapist notes some change in oral motor or swallowing function. For example, when a patient at risk for aspirating thin liquids before the swallow regains better oral control and no longer grossly exhibits a delayed swallow, reevaluation may be scheduled. The repeat study may be much more limited and targeted to a specific question in many cases.

POSITIONING DURING VIDEOFLUOROSCOPY

With compensatory techniques, SVF should allow for several swallows of each food consistency in various feeding positions. It is important to test positions that are likely to be used by family members and not just the upright position. Feeders often compensate for a poor oral phase by having a patient recline. Neurodevelopmental therapists often advocate a side-lying position for tone reduction. The upright position with slight cervical flexion is ideal for reducing the risk of aspiration in neurogenic dysphagia. Alternative head positions also need to be evaluated. Some cases in which side lying was preferred because it led to less coughing proved to be associated with an increase in the amount of aspiration when studied radiographically. Aspiration became "more silent" as the child became more relaxed. Circumstances in which supine feeding positions are preferred have been described in other studies.[16,31]

Having proper equipment in the radiology suite may help to achieve optimal positioning for swallowing studies. For children and adults, there are specialized chairs for positioning.[10] It may be possible to use a child's car seat on the platform of an x-ray table in some cases. Often, positioning will have to be improvised, making use of whatever chairs, bolsters, wedges, and straps that are available. A high back or headrest is helpful for a person with limited head and trunk control. Patients who are able to stand for the study may do so if it is convenient. Complete immobilization is neither necessary nor desirable for a successful study and is to be avoided.

CONTRAINDICATIONS

Low level of consciousness, poor cooperation, or inability to follow commands are absolute contraindications to SVF. Infants can be successfully studied as well as some individuals at Rancho Los Amigos level III or a higher level of neurologic recovery from coma. The ability to perform voluntary rather than solely passive compensatory maneuvers is limited in these patients.

COMPLICATIONS

Videofluoroscopy is considered a low-risk procedure. Risk of aspiration during the procedure can be minimized by two factors: (1) the amount of food used for an initial trial of any consistency is kept small and (2) suction and oxygen equipment should be available. One milliliter of fluid allows adequate visualization of a swallow, especially in a child. Two milliliters is necessary for semisolids. Few individuals have a combination of disordered swallowing physiology, total inability to compensate, and

severe medical risks that preclude using even tiny amounts of some consistency of foodstuff orally.

Radiation exposure to the patient and medical personnel should be monitored. Five minutes of fluoroscopy time is routine and should be achievable by an experienced team.

CONSIDERATIONS IN CHILDREN

There are differences in swallowing physiology and anatomy in children that should be appreciated. It is essential that foods be presented in a developmentally appropriate manner. An infant's tongue is relatively large compared to the total oral cavity, and the hyoid and laryngeal structures are relatively high. Suckle feeding is the normal pattern for infants and is normally gradually superseded by voluntary chewing and swallow initiation beginning in the second half of the first year and becoming completely adult in pattern by age 3 or 4 years. The anatomy of infants favors the suckle pattern, and, if neurologic maturation does not occur in children and suckling persists, increasing difficulties may occur as the anatomy changes even if neurologic status is not deteriorating. The distinctive features of suckling on videofluoroscopy include repeated stripping action of the tongue before each swallow, which may lead to some vallecular pooling as a normal finding; more frequent swallows; more filling of the esophagus before clearing; and the critical importance of the suck-swallow-breathe coordination cycle. It is essential to assess the effects of fatigue and especially to pay attention to the last swallow before respiration in each cycle since this is where breakdown of coordination and resultant aspiration is most likely to occur.[22,23]

REFERRAL FOR SURGERY

Surgery is usually indicated any time there are recommendations for alternative feeding methods because chronic nasogastric or orogastric tubes have high rates of local tissue trauma and reflux-related complications. Logemann's stated limit for nonsurgical tube feedings is 3 months, with exceptions for a patient who can learn to perform or tolerate repeated placement and removal of the tube between meals.[27]

If the swallowing study suggests the individual can tolerate at least small amounts of thickened liquids, total oral nutrition may be possible if eating is functionally a reasonable activity. Adequate intake of calories, protein, and fluid is usually difficult on semisolids alone. The time and effort necessary for eating also must be considered for individual patients. Recommendations based only on SVF occasionally reduce the time and effort involved at mealtime and usually do not increase or decrease it significantly.[16,31] A nutritionist can help to select palatable foods of the desired consistencies with higher caloric density as needed. Foods can be thickened with a commercial product such as Dia-Foods "Thick-It" or by using naturally thicker foods such as nectars instead of juices or thick milk shakes. Recipe manuals for modified diets are available.[7]

If the SVF is unrevealing, additional studies may be recommended to search for the cause of persistent symptoms. As noted earlier, gastroesophageal reflux may cause respiratory symptoms in the absence of any swallowing disorder. Gastric, duodenal, or esophageal disease may cause painful swallowing. If alternate feeding methods are to be considered, testing should be performed to assess for gastroesophageal reflux, especially in children, for whom an antireflux procedure is frequently indicated at the time of gastrostomy surgery. Some authors report an association of cricopharyngeal dysfunction with reflux. Radionuclide scanning, esophageal pH probe, or endoscopy may be considered for further evaluation. Computed tomography or magnetic resonance imaging may be necessary to delineate anatomic structures in greater detail than can be appreciated on any dynamic or functional study. Such techniques are essential in diagnosis and management of preoperative or postoperative cases of head and neck cancer.[20,35]

ALTERNATIVE STUDIES

Other methods of assessing the swallow have been used in attempts to be more physiologic and reduce radiation exposure. Cervical auscultation, ultrasound, and endoscopy are the most widely reported. Auscultation may, in selected patients, permit follow-up of timing of velopharyngeal closure or triggering of the swallow. It also may provide clues to the occurrence of aspiration if specific sounds can be identified and correlated with swallowing events for the individual.[38] However, gurgling or "wet hoarse" sounds can result from retained pharyngeal or nasopharyngeal material and do not always indicate laryngeal penetration.[25] Ultrasound evaluation has the advantage of being portable to the bedside and, like auscultation, is noninvasive and requires no radiation. The transducer is placed under the chin and may cover a field

from tongue tip to epiglottis in a sagittal plane. Larger adults may need to be repositioned slightly. A coronal plane image can capture vocal fold and cord movement. It can definitely supplement bedside evaluation of the oral phase. However, it is limited in delineating the amount and timing of aspiration.[39] Endoscopy, usually with a flexible endoscope inserted from above the nasopharynx, also can provide information without radiation exposure but requires specialized equipment and expertise in operation. Its chief limitation is that, when upper pharyngeal constriction is not severely impaired, the remainder of the swallow is obscured from view. For example, vocal cord movement during breathing or phonation may be seen, but closure during a swallow and the presence of aspiration during or immediately after a swallow generally will not be directly visible.

CONCLUSION

Involvement of the clinician in SVF may be of great benefit to individual patients, the rehabilitation team, or the dysphagia program. SVF, when performed well, provides an excellent opportunity to obtain detailed information about swallowing function. Thorough study and understanding of swallowing physiology techniques involved in SVF are essential for the clinician to make an optimal contribution to the evaluation and rehabilitation of this most essential human function.

REFERENCES

1. Agency for Health Care Policy and Research: Post-Stroke Rehabilitation. Clinical Guideline Number 16. Washington, DC, AHCPR, 1995, AHCPR publication no. 95-0062.
2. American Gastroenterological Association Clinical Practice and Practice Economics Committee: AGA technical review on management of oropharyngeal dysphagia. Gastroenterology 116:455-478, 1999.
3. American Speech-Language-Hearing Association Special Interest Division 13: Swallowing and Swallowing Disorders: Clinical Indicators for Instrumental Assessment of Dysphagia. Rockville, MD, ASHA, 1998.
4. Bach JR: Guide to the Evaluation and Management of Neuromuscular Disease. Philadelphia, Hanley & Belfus, 1999.
5. Beck TJ, Gayler BW: Radiation in video-recorded fluoroscopy. In Jones B, Donner MW (eds): Normal and Abnormal Swallowing: Imaging in Diagnosis and Therapy. New York, Springer-Verlag, 1991.
6. Briani C, Marcon M, Ermani M, et al: Radiological evidence of subclinical dysphagia in motor neuron disease. J Neurol 245:211-216, 1998.
7. Campalans NM, VanBiervliet A: Educational materials for the dysphagia diet: Development and evaluation. J Am Diet Assoc 92(Suppl):A110, 1992.
8. Campbell A: Tube feeding: Parental perspective. Exceptional Parent 36–40, April 1988.

9. Christiansen JR: Development approach to pediatric neurogenic dysphagia. Dysphagia 3:131–134, 1989.

10. Cox MS, Petty J: A videofluoroscopy chair for the evaluation of dysphagia in patients with severe neuromotor disease. Arch Phys Med Rehabil 72:157–159, 1991.

11. Cunningham ET, Donner MW, Point SM, et al: Anatomical and physiological overview. In Jones B, Donner MW (eds): Normal and Abnormal Swallowing: Imaging in Diagnosis and Therapy. New York, Springer-Verlag, 1991.

12. Darrow DH, Harley CM: Evaluation of swallowing disorders in children. Otolaryngol Clin North Am 31:405-418, 1998.

13. DeVito MA, Wetmore RF, Pransky SM: Laryngeal diversion in the treatment of chronic aspiration in children. Int J Pediatr Otorhinolaryngol 18:139–145, 1989.

14. Dodds WJ, Stewart ET, Logemann JA: Physiology and radiology of the normal oral and pharyngeal phases of swallowing. Am J Roentgen 154:953–963, 1990.

15. Donner MW, Bosma JF, Robertson DL: Anatomy and physiology of the pharynx. Gastrointest Radiol 10:196–212, 1985.

16. Griggs CA, Jones PM, Lee RE: Videofluoroscopic investigation of feeding disorders of children with multiple handicap. Dev Med Child Neurol 31:303–308, 1989.

17. Groeher M: Dysphagia Diagnosis and Management. Stoneham, MA, Butterworth, 1984.

18. Henson D, White L, Hedburg V: Report writing made easy: Combining radiologist and SLP's swallow study reports [poster]. Annual Meeting of the Arkansas Speech-Hearing-Language Association, October 1993.

19. Jaffe KM, McDonald CM, Haas J, et al: Symptoms of upper gastrointestinal dysfunction in Duchenne muscular dystrophy: Case-control study. Arch Phys Med Rehabil 71:742–744, 1990.

20. Jones B, Donner MW: The tailored examination. In Jones B, Donner MW (eds): Normal and Abnormal Swallowing: Imaging in Diagnosis and Therapy. New York, Springer-Verlag, 1991.

21. Kasprisin AT, Clumeck H, Nino-Murcia M: Efficacy of rehabilitative management of dysphagia. Dysphagia 4:48–52, 1989.

22. Kramer SS: Special swallowing problems in children. Gastrointest Radiol 10:241–250, 1985.

23. Kramer SS: Swallowing in children. In Jones B, Donner MW (eds): Normal and Abnormal Swallowing: Imaging in Diagnosis and Therapy. New York, Springer-Verlag, 1991.

24. Langmore SE, Logemann JA: After the bedside swallowing examination. What next? Am J Speech Lang Pathol 1:13–20, 1991.

25. Linden P, Siebens AA: Dysphagia: Predicting laryngeal penetration. Arch Phys Med Rehabil 64:281–284, 1983.

26. Logemann JA: Evaluation and Treatment of Swallowing Disorders. San Diego, College-Hill, 1983.

27. Logemann JA: Manual for the Videofluorographic Study of Swallowing. London, Taylor & Francis, 1986.

28. Logemann JA: Treatment for aspiration related to dysphagia: An overview. Dysphagia 1:34–38, 1986.

29. Mann G, Hankey GJ, Cameron D: Swallowing function after stroke: Prognosis and prognostic factors at 6 months. Stroke 30:744–748, 1999.

30. Morris SE: Development of oral-motor skills in the neurologically impaired child receiving non-oral feedings. Dysphagia 3:135–154, 1989.

31. Morton RE, Bonas R, Minford J, et al: Videofluoroscopy in the assessment of feeding disorders of children with neurological problems. Dev Med Child Neurol 35:388–395, 1993.

32. Muz J, Mazog RH, Borrero G, et al: Detection and quantification of laryngotracheopulmonary aspiration with scintigraphy. Laryngoscope 97:1180–1185, 1987.

33. Palmer JB, DuChane AS, Donner MW: Role of radiology in the rehabilitation of swallowing. In Jones B, Donner MW (eds): Normal and Abnormal Swallowing: Imaging in Diagnosis and Therapy. New York, Springer-Verlag, 1991.

34. Perie S, Laccourreye L, Flahault A, et al: Role of videoendoscopy in assessment of pharyngeal function in oropharyngeal dysphagia: Comparison with videofluoroscopy and manometry. Laryngoscope 108:1712–1716, 1998.

35. Point SW, Bryan RN, Cunningham ET: Integrated approach to cross-sectional imaging and dysphagia. In Jones B, Donner MW (eds): Normal and Abnormal Swallowing: Imaging in Diagnosis and Therapy. New York, Springer-Verlag, 1991.

36. Robbins J, Sufit R, Rosenbeck J, et al: A modification of the modified barium swallow. Dysphagia 2:83–86, 1987.

37. Smithard DG, O'Neill PA, Park C, et al: Complications and outcome after acute stroke: Does dysphagia matter? Stroke 27:1200–1204, 1996.

38. Smith D, Hamlet S, Jones L: Acoustic technique for determining timing of velopharyngeal closure in swallowing. Dysphagia 5:142–146, 1990.

39. Sonies BC: Ultrasound imaging and swallowing. In Jones B, Donner MW (eds): Normal and Abnormal Swallowing: Imaging in Diagnosis and Therapy. New York, Springer-Verlag, 1991.

40. Strauss D, Kastner T, Ashwal S, White J: Tubefeeding and mortality in children with severe disabilities and mental retardation. Pediatrics 99:358-362, 1997.

41. Zenner PM, Losinski DS, Mills RH: Using cervical auscultation in the clinical dysphagia examination in long-term care. Dysphagia 10:27-31, 1995.

42. Zerilli KS, Stefans VA: Pediatric swallowing videofluoroscopy one year follow-up [abstract]. Dev Med Child Neurol 31(Suppl 5), 1989.

43. Zerilli KS, Stefans VA, DiPietro MA: Protocol for the use of videofluoroscopy in pediatric swallowing dysfunction. Am J Occup Ther 44:441–446, 1990.

8

Urologic Diagnostic Testing

Inder Perkash, M.D.

Neurologic lesions of the brain, spinal cord, or peripheral nerves invariably lead to voiding dysfunctions. Often there is either partial or complete retention of urine or some degree of incontinence. Intracranial lesions such as head injury, cerebrovascular accident, Alzheimer's disease, and brain tumors can lead to hyperreflexic bladder that causes patients to void frequently with smaller volumes of urine. However, in the early phase after the injury or cerebrovascular accident, urine may even be retained.[12] In the rehabilitation of such patients, it is therefore important to evaluate voiding dysfunction so that a management plan can be developed for long-term care.

ANATOMY

The micturition reflex center in the brain has been localized in the pontine mesencephalic reticular formation in the brain stem[2,5] with interconnection to and from the frontal lobe and cortical and other subcortical areas. Efferent axons from the pontine micturition center travel down the spinal cord in the reticulospinal tract to the detrusor motor nuclei located in the sacral 2, 3, and 4 segments in the sacral gray matter. The reticulospinal tracts are in close proximity to the pyramidal tracts in the lateral column of the spinal cord. Sacral 3 and 4 nuclei have major innervation to and from the detrusor muscle through the pelvic parasympathetic nerves. The sacral 2 spinal segment has a major contribution to the external urethral sphincter through pudendal nerves, which arise from S2, S3, and S4 motor nuclei in the sacral cord (conus) as well. The external urethral sphincter surrounds the membranous urethra and also extends up and around the lower part of the prostatic urethra. Thus, there are two sphincters, one at the bladder neck, which is involuntary, and one around the prostatic and membranous urethra, which is essentially voluntary (external striated sphincter).

Lesions

Lesions below the pons produce detrusor sphincter dyssynergia; however intracranial lesions above the pons usually produce detrusor hyperreflexia wherein the bladder empties at a lower volume (a low-threshold detrusor reflex). It has been well established that spinal cord disconnection from the brain with lesions involving pyramidal tracts will lead to loss of voluntary relaxation of the striated urethral sphincter that surrounds the lower part of the prostatic urethra.

In transection of spinal cord (lesions below the pons with detrusor sphincter dyssynergia), urine is usually retained because bladder contraction leads to simultaneous contraction of the external urethral sphincter. Tetraplegics and paraplegics with lesions above T5 also exhibit autonomic dysreflexia, which is associated with detrusor sphincter dyssynergia.[1,7] Voiding is therefore incomplete and often associated with detrusor hyperreflexia and high intravesical pressure. It is known that high, sustained intravesical pressure (more than 40–50 cm of water) can lead to vesicoureteral reflux.[6] The presence of vesicoureteral reflux in patients with spinal cord injury (SCI) is risky because the higher incidence of bladder infection in these patients invariably leads to pyelonephritis and renal stone disease.

The neurogenic bladder resulting from spinal cord lesions (e.g., injury, inflammation) may not empty adequately due to two key factors: lack of adequate voluntary control to contract the bladder and lack of voluntary control to relax the external urethral sphincter. Any attempted voiding is associated with detrusor sphincter dyssynergia. Often, the detrusor muscle is also weak due to either nerve root lesions or overdistention of the bladder.

URODYNAMIC EVALUATION

Urodynamic studies play a vital role in the examination of suspected neurologically impaired patients with known or suspected neuromuscular dysfunction of the bladder. This may be associated with a known definable or unknown neurologic lesion. The urodynamic evaluation is multipurpose: (1) to determine if the neurogenic dysfunction exists, (2) to recognize and define urodynamic abnormalities such as detrusor hyperreflexia, areflexia, and detrusor sphincter dyssynergia (DESD), (3) to determine the maximum voiding pressure, (4) to determine the appropriate therapy based on the patient's disability and motivation for therapy, and (5) to titrate and evaluate drug therapy to improve voiding.

URODYNAMIC TECHNIQUES

Cystometric Examination

Cystometrogram (CMG) involves filling the bladder with air or water at body temperature. It also may be carried out with radiographic contrast in the bladder for both voiding cystogram and cystometrogram or combined cinefluoroscopic studies. Similar studies also may be performed under ultrasonic control to provide visualization of the dynamic contraction of the bladder while intravesical pressures are being recorded through a small catheter connected to a strain gauge or a simple manometer.

For cystometric studies, a French size 7 or 10 triple-lumen catheter (Fig. 8-1) is used to fill the bladder and simultaneously record the pressure. Before filling the bladder, the clinician instructs the patient to relax and tell when he or she has a "feeling" of filling and when he or she has the desire to void. The patient is then instructed to void. A paraplegic or quadriplegic patient cannot stand and void; ambulatory patients are asked to stand and void so that voiding pressures can be determined. In normal persons, the first sensation of fullness is usually perceived when the bladder is filled with 100 ml of fluid; there is a desire to void when the bladder is filled with about 300–400 ml of fluid. During filling of the bladder, the intravesical pressure is usually around 20 cm water; however, if the bladder is fibrosed this pressure may rise steeply and the bladder is then considered noncompliant. Maximum voiding pressures on attempted voiding are noted. Postvoid residuals are checked before and after cystometric examination. In patients with neurogenic bladder dysfunction, about 100 ml of postvoid residual is considered acceptable. Cystometric study thus is used to assess bladder sensation, compliance, and maximum voiding pressures.

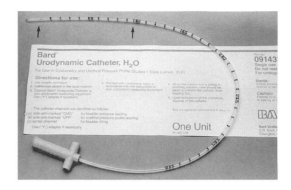

FIGURE 8-1. A triple-lumen catheter (Bard). The arrows indicate two holes, one near the tip for sensing bladder pressure and the other 10 cm from the tip for sensing urethral pressure.

The International Continence Society has classified the detrusor as either normal, hyperreflexic, or hyporeflexic based on the CMG. The hyperactive disorder is characterized by involuntary detrusor contractions that may be spontaneous or provoked by rapid filling. When involuntary detrusor contractions are due to neurologic disorders, the condition is called detrusor hyperreflexia. In the absence of a demonstrable neurologic etiology, involuntary detrusor contractions are defined as detrusor instability. The absence of a detrusor contraction, particularly in females, during CMG is not considered to be abnormal unless there are other clinical or urodynamic findings to substantiate the presence of lower motor neuron disease. In patients with spinal cord injury, suprapubic tapping can initiate voiding. It also is important to record blood pressure during the bladder filling, particularly in tetraplegic patients, to find out if patients are prone to autonomic dysreflexia.

An example of a multiple-channel urodynamic study is shown in Figure 8-2. The CMG shows a rise of 50 cm of water in intravesical pressure with the bladder filled to 300 ml. This is a true detrusor pressure because there is very little change in the rectal pressure. Tracings 6 and 1 show a simultaneous reduction in EMG activity with the rise in intravesical pressure (CMG), indicating the lack of detrusor-sphincter dyssynergia. If seen in normal persons, the sustained rise in the intravesical pressure (tracing 1) would indicate outflow obstruction, either at the bladder neck due to nonrelaxation of the internal urethral sphincter or due to an enlarged prostate. The absence of detrusor sphincter dyssynergia in the patients with spinal cord injury who are taking high-dose baclofen (such as the patient in Figure 8-2) has been observed. Sustained rise in intravesical pressure

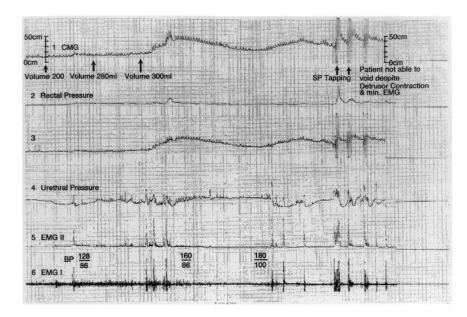

FIGURE 8-2. A multichannel urodynamic study in a tetraplegic patient. It shows simultaneous cystometrogram (CMG) (*top tracing*), rectal pressure (*second tracing*), subtracted pressure (CMG minus rectal pressure) indicating true detrusor pressure (*third tracing*), and urethral pressure (*fourth tracing*). EMG I is a true EMG with motor units, and EMG II is an integrated EMG activity of the external urethral sphincter. The CMG (*top tracing*) shows sustained bladder contraction with minimal EMG activity (*sixth tracing*). Even after suprabubic tapping, a minimal increase in EMG activity of the external urethral sphincter is noticed. Reduced EMG activity is explained on the basis of a high-dose baclofen taken by the spinal cord–injured patient during the study. A rise in blood pressure from 120/86 to 180/100 during bladder filling is indicative of autonomic dysreflexia, which is most often associated with detrusor sphincter dyssynergia. (From Perkash I: Long-term urologic management with spinal cord injury. Urol Clin North Am 20:423, 1993, with permission.)

over 40 cm of water can lead to vesicoureteral reflux.[6] Such patients on intermittent catheterization therefore need anticholinergic drugs to reduce bladder pressure. Another example of a multichannel study (Fig. 8-3) shows in the top tracing (CMG) pressures of 70–80 cm water and a sustained rise in intravesical pressure associated with marked increase in EMG activity of external urethral sphincter, indicating detrusor sphincter dyssynergia.

Uroflow (Act of Micturition)

In the able-bodied, the measurement of urinary flow rate is most frequently used as a screening procedure for the diagnosis of bladder outlet obstruction. However, it is not used in patients with spinal cord injury and other neurologic disorders because it is often difficult to evoke a flow rate.

Suprapubic tapping over the bladder region 15–20 times often leads to micturition in patients with spinal cord injury. It is usually intermittent, which does not give an easily measured flow rate. Intermittent flow rate, however, is indicative of the existence of detrusor sphincter dyssynergia, since the dyssynergic urethral sphincter relaxes intermittently. Therefore, patients with spinal cord injury can be

evaluated at the bedside: the bladder is first palpated and then suprapubicly tapped to empty it. If, following this procedure, the bladder empties easily with a good stream and without the patient becoming dysreflexic, and no significant rise in blood pressure occurs, chances are that the patient is voiding satisfactorily.

Bladder outlet obstruction due to a bladder neck ledge,[9] enlarged prostate, or detrusor sphincter dyssynergia is associated with a diminished uroflow, but usually with a sustained detrusor contraction and high intravesical pressure (see Figs. 8-2 and 8-3). On the other hand, impaired detrusor contractility is characterized by a diminished flow rate and a low pressure detrusor contraction that is poorly sustained. Even a normal uroflow may not always exclude bladder outlet or sphincteric obstruction in incomplete spinal cord lesions. Therefore, uroflow is not of great clinical value as a single examination.

Electromyography of the External Urethral Sphincter

Simultaneous cystometrographic study and electromyography (EMG) of the external urethral sphincter is important to diagnose detrusor external sphincter dyssynergia. A triple-lumen catheter is

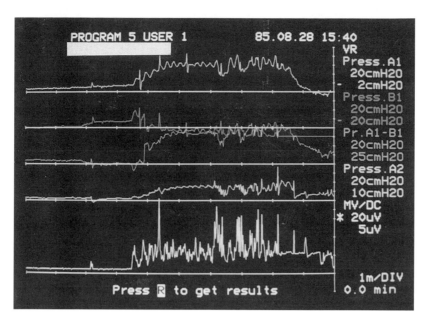

FIGURE 8-3. A simultaneous CMG demonstrating a sustained rise in intravesical pressure (*top tracing*) and increased EMG activity of the external urethral sphincter indicating detrusor sphincter dyssynergia.

used for filling the bladder and for recording intravesical and intraurethral pressures. Disposable concentric needles (Medtronic, Shoreview, MN) with a diameter of 0.46 mm (or 23 gauge) are inserted about 1.5 cm anterior to the anal verge and aimed at the tip of the prostate and guided with the finger in the rectum. Surface electrodes can be used for the EMG in patients who have intact sensation in the perineum. The bladder is filled with air or water for cystometric studies. Intra-abdominal pressures are recorded with a rectal balloon, and EMG activity of the external urethral sphincter is monitored simultaneously. In the relaxed state, the normal external sphincter is generally electrically silent with only infrequent low-amplitude motor units (fewer than 200 µV). With progressive bladder filling, there usually is an increase in external urethral sphincter EMG activity and bladder contraction that reaches a maximum just prior to voiding. An increase in EMG activity usually accompanies cough, straining, or movement. The beginning of a voluntary detrusor contraction is marked by relaxation of the external urethral sphincter in a normal person. When this happens, the sphincter EMG becomes electrically silent and the maximum urethral pressure drops dramatically (Fig. 8-4). Sphincter relaxation persists through the

FIGURE 8-4. The study shows CMG, rectal pressures, and EMG of the external urethral sphincter in a patient with incomplete spinal cord lesion. This patient had a desire to void at 220 ml (normal around 100 ml). He was able to hold his urine by contracting his external urethral sphincter and was able to relax his sphincter (shown by reduced EMG activity of the external urethral sphincter).

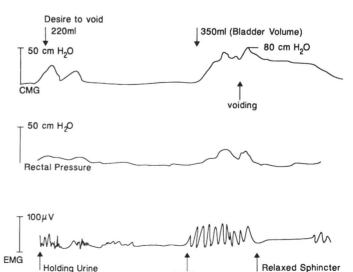

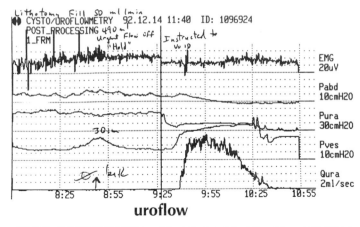

uroflow

CYSTO/UROFLOWMETRY   92.12.14 11:42   ID: 1096924
POST_PROCESSING

Results of UROFLOWMETRY

Delay Time	0:12 min:sec
Voiding Time	0:55 min:sec
Flow Time	0:55 min:sec
Time to Max Flow	0:16 min:sec
Max Flow Rate	14.9 ml/sec
Average Flow Rate	8.0 ml/sec
Voided Volume	486 ml
Residual Volume	2 ml
Pdet at Max Flow	40 cmH2O

FIGURE 8-5. Multichannel studies and computer-generated results in a patient with urge incontinence. CMG (Pves) shows uninhibited contraction during the filling phase when the patient leaked urine as shown by the small arrow at point 8:55. This action indicates an unstable bladder.

detrusor contraction, and, at the end of voiding, electromyographic activity resumes.

Cysto-uroflowmetry

Multichannel studies use a triple-lumen catheter in the bladder and a rectal catheter to determine rectal pressure, which also indicates abdominal pressure. The bladder is filled with water through one channel. The second channel records pressure through transducers, and the third channel (with a side hole) records urethral pressure. Pressure flow studies can provide bladder pressures (Pves) and corresponding urine flow rates (Qura). True detrusor (Pdet) can be determined by subtracting rectal pressure (Pabd) from bladder pressure (Pves).

An illustrated study is shown in Figure 8-5 in a woman whose bladder was filled to 490 ml and who had an urgent desire to void and also an uninhibited bladder contraction with intravesical pressure rising to 30 cm of water. When instructed to void, she had a sharp bladder contraction with intravesical pressure (Pdet) rising 40–50 cm of water (illustration) with continued, reduced EMG activity of the external

urethral sphincter. This was accompanied by significant voiding and urine flow rate as shown in the lowest tracing (Qura). The results of uroflowmetry are shown in Figure 8-5. The patient voided 486 ml with a residual of 2 ml. Because she had shown uninhibited detrusor contraction during the filling phase, she was given a small dose of anticholinergic to control her uninhibited contraction and leakage of urine.

Urethral Pressure Profilometry

The urethral pressure profile (UPP) represents the lateral closure pressure along the length of the urethra. It usually is studied with a multichannel catheter. Profilometry, with a pull-through technique, provides graphic representation of the lateral pressure along the length of the urethra (Fig. 8-6). Currently, the practiced technique has been adapted from Brown and Wickham.[3] The functional length of the urethra can be measured. These studies are done with an empty bladder. If the bladder contraction occurs other than "Pura-dif," it is calculated by subtracting bladder pressure (Pves) from Pura to

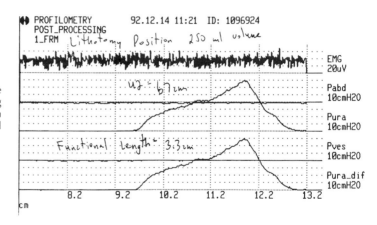

FIGURE 8-6. Urethral pressure profile of the same patient as in Figure 8-5. The upper tracing (Pura) and Pura-dif indicate a functional length of urethra being 3.3 cm, which is within normal limits.

give true urethral pressures (Fig. 8-6). For static UPP, one of the holes meant for sensing the pressure is positioned in the middle of the posterior urethra. A triple-lumen catheter, commonly used for such studies, is shown in Figure 8-1. It has a terminal hole 1 cm from the tip for filling the bladder and another side hole at 10 cm to sense the urethral pressure. Other sophisticated techniques using a microtransducer mounted at the tip of the urethral catheter have been used over the more simple and less expensive perfusion catheter systems. These microtransducer catheters are expensive, fragile, and difficult to insert in the male urethra. They also are prone to distortional errors due to the curvature and length of the transducer catheter. While the bladder is gradually filled for CMG, both intravesical and urethral pressures can be simultaneously recorded. In patients with neurologic lesions of the spinal cord, when the bladder contracts, the rise in urethral pressure along with increased EMG activity of the external urethral sphincter is indicative of detrusor sphincter dyssynergia.

Micturitional Urethral Pressure Profile

Profilometry can be combined with simultaneous voiding. The micturitional urethral pressure profile (MUPP) thus obtained is useful for defining not only the presence of a bladder outlet obstruction but the site of the obstruction as well. The examination is performed by slowly withdrawing the urethral port of the catheter through the urethra during micturition. Normally, the bladder and the entire proximal urethra are approximately isobaric during micturition. When an obstruction exists, there is an immediate drop in pressure distal to the point of obstruction. Unless urethral pressures are monitored and measured with fluoroscopic or ultrasound control, the obstruction could appear to

be the bladder neck. Regardless of the recording technique, used alone without visualization, it is impossible to determine the exact site of the anatomic vesical neck. Thus, when the proximal urethra is nonfunctional, the first rise in pressure does not occur at the site of the vesical neck but in the more distal urethra. Consequently, one may conclude erroneously that this finding represents a vesical neck obstruction.

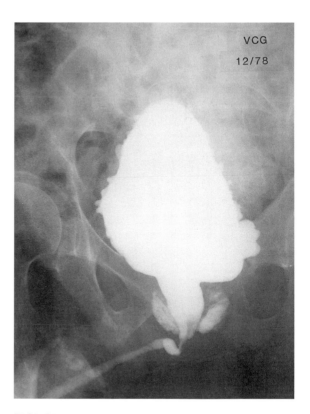

FIGURE 8-7. Voiding cystometrogram in a patient with spinal cord injury shows trabeculated bladder, wide open bladder neck, dilated prostatic urethra, prostato-ejaculatory reflux, and narrow external urethral sphincter, indicating bladder outflow obstruction due to detrusor sphincter dyssynergia.

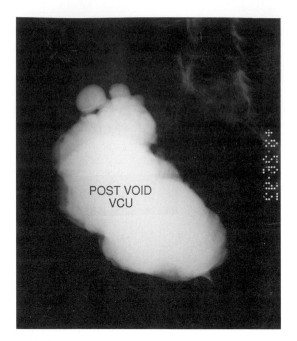

FIGURE 8-8. Postvoid film after voiding cystogram shows excessive postvoid residual, trabeculated bladder, and voiding multiple bladder diverticula.

Voiding Cystourethrography and Video-Urodynamics

Measurement of the bladder and urethral pressures and simultaneous fluoroscopic or sonographic visualization are useful for the detection of both anatomic and physiologic abnormalities. In radiographic studies, contrast is used as the infusant. The

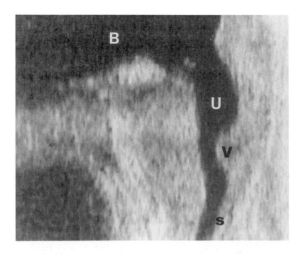

FIGURE 8-9. Sonographic voiding cystogram demonstrating the bladder (*B*) and wide open bladder neck and prostatic (*U*) and membranous urethra. Verumontanum (*V*) is seen prominently in the middle of the posterior urethra. The lower part of the urethra is slightly narrow and is surrounded by external urethral sphincter (*S*).

bladder is catheterized with a triple-lumen urodynamic catheter to simultaneously measure intravesical and urethral pressures. The third lumen is used to fill the bladder. The voiding events on fluoroscopic examination are visualized intermittently, and representative events are recorded on videotape. The bladder is filled until an involuntary detrusor contraction occurs, the patient is asked to void voluntarily, or leakage of the infusant occurs at the urethral meatus, which gives a leak pressure. Bladder outlet obstruction is characterized by a high voiding pressure and low flow. If obstruction is suspected but the site of the obstruction is not clear, the combination of radiographic visualization and MUPP may provide a definitive answer.

Voiding cystourethrography (VCUG) is useful to help define vesicoureteral reflux presence of the bladder with diverticula, trabeculation, prostato-ejaculatory reflux, detrusor sphincter dyssynergia (Fig. 8-7), and postvoid residual urine (Fig. 8-8). The site of outflow obstruction at the bladder neck or in the urethra also may be visualized on voiding films. The presence of prostato-ejaculatory reflux, as seen in Figure 8-7, is indicative of obstruction distal to the ejaculatory duct openings in the urethra due to bladder-external urethral sphincter dyssynergia. In Figure 8-7 the external urethral sphincter is almost closed between the prostate and bulbous urethra. Such patients develop repeated urinary tract infections and epididymo-orchitis. They do not respond well to conservative management with intermittent catheterization. Transurethral sphincterotomy is indicated to prevent recurrent epididymo-orchitis.

Ultrasonography in Urodynamics

Several recent reports have shown encouraging results using ultrasound as an alternative to fluoroscopy for urodynamics.[8,11] Longitudinal real-time imaging of the posterior urethra in a sagittal plane can be achieved during voiding. Using a transrectal linear array sonographic probe, the bladder neck and posterior urethra, including bulbous urethra, can be visualized without the use of dye. Urine itself provides good contrast for sonographic studies. An example of this is shown with a wide open bladder neck, posterior urethra, and bulbous urethra (Fig. 8-9). Bladder neck obstruction is easily visualized on sonography. Secondary bladder neck obstruction due to a ledge in patients with spinal cord injury has been reported.[3] Recognition of this obstruction is important because intermittent catheterization may be difficult in these patients

(Fig. 8-10). Sonographic voiding cystourethrogram shows bladder neck obstruction due to a ledge (shown as arrow) posteriorly at the bladder neck. These ledges are believed to be a complication in patients with detrusor sphincter dyssynergia who are on long-term intermittent catheterization.[8] The presence of a bladder neck ledge invariably leads to difficulty in catheterization with a plain catheter. A coudé tip catheter is more effective for intermittent catheterization.

Combined synchronous, ultrasonographic, and urodynamic monitoring is feasible (Fig. 8-11). This study could be done in lieu of a cineradiographic study combined with simultaneous urodynamics. It has been shown that simple insertion of a catheter by touching the bladder neck ledge can result in bladder contraction and wide-open bladder neck[9,10] (see Fig. 8-11) with a wide-open bladder neck and posterior urethra. It is therefore important to catheterize such patients carefully[11] and not stimulate the bladder neck to produce bladder neck stimulated cystometrogram.[9] Persistent narrowing of the membranous urethra on ultrasound imaging and elevated detrusor pressure is consistent with DESD in a complete suprasacral spinal cord injury. The main advantage of the sonographic study over cineradiographic studies is the lack of radiation exposure for the patients. However, bladder shape, trabeculation, diverticula, and vesicoureteral reflux are difficult to visualize on sonography alone.

Ultrasonographic Studies of Kidneys

Renal sonography is useful in detecting hydronephrosis of the kidneys with dilated pelvicaliceal system, stones, or other filling defects in the

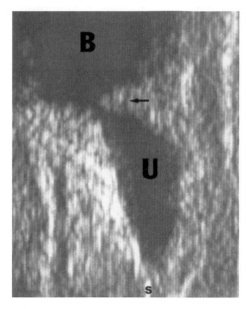

FIGURE 8-10. Transrectal sonographic voiding study showing a bladder neck obstruction (*arrow*) due to a bladder neck ledge. The bladder is seen as black (*B*). The prostatic urethra (*U*) is dilated, and the external sphincter is closed (*S*).

renal pelvis. In following patients with spinal cord injury to detect early hydronephrosis, sonography is noninvasive and eliminates yearly intravenous pyelographic studies that once were used frequently.

Intravenous Pyelography

Intravenous pyelography (IVP) is indicated to rule out stone disease and hydronephrosis and to define anatomic configuration of the pelvicaliceal system. Because routine, once yearly, IVP in patients with spinal cord injury leads to a high dose of

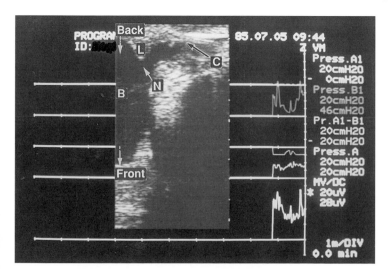

FIGURE 8-11. A multichannel urodynamic study combined with sonography. The bladder (*B*), bladder neck (*N*), bladder neck ledge (*L*), and urethral catheter (*C*) are shown. The bladder neck is wide open, which occurred after the bladder neck was touched with the urethral catheter. (From Perkash I, Wolfe V: Detrusor hyperreflexia and its relationship to posterior bladder neck sensory mechanism in spinal injured patients. Neurourol Urodyn 10:125–133, 1991, with permission.)

radiation exposure, it has been widely replaced with kidney sonographic studies. If a stone is suspected, IVP is necessary for localization and for treatment with extracorporeal shockwave lithotripsy.

Nuclear Scanning of the Kidneys

Radioisotope renography in patients with spinal cord injury has been found to be useful for follow-up screening.[12] The most common abnormality is the delay of isotope excretion. Renal plasma flow is calculated, and reduction in flow of 20% or more is believed to be significant in patients with spinal cord injury. This indicates that urodynamic studies are needed to rule out any outflow obstruction at the bladder neck due to ledge, median lobe, or the presence of detrusor sphincter dyssynergia.

SUMMARY

Neurophysiologic dysfunctions of the bladder can best be evaluated by urodynamic studies. If not carried out carefully, however, studies may give erroneous results. Selection of an appropriate size of urodynamic catheter, careful introduction of the catheter without irritating the bladder neck region, and fluid introduction at 37°C (isothermic to body) are important prerequisites to achieve true results. Sonographic studies are much less invasive than the studies using a catheter, dyes, and radiographs, but they do not provide complete information and are therefore useful only as a screening modality.

REFERENCES

1. Bors E, French JD: Management of paroxysmal hypertension following injuries to cervical and upper thoracic segments of the spinal cord. Arch Surg 64:803, 1952.
2. Bradley WE, Timm GW, Scott FB: Innervation of the detrusor muscle and urethra. Urol Clin North Am 1:3–27, 1974.
3. Brown M, Wickham JEA: The urethral pressure profile. Br J Urol 41:211, 1969.
4. Burney TL, Senapati M, Desai S, et al: Acute cerebrovascular accident and lower urinary tract dysfunction: A prospective correlation of the site of brain injury with urodynamic findings. J Urol 156:1748–1750, 1996.
5. Denny-Brown D, Robertson EG: On the physiology of micturition. Brain 56:149, 1933.
6. McGuire EJ, Woodwide JR, Borden TA, et al: Prognostic value of urodynamic testing in the myelodysplastic patient. J Urol 126:205–209, 1981.
7. Perkash I: Detrusor-sphincter dyssynergia and dyssynergic responses: Recognition and rationale for early modified transurethral sphincterotomy in complete spinal cord injury lesions. J Urol 120:469–474, 1978.
8. Perkash I, Friedland GW: Posterior ledge at the bladder neck: The crucial diagnostic role of ultrasonography. Urol Radiol 8:175–183, 1986.
9. Perkash I, Friedland GW: Transrectal ultrasonography of the lower urinary tract: Evaluation of bladder neck problems. Neurourol Urodynam 5:299–306, 1986.
10. Perkash I, Wolfe V: Detrusor hyperreflexia and its relationship to posterior bladder neck sensory mechanism in spinal injured patients. Neurourol Urodynam 10:125, 1991.
11. Shapeero G, Friedland GW, Perkash I: Transrectal sonographic voiding cystourethrography: Studies in neuromuscular dysfunction. AJR 141:83–90, 1983.
12. Tempkin A, Sullivan G, Paldi J, et al: Radioisotope renography in spinal cord injury. J Urol 133:228–230, 1985.

9

Removable Rigid Dressings

Randall Smith, M.D., and Russell R. Bond, D.O.

The removable rigid dressing (RRD) is an outgrowth of the immediate postsurgical prosthesis and rigid dressing. It has many of the advantages and benefits of its predecessors and can be placed postoperatively by the physician. It also may be removed and replaced by a surgeon who wishes to inspect the wound, or by the patient when bathing and conditioning the skin. The RRD is easily made by a physician or therapist, and the cost of materials is minimal. The physician will find that using the RRD is probably the most convenient way to protect and shape the residual limb before fitting the prosthesis.

The concept of the immediate postsurgical prosthesis was developed by Berlemont in the late 1950s[1] and was introduced by Weise at an international conference in Germany in 1966.[16] Dr. Weise was invited to present his method to physicians in the United States. Subsequently, the concept was accepted by many American physicians interested in amputation surgery. Dr. Ernest Burgess and others have done an excellent job of describing the manufacture of the immediate postsurgical prosthesis and its use in clinical practice.[2,3]

DEVELOPMENT OF THE REMOVABLE RIGID DRESSING

Weise's postsurgical prosthesis is composed of a plaster socket made over the residual limb in the operating room with provisions made for wound drainage, relief of pressure over bony prominences, suspension, and weight bearing. The socket is supracondylar, enabling it to hold the knee in extension. A metal pylon with a prosthetic foot is attached in the operating room a day or so after surgery, when weight bearing begins. Typically, prosthetists are involved in making the immediate postsurgical prosthesis. Considerable skill is required to prevent injury and to assure that the patient will be comfortable under weight bearing

conditions. Many reports have documented the safety and benefits of this procedure.[2,5,7] Benefits include wound healing, comfort, shaping of residual limb, early ambulation, and a positive psychological outlook with regard to rehabilitation.[3]

Omission of the foot and pylon results in a rigid plaster dressing extending above the knee. This dressing is not easily removable but can be placed by the surgeon in the operating room and replaced on a weekly basis in the clinic or on the ward. The prosthetist is not necessarily required because there is no pylon or foot to align. The dressing can be used when a patient is nonambulatory or when there is concern that weight bearing may injure the residual limb. Cummings evaluated 153 patients fitted with the rigid dressing.[4] He felt that early ambulation and discharge from the hospital were "fringe benefits" for certain capable patients but that the rigid dressing might be most valuable in the elderly, senile, disoriented, or diabetic patient with potential to ambulate. Benefits of wound healing, edema control, protection, and comfort of the residual limb were justification enough to use a rigid dressing for all patients. Mooney et al. reported successful management of below-knee vascular amputees with a thin plaster dressing that was not designed to bear weight but to control edema and prevent knee contracture.[8] A plaster cast with pylon was added later. The interval between surgery and use of the prosthesis was less than 6 weeks in unilateral amputees. Wound healing and eventual level of function were not lowered. Other studies in vascular amputees have clearly demonstrated improved wound healing with non–weight bearing rigid plaster dressing.[9,11]

Regardless of the documented success of postsurgical rigid plaster dressings, many surgeons are reluctant to use this device. Often care of the amputee begins long before wound healing is complete. Most surgeons have no objection to the application of a rigid dressing at this time provided that it allows inspection of the wound.

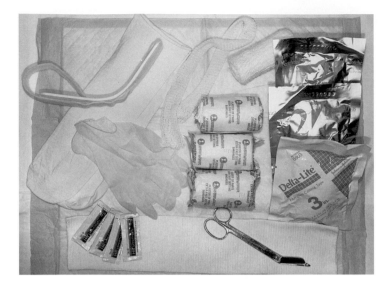

FIGURE 9-1. Materials needed to fabricate the RRD: supracondylar cuff (*upper left*), one-ply socks (*left*), plaster and fiberglass casting materials (*right*), scissors, gloves, and cast padding.

In 1977, Dr. Yeongchi Wu developed a technique for making a below-the-knee rigid dressing that was removable.[17] One of his patients who had fared well with a rigid dressing developed sores on the residual limb after the rigid dressing had been removed and an Ace wrap applied.[18] The RRD that resulted was made of plaster and extended just below the knee. It was covered by tubular stockinette that was held in place above the knee by a supracondylar cuff.

This dressing could be made within an hour; it provided protection for the wound and the residual limb; it was safe and effective in shaping the residual limb; and it allowed frequent inspection of the wound. It is for these reasons that the RRD has become a particularly useful procedure in the postoperative management of the below-knee amputee.

FABRICATION OF THE REMOVABLE RIGID DRESSING

The materials needed (Fig. 9-1) and a step-by-step technique for making the rigid dressing are outlined in Tables 9-1 and 9-2 and discussed below. Our technique generally follows that of Wu.[17,18] Variations in the technique are presented at the end of this section.

Padding

With the postoperative rigid dressing, the bony prominences are protected with felt padding, but in the RRD, these areas are protected by relief that is provided by placing cotton padding over these areas before applying the plaster. The padding is removed

after the plaster dries, leaving the proper relief on the inside of the dressing. The same principle is used to prevent any proximal narrowing of the dressing. If any proximal part of the dressing is smaller in circumference than the more distal portion of the residual limb, the dressing will not be removable. It is almost always necessary to pad the area below the medial tibial flare. Consequently, a bulbous distal end will no longer prevent removal of the rigid dressing.

The cotton padding is placed between two layers of socks—either one-ply stump socks or tube socks. The outer sock adheres to the plaster and is removed with the rigid dressing.

Applying the Plaster

Two 4-inch rolls of fast-set plaster are typically used to make the rigid shell. The plaster is soaked in water and applied gently over the residual limb. Care must be taken to avoid ridges and to avoid

TABLE 9-1. Materials and Equipment

One-ply stump socks or tube socks with the elastic removed, two each

Cotton cast padding

Two rolls of 4-inch fast-set plaster *or*
Two rolls of 2-inch synthetic casting tape

Four-inch tubular stockinette, about 18 inches long *or*
Elastic tubular netting, size 7, 18 inches long

Layers of 3-inch Hexcelite, 12–18 inches long *or*
2- to 3-inch wide casting tape

Bandage scissors
Rubber gloves
Lubricating jelly

compressing the cotton padding. The dressing is extended to just below the patella anteriorly, while posteriorly the trim line needs to be lower, making room for the hamstring tendons during knee flexion.

It is advisable to start at the proximal trim line and wrap distally. Covering the distal end of the residual limb is tricky. Going back and forth over this area and then securing the folded ends of the loops with circumferential wraps works well. One may also cut strips to reinforce the distal end, which is necessary if weight bearing is planned. The one-ply cast sock upon which the plaster was rolled is folded back over the proximal edge of the dressing, trimmed, and secured with more plaster. Ten minutes are allowed for drying. The dressing should be marked anteriorly, in line with the patella so the amputee can properly replace the RRD.

Newer materials such as synthetic casting tape have also been used to make RRDs. The use of these materials and modifications of the basic technique are discussed below.

Suspension

The RRD is suspended by covering the dressing with stockinette. A knot is tied on one end of the stockinette, and the other end is pulled up over the knee. A supracondylar cuff is placed over the stockinette just above the femoral condyles, and the upper end of the stockinette is folded back over the cuff. Elastic tubular netting used to secure surgical dressings makes a good substitute for the stockinette and provides some distal pressure on the distal end of the limb.

The cuff is usually made from a thermoplastic material such as Hexcelite. Several layers are warmed in a hydroculator and cut in strips approximately 3 inches wide and long enough to fit around the supracondylar area of the thigh but not touch or overlap posteriorly. The cuff is molded with the hands as it cools. Pressure with the palm of the hand just above the medial femoral condyle makes a depression in the cuff that will help to prevent the cuff from slipping distally. Fiberglass cast tape also may be used. In both cases, the edges need trimming to eliminate sharp corners. Traditionally, the cuff is secured by a Velcro closure attached to the cuff between the layers of Hexcelite. A band of Velfoam wrapped around the cuff and fastened with Velcro hook material also works well and is simple. Most occupational therapy departments will have the above supplies available (see Table 9-1).

TABLE 9-2. Making the Rigid Removable Dressing Step by Step

Preparation
1. Cover the limb with snug-fitting stump sock or tube sock.
2. Place 3–4 layers of cast padding over the fibular head and along the shaft of the tibia. Place extra padding over the distal end of the tibia.
3. Fill the depression below the medial tibial flare and make circumferential wraps, if necessary, to produce a more or less conical shape.
4. Roll a stump sock or tube sock over the padding.
5. Pull up on the socks and secure them proximally with tape.

Manufacture
1. Wet the plaster in the package.
2. Roll the plaster circumferentially below the patella anteriorly and below hamstring tendons posteriorly.
3. Roll the plaster in a figure-8 pattern or in back and forth layers to cover the distal end.
4. Trim the outer sock 2 inches above the proximal trim line and fold back over the edge of the plaster; secure this with another wrap of plaster.
5. Mark the midpatellar line.
6. Allow 10 minutes to dry.
7. Remove and inspect inside of the dressing for bumps or ridges. The padding is discarded.

Suspension
1. Soften layers of Hexcelite in 71°C water and cut to length. Reheat Hexcelite and mold to supracondylar area, protecting the skin with plastic wrap *or* Fold three or four layers of 3-inch synthetic casting tape lengthwise to the appropriate length and mold over the supracondylar area as noted in the text.
2. Tie a knot in the bottom of the stockinette or elastic netting, and pull it over the dressing and residual limb to above the knee.
3. Apply the cuff over the stockinette and then fold the stockinette back over the cuff.

Inspection and Training
1. Look for bumps and ridges on the inner surface.
2. Look for reddened areas on the residual limb after 30 minutes and throughout the first day.
3. Ask amputee to demonstrate donning and doffing of the RRD.

Inspection

Even clinicians experienced in rolling plaster should not expect to make a perfect dressing on the first try. Thus, inspection of the dressing is an important step. The inside should be free of ridges or bumps, especially over bony areas. The dressing should slide on and off easily. It is imperative that the dressing be removed and the skin inspected after 30 minutes of wear and every 2 hours the first day. The amputee must be taught how to don and doff the rigid dressing, then observed to assure independence.

Variations and Modifications

Several clinicians have used synthetic casting tape to make the rigid dressing.[6,14,18] Gandhavadi points out that the porous nature of the casting tape permits good aeration of the residual limb area to prevent buildup of warmth and moisture under the dressing.[6] The light weight makes the dressing easier to suspend and less cumbersome, and the strength of the casting tape makes it suitable for some weight bearing.

When making the rigid dressing with casting tape, two 2-inch rolls will usually suffice. More care needs to be taken, however, to avoid bumps or ridges on the inside of the dressing. These can usually be avoided if the cast tape is applied to the residual limb without wetting it first. The dressing is subsequently moistened and smoothed on the residual limb by rubbing with any type of water-based cream or gel. Surgical lubricating jelly or even electrode gels are usually available and work well.

Smith and Hof have used a rigid dressing made of fiberglass cast tape that covers the end of the residual limb only.[14] It does not extend to the patellar area or even the head of the fibula. It is somewhat simpler to make but still provides protection and shrinkage for the distal end of the limb. Another option by Swanson[15] is the use of below-the-knee polyethylene semirigid dressing, which is usually done by the prosthetist using direct molded techniques. The socket is flexible, and the patient also uses a stump shrinker. The advantages include that it is lighter weight, nonporous and easier to clean when drainage occurs, and comfortable to flex (Fig. 9-2).

USES FOR THE REMOVABLE RIGID DRESSING

Wound Management

The first and foremost obvious use of the RRD is to cover the surgical wound in the operating room. In this case, the wound is covered with a nonabsorbable dressing. The removable rigid dressing is

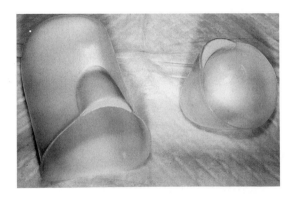

FIGURE 9-2. Two separate removable rigid dressings. Note the differences in length.

made over a sterile stump sock. The RRD protects the wound, holds soft tissue in place, and prevents edema in much the same way that the nonremovable dressing does. Alternatively, the rigid dressing can be applied at the time of the first cast change when the nonremovable rigid dressing is removed.

Many surgeons, however, do not wish to apply a rigid dressing in the operating room, opting for a traditional soft dressing with which they are familiar. Fortunately, the RRD can provide the benefits of shaping, protecting, and providing comfort to the residual limb, even when applied several days after surgery. As a consequence, the RRD is useful for the clinician in the postoperative management of the patient.

Because the RRD allows examination of the wound, it is well accepted by most surgeons. Its removability also allows physicians and nursing staff to check for pressure ulcers that may arise from improper manufacture or placement of the RRD in a patient with poor sensation.

Almost all patients and staff can learn quickly how to don and doff the RRD and apply the cuff suspension (Figs. 9-3, 9-4). The same cannot be said for wrapping with elastic bandages, which, more often than not, are applied incorrectly. Proximal circumferential constriction is common, but even more dangerous is pressure over the tibial crest.[18] Sores may develop within hours in patients who have lost pain sensation.

Protection

The importance of protecting the residual limb cannot be overemphasized. Rarely, an agitated patient will traumatize the residual limb in the early postoperative period. When serious trauma occurs, however, it usually happens after the amputee begins to transfer from bed to chair or after he or she begins to walk. Cases of severe wound dehiscence are common and have been supported in rehabilitation literature.[13] During a fall, there is a reflex extensor response that persists after an amputation. Unfortunately, this often places the weight of the amputee directly on the end of the residual limb at impact. There have even been cases of amputees getting out of bed in the night and stepping down on the missing limb. A rigid dressing will protect the amputee from this type of trauma, which, in some cases, would have led to surgical revision at a higher level. Thus, it is important that the RRD be worn nearly 24 hours a day and always during transfers and ambulation with crutches. As it turns out, after the surgical wound has healed, the term "removable rigid dressing" has less meaning and amputees will often call the RRD a stump protector.

Shaping

Shaping of the residual limb is an important component of preprosthetic management of the amputee. Postoperatively, residual limbs are edematous from the trauma of surgery and have essentially the same amount of fatty tissue and muscle that was present before the amputation. Over the next several months or years, however, the weight-bearing on soft tissues that occurs during prosthetic use causes the fatty tissue to atrophy. Additionally, in most cases, muscles in the residual limb are not used and atrophy along with other tissues. Shrinkage is quite variable but in some cases limbs may shrink 10 inches in circumference.

During the period of stump shaping, the amputee may require numerous prosthetic sockets, the cost of which is not small. If, however, shrinkage can be maximized and a "mature" shape provided to the residual limb before prosthetic fitting, the first and subsequent prosthetic sockets will fit better and fit longer.

The RRD prevents edema if applied at the time of the amputation and is effective in reducing edema when applied several days postoperatively.[10] By adding stump socks under the RRD, gentle even pressure is maintained on all parts of the residual limb. As a general guideline, one should expect one ply of socks to be added every 1–2 days for the first week or two. After 10 to 15 ply of socks are added, the residual limb will probably no longer be shaped like the RRD, and it will be time to remake the dressing. At this point, a reduction in adipose tissue and muscle mass is apparent.

The RRD also may be used along with a stump shrinker such as Compressogrip. The shrinker is applied in its normal fashion and an RRD is simply made over the elastic shrinker. The cotton padding is placed on the shrinker and covered by a stump sock before the plaster is applied. As the residual limb becomes smaller, socks are added over the stump shrinker beneath the RRD as described above. The small ring at the bottom of the elastic shrinker is over soft tissue and causes no problems.

Pressure applied to the bottom of the RRD helps to mobilize edema, which tends to develop distally. Distal pressure may be applied by placing a strop on the bottom of the RRD and pulling proximally with the patient in a seated position or by placing the rigid dressing on a stool while the amputee stands

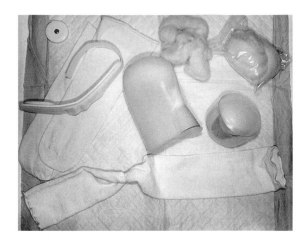

FIGURE 9-3. Materials needed for wearing the removable rigid dressing: stump shrinker (*bottom*), one-ply socks (*left*), supracondylar cuff (*left*), rigid removable dressing (*center*), and lamb's wool (*upper right*).

on the sound leg and bears some weight on the rigid dressing.[12,18]

To summarize, the RRD can be very useful in shrinking and shaping the residual limb. Despite the rigid nature of the dressing itself, its use is quite flexible. The RRD can be applied at the time of surgery or later and still be quite effective. It is easily made,

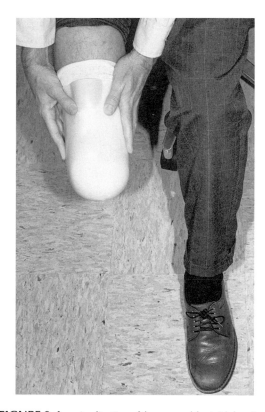

FIGURE 9-4. Application of the removable rigid dressing.

so making a new dressing for a better fit is not a problem. Distal pressure and even elastic compression can be incorporated when using the RRD. This makes the dressing quite versatile and effective in shaping the residual limb.

CONCLUSION

Postoperative rigid dressings have been shown to be safe and comfortable for the amputee. They control edema, protect the wound, and shape the residual limb better than other dressings. The RRD provides these benefits but also allows wound inspection and rapid shrinking of the residual limb. The RRD can be applied at the time of surgery, after the removal of a traditional rigid dressing, or as a first rigid dressing several days after the amputation. It can be made in 30–60 minutes with materials generally found in the hospital and is easy for amputees to don and doff. These attributes make the RRD dressing a suitable alternative to the traditional rigid dressing and an improvement over traditional soft dressings.

REFERENCES

1. Berlemont M, Weber R, Willot JP: Ten years of experience with the immediate application of prosthetic devices to amputees of the lower extremities on the operating table. Prosthet Int 3:8, 1969.
2. Burgess EM, Romano RL: The management of lower extremity amputations using immediate postsurgical prostheses. Clin Orthop 57:137–146, 1968.
3. Burgess EM, Romano RL, Zettl JH: The management of lower extremity amputations surgery. Washington, DC, U.S. Government Printing Office, TR-10-G, 1969.
4. Cummings V: Immediate rigid dressing for amputees: Advantages and misconceptions. N Y State J Med 74:980–983, 1974.
4a. Esquenazi A, Meier RH: Rehabilitation in limb deficiency. 4. Limb amputation. Arch Phys Med Rehabil 77:S18–S28, 1996.
5. Folsom D, King T, Rubin JR: Lower extremity amputation with immediate postoperative prosthetic placement. Am J Surg 164:320–322, 1992.
6. Gandhavadi B: Porous removable rigid dressing for complicated below-knee amputation stumps. Arch Phys Med Rehabil 68:51–53, 1987.
7. Kitowski VJ, Appel MF, Haslam T: Prosthetic fitting immediately after below-knee amputation. South Med J 68:739–742, 1975.
8. Mooney V, Harvey JP, McBride E, Snelson R: Comparison of postoperative stump management: Plaster vs. soft dressings. J Bone Joint Surg 53A:241–249, 1971.
9. Mooney V, Wagner FW, Waddell J, et al: The below-the-knee amputation for vascular disease. J Bone Joint Surg 58A:365–368, 1976.
10. Mueller MJ: Comparison of removable rigid dressings and elastic bandages in preprosthetic management of patients with below-knee amputations. Phys Ther 62:1438–1441, 1982.
11. Nicholas GG, DeMuth WE: Evaluation of the use of the rigid dressing in amputation of the lower extremity. Surg Gynecol Obstet 143:398–400, 1976.
12. Parhad A, Gervais B, Wu Y: Beyond the rigid dressing: Preprosthetic ambulation of the below-knee amputee. Am Correct Ther J 37:66–89, 1983.
13. Richter KJ, Hurvitz EA, Girardot K: Rigid removable dressing in a case of poor wound healing. Arch Phys Med Rehabil 69:128–129, 1988.
14. Smith RD, Hof JJ: Lightweight rigid dressing for below-knee amputations. Arch Phys Med Rehabil 69:793, 1988.
15. Swanson VM: Below-knee polyethylene semi-rigid dressing. J Prosthet Ortho 5:30–35, 1993.
16. Weiss MA, Gielzynski A, Wirski J: Myoplasty-immediate fitting-ambulation. Proceedings of Sessions of the World Commission on Research in Rehabilitation, Tenth World Congress of the International Society, Wiesbaden, Germany, 1966.
17. Wu Y, Keagy RD, Krick H, et al: An innovative removable rigid dressing technique for below-the-knee amputation. J Bone Joint Surg 61A:724–729, 1979.
18. Wu Y, Krick H: Removable rigid dressing for below-knee amputees. Clin Prosthet Orthot 11:33–44, 1987.

10

Serial Casting

David L. Nash, M.D.

Serial casting is a technique of contracture treatment that has been used successfully in a number of clinical conditions. One might consider it an aggressive nonoperative form of management that requires an understanding of the pathologic process that is contributing to the contracture development. It also requires a commitment to the close monitoring of the progress and potential side effects of the casting interventions and to the time, resources, and knowledge to apply and remove multiple casts. Because serial casting most often is indicated for patients with many other medical, rehabilitation, and sometimes surgical care issues, the decision to perform serial casting and the implementation of the intervention are usually a team process involving one or more physicians and a physical or occupational therapist. Serial casting is just one of many clinical tools that can be used to manage the effects of spasticity on a joint and prevent or treat a joint contracture. The intent of this chapter is to review the principles and practice of serial casting as they have been applied to patients with spasticity and contractures of upper and lower limb joints.

CONTRACTURES AND SPASTICITY

Contractures result from the shortening of periarticular connective tissue, particularly in muscle, joint capsules, and scars, but if contractures persist they eventually include other soft tissues such as skin, ligaments, tendons, and neurovascular structures. Shortening of these tissues occurs over time if a joint is allowed to remain in a constant position.[22] Perry emphasizes that "contractures must be recognized as an unnecessary complication" and that "the prevention of contractures and deformities must be a deliberate component of the therapeutic program for the patient with prolonged disability such as arthritis, paralysis or severe injury."[19]

Spasticity has been defined as a condition associated with a persistent increase in the involuntary reflex activity of a muscle in response to stretch and often associated with one or more of four features: hypertonia, hyperactive deep tendon reflexes, clonus, and spread of reflex responses beyond the stimulated muscle.[12] Spasticity secondary to a cerebral lesion such as a traumatic brain injury or cerebral palsy[14] often predisposes to flexion contractures of the elbows and equinus and knee flexion contractures in the lower extremities. One study of 75 consecutive patients hospitalized with traumatic head injury found 84% developed at least one clinically significant joint contracture, with contractures of the ankle occurring in 76% and of the elbow in 44% of the patients.[25]

The literature documenting the use and effectiveness of serial casting in conditions associated with spasticity and contracture is fairly limited. Clinical conditions studied include traumatic brain injury and cerebral palsy. The majority of these studies are descriptive—case reports and clinical series of patients without experimental control comparisons.

SERIAL CASTING IN PATIENTS WITH TRAUMATIC BRAIN INJURY

One of the early physical management challenges in patients with severe brain injury is that of pathologic tone management because of its potential to cause permanent contracture and deformity. If not prevented, these contractures and deformities have the potential to slow the acute and postacute rehabilitation process and interfere with functional recovery. Serial casting has been used in both the acute intensive care setting and the acute and postacute rehabilitation settings primarily to assist patients in regaining lost range of motion. Serial casting also has been used to try to decrease spastic tone[2,3,6] and facilitate gait retraining[26] in patients with traumatic brain injury (TBI).

Spastic equinus foot with ankle posturing and contracture is the most common deformity in TBI patients that may benefit from serial casting.[3] Lower extremity serial casting was used in 21% (42 of 201) of TBI patients admitted to a rehabilitation center following transfer from acute medical care. Thirty-nine of the 42 patients were treated with short leg casts. The mean time from injury to initial casting was about 3 months, with an average duration of casting of 4–5 weeks and a range of 7–92 days. Some of the casts were applied to assist in managing tone and improving range of motion (ROM). An average ROM gain of about 20° was reported for patients whose casting was designed exclusively for improving ROM.

Serial casting also has been reported to be used effectively in the acute intensive care setting following TBI.[2,6,16] In a series of 10 TBI patients reported by Conine,[6] initial casting was performed 2–14 days following head injury. The patients averaged five casts, requiring a duration of 1 month of serial cast application. The average gain in ROM was 20°; two patients failed to improve and one worsened in spite of casting. Because only limited data were presented, it is difficult to make direct comparisons of the relative effectiveness of early casting[6] with post-acute casting,[3] but a crude comparison suggests similar ROM gains and duration of casting treatment.

It is common practice to bivalve the final cast once the desired gains in ROM have been achieved. Imie reported six TBI patients who underwent serial casting with bilateral short leg casts.[16] In order to compare the effects of bivalved casts with nonbivalved casts, one randomly selected serial cast was bivalved in each patient. Imie reported significantly greater improvement in ROM and significantly fewer problems with skin breakdown in the ankles treated with nonbivalved casts.

KNEE AND ELBOW DROPOUT CASTS

Serial casting also has been successfully applied to spastic knee[1,3,5] and elbow[1,3,17] flexion contractures. Because the knee and elbow are more hinge-like in their primary plane of motion, dropout casts have been used as an alternative to cylinder style casts for both the elbow and knee.[1,3,17] For a knee flexion contracture, a dropout cast is applied as a cylinder cast and subsequently cut to remove a portion either over the anterior lower leg or the anterior thigh so that the posterior portion acts as a flexion stop. With proper positioning the dropout cast can take advantage of gravity to provide periodic prolonged stretches to the tight flexors. In a similar manner, a long arm cylinder cast is applied

to an elbow flexion contracture and cut out to expose the extensor portion of the upper or lower arm. Because some joint motion generally occurs between cast changes, less joint stiffness is observed at the time of cast change. In addition, some clinicians have combined the dropout casting technique with neuromuscular electrical stimulation (NMES), claiming additive benefits in overcoming flexion contracture by periodically stimulating the extensor muscle groups.[1] In theory, the NMES not only applies an extensor muscle–induced stretch at the joint but also may provide some temporary reflex inhibition of the antagonist spastic flexor muscles.

INHIBITIVE (TONE-REDUCING) CASTS

Short leg casts with special features designed to decrease abnormal tone and therefore improve gait characteristics have been described as an adjunct to neurodevelopmental therapy (NDT) in children with cerebral palsy.[9,23,24] The theory that these casts are helpful is based on the premise that a "balanced secure support under the dynamic arch systems and stable midline forefoot, subtalar, and ankle control" will reduce excessive reflex and tone responses during standing and gait and secondarily allow for more effective NDT to train more normal patterns of motor control and mobility.[2] Sussman hypothesized that two primary factors promote balance and mobility gains in therapy with "tone-reducing casts."[23] First, gains may be achieved by inhibiting abnormally strong plantar grasp reflexes by supporting the toes in slight dorsiflexion in the casts. The second factor is based on the theory that the cast provides greater stability at the ankle, which in turn decreases stimulus for excessive reflex motor response. In a study comparing the effects of "tone-reducing" casts with standard short leg walking casts in children with cerebral palsy, Hinderer et al. demonstrated a significantly better stride length with the tone-reducing casts along with other subjective differences.[13] This result suggests that the therapeutic benefits of the casting are not entirely caused by providing ankle stability. Brouwer et al. demonstrated that increased reflex threshold following serial casting was associated with gains in ankle dorsiflexion in children with cerebral palsy.[4] Another study failed, however, to show any radiologic difference in bony alignment of children with cerebral palsy standing in their "inhibitory casts" compared to standing barefoot. Duncan and Mott emphasize the role of "inhibitory casts" in reducing input to certain reflexogenic areas of the feet that in turn trigger overactive tonic reflexes.[9] Watt et al. found that the primary effect of "inhibitive casting" was to increase dorsiflexion in spastic children; however, the gains were lost after 5 months, even though rigid ankle-foot orthotics were used after the 3 weeks of casting.[24a] The critical features and mechanisms of action that seem to make inhibitive casts at least a temporary beneficial adjunct to therapy in spastic children remains unclear. These casts are often used by practitioners not only for the "tone-reducing" qualities, but also to treat equinus contractures with serial casting.

BOTULINUM TOXIN: ADJUNCT OR ALTERNATIVE

It has become common practice with some physicians who treat focal spasticity with botulinum toxin injections to use serial casting to further reduce tone and gain ROM. To date, this author has not found any literature reporting on the combined effects of the two interventions. Two studies, however, have compared botulinum toxin injections with serial casting to treat dynamic spastic equinus deformities in children with cerebral palsy. In a prospective randomized trial Corry et al. found comparable results in tone reduction and improvements in gait analysis measures, but benefits persisted longer with botulinum toxin intervention compared to the serial casting at 12 weeks postintervention.[7] In a similar study, Flett et al. reported on a prospective, randomized single-blind controlled study of children with spastic cerebral palsy treated with botulinum toxin or serial casting for dynamic spastic equinus.[11] They found comparable benefit at 6 months with the two treatment groups but noted the parents' preference for the botulinum toxin injection over serial casting because of the inconvenience of serial casting. Further studies may help clarify the circumstances when combined casting and botulinum toxin are indicated. Until then, clinical judgment and experience must guide the practitioner.

INDICATIONS FOR SERIAL CASTS

Serial casting should be considered when there is a failure to achieve or maintain functional ROM of a peripheral joint such as the ankle, knee, or elbow with traditional ROM and stretching exercises and resting splints. When one identifies the potential for developing significant joint deformity and contracture secondary to severe spasticity that is not responding well to medical and physical measures, serial casting should be considered. In patients with TBI it is generally believed that the earlier the serial casting is initiated, the more effective it will be in restoring functional ROM.[2,3] Serial casting is most effective when the patient is still showing signs of neurologic recovery and when the loss of ROM is primarily due to spasticity rather than other possible factors, such as heterotopic ossification, healing fracture, or ligamentous injury.[3]

CONTRAINDICATIONS

The skin must be free from lesions that might worsen or become infected when hidden from view and denied frequent wound care and observation.[3] Serial casts should be avoided in patients with skin that appears particularly vulnerable, such as the very thin skin of individuals who chronically take corticosteroids or the mottled or pale and cool skin of those with severe peripheral vascular disease. Although not well documented in the literature, concern has been expressed by some that serial casting possibly may increase hypertension or intracranial pressures, particularly in acutely injured and agitated TBI patients.[3] It is essential in patients with acute brain injury that the primary physician agree with any plans to perform serial casting. If the limb, particularly an upper extremity limb, is required for monitoring vital signs or administering medications, the priority obviously is medical management, and serial casting must be postponed.[2] ROM limited by acute heterotopic ossification should be treated with ROM exercises rather than immobilization.

GUIDELINES FOR CASTING

Several helpful resources detail preparation for casting and application of the cast itself.[8,10,15,18] One should always consider the indications, contraindications, and potential alternative options before engaging in serial casting. Once it has been decided to recommend serial casting, the clinician needs to explain the procedure, its purpose, and its goals to the patient and family. The local informed consent procedure must be followed. If the patient is agitated when the cast is applied, some type of sedation may be helpful. Sometimes, initial casts can be applied when the patient is under general anesthesia that has been given for another procedure, such as a tracheotomy, gastrostomy, or surgical wound management.

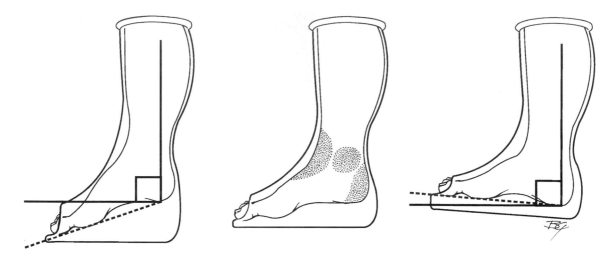

FIGURE 10-1. Serial short leg casts depicting a reduction of plantar flexion contracture of 20° to a final holding cast at 5° of dorsiflexion. Several intermediate casts between the initial and final holding cast may be required to achieve a gradual lengthening of the contracted gastrocsoleus muscle.

Lower Extremity Serial Casts

The spastic equinus deformity is the most common deformity to be treated by serial casts. The patient needs to be positioned as comfortably as possible, which is often supine with hips and knees flexed for short leg casting. Some prefer the patient to be prone with the knee flexed 90° or sitting, if tolerated. Gentle stretching and ROM exercises immediately prior to casting help to achieve optimal positioning. When severe spasticity limits even a mild reduction in the equinus posturing, casting with conscious sedation or general anesthesia may be required. Other alternatives include a temporary tibial nerve block with bupivacaine or a more prolonged effect with a phenol motor point or tibial nerve block. Botulinum toxin, if injected to reduce tone prior to casting, is best given a week to 10 days before casting, whereas the effects of bupivacaine and phenol are more immediate and casting can directly follow these procedures. Depending on the patient's ability to cooperate, one or two assistants will be indispensable during the procedure. The short leg cast is started by applying a stockinette extending from the knee to several inches beyond the toes. Cotton padding is rolled up the leg from the toes to about 2 or 3 cm below the level of the fibular head, and the procedure is repeated to create two layers. Additional foam or felt padding may be added around bony prominences,[8] with the extra padding fixed between layers of cotton roll padding. Before beginning to apply the plaster, it is essential to reassess hindfoot and forefoot alignment. It is

important to correct the hindfoot to subtalar neutral and try to achieve midtarsal neutral alignment before exerting any significant dorsiflexion stretch. If the alignments are difficult to establish and hold, the casting process can be divided into two steps. First, a slipper cast is applied in an attempt to establish some correction toward subtalar and midtarsal neutral. The plaster is allowed to begin to set before a slight amount of dorsiflexion stretch is applied and the plaster extended up the leg.[6] After two or three layers of plaster are applied, the top and bottom stockinette are trimmed back and rolled back onto the cast and covered with plaster 3-inch by 15-inch splints, leaving exposed the padded rolled stockinette edge at the proximal and distal extremes of the cast. Serial short leg casts are depicted in Figure 10-1.

If ankle plantar flexors and knee flexors are equally affected by spasticity and contracture, a long leg cast can be made to incorporate both the knee and the foot. A cylinder cast extending from just proximal to the ankle up the leg to the proximal thigh can be used for an isolated knee flexion contracture. Dropout casts of the lower extremity can be made by cutting out the anterior thigh or leg portion of a cylinder cast as described.

Upper Extremity Casts

Elbow flexor spasticity and contracture can be treated with long arm cylinder casting.[3] The patient is positioned supine, the elbow flexors are stretched, and ROM is provided to the shoulder and hand prior to initiating casting. The arm is positioned in

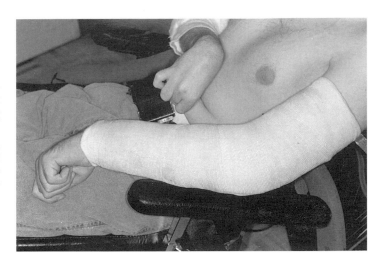

FIGURE 10-2. A 32-year-old man with an old right hemiparesis from a childhood traumatic brain injury suffered a superimposed left hemiparesis from an intracranial hemorrhage as an adult. A spastic elbow flexion contracture of 2 years' duration limited some residual function in the left hand. A phenol musculocutaneous nerve block followed by serial casting reduced the contracture by 50% and helped improve function and ease of care. The photo shows the final holding cast before it was bivalved.

slight abduction with the elbow extended and slightly supinated to the degree that can be comfortably tolerated by the patient and maintained by the individual assisting with the casting. A stockinette is rolled up the arm, covering the wrist to the axilla. Three-inch cotton padding is applied next, winding around the arm from the wrist to the axilla and overlapping the edges. Extra padding is then added around bony prominences, including the olecranon process and the humeral condyles. This is then covered with another layer of cotton padding. A 4-inch plaster roll is moistened and applied over the cotton padding. While the plaster is still wet, it is smoothed and gently molded to the arm's contours while the assistant maintains the relative extension and supination. The proximal and distal ends of the stockinette are rolled back onto the cast and incorporated into the cast by applying moistened 3-inch by 15-inch plaster splints around each end of the cast. While the cast is setting, it is important to maintain the desired positioning without applying any squeezing pressure with the fingers over the cast that would create an undesirable point of increased pressure to the skin beneath the cast.

In some circumstances it may be desirable to incorporate the wrist and hand into the cast to provide prolonged stretch to tight wrist and finger flexors.[3] Short arm casts can be used if the elbow is not as tight as the wrist and can be maintained with conventional ROM and stretching.

Cast Monitoring and Changes

Following application of the initial cast, fingers or toes distal to the casts are monitored for discoloration. If discoloration suggestive of circulation compromise persists longer than 30 minutes, the cast should be removed and reapplied.[3] The casts should be protected from deforming forces for 24 hours, particularly weight bearing on a lower extremity plaster cast. Fiberglass casts achieve their full strength more quickly and can tolerate weight bearing shortly after application. The casts are generally changed approximately weekly with a brief period of therapeutic ROM and joint mobilization prior to fabricating the next cast. Casting is continued until the goal ROM has been reached or gains from the casting seem to have reached a plateau. Four or five cast changes are common. The final cast, often referred to as a holding cast, is often left in place 10–14 days and then bivalved so that it can be used as a night splint (Fig. 10-2). If needed, it can be worn on a scheduled basis throughout the day to maintain ROM. There usually is a prolonged need for a positioning aid for the extremity in order to maintain the gains in ROM. A light-weight orthoplast splint or polypropylene orthosis can be fabricated for this purpose.

CONCLUSION

Serial casting is a useful but labor-intensive adjunct to the treatment of clinically and functionally significant spasticity and contracture of the upper and lower extremities. Careful patient selection and clearly defined objective therapeutic goals are essential. Rehabilitation team members with casting skills can clearly contribute significant expertise within the full spectrum of comprehensive rehabilitation services.

REFERENCES

1. Baker LL, Parker K, Sanderson D: Neuromuscular electrical stimulation for the head injured patient. Phys Ther 63:1967–1974, 1983.

2. Barnard P, Dill H, Eldredge P, et al: Reduction of hypertonicity by early casting in a comatose head-injured individual. Phys Ther 64:1540–1542, 1984.

3. Booth BJ, Doyle M, Montgomery J: Serial casting for the management of spasticity in the head-injured adult. Phys Ther 63:1960–1966, 1983.

4. Brouwer B, Wheeldon RK, Stradiotto-Parker N, Allum J: Reflex excitability and isometric force production in cerebral palsy: The effect of serial casting. Dev Med Child Neurol 40:168–175, 1998.

5. Cherry DB, Weingand GM: Plaster drop-out casts as a dynamic means to reduce muscle contracture. Phys Ther 61:1601–1603, 1981.

6. Conine TA, Sullivan T, Mackie T, Goodman M: Effect of serial casting for the prevention of equinus in patients with acute head injury. Arch Phys Med Rehabil 71:310–312, 1990.

7. Corry IS, Cosgrove AP, Duffy CM, et al: Botulinum toxin A compared with stretching casts in the treatment of spastic equinus: A randomized prospective trial. J Pediatr Orthop 18:304–311, 1998.

8. Cusick BD: Serial Casts: Their Use in Management of Spasticity-Induced Foot Deformity, revised ed. Tucson, Therapy Skill Builders, 1990, pp 1–105.

9. Duncan WR, Mott DH: Foot reflexes and the use of the "inhibitive cast." Foot Ankle 4:145–148, 1983.

10. Feldman PA: Upper extremity casting and splinting. In Glenn MB, Whyte J (eds): The Practical Management of Spasticity in Children and Adults. Philadelphia, Lea & Febiger, 1990, pp 149–166.

11. Flett PJ, Stern LM, Waddy H, et al: Botulinum toxin A versus fixed cast stretching for dynamic calf tightness in cerebral palsy. J Paediatr Child Health 35:71–77, 1999.

12. Gans BM, Glenn MB: Introduction. In Glenn MB, Whyte J (eds): The Practical Management of Spasticity in Children and Adults. Philadelphia, Lea & Febiger, 1990, p 1.

13. Hinderer KA, Harris SR, Purdy AH, et al: Effects of "tone-reducing" vs. standard plaster-casts on gait improvement of children with cerebral palsy. Dev Med Child Neurol 30:370–377, 1988.

14. Hoffer MM, Knoebel RT, Roberts R: Contractures in cerebral palsy. Clin Orthop 219:70–77, 1987.

15. Hylton N: Dynamic casting and orthotics. In Glenn MB, Whyte J (eds): The Practical Management of Spasticity in Children and Adults. Philadelphia, Lea & Febiger, 1990, pp 167–200.

16. Imie PC, Eppinghaus CE, Broughton AC: Efficacy of non-bivalved and bivalved serial casting on head injured patients in intensive care. Phys Ther 66:748, 1986.

17. King TI: Plaster splinting as a means of reducing elbow flexion spasticity: A case study. Am J Occup Ther 36:671–673, 1982.

18. Leahy P: Precasting work sheet—an assessment tool: A clinical report. Phys Ther 68:72–74, 1988.

19. Perry J: Contractures: A historical perspective. Clin Orthop 219:8–14, 1987.

20. Ratcliff R, Kempthorne P: Temporary tibial nerve block: Adjunct to inhibitory plasters in the physiotherapy management of equinus in severely head-injured children. Austr J Physiother 29:119–125, 1983.

21. Ricks NR, Eilert RE: Effects of inhibitory casts and orthoses on bony alignment of foot and ankle during weight-bearing in children with spasticity. Dev Med Child Neurol 35:11–16, 1993.

22. Stolov WC, Thompson SC: Soleus immobilization contracture in the baboon [abstract]. Arch Phys Med Rehabil 60:556, 1979.

23. Sussman MD: Casting as an adjunct to neurodevelopmental therapy for cerebral palsy. Dev Med Child Neurol 25:804–805, 1983.

24. Sussman MD, Cusick B: Preliminary report: The role of short-leg, tone-reducing casts as an adjunct to physical therapy of patients with cerebral palsy. Johns Hopkins Med J 145:112–114, 1979.

24a. Watt J, Sims D, Harckham F, et al: A prospective study of inhibitive casting as an adjunct to physiotherapy for cerebral-palsied children. Dev Med Child Neurol 28:480–488, 1986.

25. Yarkony GM, Sahgal V: Contractures: A major complication of craniocerebral trauma. Clin Orthop 219:93–96, 1987.

26. Zachazewski JE, Eberle ED, Jeffries M: Effect of tone-inhibiting casts and orthoses on gait. Phys Ther 62:453–455, 1982.

11

Shoulder and Chest Wall Blocks

Ted A. Lennard, M.D., and Daniel Y. Shin, M.D.

Nerves of the proximal upper extremity, trunk, and head are easily accessible to percutaneous block procedures. Blocks in many of these specific areas carry risks of pneumothorax because of the proximity of the pleural cavity to the regional anatomy. This is especially true with intercostal, suprascapular, thoracodorsal, pectoral, and lower subscapular blocks. Therefore, blocks in this region require the clinician to have a thorough knowledge of shoulder, neck, and chest wall anatomy.

SUPRASCAPULAR NERVE

The suprascapular nerve originates from the superior trunk of the brachial plexus and contains fibers from the fifth and sixth cervical nerve roots. It enters the supraspinous fossa below the transverse scapular ligament after passing obliquely deep to the trapezius and omohyoid muscles. The nerve innervates the supraspinatus muscle and gives branches to the glenohumeral and acromioclavicular joints as well as the conoid, trapezoid, and coracoacromial ligaments. The nerve passes around the spinoglenoid notch to terminate in the infraspinatus muscle. It also carries sympathetic innervation to the joint capsule.

Therapeutic or diagnostic injections can be performed to block the suprascapular nerve. Anesthetic injections with or without corticosteroids can be used to treat suprascapular neuropathies, cancer pain, and postoperative shoulder pain, especially after acromioplasty.[4,6,10,12] These injections also may be useful to facilitate glenohumeral range of motion in patients with adhesive capsulitis with or without superimposed reflex sympathetic dystrophy.[13]

Suprascapular Nerve Block Technique

Granirer originally described a suprascapular nerve block technique using a posterior approach.[5] A point is identified on the scapular spine 2 inches from the lateral border of the acromion. The needle is inserted $\frac{1}{2}$ inch superior to this point into the supraspinatus fossa (Fig. 11-1) and is advanced until bone is contacted and then withdrawn several millimeters and angled approximately 15° cephalad.

An alternative posterior approach involves dividing the scapular spine into thirds and dropping a perpendicular line at the junction of the middle and outer third. The scapular notch lies 1–2 cm superior to this point of intersection. The needle is advanced about 2 inches until bone is contacted. The needle can be adjusted until the suprascapular notch is identified and 8–10 ml of solution can be injected.

An anterior approach described by Wassef can be performed with the patient in the supine or sitting position.[13] The point of entry of the needle is at the anteromedial border of the trapezius muscle where it attaches to the lateral third of the clavicle. The needle is inserted above the clavicle and advanced posteriorly with a slight downward and medial projection.

Pneumothorax is the most serious complication of suprascapular nerve block. In skilled hands, its incidence is reported to be less than 1% from the posterior approach, and it is even less common from the anterior approach.[7]

THORACODORSAL NERVE

The thoracodorsal nerve originates from the posterior cord of the brachial plexus and is composed of fibers from the C6, C7, and C8 nerve roots (Fig. 11-2). As it exits the posterior cord, it travels adjacent to the subscapular artery along the posterior wall of the axilla where it terminates into the latissimus dorsi muscle.

The latissimus dorsi muscle is one of the strongest humeral adductors and also assists in humeral internal rotation and extension. A thoracodorsal nerve block is useful to reduce spasticity that results in a shoulder adduction and internal rotation deformity.

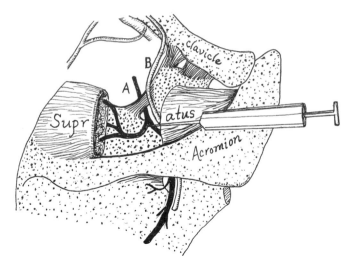

FIGURE 11-1. Technique for blocking the suprascapular nerve. *A*, Suprascapular nerve. *B*, Suprascapular artery.

This block is often used in conjunction with blocks of the pectoral and lower subscapular nerves.

Thoracodorsal Nerve Block Technique

The thoracodorsal nerve can be blocked in the anterior axillary region. A midaxillary line is drawn that intersects with a perpendicular line 1.5 inches above the nipple line (Fig. 11-3). Using a surface stimulator, the nerve is located at the intersection of these lines between the latissimus dorsi and the chest wall. The latissimus dorsi muscle can be esasily separated from the lateral chest wall because the nerve passes between these two structures. The needle is inserted anterior to the latissimus dorsi muscle in a posteriorly directed orientation. Caution is necessary to prevent introduction of the needle into the pleural cavity or into the subscapular

artery that travels with the nerve. The nerve may be approached more precisely with the use of a nerve stimulator, watching for strong humeral adduction with current less than 2 mA.

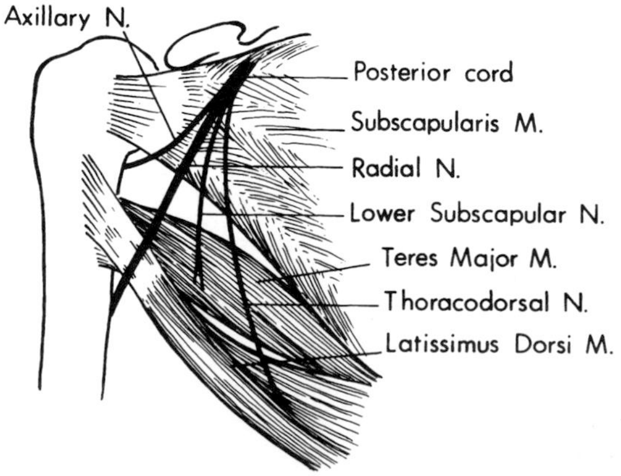

LOWER SUBSCAPULAR NERVE

The lower subscapular nerve (LSN) originates from the posterior cord of the brachial plexus and contains fibers from the C5 and C6 spinal nerves (see Fig. 11-2). The LSN initially enters the axillary portion of the subscapularis muscle and later terminates in the teres major muscle (Fig. 11-4). This latter muscle primarily acts as an internal rotator and adductor of the humerus. The teres major muscle, in combination with the pectoralis major and latissimus dorsi muscles, is partly responsible for spasticity-induced shoulder adduction deformities.

Lower Subscapular Nerve Block Technique

The LSN can be localized along the axillary border of the scapula at the midpoint between the acromion and the inferior angle of the scapula. The needle is advanced immediately adjacent to the bone and directed parallel to the chest wall in an anterior and lateral direction (see Fig. 11-4). The combination use of both surface and Teflon-coated needle electrodes facilitates this procedure.

MEDIAL AND LATERAL PECTORAL NERVES

The medial (MPN) and lateral (LPN) pectoral nerves are small in size and are purely motor nerves

Axillary N.

Posterior cord

Subscapularis M.

Radial N.

Lower Subscapular N.

Teres Major M.

Thoracodorsal N.

Latissimus Dorsi M.

FIGURE 11-2. A posterior view of the posterior cord of the brachial plexus and its branches: axillary, radial, lower subscapular, and thoracodorsal nerves with the scapula removed.

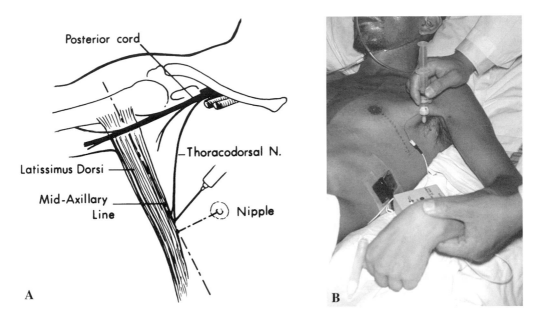

FIGURE 11-3. *A,* The thoracodorsal nerve (anterior chest view) takes its origin from the posterior cord of the brachial plexus. Note the needle tip above and lateral to the nipple level. *B,* The needle is advanced perpendicular to the anterior chest but lateral to the ribs.

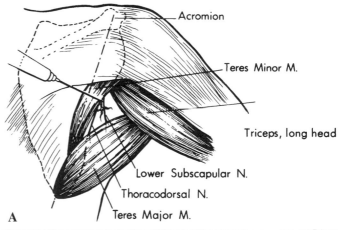

FIGURE 11-4. *A,* The lower subscapular nerve (posterior shoulder view with the scapula shown in dotted lines) is visualized in its relation to the thoracodorsal nerve and teres major. *B,* Lower subscapular nerve block technique.

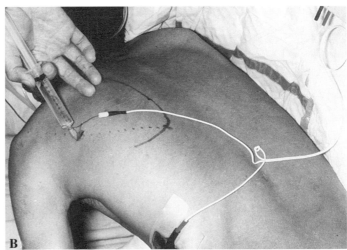

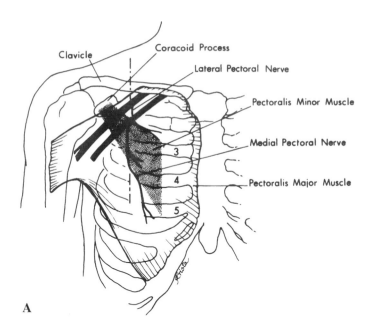
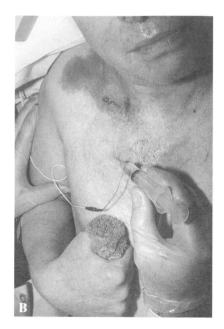

FIGURE 11-5. *A,* The key to pectoral nerve blocks is the physician's ability to accurately locate the pectoralis minor muscle. *B,* Note the needle angle in comparison to the chest wall.

(Fig. 11-5). MPN is a branch of the medial cord of the brachial plexus that originates from the C8 and T1 spinal roots. This nerve innervates the pectoralis minor muscle (Pmm) and emerges from its infero-lateral border to innervate the lower portion of the pectoralis major muscle (PMM). The remaining clavicular head of the PMM is innervated by the LPN. This nerve is a branch of the lateral cord of the brachial plexus originating from the C5, C6, and C7 spinal roots. It emerges from the superior border of the Pmm immediately below the midclavicle prior to innervating the PMM.

The PMM is partly responsible for humeral ad-duction and internal rotation movements while the Pmm depresses and rotates the scapula. Therefore, in cases of spasticity affecting these muscles, shoul-der adduction and internal rotation deformities result. This deformity creates problems with axil-lary hygiene, upper extremity dressing, positioning, and shoulder pain.

Medial Pectoral Nerve Block Technique

When performing pectoral nerve blocks, accu-rate anatomic landmarks must be identified on the anterior chest wall. Outlining the borders of the Pmm on the skin is the key to a successful block. This muscle originates from the outer surfaces of the third, fourth, and fifth sternocostal margins and inserts into the coracoid process. The MPN can be located using a surface stimulator at the intersection of the lower border of the Pmm and a perpendicular line drawn from the midclavicle. Once located with surface stimulation, a needle is introduced in a plane parallel to the muscle. To avoid inadvertent in-trapleural injection, the needle should not be ad-vanced perpendicular to the chest wall.

Lateral Pectoral Nerve Block Technique

With the lateral pectoral nerve block technique, the LPN becomes exposed at the superior margin of the Pmm. If the same midclavicular line described in the MPN block is extended perpendicularly across the Pmm superiorly, the LPN can be located. Recognizing the Pmm attachment sites is essential for an accurate block. A surface stimulator is useful, and once the nerve is identified, the needle is in-serted in a posteriorly and superiorly directed angle. As in the MPN block, caution is advised with needle advancement to avoid intrapleural injection. Needle advancement in blocking both the MPN and LPN should not occur in a perpendicular plane to the chest wall. This avoids penetration into the pleural cavity and subsequent pneumothoraces.

MUSCULOCUTANEOUS NERVE

The musculocutaneous nerve (MCN) originates from the lateral cord of the brachial plexus and is

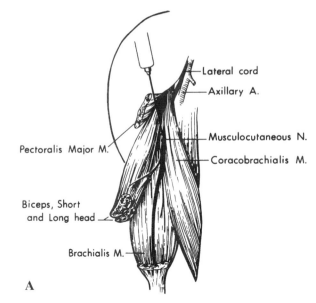

FIGURE 11-6. *A*, The musculocutaneous nerve is shown behind the pectoralis major tendon and in the substance of coracobrachialis muscle. *B*, Musculocutaneous nerve block technique. The arm is held in abduction by an assistant while the physician advances the needle. The block stimulator rests on the patient's chest.

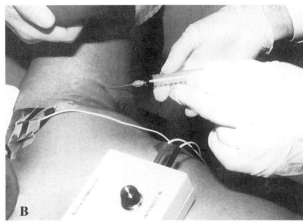

composed of fibers from the C5, C6, and C7 spinal nerve roots. It exits the lateral cord just proximal to the origin of the median nerve. The MCN travels obliquely downward and laterally to supply the coracobrachialis, biceps, and brachialis muscles (Fig. 11-6). A small branch often supplies the elbow joint, but the main MCN terminates to supply the skin of the radial surface of the forearm, often extending to the dorsum of the wrist.

Musculocutaneous Nerve Block Technique

The MCN is easily blocked with an axillary approach. A needle is inserted below the tendon of the pectoralis major muscle adjacent to its insertion into the humerus and anterior to the axillary artery. The needle is advanced parallel to the arm and toward the coracoid process. The tip of the needle will lie first in proximity to the median nerve, as noted by a contraction of the wrist and finger flexors when a nerve stimulator is used. With additional needle advancement of approximately 1 cm, the needle tip should be near the MCN and confirmed with a visible contraction of the biceps when using a nerve stimulator. The needle should remain anterior to the axillary artery.

An alternative approach can be performed while the humerus is in abduction. The axillary artery is palpated posteriorly, and a needle is inserted perpendicular to the coracobrachialis muscle immediately posterior to the pectoralis major tendon (see Fig. 11-6). The MCN is anterior and lateral to the axillary neurovascular sheath at this location and approximately 2 cm in depth within the coracobrachialis muscle.

In patients with marked internal rotation and adduction deformities of the humerus, normal anatomic landmarks can be difficult to palpate. In this event, inadvertent injection into the axillary artery is possible, although rare. This complication can be avoided by careful palpation of the axillary pulse during advancement of the needle.

SPINAL ACCESSORY NERVE

The spinal accessory, or eleventh cranial nerve, is composed of two parts: a spinal portion that innervates the trapezius and sternocleidomastoid (SCM) muscles and an accessory portion that joins the vagus nerve. This nerve divides after its exit from the jugular foramen with the spinal portion emerging adjacent to the transverse process of the atlas. This spinal portion reaches the upper SCM muscle, later emerging from its posterior surface at the junction of the superior and middle thirds. It then traverses the posterior cervical triangle to innervate the trapezius muscle about 5 cm above the clavicle. Branches from the C3 and C4 ventral rami also innervate the trapezius muscle while those from the C2 innervate the SCM.

When these nerves are blocked, these muscles relax and can be stretched in disorders such as myofascial pain syndromes and torticollis, thus facilitating physical therapy. An anesthetic block could predict the effect of surgical denervation of the nerve or section through the muscle in cases of torticollis.

Spinal Accessory Nerve Block Technique

The spinal portion of the spinal accessory nerve can be easily blocked anywhere along its course on the posterior cervical triangle. The most common area is immediately posterior to the SCM at the junction of the middle and superior third of the muscle belly (Fig. 11-7). The needle is advanced to the depth of the posterior aspect of the SCM muscle, and 8–10 ml of solution can be injected. Only the trapezius muscle will be affected with this technique, sparing the SCM muscle.

Ramamurthy et al. have described blocking the nerve in the substance of the SCM muscle.[9] A 23-gauge, 2.5-cm needle is introduced 2–3 cm inferior to the tip of the mastoid process and advanced into the belly of the SCM. About 5–10 ml of anesthetic can be injected. This technique blocks both the SCM and trapezius muscles.

Because of the close proximity of the lesser occipital nerve to the block location when performing the injection within the substance of the SCM, this nerve is often blocked, resulting in numbness behind the ear. One should expect movement changes around the neck for the life of the anesthetic (i.e., inability to turn the neck or elevate the shoulders).

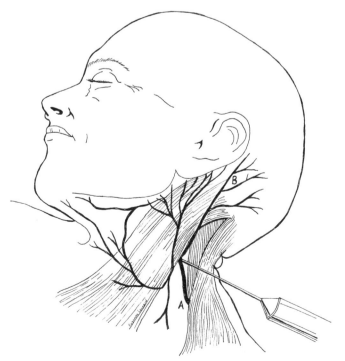

FIGURE 11-7. Block technique of the spinal accessory nerve. *A*, Spinal accessory nerve. *B*, Lesser occipital nerve. Note the proximity of the needle tip.

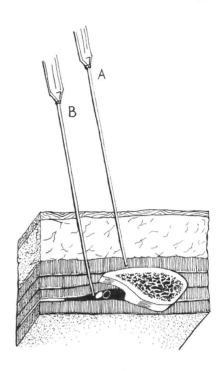

FIGURE 11-8.   Intercostal nerve block technique. Needle (*A*) initially contacts bone and is slowly moved inferior (*B*) to the subcostal groove. (Adapted from Thompson GE, Moore DC: Celiac plexus, intercostal, and minor peripheral blockade. In Cousins MJ, Bridenbaugh PO (eds): Neural Blockade in Clinical Anesthesia and Management of Pain, 2nd ed. Philadelphia, J.B. Lippincott, 1988, p 514.)

INTERCOSTAL NERVE

Intercostal nerves originate as anterior divisions of the first through twelfth thoracic spinal nerves. These paired nerves vary depending on their spinal level, but most divide into four branches. Initially, they communicate with the sympathetic chain by way of a gray rami communicans branch. Three cutaneous branches—lateral, posterior, and anterior—supply sensation to skin and nearby muscles, including the internal and external intercostal muscles. Collectively, the three branches supply sensation to the abdominal and chest wall, including breast tissue, in distinct segmental distributions. In the lower thoracic region, intercostal nerves supply motor branches to the abdominal musculature. The intercostal nerves lie in the costal groove on the inferior surface of the rib adjacent to the intercostal artery and vein.

A block of an intercostal nerve can be used to treat the pain of herpes zoster, rib fractures, and intercostal neuropathies. It can be helpful in the diagnosis of unusual abdominal or chest wall pain. In postoperative thoracotomy, physical therapy can be facilitated.

Intercostal Nerve Block Technique

With the patient semiprone or in the lateral decubitus position and the intended block region upward, the lateral mass of the paraspinal muscles is identified.

At the intersection of the rib margins and the paraspinal muscles, the lower border of the rib is palpated. Meticulous technique is required to properly locate these rib landmarks. A ¾- to 1-inch, 22- or 25-gauge needle can be inserted over the rib and directed about 20° cephalad. Longer needles may be necessary in obese patients. Once the needle contacts bone, it can be slowly walked off the inferior border of the rib. Manually retracting the skin superiorly prior to needle puncture allows the needle to automatically move inferior once the needle contacts bone. This maneuver reduces needle motion and rotation. Once the lower rib margin is identified, the needle can be advanced 2–3 mm into the subcostal groove (Fig. 11-8). About 3–5 ml of anesthetic is usually injected.

The most common problem with intercostal blocks occurs when an injection is given too superficially. This can be avoided with the correct technique and proper advancement of the needle tip. Vigorous needle advancement or probing should be avoided because of the risk of pneumothorax—the most serious complication with intercostal nerve blocks. Local absorption of anesthetics may cause systemic toxicity and can be potentially serious. Careful postprocedure monitoring is necessary to detect these complications.

SUPRAORBITAL NERVE

The supraorbital nerve (SON) originates from the frontal branch of the purely sensory ophthalmic

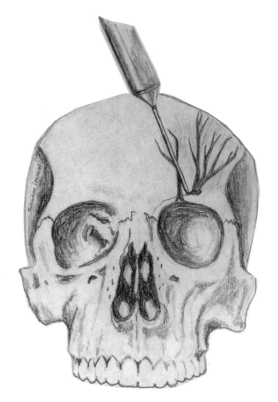

FIGURE 11-9. Block technique for the supraorbital nerve. The needle tip is adjacent to the nerve. (Adapted from Katz J (ed): Atlas of Regional Anesthesia, 2nd ed. East Norwalk, CT, Appleton & Lange, 1994, p 9.)

nerve. At the base of the orbit the frontal nerve divides into the supratrochlear and supraorbital branches. The supraorbital branch penetrates the supraorbital foramen where it gives off fibers to the upper eyelid. It ascends through the supraorbital notch where it divides into the medial and lateral terminal branches (Fig. 11-9). These terminal branches innervate the skin of the forehead as far posterior as the occiput. Other branches supply the pericranium of the frontal and parietal bones.

An SON block is useful for anesthesia for procedures involving the upper forehead region. Treatment for tic douloureux and the differential diagnosis of headaches are other uses.[2]

Supraorbital Nerve Block Technique

With the patient supine and the forehead exposed, the upper border of the orbit is identified. The supraorbital notch is located in the upper orbit adjacent to the brow, usually in a direct line above the pupil. A ⅜- or ½-inch needle of 25 or 27 gauge in diameter is directed toward the supraorbital notch. Paresthesias from the supraorbital nerve may

be encountered during needle advancement, verifying accurate placement. If bone is contacted first, the needle can be directed in a fan-like direction, and 2–4 ml of anesthetic solution is injected.

GREATER AND LESSER OCCIPITAL NERVES

The greater occipital nerve (GON) is the largest branch of the C2 dorsal ramus and curves around the border of the obliquus inferior muscle and crosses deep to the semispinalis capitis. It emerges above the superior nuchal line, about one-third of the way between the occipital protuberance and the mastoid process (Fig. 11-10). It receives communicating branches from the third occipital nerve and may send a branch to the semispinalis capitis muscle. The nerve enters the scalp above the aponeurotic sling between the SCM and trapezius muscles, thereby rendering it safe from trapezius spasm.[1] It ultimately supplies sensation to the skin of the occiput and temporal region, extending across the vertex toward the forehead and into the auricle. The posterior occipital artery accompanies the nerve in the scalp.

The lesser occipital nerve (LON) supplies sensation to the lateral occipital region, including the posterior portion of the ear. This nerve originates from the C2 and C3 ventral rami and emerges superficially at the posterior border of the upper SCM muscle (see Fig. 11-10).

Primary neuropathies of the GON have been reported but are believed to be rare causes of occipital neuralgia.[14] The pain generator in most cases of occipital neuralgia is believed to be the upper cervical facet joints; therefore, treatment directed at these structures is advocated (see chapter 28). It appears that cervical spine strains such as whiplash injuries would injure the atlantoaxial joints rather than the C2 nerves. Nevertheless, GON blocks can be performed easily at the bedside with very little risk to the patient and can help differentiate various types of headaches.[2,3,8,11]

Greater Occipital Nerve Block Technique

The patient's occipital protuberance and mastoid process are identified by palpation on the involved side of the skull. An imaginary horizontal line above the base of the skull connecting these two bony landmarks is identified. The greater occipital nerve lies on the medial third of this line. The posterior

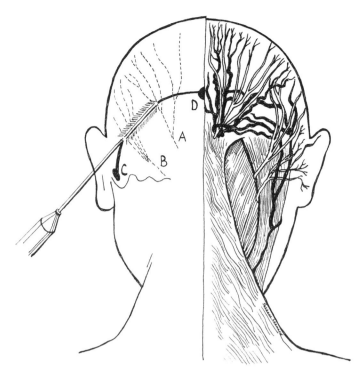

FIGURE 11-10. Block technique for the greater (A) and lesser (B) occipital nerves. Key landmarks include the mastoid process (C) and occipital protuberance (D). Note the vascularity on the right side of the head. (Adapted from Murphy TM: Somatic blockade of the head and neck. In Cousins MJ, Bridenbaugh PO (eds): Neural Blockade in Clinical Anesthesia and Management of Pain, 2nd ed. Philadelphia, J.B. Lippincott, 1988, p 552.)

occipital artery can be palpated adjacent to this nerve as it traverses the superior nuchal line. Using clean technique, a 25-gauge needle is injected into the subcutaneous tissue down to the occipital bone and is slightly withdrawn. The medication is injected in a fan-like manner medially and laterally (see Fig. 11-10). Immediate anesthesia will be noted locally and soon in the nerve's distribution.

Lesser Occipital Nerve Block Technique

Similar to the GON block, the LON can be blocked in the posterior scalp region. The imaginary line described above between the mastoid process and the occipital protuberance can be visualized. The junction of the middle and outer third of this line directly above the superior nuchal line is located. A small 25-gauge needle is advanced down to the bone, and solution is injected. Branches from the GON also will be blocked with this technique.

REFERENCES

1. Bogduk N: The anatomy of occipital neuralgia. Clin Exp Neurol 17:167–184, 1981.
2. Bovim G, Sand T: Cervicogenic headache, migraine without aura and tension-type headache: Diagnostic blockade of greater occipital and supra-orbital nerves. Pain 51:43–48, 1992.
3. Choi YK, Liu J: The use of 5% lidocaine for prolonged analgesia in chronic pain patients: A new technique. Reg Anesth 23:96–100, 1998.
4. Fouch RA, Abram SE, Hogan QH: Neural blockade for upper extremity pain. The painful hand. Hand Clin 12:791–800, 1996.
5. Granirer LW: A simple technic for suprascapular nerve block. N Y U State J Med 51:1048, 1951.
6. Meyer-Witting M, Foster JMG: Suprascapular nerve block in the management of cancer pain [letter]. Anaesthesia 47:626, 1992.
7. Moore DC: Regional Block, 4th ed. Springfield, IL, Charles C Thomas, 1965, pp 300–303.
8. Plum F: Diagnostic nerve block for headache? [abstract and commentary]. Neurology Alert, (Jan):33–34, 1993.
9. Ramamurthy S, Akkineni S, Winnie A: A simple technique for block of the spinal accessory nerve. Anesth Analg 57:591–593, 1978.
10. Risdall JE, Sharwood-Smith GH: Suprascapular nerve block. New indications and a safer technique [letter]. Anaesthesia 47:626, 1992.
11. Sanchez CA: Nerve blocks for the relief of chronic headaches [abstract]. Reg Anesth 18:45, 1993.
12. Torres-Ramos FM, Biundo JJ: Suprascapular neuropathy during progressive resistive exercises in a cardiac rehabilitation program. Arch Phys Med Rehabil 73:1107–1111, 1992.
13. Wassef MR: Suprascapular nerve block: A new approach for the management of frozen shoulder. Anaesthesia 47:120–124, 1992.
14. Weinberger LM: Cervico-occipital pain and its surgical treatment: The myth of the bony millstones. Am J Surg 135:243–247, 1978.

12

Arm, Forearm, and Hand Blocks

Charles C. Mauldin, M.D., and D. Wayne Brooks, M.D.

Arm, forearm, and hand blocks require meticulous technique and can be challenging to those unfamiliar with the regional anatomy. Blocks in this region generally should be performed with small, short bevel needles with the least volume of solution necessary. Electrical stimulation at the surface or needle tip is often helpful to minimize probing and volume injected, especially with deep injections. One must be familiar with the common anatomic variations[23] of the upper extremity in order to understand the otherwise unexpected result that may be seen with these blocks.

This chapter explains common approaches to arm, forearm, and hand blocks commonly performed in clinical practice. Volumes indicated in this chapter are for anesthetic solutions alone; volumes of corticosteroids usually are lower.

CUTANEOUS NERVES OF THE FOREARM

Sensation to the forearm is supplied by three nerves: the medial (MACN), lateral (LACN), and posterior (PACN) antebrachial cutaneous nerves. Diagnostic blocks to these nerves often are used because their distributions overlap significantly, interfering with the clinical diagnosis. Neuropathies involving these cutaneous nerves can occur spontaneously or secondary to acute or repetitive injury. Initial conservative management may include injections of these nerves at the site of inflammation with corticosteroid and/or anesthetic solution, which often hastens resolution.[1] Chemical neurolysis may be considered for more permanent relief of painful neuropathy.

Medial Antebrachial Cutaneous Nerve

The MACN carries fibers from the C8 and T1 roots via the medial cord of the brachial plexus. At the junction of the middle and lower third of the medial arm, the nerve exits the deep fascia between the biceps and triceps muscles and is accompanied

by the basilic vein. The MACN then divides into its anterior and ulnar branches, ultimately supplying sensation to the medial forearm.

Medial Antebrachial Cutaneous Nerve Block Technique

With the medial arm exposed, mark the midpoint between the biceps tendon and the medial epicondyle at the elbow crease. Insert a needle subcutaneously at a point approximately 5–6 cm superior to the mark along the inferomedial border of the biceps muscle. Figure 12-1 shows an alternative localizing procedure. Inject 5–7 ml of solution with a $\frac{5}{8}$-inch, 25- to 27-gauge needle in a fan-like manner anterior to posterior across the path of the nerve. An inadequate block will occur if the injection is given beneath the brachial fascia.

Lateral Antebrachial Cutaneous Nerve

The LACN is derived from the C5 and C6 spinal roots and is the terminal cutaneous branch of the musculocutaneous nerve. At the elbow, the LACN runs under the lateral border of the biceps beneath the deep brachial fascia on top of the brachialis muscle. The nerve courses the antecubital fossa and becomes subcutaneous as it pierces the brachial fascia lateral to the biceps tendon at the elbow crease.[1] The nerve often pierces the brachial fascia 5–10 cm above the elbow crease. At the subcutaneous level, it divides into the anterior and posterior branches, supplying sensation to the skin of the lateral forearm.

Lateral Antebrachial Cutaneous Nerve Block Technique

With the elbow extended, mark the intersection of the elbow crease and biceps tendon. Insert the needle subcutaneously just lateral to the mark, and inject 3–5 ml of solution with a 1-inch, 25- to 27-gauge needle. As an alternative, a subcutaneous

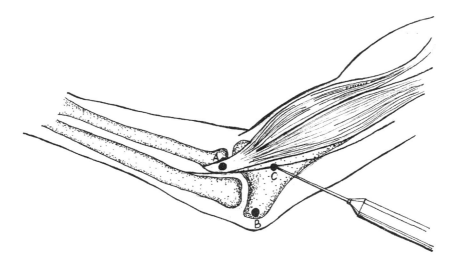

FIGURE 12-1. Medial antebrachial cutaneous nerve block. Inject (C) in the location that forms an equilateral triangle with the medial biceps tendon (A) and the medial epicondyle (B). The elbow should be in about 45° of flexion for the procedure.

field block can be performed extending from where the biceps tendon inserts into the radius to approximately two-thirds the distance to the lateral epicondyle.

An inadequate block results if the solution is injected on the wrong side of the brachial fascia. This easily can occur when one considers the exit point variability of the LAC nerve from the brachial fascia. Blocks of this nerve above the elbow crease could be made just deep to the fascia and subcutaneous with the same needle insertion to help ensure that the nerve is infiltrated.[25] Many subcutaneous vessels lie in this area, and care should be taken to avoid intravascular injection.

Posterior Antebrachial Cutaneous Nerve

The PACN originates from the radial nerve at the level of the humeral spiral groove, carrying fibers from the C5–C8 nerve roots. The nerve passes through the brachial fascia about 8 cm above the elbow and descends behind the lateral epicondyle of the humerus, where it often becomes palpable. The PACN supplies sensation to the skin of the posterior forearm proximally to the wrist.

Posterior Antebrachial Cutaneous Nerve Block Technique

With the patient's posterior arm exposed, insert a 2-inch, 25-gauge needle perpendicular to the skin directly over the lateral epicondyle, and infiltration of 3–5 ml is made subcutaneously extending 2–3 cm toward the olecranon.

MEDIAN NERVE

The median nerve innervates the muscles of the forearm flexor group, excluding the flexor carpi ulnaris and ulnar portion of the flexor digitorum profundus. In the hand, the nerve normally supplies the lumbricales to the index and middle fingers and all the muscles of the thenar eminence except for a portion of the flexor pollicis brevis. On the palmar surface, its normal cutaneous innervation includes the medial part of the thenar eminence, the central depressed area of the palm, and the lateral 3½ digits. Dorsally, its distribution of sensation includes the distal phalanges and the nail beds of the lateral 3½ digits.

Median Nerve at the Elbow

The median nerve arises from the union of the medial and lateral cords in the axilla and is supplied by the C5–T1 spinal roots. The nerve leaves the axilla and descends the arm adjacent to the brachial artery. At the elbow, the nerve lies just medial to the brachial artery. This artery divides into its ulnar and radial branches high in the arm in 15% of people,[23] thereby distorting normal anatomic landmarks. At the flexor crease, the nerve passes midway between the medial epicondyle and the biceps tendon. In the forearm, the nerve innervates the pronator teres muscle before passing through its two heads.

Median Nerve Block Technique at the Elbow

With the elbow extended, mark the intersection of the elbow crease and the biceps tendon. Just superior and medial to this mark, palpate the brachial artery. While palpating the artery to avoid intravascular injection, a 1½-inch, 23- to 25-gauge needle is inserted subcutaneously just medial to the artery. Once through the skin, direct the needle slightly lateral and advance it slowly toward the nerve to a depth slightly deeper than the artery. If desired, use a nerve stimulator while observing for wrist and finger flexion to ensure close proximity of the nerve. A median nerve block at the elbow level will affect all of the median innervated muscles and its entire cutaneous distribution.

Median Nerve at the Pronator Teres Muscle

The median nerve can become entrapped as it passes through the two heads of the pronator muscle, causing a neuropathy commonly referred to as the pronator syndrome. This syndrome also may be caused by a thickened lacertus fibrosus, by a thickened flexor superficialis arch, and by the median nerve passing below the pronator heads.[5,11,21] The symptoms and findings of the pronator syndrome vary and are often vague, with the most consistent finding being tenderness over the pronator muscle.[5,11,21] Any portion of the median nerve can be affected, but the anterior interosseous nerve branch is usually spared.[21]

Median Nerve Block Technique at the Pronator Teres Muscle

At the elbow crease make a mark at the midpoint between the medial epicondyle and the biceps tendon. Insert a 1½-inch, 23- to 25-gauge needle into the pronator teres muscle approximately 2–2.5 cm below the mark or at the point of maximal tenderness in the muscle (Fig. 12-2). Confirm needle placement using a nerve stimulator to provoke contractions of the wrist and finger flexors, and inject 3–5 ml of solution. If using a nerve stimulator, direct stimulation of the pronator teres muscle will occur, erroneously suggesting the needle tip is close to the median nerve. A block at this site can affect all median motor and sensory innervations.

When using corticosteroid solutions for the treatment of pronator syndrome, perform the injection in a fan-like manner, superior to inferior, to improve the likelihood the solution contacts the area of compression. The proximity of the needle tip to the nerve should be rechecked with the stimulator each time the needle is repositioned.

Anterior Interosseous Nerve

The anterior interosseous nerve (AIN) is the largest branch of the median nerve. In the cubital fossa, the AIN branch arises posteriorly soon after the median nerve passes between the two heads of the pronator teres. It descends on the volar surface of the interosseous membrane along with the anterior interosseous branch of the ulnar artery. Near its origin, the AIN supplies branches to the radial portion of the flexor digitorum profundus (FDP) muscle. Descending toward the wrist, the nerve innervates the flexor pollicis longus (FPL) and pronator quadratus (PQ) muscles and then terminates in articular branches to the wrist and intercarpal joints.

Anterior interosseous nerve syndrome is an entrapment neuropathy that causes weakness in the FDP, FPL, and PQ muscles. Injury to the terminal

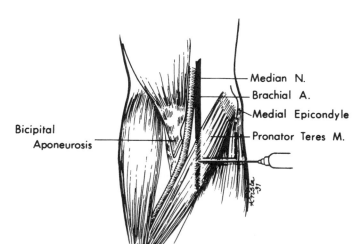

Bicipital
Aponeurosis

Median N.
Brachial A.
Medial Epicondyle
Pronator Teres M.

FIGURE 12-2. Median nerve block at the pronator teres muscle. Note the relationship between the nerve and artery above the elbow in reference to blocks at that site.

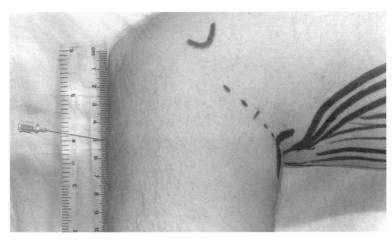

FIGURE 12-3. Needle entry site for proximal anterior interosseous nerve block. The first muscle penetrated is the flexor digitorum profundus.

sensory fibers can cause dull aching volar wrist pain.[6] An extensive list of etiologies of AIN syndrome has been described by Wertsch.[26]

Proximal Anterior Interosseous Nerve Block Technique

With the posterior elbow exposed and the forearm in neutral rotation, mark the skin over the posteromedial aspect of the ulna approximately 5 cm distal to the tip of the olecranon (Fig. 12-3). Insert a 2-inch, 25-gauge needle just medial to the mark at a depth of about 3.5 to 5 cm, directing it toward the biceps tendon insertion at the radius. The needle should be in the AIN innervated portion of the FDP. A nerve stimulator is essential with this technique and after needle position is verified, 3–5 ml of solution can be injected.

Phenol nerve blocks of the AIN for flexor spasticity of the hand should not cause paresthesias. Care must be taken to avoid accidental injection of the main branch of the median nerve (Fig. 12-4). Stimulation of the main branch of the median nerve at this level would cause flexion of digits 2 through 5, flexion of the wrist, and paresthesias in the median cutaneous distribution, but it would not activate the PQ muscle. As an alternative approach, the main branch of the median nerve could be initially located with deeper needle penetration and the AIN found with gentle needle withdrawal while using a nerve stimulator.

In 30% of people, the AIN will innervate the flexor digitorum superficialis muscle.[21] A Martin-Gruber median-to-ulnar anastomosis usually arises from the AIN,[21] and blocks in this situation may affect intrinsic hand muscles, which may not be desired. Because of these abnormalities, temporary blocks with anesthetic agents should be performed before any chemical neurolysis.

Distal Anterior Interosseous Nerve Block Technique

With the patient's dorsal forearm exposed, make a mark on the skin at the point between the middle and distal thirds along a line from the olecranon to the radial styloid process. At the mark, insert a 2-inch, 25-gauge needle and advance it until it is between the radius and ulna bones. The needle tip will be in close proximity to the AIN as soon as the interosseous membrane is pierced (Fig. 12-5). Determine proximity by using a nerve stimulator and observing for PQ contraction. The patient may also complain of an aching pain in the volar wrist. If

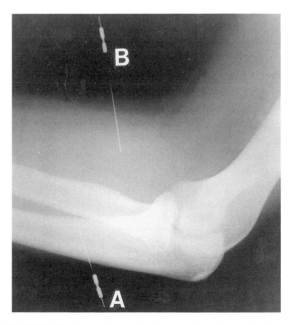

FIGURE 12-4. Radiograph showing the relationship between the anterior interosseous (A) and the median nerve (B). The needle tip is adjacent to the corresponding nerve and was confirmed by nerve stimulation.

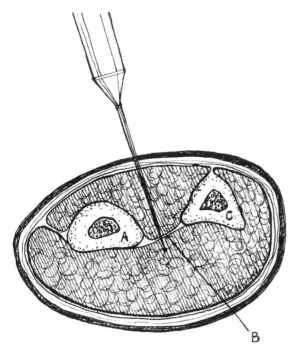

FIGURE 12-5. Distal anterior interosseous nerve block. After carefully avoiding extensor tendons, direct the needle between the radius (*A*) and the ulna (*C*). Puncture of the interosseous membrane (*B*) usually can be felt.

the needle is positioned too deep, the electrical stimulation will cause thumb flexion; if too superficial, it will cause finger and/or wrist extension. Take care to avoid penetrating the extensor tendons and to avoid injecting into the anterior or posterior interosseous vessels. Inject 5 ml of solution after maximal PQ contraction is obtained. Blocking the distal AIN from a volar approach has been described but can be more difficult due to the increased number of tendons and vessels that may be encountered. A distal AIN block can be useful when evaluating difficult volar wrist pain.

Median Nerve at the Wrist

At the wrist, the median nerve is invested by the ulnar bursa and is accompanied by the tendons of the FPL, FDP, and the flexor digitorum superficialis (FDS) muscles. It travels between but deep to the flexor carpi radialis (FCR) and palmaris longus (PL) tendons. The nerve is usually the most superficial structure coursing beneath the flexor retinaculum in the area referred to as the carpal tunnel.

Median nerve blocks at the wrist usually are indicated for the treatment of carpal tunnel syndrome (CTS), but they also may be used to treat pain in a median nerve distribution within the

hand. Conservative treatment of CTS, including corticosteroid injections, splinting, and activity modification, has been used for more than 40 years.[18] In general, CTS that exhibits mild, intermittent signs and symptoms of short duration usually responds well to conservative treatment.[16,17,24] However, advanced cases of CTS—with constant symptoms, weakness, atrophy, and electromyographic evidence of denervation—are unlikely to respond to this form of treatment.[5]

Median Nerve Block Technique at the Wrist

Although the injections are commonly referred to as carpal tunnel injections, solution is actually injected into the ulnar bursa proximal to the carpal tunnel. Many injection techniques have been described for treating CTS.[3,12,14]

With the patient's forearm supinated, insert a ⅝-inch, 27-gauge needle proximal to the distal wrist crease and ulnar to the PL tendon. About 2–20% of people lack a PL muscle,[23] and in such cases the midpoint between the ulna and radial styloid processes can be used as a reference point. Direct the needle dorsally and angle it 30° distally to a depth of about ⅝ inches

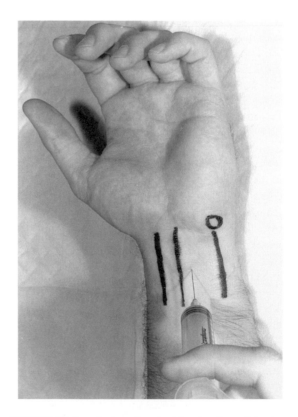

FIGURE 12-6. Preferred method for ulnar bursa injection. Needle puncture is just ulnar to the palmaris longus tendon. The circle is over the pisiform bone.

or upon contact with a tendon. Confirm placement by moving the needle with gentle passive finger extension. Inject 2 ml of volume slowly, and then use active finger flexion and extension for 1–2 minutes to distribute the solution throughout the ulna bursa[14] (Figs. 12-6 and 12-7). Increased pain during injection is rare and should alert the physician to abnormal needle placement.

An alternative technique involves inserting a 1½-inch, 25-gauge needle 1 cm proximal to the distal wrist crease, ulnar to the PL tendon. The needle is angled 45–60° distally and is advanced 1 cm until it pierces the flexor retinaculum. Solution is injected after advancement of the needle an additional 1 cm. With this technique, the injection should occur under the transverse carpal ligament. This technique causes pain when the nerve is injected or when the additional volume is not tolerated in a space that is already too tight. If significant pain is encountered that cannot be controlled by very slow injection and changes in needle placement, the procedure should be abandoned. Anesthetics should not be used to dilute the corticosteroid so that nerve injection can clearly be recognized. Numbness, however, is anticipated from this injection and serves to prove proper placement. It usually lasts no more than 2 hours.

Local tenderness and superficial hematomas at the injection site are common after carpal tunnel injections. Intraneural corticosteroid injections that cause nerve damage requiring surgical debridement have been reported.[8] Persisting or worsening pain and numbness or swelling that lasts more than 48 hours after injection indicates that nerve injection or neurotoxic injury is likely.[12,22]

Recurrent Motor Branch of the Median Nerve

The median nerve enters the palm under the flexor retinaculum radial to the PL tendon and gives off the recurrent motor branch just distal to the transverse carpal ligaments, but occasionally it pierces through the ligament. Although there are many variations, most commonly the recurrent motor branch innervates the abductor pollicis brevis, opponens pollicis, and superficial head of the flexor pollicis brevis (Fig. 12-8).

A block of the recurrent motor branch can be used to help evaluate and treat thumb-in-hand spasticity. This block can potentially affect other intrinsic hand muscles if the patient has a Riche-Cannieu anastomosis between the recurrent branch of the median and the deep branch of the ulnar nerve or if there are other anatomic variations.

Recurrent Motor Branch Block Technique

With the patient's palm positioned upward, make a mark at the intersection of the radial border of the third metacarpal and Kaplan's cardinal line. This line is parallel to the proximal palmar crease beginning at the apex of the first web space. Use a nerve stimulator to localize the nerve, observing for opposition, abduction, and proximal phalanx flexion movements of the thumb. Slowly insert a 1-inch, 25- to 27-gauge needle, and inject 2 ml of solution.

ULNAR NERVE

The ulnar nerve innervates the majority of intrinsic hand muscles, excluding the median innervated thenar and the two most radial lumbrical muscles. In the forearm, the ulnar nerve supplies the flexor carpi ulnaris and ulnar portion of the flexor digitorum profundus muscles. Its cutaneous distribution is to the ulnar aspect of the distal forearm, wrist, and hand. In the hand on the volar surface, the ulnar nerve supplies sensation to the ulnar aspect of the

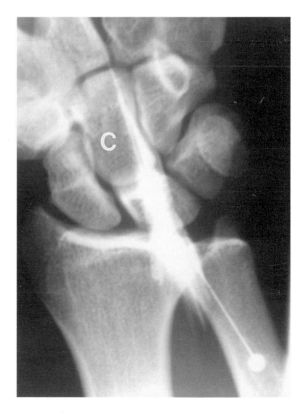

FIGURE 12-7. Radiograph showing free flow of dye as far as the distal capitate bone (C) after ulnar bursa injection of 1.5 ml.

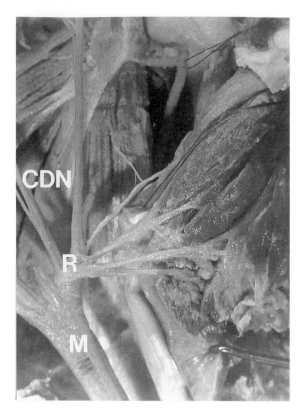

FIGURE 12-8. The recurrent thenar branches (*R*) arising from the median nerve (*M*) just distal to the transverse carpal ligament (removed). The proximity of the common digital nerve to the thumb (*CDN*) is of concern in neurolytic blocks (From Zancolli EA, Cozzi EP: Atlas of Surgical Anatomy of the Hand. New York, Churchill Livingstone, 1992, pp 263–325, with permission.)

palm and the entire fifth and ulnar half of the fourth digits. Dorsally, the nerve supplies sensation to the medial aspect of the hand, the entire fifth finger, the entire fourth finger except for the radial aspect of the distal phalanx, and the ulnar one-half of the middle finger to about the distal interphalangeal joint. There is no site along the nerve where selective blocks of motor branches can be achieved without potentially affecting sensation.

Blocks of the ulnar nerve are used as part of conservative treatment of mild compression or entrapment neuropathies at the elbow and wrist.[17] Acute or subacute compression neuropathies—as seen from trauma to the elbow or to more prolonged compression during a phase of illness or anesthesia—or entrapment at the cubital tunnel or Guyon's canal usually respond well to conservative care.[6a] Chronic ulnar neuropathies and those associated with intrinsic atrophy and denervation on electromyographic studies will not respond well to conservative treatment.

Ulnar Nerve at the Elbow

The ulnar nerve is formed from the C8 and T1 spinal roots and is the major terminal branch of the medial cord of the brachial plexus. At the elbow, the nerve travels between the borders of the triceps and brachialis muscles, soon emerging to lie within the ulnar groove where it becomes palpable. The nerve descends through the cubital tunnel that is formed by the fibroaponeurotic triangular or arcuate ligament, two heads of the flexor carpi ulnaris (FCU), and the medial collateral ligament. An ulnar nerve branch to the FCU muscle runs adjacent to the main nerve in the groove and rarely is involved in neuropathies at the elbow.

Ulnar Nerve Block Technique at the Elbow

With the patient's medial arm and elbow exposed, mark the ulnar nerve between the triceps and brachialis muscle approximately 5 cm above the medial epicondyle (Fig. 12-9). It should be on a line between the epicondyle and the apex of the axilla. Insert a 1–2-inch, 25-gauge needle subcutaneously at this point perpendicular to the humerus. If the nerve is not palpable, inject (beneath the subcutaneous fat) in a fan-like manner across the expected path of the nerve, or use a nerve stimulator and observe for wrist flexion and intrinsic hand

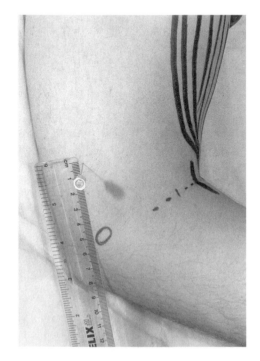

FIGURE 12-9. Ulnar nerve block above the elbow. The circle is over the medial epicondyle.

movements to assure close proximity to the nerve. In either case, inject 5–8 ml of solution.

An alternative ulnar nerve block may be performed within the ulnar groove. With the patient's posteromedial elbow exposed, palpate and mark the medial epicondyle. While pinching and retracting the redundant skin over the groove, insert the needle at the medial epicondyle, aiming just below and anterior to the tip of the olecranon. As an alternative, one can gently stabilize the nerve between a finger and the olecranon and insert a needle subcutaneously between the finger and the medial epicondyle.

While in the groove, the ulnar nerve is tightly confined, thereby increasing the risk of injury at this site. Injections at this site should be reserved for corticosteroid solutions for treatment of compression neuropathies, both within the groove and cubital tunnel. Injection solution should be limited to less than 5 ml. Limiting the use of anesthetic agents in the groove, which could mask paresthesias, also will reduce the risk of nerve injury.

An ulnar nerve block above the ulnar groove is considered safer than within the groove. In this location, less risk of direct nerve injury by the needle and greater volumes of solutions, including anesthetic agents, can be safely used. Blocks from the ulnar groove and above will affect the entire motor and sensory distribution of the nerve. Because the sensory distribution of the ulnar nerve is at the wrist and hand, anesthetic blocks need not be performed at the elbow unless block of the dorsal ulnar cutaneous nerve distribution is necessary.

Ulnar Nerve at the Wrist

At the wrist, the ulnar nerve lies directly below the tendon of the FCU just proximal to the pisiform bone. At this point, the nerve lies on the ulnar side of and deep to the ulnar artery. The nerve at this level has given off its palmar and dorsal cutaneous branches. As the nerve passes radial to the pisiform, it enters the ulnar tunnel, commonly referred to as Guyon's canal. The borders of this canal are the pisiform bone medially and proximally and the hook of the hamate bone laterally and distally. The roof is formed by the thickening of the deep forearm fascia and the floor by the thick transverse carpal ligament. Within the canal, the nerve bifurcates into its terminal deep (motor) and the superficial (sensory) branches. The ulnar artery travels through the canal with the nerve. The deep branch supplies the muscles of the hypothenar compartment, the interosseous muscles, the medial two

lumbricals, the adductor pollicis, and a portion of the flexor pollicis brevis. The superficial branch supplies the palmaris brevis and digital sensory branches to the fifth finger and the ulnar half of the fourth finger.

Ulnar Nerve Block Technique at the Wrist

Ulnar nerve block at the wrist is more reliable and carries fewer risks of complications than a block at the elbow. With the volar wrist exposed, palpate and mark the pisiform bone and FCU tendon. The ulnar nerve can be blocked from either a volar or ulnar approach.

With the volar approach, insert a 1-inch, 25- to 27-gauge needle to either side of the FCU tendon about 1 cm proximal to the pisiform bone. Inject 2–5 ml of solution into the tissue between the tendon and the distal ulna.

With the ulnar approach, introduce a similar size needle subcutaneously at the medial wrist and direct it radially until the needle tip lies under the FCU tendon. Inject 2–5 ml of solution. The needle can be withdrawn and repositioned subcutaneously and an additional 1–2 ml of solution can be injected on the ulnar side and well onto the dorsum of the wrist. This blocks the dorsal cutaneous branch of the ulnar nerve. With the ulnar approach, there is a reduced chance of puncturing the ulnar artery in comparison to the volar approach. However, if the needle is inserted anterior to the neurovascular bundle and thus anterior to the thick fascial layer, the block may be ineffective (Fig. 12-10).

Ulnar Nerve Block Technique at Guyon's Canal

First, palpate and mark the pisiform bone and the hook of the hamate. The motor branch of the nerve may be palpable in the canal between these marks. Insert a 2-inch, 25-gauge needle at the distal wrist crease to the radial side of the pisiform bone and angled sharply distally so that its tip lies just ulnar to the palpable hook of the hamate (Figs. 12-10 and 12-11). Inject 1 ml of solution very slowly. Compression neuropathies in Guyon's canal are infrequent but are seen more often in occupations that require frequent hand tool use and in recreational activities such as biking and golf.[5] Similar to the ulnar nerve in the ulnar groove, the nerve is also in a confined space in Guyon's canal. For this reason, injections into Guyon's canal should be considered primarily for injections of corticosteroid solution for treatment of nerve compression at this site.

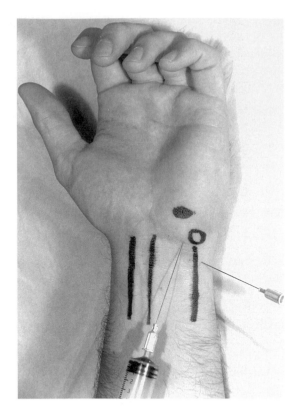

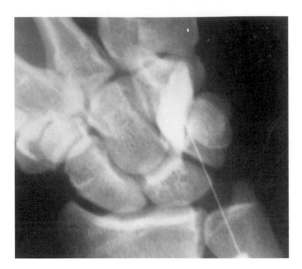

FIGURE 12-11. Radiograph showing dye pattern after injection of 1 ml into Guyon's canal by the technique shown in Figure 12-10.

FIGURE 12-10. Approaches for two ulnar nerve blocks. The needle with syringe attached demonstrates the puncture for block at Guyon's canal. The circle is over the pisiform bone and the solid mark over the hook of the hamate. The second needle demonstrates the puncture site for an ulnar nerve block at the wrist, ulnar approach.

RADIAL NERVE

The radial nerve is a terminal branch of the posterior cord of the brachial plexus formed from the C5–C8 spinal roots. The radial nerve innervates the posterior arm and forearm compartment muscles and often the lateral portion of the brachialis muscle.[21] It supplies sensation to the posterior forearm, lateral thenar eminence and dorsum of the hand, and the dorsal aspect of the lateral 2½ fingers. It also supplies articular branches to the elbow and wrist.

Distal radial neuropathies that occur near the origin of the posterior interosseous nerve (PIN), often called radial tunnel or supinator syndrome, and the superficial radial nerve near the wrist have been well described.[21] Entrapment of the distal PIN has been reported to cause dorsal wrist pain.[4] Initial management of mild radial compression neuropathies should be conservative, which can include corticosteroid injections. Pain relief after a diagnostic nerve block of the proximal PIN has been shown

to be a good indicator of a successful outcome from surgical decompression.[19]

Radial Nerve at the Arm

In the arm, the radial nerve pierces the lateral intermuscular septum approximately 10 cm above the elbow crease at the lateral side of the arm where it is prone to injury. It crosses anterior to the lateral epicondyle after lying between the brachialis and brachioradialis muscles. In the arm, the radial nerve supplies motor branches to the brachioradialis and extensor carpi radialis longus muscles. It also gives off the PACN.

Radial Nerve Block Technique at the Arm

With the patient's lateral arm exposed, locate the skin over the humerus at the point between the middle and distal one third on a line between the lateral epicondyle and the tip of the acromion process. This point lies between the muscle bellies of the biceps and triceps and is located about 15 cm proximal to the tip of the olecranon. The nerve often can be palpated in thin individuals. Insert a 1-inch, 25-gauge needle at this point, and advance it until bone is contacted. If a nerve stimulator is used, elbow flexion and wrist extension will be visualized. About 4–7 ml of solution may be injected.

A radial block at the elbow affects all radial innervated muscles except for the elbow extensors. This includes the brachioradialis, extensor carpi radialis longus and brevis, and the muscles innervated by the PIN and all radial sensory innervations.

Radial Nerve at the Elbow

In the cubital fossa, the radial nerve divides into the PIN and the superficial radial nerve between the brachialis and brachioradialis muscles. Prior to this division, motor branches to the brachioradialis (BR) and extensor carpi radialis longus (ECRL) are formed. A motor branch to the extensor carpi radialis brevis (ECRB) arises from the superficial radial nerve in most cases.[21] After giving off branches to the supinator, the PIN passes through the arcade of Frohse between the deep and superficial heads of the supinator muscle where it may become entrapped, referred to as supinator syndrome. The PIN then passes distally along the dorsum of the forearm to terminate in articular branches to the dorsum of the carpus.

Radial Nerve Block Technique at the Elbow

With the patient's anterior elbow exposed, mark a point at the elbow crease between the lateral border of the biceps tendon and the medial border of the BR muscle. The nerve is blocked as it crosses the anterior aspect of the lateral epicondyle close to the humerus (Fig. 12-12). Insert a 2-inch, 25-gauge needle at the mark and direct it posterior until bone is contacted at the lateral margin of the epicondyle. Withdraw the needle 0.5–1.0 cm and inject approximately 2 ml of solution. Withdraw the needle to the skin and redirect it slightly more medial, and advance it again until bone is contacted. The use of a nerve stimulator will prevent excessive probing and help localize the tip of the needle. Varying degrees of effect will be noted on the BR and ECRL muscles with a radial nerve block at the elbow and in the arm. The PACN should not be affected with either of these two blocks.

Posterior Interosseous Nerve Block Technique at the Elbow

Locate the most distal point of the insertion of the biceps tendon on the radius, about 2–3 cm below the elbow crease. With the forearm pronated, insert a 2-inch, 25-gauge needle 1 cm lateral to this point just medial to the BR muscle. Using a palpating finger on the posterior aspect of the ulna about 5 cm from the olecranon as a guide, advance the needle to the surface of the ulna. With the use of a nerve stimulator, the PIN can be quickly located by observing for finger extension at a low stimulus intensity. Inject 2–5 ml of solution. This block can be used in suspected cases of supinator syndrome and forearm and wrist spasticity.

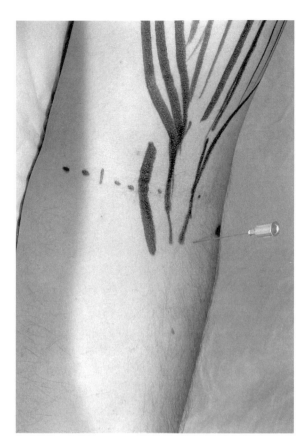

FIGURE 12-12. Radial nerve block at the supinator muscle. Note that the needle entry is between the biceps tendon and the brachioradialis muscle.

Distal Posterior Interosseous Nerve

In the dorsal forearm, the PIN emerges with the posterior interosseous artery in the interval between the deep and superficial muscles of the forearm extensor group. Lying on the dorsal aspect of the interosseous membrane, the nerve courses toward the wrist and passes deep to the extensor pollicis longus muscle. At the wrist, it terminates as a small gangliform enlargement from which branches supply the intercarpal joints.

Distal Posterior Interosseous Nerve Block Technique

With the patient's distal dorsal forearm exposed, insert a 2-inch, 25-gauge needle 3 cm proximal and 1 cm ulnar to Lister's tubercle. Slowly advance the needle to the depth of the interosseous membrane. Inject solution across the nerve's path.[4] This block can be useful when evaluating difficult pain disorders of the wrist.

Radial Nerve at the Wrist

Radial nerve blocks at the wrist are used to interrupt the terminal cutaneous branches that supply the radial side of the dorsum of the hand and the proximal parts of the radial 3½ digits. Although uncommon, isolated compression neuropathies of the cutaneous branch of the radial nerve, referred to as cheiralgia paresthetica, can occur from acute injury or from prolonged compression, i.e., watchband. Local injection of corticosteroids may be an effective treatment.

The superficial radial nerve descends to the wrist along the lateral side of the forearm behind the BR muscle. The nerve pierces the deep fascia and becomes superficial as it emerges from the posterior border of the BR just proximal to the muscle's insertion. At this location, the nerve is most likely to be injured. Once superficial, it divides into dorsal digital nerves supplying the thenar eminence, dorsum of the first, second, and the radial side of the third digit.

Superficial Radial Nerve Block Technique

With the forearm pronated, locate the anatomic snuffbox and mark its bordering tendons: extensor pollicis longus (EPL) and brevis (EPB). Take a point over the EPL tendon adjacent to the base of the first metacarpal where the nerve is often palpable. Direct the needle proximally along the tendon as far as the dorsal radial tubercle. Inject 2 ml of solution superficially. Withdraw the needle to the skin and redirect it across the snuffbox just past the EPB tendon, and inject an additional 2–3 ml of solution.

DIGITAL NERVES

Anesthetic digital blocks for minor procedures of the fingers are common. Compression neuropathies of the common digital nerves can occur at the intermetacarpal ligaments and can be treated with digital blocks. Neuropathies of proper digital nerves, sometimes referred to as digitalis paresthetica, can be caused by acute or repeated trauma; this condition is commonly known as "bowler's thumb" when it occurs in the thumb.

The common digital nerves are derived from the median and ulnar nerves and divide in the distal palm into the volar digital nerves to supply the adjacent sides of the fingers, palmar aspect, tip, and nail bed area. These main digital nerves are accompanied by the digital vessels and run on the ventromedial and ventrolateral aspects of each finger beside the flexor tendon sheath. Small dorsal digital nerves derived from the radial and ulnar nerves supply the back of the fingers as far as the distal joint. These run on the dorsomedial and dorsolateral aspect of the fingers.

Digital Nerve Block Technique

Insert a 2-inch, 25-gauge needle at a point on the dorsolateral and dorsomedial aspect of the base of the finger and direct it anteriorly to slide past the base of the phalanx. Advance the needle until noting the resistance of the palmar dermis or the pressure on a "protective" finger placed under the patient's finger and directly opposite the needle path. Inject about 1 ml of solution while withdrawing the needle 2–3 mm to block the volar nerve, and inject 0.5–1 ml just under the point of entry to block the dorsal nerve. The volar digital nerves can also be approached from the sides of the finger, which is useful for index and little fingers and is less painful.

An alternative technique is to block the digits from the bifurcation of the common digital nerve at the metacarpal heads. With the fingers widely abducted, insert the needle into the web 2–3 mm dorsal to the junction of the web and palmar skin. Direct the needle straight back toward the hand in line with the extended fingers to a depth of about 1.5 cm, and inject 1–2 ml of solution. Redirection to block the dorsal nerves can easily be performed from the same point of entry.

A new single injection technique appears to be a simple and effective option for anesthesia of the volar digital nerves.[13] Two milliliters of anesthetic are injected subcutaneously over the flexor tendon just distal to the A-1 pulley. Dorsal digital nerve block may occur as well.

A thumb block can be performed by blocking the radial and median nerves at the wrist or with a circumferential infiltration block or "ring block." Another option for the median portion of the block is to inject the common digital nerve to the thumb with a single injection in the palm. With the thumb in palmar abduction, enter the skin in the fascial plane between the flexor pollicis brevis and the adductor pollicis 1–2 cm proximal to the margin of the skin web. Direct a 1-inch, 25- to 27-gauge needle toward the medial margin of the first metacarpal somewhat perpendicular to the skin at the site of entry and gently advance it until its tip rests upon the palmar fascia. Inject 1–2 ml of solution.

These described blocks are for anesthesia. If using corticosteroids, direct the injection at the site of compression or palpable neuroma. The use of epinephrine with digital blocks is not advised.

REFERENCES

1. Bassett FH, Nunley JA: Compression of the musculocutaneous nerve at the elbow. J Bone Joint Surg 64A:1050–1052, 1982.
2. Bonica JJ: Causalgia and other reflex sympathetic dystrophies. In Bonica JJ (ed): The Management of Pain. Philadelphia, Lea & Febiger, 1990, pp 220–241.
3. Bridenbaugh LD: The upper extremity: Somatic blockade. In Cousins MJ, Bridenbaugh PO (eds): Neural Blockade in Clinical Anesthesia and Management of Pain, 2nd ed. Philadelphia, J.B. Lippincott, 1988, pp 387–417.
4. Carr D, Davis P: Distal posterior interosseous nerve syndrome. J Hand Surg 10A:873–878, 1985.
5. Dawson DM, Hallett M, Millender LH (eds): Entrapment Neuropathies, 2nd ed. Boston, Little, Brown & Co., 1990, pp 64–67.
6. Dellon AL, MacKinnon SE, Daneshvar A: Terminal branch of anterior interosseous nerve as source of wrist pain. J Hand Surg 9B:316–322, 1984.
6a. Dellon AL, Hament W, Gittelshon A: Nonoperative management of cubital tunnel syndrome. Neurology 43:1673–1677, 1993.
7. Ditmars DM Jr: Local and regional block anesthesia for the upper extremity. In Kasdan ML (ed): Occupational Hand and Upper Extremity Injury and Diseases. Philadelphia, Hanley & Belfus, 1991, pp 143–153.
8. Frederick HA, Carter PR, Littler JW: Injection injuries to the median and the ulnar nerves at the wrist. J Hand Surg 17A:645–647, 1992.
9. Giannini F: Electrophysiologic evaluation of local steroid injection in carpal tunnel syndrome. Arch Phys Med Rehabil 72:738–742, 1991.
10. Gutman L: AAEM minimonograph #2: Important anomalous innervations of the extremities. Muscle Nerve 16:339–347, 1993.
11. Hartz CR, Linscheid RL, Gramse RR, Daube JR: The pronator syndrome: Compressive neuropathy of the nerve. J Bone Joint Surg 63A:885–890, 1981.
12. Kasten SJ, Louis DS: Carpal tunnel syndrome: A case of median nerve injection injury and a safe and effective method for injecting the carpal tunnel. J Fam Pract 43:79–82, 1996.
13. Low CK, Vartany A, Engstrom JW, et al: Comparison of transthecal and subcutaneous single-injection digital block techniques. J Hand Surg 22A:901–905, 1997.
14. Minamikawa Y, Peimer CA, Kambe K, et al: Tenosynovial injection for carpal tunnel syndrome. J Hand Surg 17A:178–181, 1992.
15. Olson IA: The origin of the lateral cutaneous nerve of forearm and its anesthesia for modified brachial plexus block. J Anat 105:381–382, 1969.
16. Özdogan H, Yazici H: The efficacy of local steroid injections in idiopathic carpal tunnel syndrome: A double-blind study. Brit J Rheumatol 23:272–275, 1984.
17. Pechan J, Kredba J: Treatment of cubital tunnel syndrome by means of local administration of corticosteroids: II. Long-term follow-up. Acta Univ Carol [Med] (Praha) 26:135–140, 1980.
18. Phalen GS: The carpal-tunnel syndrome: Seventeen years experience in diagnosis and treatment of six hundred forty-four hands. J Bone Joint Surg 48A:211–228, 1966.
19. Ritts GD, Wood MB, Linscheid RL: Radial tunnel syndrome. Clin Orthop 219:201–205, 1987.
20. Rosenbaum RB, Ochoa JL: Nonsurgical treatment of carpal tunnel syndrome. In Rosenbaum RB, Ochoa JL (eds): Carpal Tunnel Syndrome and Other Disorders of the Median Nerve. Boston, Butterworth-Heinemann, 1993, pp 251–256.
21. Spinner M: Injuries to the Major Branches of Peripheral Nerves of the Forearm. Philadelphia, W.B. Saunders, 1978, pp 162–192.
22. Tavares SP, Giddins GEB: Nerve injury following steroid injection for carpal tunnel syndrome. J Hand Surg 21B:208–209, 1996.
23. Tountas CP, Bergman RA: Anatomic Variations of the Upper Extremity. New York, Churchill Livingstone, 1993, pp 211–240.
24. Urbaniak JR, Desai SS: Complications of nonoperative and operative treatment of carpal tunnel syndrome. Hand Clin 12:325–335, 1996.
25. Visconi CM, Reese J, Rathmell JP: Medial and lateral antebrachial cutaneous nerve blocks. Reg Anesth 21:2–5, 1996.
26. Wertsch JJ: AAEM case report #25: Anterior interosseous nerve syndrome. Muscle Nerve 15:977–983, 1992.

13

Proximal Lower Extremity Blocks

Ted A. Lennard, M.D., and Daniel Y. Shin, M.D.

Lower extremity peripheral nerves can be selectively blocked with a good understanding of lumbar, pelvic, and gluteal anatomy. Their usefulness in practice is directed primarily toward hip and knee spasticity that affects gait patterns, sitting posture, and transfer. As with other nerve blocks, they are also useful in differentiating pain disorders and providing anesthesia for procedures in this region of the body.

SOMATIC LUMBAR NERVE BLOCK

Somatic lumbar nerves can be blocked after their exit from the intervertebral foramen outside the epidural space. This is in contrast to the selective epidural nerve root blocks discussed in chapter 30 that intentionally places medication into the epidural space. These somatic nerves innervate distal myotomes and transmit sensation to large peripheral areas. Therefore, a block at this level would be expected to affect multiple distal structures.

Meelhuysen performed phenol lumbar somatic blocks in an effort to avoid the complications of intrathecal blocks and to yield a selective effect upon spastic hip and knee flexors in paraplegics.[10] Hip flexor spasticity was treated by injecting the L2, L3, and L4 nerves. Knee flexor spasticity was treated by injecting the L5 and S1 nerves. Each nerve was blocked at its emergence from the intervertebral foramen using a nerve stimulator. Of the 31 blocks, 21 yielded partial muscle relaxation with electrical evidence of denervation.

Lumbar somatic nerve blocks are technically more cumbersome than intrathecal procedures but have the advantage of high selectivity. A single paravertebral nerve block may result in loss of spasticity in several different muscle groups and changes in sensation in the corresponding dermatome.

Technique

The lumbar somatic nerves can be blocked with the patient in the prone or the lateral decubitus position with the intended block side up. The patient's lumbar spinous processes are palpated and marked on the skin. A horizontal line is extended 3 cm lateral from the superior edge of the spinous process. This line corresponds with the transverse process. A needle is directed perpendicular to the skin at the end of this line and advanced until the transverse process is contacted (Fig. 13-1). Once bone is contacted, the needled is slid over the superior surface of the transverse process and advanced an additional 2–4 cm. The lumbar somatic nerve can be blocked at this location with 3–7 ml of solution, depending on the agent injected. If precise diagnostic information is desired, only 1–2 ml of solution may be required.

Alternatives to somatic blocks to control hip flexor spasticity can be performed by blocking the direct innervation to the psoas major muscle. The femoral nerve not only innervates this muscle, but also directs spinal branches from the L2 and L3 spinal nerves (Fig. 13-2). These latter nerves can be blocked within the L4 and L5 interspaces. A needle is inserted 1 cm medial to the tip of both the L4 and L5 transverse processes and advanced 1–2 cm (Fig. 13-3). The nerve to the psoas major muscle lies immediately anterior to this point. The L2 and L3 nerve fibers contributing to the femoral nerve pass posterolateral to these nerves to the psoas muscle, and the fibers supplying the obturator nerve are located posteromedially (Fig. 13-4). When using a nerve stimulator, if contraction of the quadriceps muscle is observed during a block of these spinal nerves to the psoas major muscle, the needle should be withdrawn and redirected anteromedially.

Control of hip flexor spasticity originating from the psoas major muscle also may be accomplished by injecting solution directly into the psoas muscle.

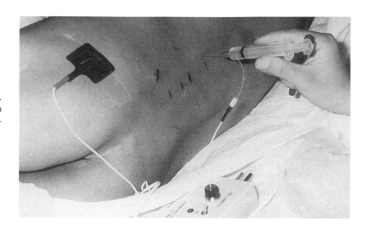

FIGURE 13-1. Lumbar somatic nerve block. The needle is placed approximately 3 cm lateral to the spinous process and advanced about 3 cm anterior to the transverse process.

This technique requires an excellent knowledge of lumbar and pelvic anatomy to avoid inadvertent needle placement into the abdominal peritoneum or adjacent vascular structures. Fluoroscopic or electromyographic (EMG) needle guidance may be helpful to determine needle depth to prevent these complications. Koyama et al. performed direct psoas major and minor intramuscular phenol blocks under ultrasonic monitoring in an attempt to reduce x-ray exposure and minimize the risk of organ and vascular injury.[8] Hip range of motion improved in all patients without significant complications. This latter technique is limited to clinicians skilled in echographic anatomy.

Most complications with lumbar somatic nerve blocks, direct psoas nerve blocks, or intramuscular psoas blocks occur as a result of misplaced needles. If the needle is advanced too deep, inadvertent puncture of major blood vessels may occur, including the aorta on the left side and inferior vena cava on the right. Also, with deep injections or when using large volumes of anesthetics, sympathetic blockade may occur. If the needle is angled too far medially, a transforaminal epidural, paramedian epidural, or subarachnoid block would be possible.

ILIOHYPOGASTRIC AND ILIOINGUINAL NERVE BLOCK

The iliohypogastric and ilioinguinal nerves are branches from the first lumbar nerves. The iliohypogastric nerve emerges from the psoas major muscle and crosses obliquely anterior to the quadratus lumborum muscle. It extends toward the iliac crest where it divides into the iliac and hypogastric branches. The iliac branch supplies sensation to the gluteal region and the hypogastric branch to the hypogastric region.

The ilioinguinal nerve arises from the first lumbar nerve just below the iliohypogastric nerve.

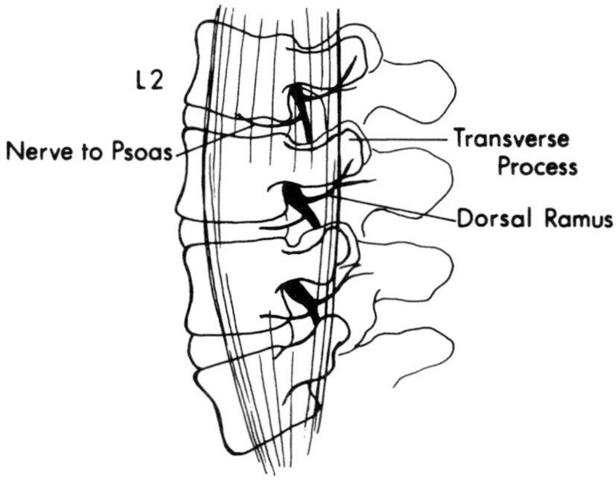

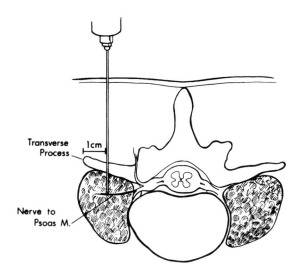

FIGURE 13-2. The direct spinal nerve branches to the psoas major muscle shown at the L2–L3 and L3–L4 intertransverse space.

FIGURE 13-3. Needle position and depth when injecting the direct spinal nerve to the psoas major muscle.

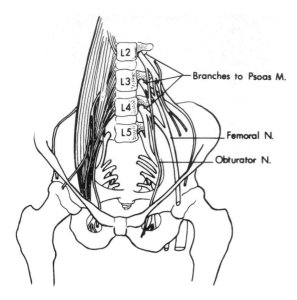

FIGURE 13-4. The lumbar plexus, branches to psoas major, and the relation of the psoas major to the femoral nerve (posterolateral) and the obturator nerve (posteromedial) at the third and fourth lumbar space.

It passes obliquely anterior not only to the quadratus lumborum muscle, but also to the iliacus muscle. The nerve innervates the internal oblique muscle and later follows the spermatic cord through the external abdominal ring. The ilioinguinal nerve ultimately supplies sensation to the proximal medial thigh, male scrotum, and female labium major.

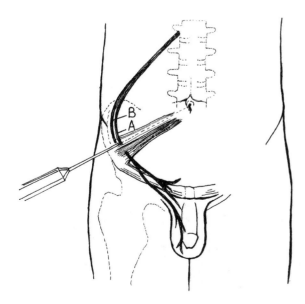

FIGURE 13-5. Block technique for the ilioinguinal (A) and iliohypogastric (B) nerve block. (Adapted from Katz J: Atlas of Regional Anesthesia, 2nd ed. East Norwalk, CT, Appleton & Lange, 1994, p 121.)

One of the primary reasons to block these nerves is to differentiate painful conditions of the medial thigh and genital regions. Treatment for primary neuropathies, entrapments, and scarring from lower abdominal surgeries such as herniorrhaphies can be other indications.

Technique

With the patient's anterior pelvis exposed, the bony landmarks of the iliac crest are identified, specifically the anterior superior iliac spine (ASIS). Two centimeters above the ASIS, a needle is injected immediately medial to the iliac crest. The needle is maintained against the iliac bone as it is advanced toward the iliacus muscle and directed medially toward the umbilicus (Fig. 13-5). With the needle tip in this position, both the ilioinguinal and iliohypogastric nerves usually can be blocked. The needle depth varies depending on the patient's size, but averages 3–5 cm.

SCIATIC NERVE BLOCK

The sciatic nerve is composed of the common peroneal and tibial nerves carrying fibers from the L4–S3 nerve roots. This nerve exits the pelvis through the greater sciatic notch just below the piriformis muscle (Fig. 13-6). It runs through the posterior thigh where it divides into the tibial and common peroneal nerves, usually within the popliteal fossa. The nerve supplies sensation to the posterior thigh, leg, and foot and motor innervation to the posterior thigh, leg, and foot muscles.

Anesthetic sciatic nerve injections are commonly used to facilitate casting of a spastic ankle or knee flexion contractures. These blocks can be used effectively to control lower extremity spasticity in patients with spinal cord injury,[4] provide anesthesia for lower extremity procedures, or assist with diagnosing lower extremity pain problems, including those at the knee.[11]

Technique

Although lateral and anterior approaches have been described to block the sciatic nerve,[3,6] the posterior approach is the most common. Labat's classic approach places the patient in the lateral decubitus position with the intended block side up.[9] The knee on the intended block side is placed in partial flexion and the heel laid to rest on the contralateral noninvolved extended extremity. One method of identifying the sciatic nerve is to extend a line between the upper aspect of the greater trochanter of the femur and the posterior superior iliac spine (PSIS). This line should coincide with the upper border of both the piriformis muscle and the sciatic notch. The sciatic nerve is located 3 cm below the midpoint of this line, where the injection site is located (Fig. 13-7).

An alternative method of locating this same injection site includes drawing a line between the greater trochanter of the femur and a point about 2 cm below the sacral hiatus. The midpoint of this line corresponds to the location of the sciatic nerve. This should also be the same spot as that located by the first line described above (Fig. 13-8). A long needle, up to 15 cm, is required to reach the sciatic nerve. When using a nerve stimulator, as the needle is advanced, a gluteus maximus muscle contraction will be observed initially. With further advancement of the needle, a knee flexion contraction should be observed as the gluteus maximus muscle contraction diminishes.

Blocking the sciatic nerve within the posterior gluteal region as described above is often difficult because of its depth. Multiple attempts at locating the nerve with frequent needle repositioning are often required. The use of Doppler ultrasound to assist with location of the sciatic nerve has been described to prevent this repeated probing.[5]

OBTURATOR NERVE BLOCK

The obturator nerve originates in the substance of the psoas major muscle from the L2–L4 spinal nerves (see Fig. 13-4). It exits the pelvis through the obturator foramen where it lies adjacent to the ob-

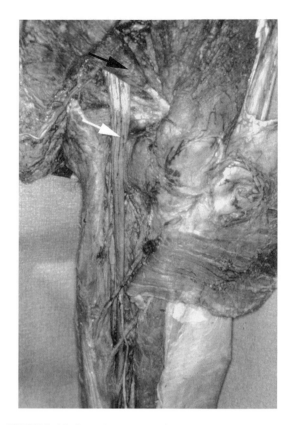

FIGURE 13-6. The course of the sciatic nerve (*white arrow*) under the piriformis muscle (*black arrow*).

turator vessels. The nerve divides into the anterior and posterior branches at the external obturator muscle. The anterior branch innervates the adductor brevis, gracilis, adductor longus, and in some cases the pectineus muscle (Fig. 13-9). It also gives a branch to the hip joint and supplies sensation to the medial thigh. The posterior branch innervates the external obturator, adductor magnus, and occasionally

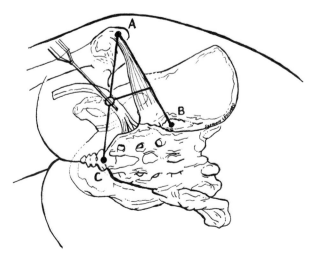

FIGURE 13-7. Landmarks for a sciatic nerve block. *A*, Greater trochanter of the femur; *B*, posterior superior iliac spine (PSIS); *C*, a point 2 cm below the sacral hiatus.

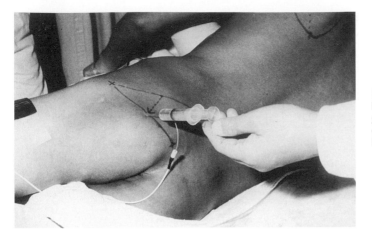

FIGURE 13-8. Landmarks for a sciatic nerve block. The upper line connects the PSIS with the greater trochanter of the femur. The lower line connects the greater trochanter with a point 2 cm below the sacral hiatus.

the adductor brevis muscles. The posterior branch often sends a branch to the knee joint. Both the anterior and posterior branches of the obturator nerve lie almost at the same sagittal plane separated by the adductor brevis muscle. The posterior branch lies at a deeper plane than the anterior branch.

The obturator nerve is frequently blocked in cases of adductor spasticity (Figs. 13-10, 13-11, and 13-12). This can facilitate perineal hygiene, positioning, and lower extremity dressing. Scissoring gait patterns can also be improved. The block also can be used to differentiate hip and knee pain.

Technique

The main branch of the obturator nerve can be blocked at its exit from the obturator foramen. A block at this level would affect both the anterior and posterior branches. The patient is first placed in the supine position with the hip abducted and externally rotated. Attempts are made to palpate the obturator foramen and nearby bony landmarks, especially the pubic tubercle, ischial tuberosity, and symphysis pubis. Delineating each of these landmarks may be difficult depending on the patient's size and any deforming hip contractures that may be present. After locating the pubic tubercle, the needle is placed in the skin 2 cm below and 2 cm lateral to this bony landmark. The needle is advanced in a slight medial direction until the bony ridge of the pubic bone is contacted. The needle is withdrawn slightly and redirected in a more superior and lateral position until the superior bony border of the obturator foramen is contacted. It is important to "walk" the needle around the superomedial border of the obturator foramen, contacting bone. This gives a good indication of the depth of the obturator nerve and vessels and avoids inadvertent puncture into organs medial and superior to this point, such as the bladder and vagina. Once the needle is in a superior position

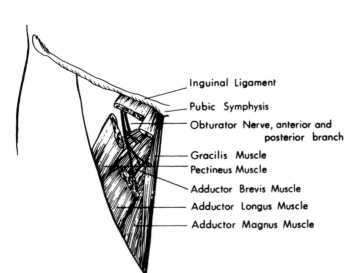

Inguinal Ligament

Pubic Symphysis

Obturator Nerve, anterior and
          posterior branch

Gracilis Muscle

Pectineus Muscle

Adductor Brevis Muscle

Adductor Longus Muscle

Adductor Magnus Muscle

FIGURE 13-9. Anterior and posterior branches of the obturator nerve. Note that these branches are separated by the adductor brevis muscle.

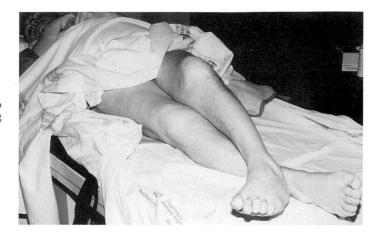

FIGURE 13-10. Adductor spasticity prior to an obturator block causes poor bed positioning and difficult perineal hygiene.

against bone, it is slowly directed posteriorly and "walked" through the obturator foramen. About 8–12 ml of solution can be injected; however, caution should be exhibited during infusion to avoid vascular injection.

An alternative approach involves blocking the anterior and posterior branches separately, but more distal. This technique can provide a more specific block while reducing the risk of vascular or organ puncture with the more proximal block. The anterior branch can be blocked by inserting a needle on the anterolateral surface of the adductor longus muscle 3–7 cm from the pubic tubercle (Fig. 13-13). The muscle bellies of the adductor longus and brevis can be "gripped" in most patients close to the pubic tubercle, thereby providing an important landmark. The needle is directed posteriorly to the adductor longus muscle and slowly advanced. It is stopped on the posterior surface of the adductor longus muscle to block the anterior branch. About 5–8 ml of anesthetic solution can be injected. The needle can be advanced through the adductor brevis

muscle to its posterior border where the posterior branch of the obturator nerve can be blocked. This branch lies between the adductor brevis and adductor magnus muscles. Again, 5–8 ml of anesthetic solution can be injected. The use of a nerve stimulator makes this block quick and simple.

Common pitfalls to both approaches of the obturator block include a misplaced needle secondary to an improper needle angle, especially with the distal block. The majority of patients receiving an obturator block have adductor spasticity resulting in hip adduction and rotation deformities. These deformities distort the normal anatomic relationships and make this block more challenging and often more frustrating to less experienced clinicians.

FEMORAL NERVE BLOCK

The femoral nerve is composed of fibers from the L2, L3, and L4 nerve roots. It enters the anterior thigh posterior to the inguinal ligament and anterior to the iliopsoas muscle. While in the femoral triangle, the

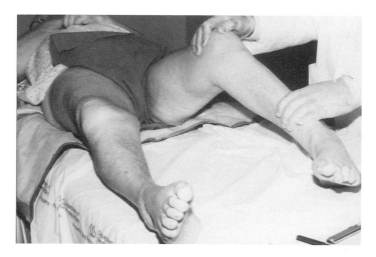

FIGURE 13-11. Marked improvement in bed positioning following bilateral phenol obturator blocks in the same patient as in Figure 13-10.

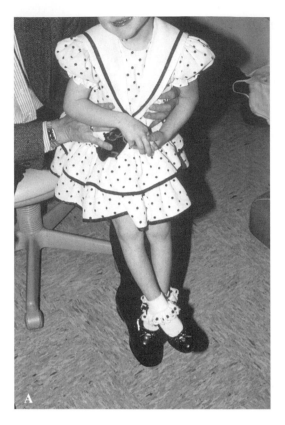 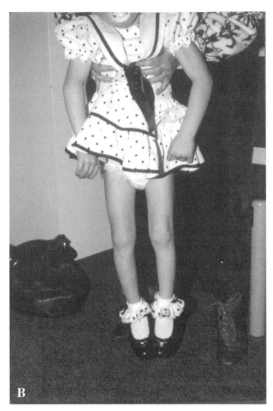

FIGURE 13-12.   Obturator block before (A) and after (B) in a pediatric patient. Sitting and standing postures are significantly improved.

nerve lies lateral to the femoral artery and vein. At the level of the inguinal ligament, the nerve divides into two parts: anterior and posterior branches. The anterior branch supplies sensation to the anterior and medial thigh and often a muscular branch to the sartorius muscle. The posterior branch innervates the remaining

muscles in the anterior compartment of the thigh and knee joint and terminates as the saphenous nerve.

The femoral nerve can be blocked in cases of severe knee extensor spasticity in the nonambulatory patient, which may interfere with sitting. As with other blocks, pain problems in its sensory distribution

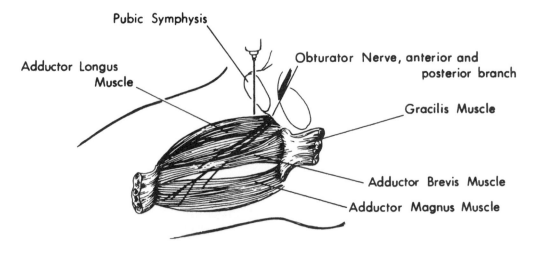

FIGURE 13-13.   The obturator nerve at its exit from the obturator foramen. Note the angle of the needle to the hemipelvis.

and anesthetic injections for procedures are other common indications to performing this block.[11]

Technique

The femoral nerve can be easily blocked within the femoral triangle.[7] With the patient supine, the femoral artery is palpated just below the inguinal ligament. This ligament can be visualized by drawing a line connecting the anterosuperior iliac spine and the pubic symphysis. While the second and third digits of the nondominant hand palpate the femoral artery, a needle is slowly advanced perpendicular to the skin in the direction of the femoral nerve immediately lateral to the artery (Fig. 13-14). The needle is advanced through the fascia lata and fascia iliaca, at times causing pain. One can often feel a loss of resistance as the needle advances through these fascial layers. Because an inadequate block occurs if the needle is placed outside of the fascia iliaca, proper depth is essential. If a nerve stimulator is used, one quickly identifies knee extension and hip internal rotation. Up to 15 ml of volume can be injected after careful aspiration is performed.

LATERAL FEMORAL CUTANEOUS NERVE BLOCK

The lateral femoral cutaneous nerve provides sensation to the anterior, lateral, and posterior aspect of the thigh. This purely sensory nerve originates from the L2 and L3 nerve roots. Deep in the pelvis, it emerges from the psoas major muscle where it passes adjacent to the iliacus muscle and posterior to the inguinal ligament near the ASIS. The nerve passes over the sartorius muscle, becomes superficial 12 cm inferior to the ASIS where it terminates into smaller branches that supply the skin of the thigh.

Lateral femoral cutaneous nerve blocks can be performed in suspected cases of neuropathic pain originating from this nerve. In cases of entrapment, such as meralgia paresthetica, a mixture of anesthetic and corticosteroids can be injected. As expected, this nerve is commonly blocked in conjunction with other peripheral nerves to provide anesthesia for thigh procedures.

Technique

With the patient's anterior pelvis exposed, the ASIS and the inguinal ligament are identified. A needle is placed perpendicular to the skin approximately 1 inch medial to the ASIS and inferior to the inguinal ligament. The needle is advanced into the soft tissue about 1 inch, but this varies depending on the patient's size. At times, paresthesias may be elicited, thereby verifying needle placement. Once needle placement is satisfactory, 5–10 ml of solution can be injected.

INFERIOR GLUTEAL NERVE BLOCK

The inferior gluteal nerve innervates the gluteus maximus muscle, the most powerful hip extensor. The nerve arises from the posterior divisions of the lumbosacral plexus consisting of fibers from the L5, S1, and S2 nerve roots. The nerve parallels the sciatic nerve under the inferior border of the piriformis muscle and turns sharply posterolaterally toward the sacrotuberous ligament where it enters the gluteus maximus muscle. In cases of severe hip extensor spasticity that interferes with sitting, this nerve can be blocked.

Technique

To localize the inferior gluteal nerve, a needle is inserted into the center of the gluteus maximus muscle. This center point can be located by outlining the borders of this quadrilateral-shaped muscle. It originates medially from the posterior surface of the sacrum and inserts laterally into the gluteal

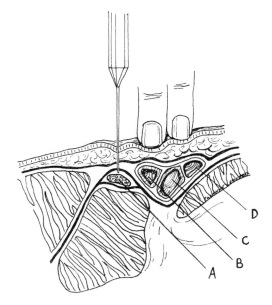

FIGURE 13-14. Cross section through the femoral triangle: nerve (A), artery (B), vein (C), and lymphatics (D). Note the needle tip adjacent to the femoral nerve.

tuberosity of the femur. The needle is slowly advanced to a depth of about 3 cm, often varying based on the patient's size. When using a nerve stimulator, a strong contraction of the gluteus maximus muscle should be observed. If any contraction is seen in the hamstring muscles, the needle should be withdrawn because the needle is close to the sciatic nerve.

REFERENCES

1. Fouch RA, Abram SE, Hogan QH: Neural blockade for upper extremity pain. The painful hand. Hand Clin 12:791–800, 1996.
2. Gray H: Gray's Anatomy, Descriptive and Surgical. New York, Bounty Books.
3. Guardini R, Waldrom BA, Wallace WA: Sciatic nerve block: A new lateral approach. Acta Anaesthesiol Scand 29:515–519, 1985.
4. Gunduz S, Kalyon TA, Dursun H, et al: Peripheral nerve block with phenol to treat spasticity in spinal cord injured patients. Paraplegia 30:808–811, 1992.
5. Hullander M, Balsara Z, Spillane W, et al: The use of Doppler ultrasound to assist with sciatic nerve blocks. Reg Anesth 16:282–284, 1991.
6. Ichiyanaghi K: Sciatic nerve block: Lateral approach with patient supine. Anesthesiology 20:601–604, 1959.
7. Khoo ST, Brown TK: Femoral nerve block: The anatomical basis for a single injection technique. Anaesth Intens Care 11:40–42, 1983.
8. Koyama H, Murakami K, Suzuki T, Suzaki K: Phenol block for hip flexor muscle spasticity under ultrasonic monitoring. Arch Phys Med Rehabil 73:1040–1043, 1992.
9. Labat G: Regional Anesthesia. Philadelphia, W.B. Saunders, 1922, pp 289–291.
10. Meelhuysen FE, Halpern D, Quast J: Treatment of flexor spasticity by paravertebral lumbarspinal nerve block. Arch Phys Med Rehabil 49:712–722, 1968.
11. Rooks M, Fleming LL: Evaluation of acute knee injuries with sciatic and femoral nerve blocks. Clin Orthop 179:185–188, 1983.
12. Tajiri K, Takahashi K, Ikeda K, Tomita K: Common peroneal nerve block for sciatica. Clin Orthop 347:203–207, 1998.

14

Leg, Foot, and Ankle Blocks

Dennis Matthews, M.D.

Lower extremity nerve blocks are used primarily for anesthesia during surgical procedures, especially when general, spinal, or epidural techniques cannot be used. Their use in clinical practice includes the diagnosis and management of pain syndromes and spasticity.[19,20] These blocks allow a more active and functional participation in therapies and can assist in orthotic management for gait training and positioning for wheelchair seating evaluations.[1]

TIBIAL AND COMMON PERONEAL NERVES

The tibial and common peroneal nerves originate as a bifurcation of the sciatic nerve, usually high in the popliteal fossa. The tibial nerve consists of fibers from the L4–S3 nerve roots and runs from the apex of the popliteal fossa with the popliteal artery to the distal border of the popliteus muscle. It then passes deep to the arch of the soleus muscle to enter into the deep posterior compartment of the leg. The tibial nerve innervates the posterior compartment muscles of the leg and supplies sensation to the lateral border and sole of the foot.

The common peroneal nerve consists of fibers from the L4–S2 nerve roots and follows the lateral border of the popliteal fossa just deep to the popliteal membrane. It then courses laterally around the neck of the fibula to supply the anterior and lateral compartment muscles of the leg and sensation to the dorsum of the foot and lateral aspect of the leg.

The tibial and common peroneal nerve are usually blocked at the level of the knee. Diagnostic or therapeutic blocks in the popliteal fossa have varying clinical applications.[8,16,21] Local blockade of the tibial and common peroneal nerves produces excellent anesthesia of the lower leg and foot[2,3,15,16,17,21,22,24] and provides good analgesia following surgery below the knee.[17] It can be used as a diagnostic block in children who have toe walking[13] or as an

adjunct to physical therapy in children with brain injury and equinus deformities.[14]

Tibial Nerve Block Technique

With the patient in the prone position, the triangular borders of the popliteal fossa are identified. The knee crease corresponds to the base, semimembranosus muscle to the medial border, and the biceps femoris muscle to the lateral border of this triangle. A perpendicular line is extended from the midpoint of the base to the apex of the triangle (Fig. 14-1). The needle is introduced perpendicular to the skin 6–7 cm proximal to the base on this line and 1 cm lateral (Fig. 14-2). The needle should be advanced midway between the skin and the femur or to a depth of approximately 3 cm. The use of a nerve stimulator to provoke a plantar flexion muscle contraction at the ankle can be helpful to better localize this nerve.[27]

Common Peroneal Nerve Block Technique

With the patient's lateral knee and leg exposed, the fibular head is identified (Fig. 14-3). The common peroneal nerve as it crosses the fibula 2–3 cm below the fibular head is palpated. The needle is slowly advanced adjacent to the nerve and small volumes of solution injected, usually fewer than 5 ml. When using a nerve stimulator, contraction of the anterior and lateral compartment muscles of the leg should be observed.

An alternative to the above technique is blocking the common peroneal nerve within the popliteal fossa (see Figs. 14-1 and 14-2). Within this fossa, the nerve lies adjacent to the biceps femoris muscle lateral to the tibial nerve. The apex of this fossa is bisected and a needle inserted on the lateral aspect of this division to a depth midway between the skin and femur, usually 0.5 cm below the popliteal membrane.

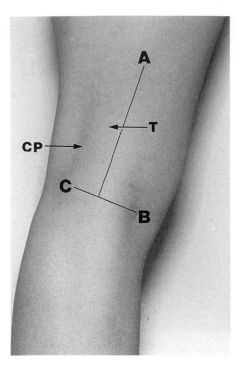

FIGURE 14-1.   The borders of the popliteal fossa are outlined (*ABC*) and the surface location of the tibial nerve (*T*) and common peroneal nerve (*CP*) are noted.

Complications with tibial and common peroneal blocks are rare. Inadvertent injection into the popliteal artery can be avoided with good technique and careful aspiration after placement of the needle. A pressure neuropathy is possible when injecting around the common peroneal nerve at the fibular head if large volumes of medication are used. Kempthorne and Brown performed 50 blocks in children with no detectable intravascular injections, popliteal hematomas, neuralgias, or persistent sensory changes.[13]

ANKLE BLOCKS

A total ankle block consists of circumferentially blocking five nerves at the level of the ankle that control sensation to the entire foot. Two major nerves, the femoral and sciatic, are represented. These nerves originate from the lumbar and sacral plexus and terminate as the posterior tibial, deep peroneal, sural, saphenous, and superficial peroneal nerves. Simultaneous blocks to each of these nerves are commonly performed to facilitate superficial operations of the foot when a tourniquet is not required. Total ankle blocks are technically difficult because five nerves must be blocked to achieve total anesthesia of the foot. Schurman describes this approach as ideal because it produces only minimal immobility of the lower extremity in addition to the desired sensory changes.[23] Individual nerves also may be blocked at the ankle to help differentiate painful foot and ankle disorders or cases of neuropathic pain.

POSTERIOR TIBIAL NERVE

The posterior tibial nerve (PTN) originates adjacent to the popliteus muscle and travels with the posterior tibial artery within the posterior compartment of the leg. At the ankle, the nerve passes through the posterior tarsal tunnel at the midpoint between the medial malleolus and calcaneus under the flexor retinaculum. It travels posterior to the posterior tibial artery within the tunnel and divides within 1 cm of the malleolar-calcaneal axis in the majority of feet.[11] The PTN innervates all posterior leg compartment muscles and supplies sensation to the ankle joint, skin of the heel, and inner sole of the

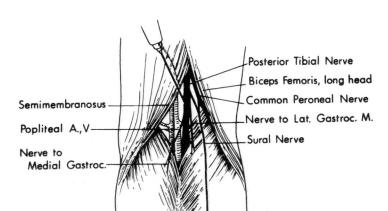

Semimembranosus

Popliteal A., V

Nerve to Medial Gastroc.

Posterior Tibial Nerve
Biceps Femoris, long head
Common Peroneal Nerve
Nerve to Lat. Gastroc. M.
Sural Nerve

FIGURE 14-2.   The popliteal fossa with its contents in relation to the posterior tibial and common peroneal nerves. The needle tip is in position to block the posterior tibial nerve.

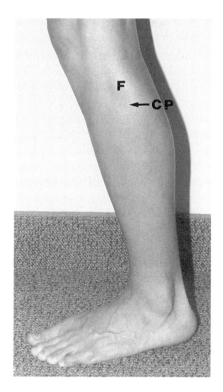

FIGURE 14-3. Lateral view of the leg with surface markings representing the fibular head (*F*) and common peroneal nerve (*CP*) well delineated.

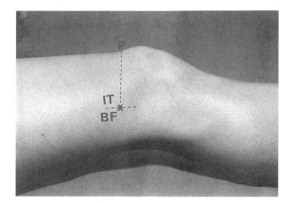

FIGURE 14-4. Lateral approach to common peroneal and tibial nerves. The upper edge of the patella (*P*) and the groove between the iliotibial tract and the tendon of the biceps femoris (*IT-BF*) are drawn on skin.

foot. The PTN terminates at the medial and lateral plantar nerves that innervate the intrinsic foot muscles and supply sensation to the entire sole of the foot and many of the tarsal and metatarsal joints.

Lateral Approach

With the patient supine, the upper edge of the patella and the groove between the iliotibial tract and the tendon of the biceps femoris are palpated and drawn on the skin (Fig. 14-4). The needle is inserted 20° to 30° posteriorly related to the horizontal plane with a slight caudal direction. The common peroneal nerve will be encountered first with dorsiflexion or eversion of the foot. Medial and posterior redirection will allow identification of the tibial nerve with plantar flexion or inversion of the foot.

The lateral approach has the advantage of being performed with the patient supine.[7,10] The technique is safe and easy and has a smaller risk of vascular puncture than the posterior approach. Both techniques accurately identify surface landmarks.

A PTN block is commonly used in podiatric medicine.[8] Tarsal tunnel surgery, removal of soft tissue masses or foreign bodies, and preinjection

therapy for painful heel conditions are a few reasons to perform this type of block.

Posterior Tibial Nerve Block Technique

With the patient's medial ankle exposed, the medial malleolus and posterior tibial artery are palpated (Fig. 14-5) at the level of the posterior tarsal tunnel. A needle can be introduced posterior to the posterior tibial artery and directed 45° anteriorly. If nerve stimulation is used, contraction of the intrinsic foot muscles will be observed.

A second approach blocks the PTN proximal to the posterior tarsal tunnel. With the patient supine and the foot elevated and externally rotated, a needle is inserted at the midpoint of a transverse line joining the upper portion of the medial malleolus with the medial edge of the Achilles tendon (Fig. 14-6). The needle is directed anterolaterally until the

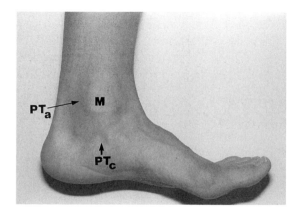

FIGURE 14-5. Medial view of the ankle and foot with surface markings representing the medial malleolus (*M*), posterior tibial artery (*PT$_a$*), and sustentaculum tali (*PT$_c$*) noted.

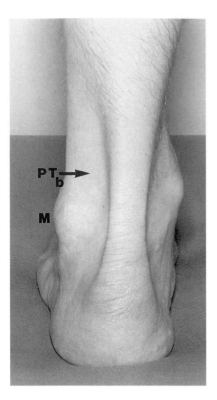

FIGURE 14-6. Posterior view of the ankle with surface markings representing medial malleolus (*M*) and the block site of the posterior tibial nerve (*PT_b*).

posterior surface of the tibia is contacted, then withdrawn 2–3 mm before solution is injected.

An alternative approach involves blocking the PTN distal to the posterior tarsal tunnel. With the medial ankle exposed, the borders of the medial malleolus and sustentaculum tali are identified (see Fig. 14-5). A needle is inserted posterior and inferior to the ridge on the sustentaculum tali, immediately below the midpoint of the medial malleolus.[25] The needle is advanced until bone is contacted and withdrawn 2 mm prior to injecting the blocking agent.

Bareither et al. identified a range for the PTN bifurcation from 2.8 cm distal to 14.3 cm proximal to the medial malleolus.[5] A PTN block performed lateral to the posterior tibial artery adjacent to the medial malleolus was unsuccessful in 20% of patients. A 96% success rate in blocking the PTN was noted when the injection site was 8 cm proximal to the medial malleolus.

DEEP PERONEAL NERVE

The deep peroneal nerve (DPN) branches from the common peroneal nerve to innervate the muscles of the anterior compartment of the leg (Figs. 14-7

and 14-8). It also innervates the extensor digitorum brevis muscle on the dorsum of the foot and supplies sensation to the ankle, tarsal, and first through fourth metatarsophalangeal joints as well as the dorsal skin between the first and second toes. The DPN lies deep to the extensor retinaculum at the anterior ankle next to the anterior tibial artery, lateral to the extensor hallucis longus (EHL) tendon within the anterior tarsal tunnel.

Deep Peroneal Nerve Block Technique

With the anterior ankle exposed, the midpoint of a line intersecting both the medial and lateral malleoli is identified (see Fig. 14-7). The anterior tibialis tendon and dorsalis pedis artery are palpated over the anterior ankle. A needle can be inserted perpendicular to the skin, just lateral to the artery and advanced 2–4 cm depending on the patient's size (see Fig. 14-8). If the artery is not palpable, the needle is placed lateral to the EHL tendon. The patient is asked to move the great toe as the physician watches for needle movement, suggesting needle placement into the substance of the EHL tendon. In this case,

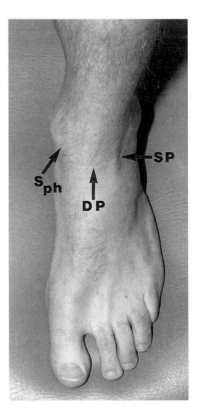

FIGURE 14-7. Anterior view of the foot and ankle depicting the surface locations of the saphenous (*S_ph*), deep peroneal (*DP*), and superficial peroneal (*SP*) nerves.

the needle position is adjusted and solution injected inferior to the extensor retinaculum.

SURAL NERVE

The sural nerve (SN) consists of fibers from the L5 and S1 nerve roots and is formed from branches of the common peroneal and tibial nerves. It arises immediately distal to the popliteal space and descends superficially within the posterior leg in the midline. The SN supplies sensation to the lateral leg and extends distally along the lateral aspect of the ankle, midway between the lateral malleolus and calcaneus, where it supplies sensation to the skin of the lateral aspect of the foot.

Sural Nerve Block Technique

A distal SN block is performed immediately posterior to the lateral malleolus. With the lateral ankle exposed, a needle is inserted midway between the lateral malleolus and calcaneus (Fig. 14-9). The needle is directed toward the posterior surface of the lateral malleolus until bone is contacted. The depth of needle placement varies, but in most patients 4–6 ml of superficially injected solution is adequate.

A proximal SN block can be easily performed in the posterior leg between the skin and the gastrocnemius muscle. The midportion of this muscle is identified and the nerve blocked in the midline 12–16 cm proximal to the upper calcaneus. The needle is advanced to the outer aspect of the gastrocnemius muscle, and 4–7 ml of solution injected.

SAPHENOUS NERVE

The saphenous nerve (SAN) is a purely sensory branch of the femoral nerve derived from the L3 and L4 nerve roots. It runs adjacent to the femoral artery until its superficial exit at the medial knee, where it supplies sensation. The nerve descends in the superficial fascia anterior to the medial malleolus with the great saphenous vein. It ultimately supplies sensation to the medial leg and foot.

Saphenous Nerve Block Technique

With the medial ankle exposed, the medial malleolus at the level of the saphenous vein is identified.[12] The SAN lies immediately medial to the anterior tibialis tendon on the anterior surface of the medial malleolus (see Fig. 14-7). A 25-gauge

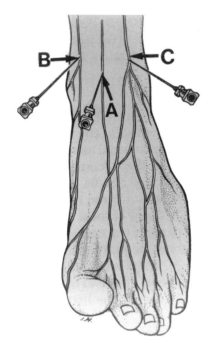

FIGURE 14-8. Anatomic drawing of the ankle and foot depicting block sites and relationships of the deep peroneal nerve (*A*), saphenous nerve (*B*), and superficial peroneal nerve (*C*). (From Carron H, Korbon GA, Rowlingson JC: Lower extremity blocks. In Carron H, Korbon GA, Rowlingson JC (eds): Regional Anesthesia: Techniques and Clinical Applications. Orlando, FL, Grune & Stratton, 1984, with permission.)

needle can be inserted at this point and 4–7 ml of solution injected (see Fig. 14-8). Needle depth should remain superficial.

An alternative proximal SAN block can be performed at the knee. A block at this location can be used to treat some cases of medial knee pain attributed to SAN entrapment.[26] With the medial knee exposed, the medial femoral condyle is palpated. Palpation of the SAN is often possible at this location, especially in thin patients. A 23- or 25-gauge needle can be inserted perpendicular to the skin at the level of the medial femoral condyle. The needle is advanced until the femur is contacted and withdrawn slightly. Injection of 4–8 ml of solution may be required.

SUPERFICIAL PERONEAL NERVE

The superficial peroneal nerve (SPN) branches from the common peroneal nerve to innervate the peroneus longus and brevis muscles of the lateral compartment of the leg. The nerve descends into the leg, where it emerges above the extensor retinaculum, supplying sensation to the skin of the dorsal foot and toes (see Figs. 14-7 and 14-9).

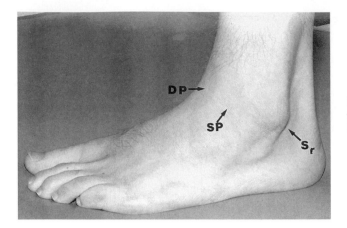

FIGURE 14-9. Lateral view of the foot and ankle depicting the surface locations of the deep peroneal (*DP*), superficial peroneal (*SP*), and sural (*S$_r$*) nerves.

Superficial Peroneal Nerve Block Technique

With the patient supine and the anterior ankle exposed, the anterior tibial artery and lateral malleolus are identified. At the level of the ankle, a needle may be inserted adjacent to the artery but anterior to the extensor retinaculum (see Fig. 14-8). A subcutaneous ridge of anesthetic solution along the skin crease will adequately block the SPN. This ridge will overlay the previously discussed subfascial injection of the deep peroneal nerve.

PLANTAR AND INTERDIGITAL NERVES

The medial and lateral plantar nerves are the terminal branches of the posterior tibial nerve. These

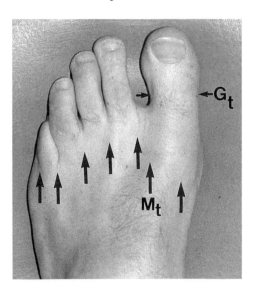

FIGURE 14-10. Dorsal view of the foot depicting the location of metatarsal (*M$_t$*) blocks (*large arrows*) and great toe (*G$_t$*) blocks (*small arrows*).

nerves innervate the intrinsic foot muscles and ultimately divide into the interdigital nerves that supply sensation to the skin of the toes. Blocks to this region are commonly performed at the level of the metatarsal heads—thus, the name "metatarsal nerve blocks." Metatarsal nerve blocks are designed to deposit solution in a ring-like form around the head of each metatarsal bone. The most common indication for these blocks is to provide anesthesia for bunionectomies and surgical removal of ingrown toenails.[3] Facilitation of digital range of motion and relief of pain from neuromas are other indications.

Metatarsal Nerve Block Technique

From a dorsal approach, a 25-gauge needle is inserted adjacent to the metatarsal head directed toward the sole of the foot. The needle is advanced to the level of the midportion of the metatarsal bone. If all toes need to be anesthetized, each intertarsal space is infiltrated; otherwise, only isolated blocks need to be performed. Separate injections are made on the sides of the first and fifth metatarsals, when indicated. Superficial skin wheals between the metatarsal bones are often necessary to provide greater comfort to the patient before injecting deeper (Fig. 14-10).

For a description of digital nerve blocks, see chapter 12.

SUMMARY

Indications for lower extremity nerve blocks in a clinician's practice include pain syndromes and spasticity. These blocks can be used effectively to allow more active and functional participation in therapies. A physician knowledgeable in the regional anatomy, indications, and block technique can safely perform these lower extremity blocks with only rare complications.

REFERENCES

1. Arendzum JH, Van Juijn H, Beckman MK, et al: Diagnostic blocks of the tibial nerve in spastic hemiparesis. Scand J Rehabil Med 24:75–81, 1992.
2. Armitage EN: Regional anesthesia in pediatrics. Clin Anaesthesiol 3:353, 1985.
3. Arthur DS, McNicol LR: Local anesthetic techniques in pediatric surgery. Br J Anaesth 58:760–778, 1986.
4. Awad EA: Injection Techniques for Spasticity. Minneapolis, 1993.
5. Bareither DJ, Genau JM, Massaro JC: Variations in the divisions of the tibial nerve: Application to nerve blocks. J Foot Surg 29:581–583, 1990.
6. Bouaziz H, Narchi P, Zetlaoui PJ, et al: Lateral approach to the sciatic nerve of the popliteal fossa combined with saphenous nerve blocks. Tech Reg Anesth Pain Manage 3:19–22, 1999.
7. Brown TCK, Schulte-Steinberg OH: Neural blockade for pediatric surgery. In Cousins MC, Bridenbaugh PO (eds): Neural Blockage in Clinical Anesthesia and Management of Pain. Philadelphia, J.B. Lippincott, 1988, pp 669–692.
8. Cohen SJ, Roenigk RK: Nerve blocks for cutaneous surgery of the foot. J Dermatol Surg Oncol 17:527–534, 1991.
9. Collins VJ: Fundamentals of Nerve Blocking. Philadelphia, Lea & Febiger, 1960.
10. Collum CR, Courtney PG: Sciatic nerve blockade by the lateral approach to the popliteal fossa. Anesth Intensive Care 21:236–237, 1993.
11. Dellon AL, Mackinnon SE: Tibial nerve branching in the tarsal tunnel. Arch Neurol 41:645–646, 1984.
12. Gurmarnik S, Hurwitz E: Saphenous and common peroneal nerve block will prevent tourniquet pain in prolonged podiatry procedures. J Foot Surg 30:319, 1991.
13. Kempthorne PM, Brown TC: Nerve blocks around the knee in children. Anesth Intens Care 12:14–17, 1984.
14. Kempthorne PM, Ratcliff RN: Temporary tibial nerve block-adjunct to inhibitory plastics in the physiotherapy management of equinus in severely head-injured children. Aust J Physiother 29:119, 1983.
15. Lofstrom B: Nerve block at the knee. In Illustrated Handbook in Local Anesthesia. Chicago, Year Book, 1969, pp 70–85.
16. McKenzie PJ, Loach AB: Local anesthesia for orthopedic surgery. Br J Anesth 58:779–789, 1986.
17. McNicol LR: Lower limb blocks in children. Anesthesia 41:27, 1986.
18. Moore DC: Regional Blocks. Springfield, IL, Charles C Thomas, 1965.
19. Moore TJ, Anderson RB: The use of open phenol blocks to monitor branches of the tibial nerve in adult-acquired spasticity. Foot Ankle 11:219–221, 1991.
20. Petrillo CR, Knoploch S: Phenol block of the tibial nerve for spasticity: A long-term follow-up study. Int Disabil Stud 10:97–100, 1988.
21. Raj PP: Clinical Practice of Regional Anesthesia. New York, Churchill Livingstone, 1991.
22. Rorie DK, Byer DE, Nelson DO, et al: Assessment of block of the sciatic nerve in the popliteal fossa. Anesth Analg 59:371–376, 1980.
23. Schurman DJ: Ankle block anesthesia for foot surgery. Anesthesia 44:342, 1976.
24. Sparks CJ, Higeleo T: Foot surgery in vanuati: Results of combined tibial, common peroneal, and saphenous nerve blocks in fifty-six adults. Anesth Intens Care 17:336–339, 1989.
25. Wasseff MR: Posterior tibial nerve block. Anesthesia 46:841–844, 1991.
26. Worth RM, Kettelkamp DB, Defalque RJ, et al: Saphenous nerve entrapment: A cause of medial knee pain. Am J Sports Med 12:80–81, 1984.
27. Zahari DT, Englund, Girolamo M: Peripheral nerve block with use of stimulator. J Foot Surg 29:162–163, 1990.

15

Peripheral Joint Injections

John P. Obermiller, M.D., and Dennis M. Lox, M.D.

Intra-articular injections are but one of the clinician's many tools for the treatment of musculoskeletal disorders. Injection should be considered an adjunct to the overall treatment plan—never the sole component of therapy. Injections may be used diagnostically as well as therapeutically and are generally "safe" when used judiciously by a skilled practitioner.

The introduction of hydrocortisone in 1951 advanced the idea for local intra-articular injections. Much of the anecdotal evidence that "steroid" injections are harmful has been found over the ensuing years to be untrue. Although a number of studies have been performed, it has not yet been proved that intra-articular corticosteroids actually destroy joints unless used in an indiscriminate manner.[4] Isolated reports disclose articular surface damage from corticosteroid therapy[1]; in others, concomitant or antecedent facts were likely to have contributed to osteonecrosis or periarticular problems.[2,5,12,18,22] These reports are disputed, and the deleterious effects of corticosteroids used under accepted guidelines are believed to be more transient.[4] The use of corticosteroids in combatting inflammatory conditions and painful arthritic conditions has, in fact, proved beneficial in some studies.[4,14]

Nevertheless, every practitioner must be mindful that complications and serious problems may arise with intra-articular injections. Thus, a basic knowledge of the pharmacokinetics of corticosteroids[6] is paramount along with awareness of the signs of any potential side effects. Of course, the specific anatomy of the joint injected must be well understood. Perhaps most basically, the physician must be able to determine which patients are most likely to benefit from intra-articular injections and at what point in the patients' treatment will they be beneficial. This chapter examines specific aspects of peripheral joint injections and describes their use in common joints.

INDICATIONS FOR INTRA-ARTICULAR STEROIDS

Understanding the rationale for the use of corticosteroids in intra-articular spaces is of primary importance. The most common use of corticosteroids in the peripheral joints is in patients with rheumatoid arthritis. These drugs are used specifically to reduce inflammation and provide relief from pain attributable to synovitis and conditions associated with rheumatoid arthritis. Corticosteroids also may be very useful in providing pain relief in long-standing osteoarthritic joints. The restoration of joint motion in conditions of adhesive capsulitis is yet another common use. Aspiration of synovial fluid for pain relief and laboratory evaluation of the synovial fluid as well as arthrography for the evaluation of joints are common diagnostic tools that facilitate the rehabilitation of painful joints.

Basically, the physician should consider the use of corticosteroid injections in the peripheral joints when comprehensive therapy, including physical therapy, nonsteroidal anti-inflammatory drugs (NSAIDs), analgesics, and other physical modalities, fail.

DRUGS: ACTION, SELECTION, DOSAGE

Corticosteroids produce significant anti-inflammatory effects. Numerous long-acting corticosteroid ester preparations are available. The most widely used corticosteroids include triamcinolone acetonide (Kenalog), triamcinolone hexacetonide (Aristospan), betamethasone sodium phosphate and betamethasone acetate (Celestone Soluspan), methylprednisolone acetate (Depo-Medrol), and dexamethasone acetate (Decadron-LA).[12] These compounds were developed to reduce undesirable hormonal side effects with less rapid dissipation from the joint. None of these corticosteroid derivatives appears to have any superiority over another; however, triamcinolone hexacetonide is the least water-soluble preparation and thus provides the longest duration of effectiveness within the peripheral joint space.[3]

Systemic absorption after peripheral joint injection occurs within 2–3 weeks. Improvement of inflammatory processes remote from the injection site demonstrates that intra-articular corticosteroids exert a systemic effect.

The practitioner's choice of a drug should be based on the intended purpose for injecting the peripheral joint. For example, for long-term suppression of an inflammatory process such as rheumatoid arthritis, the long-acting triamcinolone hexacetonide would be preferable. If the patient's condition requires faster reduction of symptoms but also a long-acting medicine, the betamethasone phosphate and acetate preparation (Celestone Soluspan) would be preferable. The short onset from the phosphate preparation and the long duration from the acetate preparation make this a desirable choice. For more rapid onset of therapy, the shorter-acting methylprednisolone acetate (Depo-Medrol) would be the drug of choice.

Estimated dosages for the peripheral joints vary widely and usually depend on the size of the joint. The larger joints, such as the knee and shoulder, respond well to a 40-mg dose of methylprednisolone acetate or the equivalent of another agent. The smaller joints, such as the elbow and ankle, respond to a 20- to 30-mg dose of methylprednisolone acetate or the equivalent. Even smaller joints, such as the acromioclavicular and sternoclavicular joints, respond to a 10- to 20-mg dose of methylprednisolone acetate or the equivalent.

The number of injections per joint is also widely variable. Commonly, joints that are injected for the purpose of reducing inflammation in rheumatoid arthritis will be injected many times over the course of the disease process. These multiple injections have been shown to cause interference with normal cartilage protein synthesis.[12] However, it has also been demonstrated that patients with long-standing rheumatoid arthritis who do not receive intra-articular corticosteroid injections have joint disuse and decreased function much sooner than those who receive the injections.[10] For the purposes of pain reduction in osteoarthritis as well as an adjunct in the mobilization of the treatment of adhesive capsulitis, injections at the rate of one per 4–6 weeks for a maximum of three injections is the most commonly accepted regimen. This regimen, of course, is subject to the patient's response to his or her overall treatment plan, of which the intra-articular corticosteroid injection is but one part.

It is usual practice to combine the corticosteroid medications with an anesthetic substance, such as procaine (Novocain) or lidocaine (Xylocaine) or the equivalent. The combined use of corticosteroids and anesthetic agents provides a larger volume of injectable material with which to bathe the joint more adequately. The added effect of analgesia is also desirable for patient comfort and for a more immediate response to treatment. Thus, the patient may obtain immediate pain relief and provide valuable feedback with which to help determine the overall rehabilitation plan. The usual anesthetic injected is lidocaine, 1% without epinephrine, with which the practitioner can provide a preliminary skin wheal and a control test before proceeding with the deeper injection. Bupivacaine (Marcaine, Sensorcaine), 0.25% or 0.5%, is also useful in providing a longer-acting analgesic effect for the patient. Use of the longer-acting bupivacaine, of course, depends on patient compliance, because the patient may "feel cured" and proceed to use the anesthetized joint indiscriminately. The dosages of lidocaine and bupivacaine also vary widely with the size of the joint. Usually, the smaller joints such as the acromioclavicular, sternoclavicular, and elbow joints would take 1–2 ml of 1% lidocaine combined with the corticosteroid. The glenohumeral, knee, and hip joints would take 2–4 ml of anesthetic agent. Bupivacaine is often preferable for non–weight-bearing joints such as the shoulder, elbow, acromioclavicular, and sternoclavicular joints, so long as these joints can be somewhat immobilized for several hours. Likewise, lidocaine is the drug of choice for injections in the weight-bearing joints such as the knee because its duration is much shorter and, thus, the joint is subject to less postinjection trauma by the seemingly compliant patient.

CONTRAINDICATIONS AND COMPLICATIONS

The clinician must be acutely sensitive to contraindications and complications of intra-articular corticosteroid therapy. Some of the most obvious contraindications include infection of the joint or of the skin overlying the joint. A patient with generalized infection also should be considered an unsuitable candidate for corticosteroid injection. Injection of corticosteroids may render a joint susceptible to hematogenous seeding from more distant skin lesions. Thus, the overall health of the patient must be assessed before considering the use of intra-articular corticosteroids.[9] Other obvious contraindications include hypersensitivity to any of the anesthetic preparations or the corticosteroids themselves. When hypersensitivity to a medication is suspected, a simple test dose should be given at the site of injection by raising a skin wheal with the indicated anesthetic and allowing time to determine any adverse effects.

Patients receiving intra-articular injections in the presence of anticoagulants would be susceptible to serious bleeding. Determination of prothrombin time is necessary before injection therapy in these patients.

Patients with a recent injury to the joint such as a ligamentous destruction or bony destruction of the underlying joint should not be subjected to corticosteroid therapy. Instead, aspiration of the joint may be indicated if there is a relatively large inflammatory effusion.[23] Soft tissue or bony tumors at or near the underlying joint would also be a major contraindication to corticosteroid injections.

Even small doses of corticosteroids with intra-articular injections may trigger episodes of hyperglycemia, glycosuria, and even electrolyte imbalance in patients with diabetes; caution must be exercised in these situations.[11]

Although rare, infections can be a serious complication.[19] Usually, such infections can be avoided by using an aseptic technique (discussed later in this chapter).[29] Infections may be quite subtle in patients with long-standing rheumatoid arthritis and in those receiving immunosuppressive agents; the most common organism is *Staphylococcus aureus*.[27,30] One must also use caution in geriatric patients and those with debilitating diseases.

Hypercorticism from systemic corticosteroid therapy may be a complication if the patient receives multiple intra-articular injections in succession or if the patient is receiving concomitant oral cortisone therapy. Corticosteroid arthropathy with avascular necrosis also has been reported[14] but is rare and has not been noted to occur after single corticosteroid injections. Joint capsule calcification is also a potential complication of multiple intra-articular corticosteroid injections.[13]

Depigmentation and subcutaneous fat necrosis occasionally occur. The depigmentation is cosmetically unacceptable, especially in darker-skinned individuals in whom it can be quite noticeable. Fat necrosis usually is not a complication in superficial joints that have minimal amounts of overlying fat

tissue. Using a small amount of lidocaine to flush the needle in order to avoid leaving a needle track of corticosteroid suspension will help to minimize this complication.

A common complication in patients with rheumatoid arthritis who are receiving corticosteroid injections in the joints is "postinjection flare" (the joint appears inflamed or even infected), which tends to subside spontaneously in 24–72 hours.[8]

TECHNIQUES FOR INTRA-ARTICULAR INJECTIONS

Once the clinician has established that a peripheral joint needs to be injected or aspirated, the specific preparation for the injection is essentially the same for all joints. Thorough understanding of the underlying anatomy is important in order to accomplish a painless injection. The optimal site for injection of the joint usually is the extensor surface at a point where the synovium is closest to the skin. Approaching the joint from the extensor surfaces allows the injection to be as remote as possible from any major arteries, veins, and nerves.[14] When the site of injection has been determined, it can be marked with the needle hub or a retracted ballpoint pen by pressing the skin to produce a temporary indentation to mark the point of entry. The skin is then prepared by cleansing a generous area with a detergent or cleaner such as an iodine-based surgical scrub. This area is then painted with an antiseptic solution and allowed to dry. Aseptic technique is always advised, including the wearing of sterile gloves so that the area to be injected may be continually palpated and the anatomy appreciated throughout the procedure. A small skin wheal may then be raised using 1% lidocaine with no epinephrine (or an equivalent anesthetic agent). A 27-gauge skin needle approximately 0.75–1.0 inch long is used with approximately 1 ml of anesthetic agent. For joints distended with fluid or those that are particularly close to the surface of the skin such as the acromioclavicular and sternoclavicular joints, the raising of a skin wheal or pre-anesthesia is usually not necessary. If a patient is particularly apprehensive about the injection procedure, one of the vapocoolant sprays such as dichlorotetrafluoroethane or ethyl chloride may provide adequate anesthesia.

After the skin wheal is raised, a 25- or 22-gauge needle approximately 1.5 inches long may be used to introduce the injectant. The needle is then slided gently into the joint, with the clinician avoiding a strong thrusting motion. Just before beginning the actual injection, the practitioner should aspirate to ensure there is no return of blood. After ascertaining the needle's position in the joint space, the injectable material should be introduced using slow, steady pressure on the plunger.

If the joint is to be aspirated before introduction of a corticosteroid, the same technique is used in preparation; however, a larger needle may be introduced, such as a 20- or even an 18-gauge needle. Again, slow, steady pressure is used when the needle is introduced into the joint. The aspirate is then withdrawn with the practitioner gently pulling the plunger on the syringe with the dominant hand, holding the syringe barrel steady with the nondominant hand. If it is suspected that not all of the aspirate has been obtained from the joint, the needle tip may be moved around within the joint, and the joint itself may be "milked," using steady pressure with the opposite hand on the joint itself by kneading the skin toward the site of aspiration. After all of the available fluid is aspirated, the needle may be left in place with the syringe removed. A separate syringe may then be attached to the aspirating needle, and the injectant may then be introduced into the joint itself. Again, a slow, gentle introduction of the injectable material is desired.

If resistance is met during the time of the injection, the needle should be readjusted so that there is no resistance. Any time the needle is readjusted, the plunger on the syringe should be withdrawn to ensure that the needle tip does not pierce a blood vessel.

After the drug or drugs have been injected, the needle is withdrawn and mild pressure is applied with a sterile gauze pad to prevent bleeding. Whenever the injected material includes corticosteroids, a slight amount of lidocaine may be used to clear the needle before withdrawal. As mentioned earlier, this technique prevents leaving a steroid track through the adipose tissue and skin, which may cause depigmentation or subcutaneous necrosis.

Psychological care of the patient is important to the success of these injections. Throughout the procedure, the patient must be coaxed to achieve muscle relaxation and reassured of the importance of the procedure. It is likewise important that the patient be reminded of the practitioner's skill with and knowledge of the procedure. After the procedure, the patient should be assessed carefully to be sure that he or she is not exhibiting a vasovagal response and that appropriate measures are taken to prevent any secondary harm, such as falling as a result of transient hypotension.

UPPER EXTREMITY JOINTS

Glenohumeral Joint

The glenohumeral joint is subject to multiple traumatic and pathologic problems more frequently than any other joint except the knee. The anatomy of the shoulder must be well understood for a relatively painless injection to be achieved. In entering the subacromial space in the shoulder, there is little anterior space for placement of the needle. A lateral or posterior approach may be more desirable.[7]

When injecting the shoulder for problems such as bicipital tendinitis, the anterior approach is necessary (Fig. 15-1). The patient is placed in a sitting position, the anterior portion of the shoulder is prepared aseptically, and, if desired, a cutaneous wheal is raised medial to the head of the humerus and just inferior to the tip of the coracoid process. It is useful to have obese patients lie supine with the forearm across the abdomen. In this position, the shoulder may be passively rotated internally and externally to identify the head of the humerus. The coracoid process is then easily palpated. The injection is thus directed in the anteroposterior plane just lateral to the coracoid process. The needle is advanced into the groove between the medial aspect of the humeral head and the glenoid. No resistance should be felt to the advancement of the needle.

The lateral approach to injection of the shoulder is sometimes useful when treating supraspinatus tendinitis (see Fig. 15-2).[7] The patient is placed in a sitting position with the arm relaxed in the lap, which increases the subacromial space. The lateralmost point of the shoulder is palpated and the needle prepared for insertion below the acromion. After aseptic preparation, the needle is directed almost perpendicularly to the skin surface, with a slight upward angle. The space is then easily entered, and no resistance should be felt with advancement of the needle.

The posterior approach to the shoulder is popular for conditions such as adhesive capsulitis as well as synovitis or chronic osteoarthritis (Fig. 15-2). The posterior approach also allows the practitioner to be out of the patient's vision, thus reducing any apprehension. The patient is placed in the sitting position with his or her arm in the lap, which allows internal rotation of the shoulder and adduction of the arm. The skin is prepared aseptically, and the site

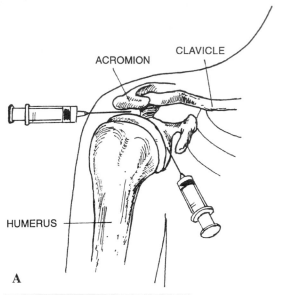

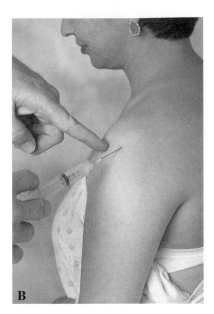

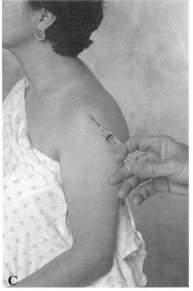

FIGURE 15-1. Internal anatomic (*A*) and approximate surface anatomic (*B*, lateral; *C*, anterior) sites for injection of the glenohumeral joint laterally and anteriorly.

of injection is palpated. The site of injection is just under the posteroinferior border of the posterolateral angle of the acromion. It is useful for the practitioner to palpate the patient's coracoid process in the anterior portion of the shoulder with the index finger. This is the point at which the needle is "aimed." The needle is then inserted approximately 1 inch below the posterolateral acromion process and directed from the posterolateral portion of the shoulder to the anteromedial portion of the shoulder toward the coracoid process. If resistance is encountered, the needle may be withdrawn slightly and angled upward. The needle will then be in the upper recess of the shoulder joint away from the head of the humerus.

Acromioclavicular Joint

The acromioclavicular joint is small and superficial (Fig. 15-3). It is occasionally swollen and usually tender during palpation when inflamed. This joint can be injected easily using a 25-gauge needle with the patient sitting or supine and the shoulder propped on a pillow. Usually, injections into this joint are for chronic pain such as occurs in shoulder separations that have not responded to noninvasive treatment.

Many times, the joint is injected for diagnostic purposes to delineate the source of pain in the shoulder, and therefore corticosteroids are not used. However, with chronic pain that does not subside

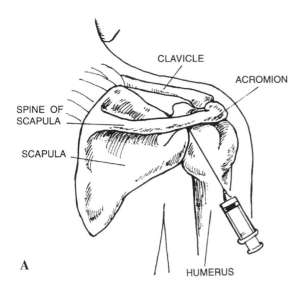

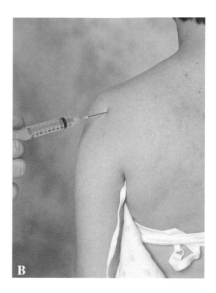

FIGURE 15-2.   Internal anatomic (*A*) and approximate surface anatomic (*B*) sites for injection of the glenohumeral joint posteriorly.

after a trial of anesthetics (such as lidocaine), corticosteroids may be used.

The joint is prepared aseptically, as described earlier. The joint is easily palpated by locating the tip of the distal clavicle and injecting from either a superior angle or an anterosuperior angle into the joint space. In a degenerative joint, many times the needle will not pass easily into the joint, which then needs to be probed gently so that the needle can be advanced just to the proximal margin of the joint's surface. It is usually not necessary to penetrate the joint any deeper.

Sternoclavicular Joint

The sternoclavicular joint is easily located just lateral to the notch of the sternum (Fig. 15-4). Many times the sternoclavicular joint is slightly dislocated, thus providing a source of pain and making it easily palpable because the proximal clavicle may be slightly elevated in relationship to the sternum. This joint is small and may be difficult to inject unless a 25- or 27-gauge needle is used. Great care should be taken that these injections into the sternoclavicular area are done superficially because immediately

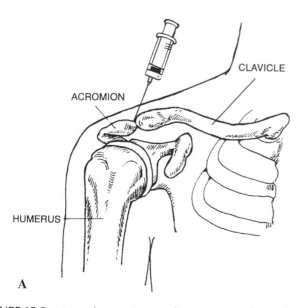

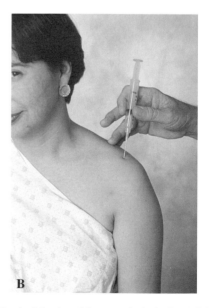

FIGURE 15-3.   Internal anatomic (*A*) and approximate surface anatomic (*B*) sites for injection of the acromioclavicular (AC) joint.

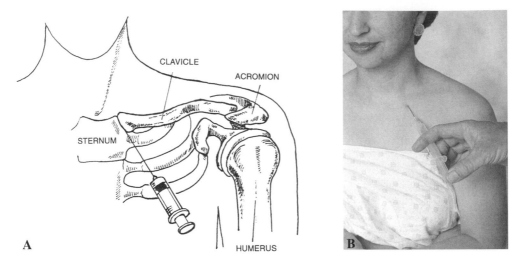

FIGURE 15-4. Internal anatomic (*A*) and approximate surface anatomic (*B*) sites for injection of the sternoclavicular joint.

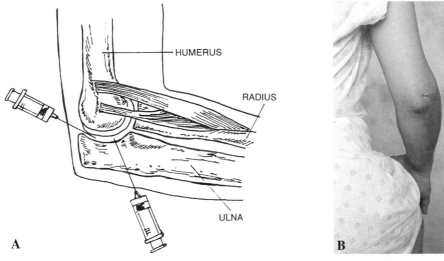

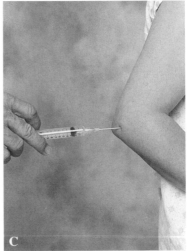

FIGURE 15-5. Internal anatomic (*A*) and approximate surface anatomic (*B*, lateral; *C*, posterior) sites for injection of the elbow laterally and posteriorly.

posterior to the sternoclavicular joint are the brachiocephalic veins.

Elbow

The elbow region is usually subject to periarticular problems, including lateral epicondylitis and medial epicondylitis; however, in this chapter, attention is directed to the joint space itself. Aspiration for problems such as synovitis in patients with rheumatoid arthritis and arthrography of the joint for delineation of multiple pathologic processes, including loose bodies, are the initial approaches to treatment.[17] Once it is determined that an intra-articular injection is needed, the practitioner must remember that the extensor surfaces of the joint are the safest places to avoid vessels and nerves. Thus, the injection should be directed to the posterolateral portion of the elbow or to the posterior portion of the elbow (Fig. 15-5). These approaches will allow the practitioner to enter the humeroulnar joint, the true elbow joint.

The patient is placed with the elbow positioned between 50° and 90° of flexion. The posterior and/or lateral skin surfaces are prepared aseptically. For the posterolateral approach, the lateral epicondyle area and the posterior olecranon area are palpated. The groove between the olecranon below and the lateral epicondyle of the humerus is located. The needle is then directed proximally toward the head of the radius and medially into the elbow joint. Again, no resistance should be felt when the needle enters the joint. Aspiration or injection of the joint may then be undertaken. The posterior approach to the elbow is relatively simple. The posterior olecranon is palpated with the lateral olecranon groove located just posterior to the lateral epicondyle. The needle is then inserted above the superior aspect of and lateral to the olecranon. It is advanced into the joint, and, again, no resistance should be felt.

Wrist

Many of the small joints of the wrist have interconnecting synovial spaces, thus making it possible to provide relief to the entire joint complex with one injection. The wrist may be infiltrated by several methods.[20,28,31] The route of entry may be influenced by the site of inflammation or desired anatomic area. The preferred method is the dorsal approach, which may be facilitated with slight flexion of the hand. This can be easily accomplished by flexing the hand over a rolled towel. The point of entry (Figs. 15-6 and 15-7) is just medial to the extensor pollicis

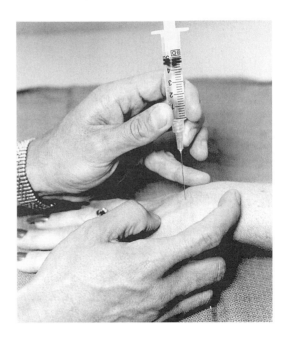

FIGURE 15-6. Dorsal wrist approach. The needle is inserted medial to the extensor pollicis longus tendon.

longus tendon in the distal aspect of the midpoint of the radius and ulna. This can be easily palpated as a depression between the radius and the scaphoid and lunate bones. The needle is placed perpendicular to the skin and inserted 1–2 cm lateral to the extensor

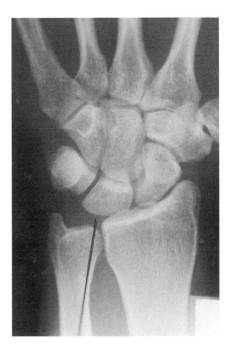

FIGURE 15-7. Anteroposterior x-ray of the wrist demonstrating proper needle placement into the wrist joint using a dorsal approach.

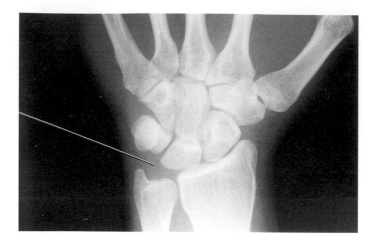

FIGURE 15-8. Anteroposterior x-ray of the wrist demonstrating proper needle placement using the ulnar approach.

pollicis longus tendon.[28] Optional approaches to the wrist include the ulnar or the dorsal snuffbox approach. With the ulnar approach, the injection is made just distal to the lateral ulnar margin in a palpable gap between the border of the distal ulna and the carpal bones (Fig. 15-8). A third approach is the dorsal aspect just medial to the anatomic snuffbox between the radius and carpal bones (Fig. 15-9). Anesthetic and corticosteroid preparations may diffuse throughout the joint and are facilitated by range-of-motion exercises following injection.[24,25] The approach used should be based on the area of maximal point tenderness or site of inflammation and specific anatomic structures underlying the region to be infiltrated, such as the scapholunate ligaments or the triangular fibrocartilaginous complex. Caution should be taken in order to arrive at an accurate diagnosis when treating a chronic condition. An underlying wrist injury with unremarkable initial radiographs may cause scapholunate dissociation, carpal instability, or avascular necrosis. These

disorders should be considered in the differential diagnosis during conservative management.

Intercarpal Joints

Injection into the intercarpal joints such as the triquetrolunate space can be accomplished by palpating the borders of the carpal bone. Palpation is easier to perform when the joint is swollen and fluctuant.[31] Fluoroscopic guidance may be necessary for precise location.

Carpometacarpal Joint

The first carpometacarpal joint or trapeziometacarpal joint is a frequent source of pain in osteoarthritis and from occupations or sports that subject the patient to undue stress. The joint may be infiltrated or aspirated from the dorsal aspect of the radial side of the carpometacarpal joint (Figs. 15-10 and 15-11) by holding the thumb in slight flexion and palpating for the point of maximal tenderness.[15,20,33] When injecting the carpometacarpal joint, care should be taken to avoid the radial artery and the extensor pollicis tendon.[32] To avoid the radial artery, the needle should be placed toward the dorsal side of the extensor pollicis brevis tendon.

Interphalangeal Joints

The proximal and distal interphalangeal joints are affected most frequently by arthritic processes. The proximal interphalangeal joint is frequently affected in rheumatoid arthritis.[27,31] These smaller joints require a small-gauge needle (25- or 27-gauge) to facilitate entry. A vapocoolant spray may be used for superficial skin anesthesia with or without a superficial skin wheal to diminish the pain on initial

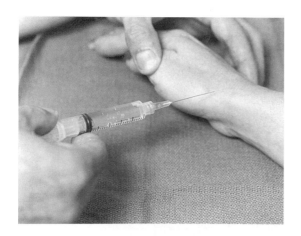

FIGURE 15-9. Needle placement adjacent to the anatomic snuffbox between the radius and carpal bones.

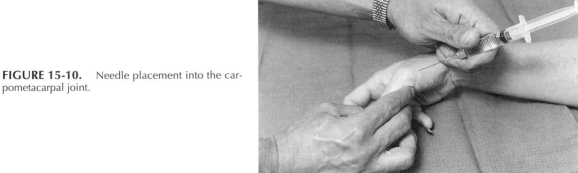

FIGURE 15-10. Needle placement into the carpometacarpal joint.

infiltration; infiltration of these smaller joints is painful.[20] Because the joint space is very small, the tip of the needle must be advanced gently into the intra-articular capsule. The joint will accommodate only a small amount of fluid, usually less than 2 ml, and overdistention should be avoided. Pericapsular and subcutaneous injections have been known to provide some beneficial effect when direct joint infiltration could not be obtained, presumably by transport of the corticosteroids to inflamed capsule and synovium.[32] The proximal and distal interphalangeal joints are infiltrated by palpating the borders of the joint and advancing a fine needle, preferably with a small syringe (2 ml) to facilitate fine motor control (Fig. 15-12). Splinting the affected joint may allow resolution of an inflammatory response.[16,21,26]

LOWER EXTREMITIES

Hip Joint

The hip joint is often difficult to infiltrate or aspirate because of its depth and the surrounding

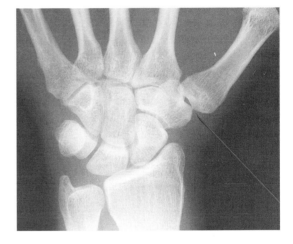

FIGURE 15-11. Anteroposterior x-ray of the hand demonstrating needle placement into the first carpometacarpal joint.

tissue. Fluoroscopic guidance with injection of contrast material is often necessary to confirm proper needle placement. This joint may be infiltrated by an anterior or lateral approach (Fig. 15-13). The

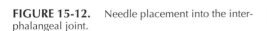

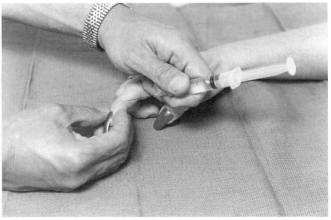

FIGURE 15-12. Needle placement into the interphalangeal joint.

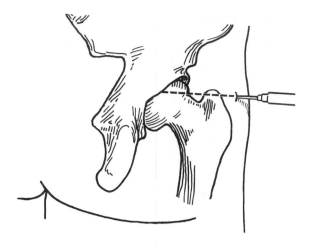

FIGURE 15-13. Lateral arthrocentesis and injection of the hip joint.

anterior approach is preferred.[28,31] With the anterior approach, the patient is in the supine position with the lower extremity externally rotated. The length of the needle will depend on the patient's size. The anatomic landmarks for the anterior approach are 2 cm distal to the anterior superior iliac spine and 3 cm lateral to the palpated femoral artery at a level corresponding to the superior margins of the greater trochanter. After superficial anesthesia is administered, the needle is advanced at an angle 60° posteromedially through the tough capsular ligaments, advanced to bone, and slightly withdrawn. This technique places the tip of the needle directly into the joint, and aspiration or injection may be performed. This approach is much simpler using fluoroscopic guidance to direct the needle posteromedially into the joint; once the capsular ligaments have been penetrated, contrast medium will confirm proper needle placement. Depending on the integrity of the joint, 2–4 ml of anesthetic and corticosteroid suspension may be introduced.

The lateral approach is performed by palpating the greater trochanter of the femur, which may be facilitated by externally rotating the lower extremity. Superficial anesthesia may be used and, again, depending on the size of the patient, the appropriate-length needle is selected. A 3- to 4-inch needle is usually sufficient; however, in large patients, longer needles may be necessary. Just anterior to the greater trochanter, the needle is advanced and walked medially along the neck of the femur until the joint is reached. Aspiration may be obtained but is more difficult with the lateral approach. The amount of fluid that may be introduced may be limited, depending on the integrity of the joint. Avascular necrosis is

a potential complication of corticosteroid injection to the hip. However, no recent cases have been reported in the literature as a direct result of this procedure.

Knee

The knee is the most commonly aspirated and injected joint in the body. It contains the largest synovial space and demonstrates the most visible and palpable effusion (when present). A patient is usually most comfortable lying supine with sufficient pillows. The knee is prepared using an aseptic technique. If a large effusion is present, whether medially or laterally, the site of entry should be over the maximal expansion of the effusion in order to cause the least discomfort during the procedure. For injections in which a large effusion is not present, the lateral, medial, suprapatellar, or anterior approach may be used (Fig. 15-14). Before injecting or aspirating the knee, the patella should be grasped between the examiner's thumb and forefinger and rocked gently from side to side to ensure that the patient's muscles are relaxed.

The medial approach to the knee is simple. First, the practitioner puts a small amount of lateral pressure on the patella, pushing it slightly medially and displacing it somewhat to increase the gap between the patella and the femur medially. The needle is then introduced about midway between the superior and inferior pole of the patella, medial to the patella and midway between the medial border of the patella and the femur. A pre-injection skin wheal may be raised with an anesthetic agent, or the skin itself may be anesthetized with a vapocoolant spray for patient comfort. As the needle is introduced into the joint space, the needle should be aspirated progressively. If no aspirate is obtained, the corticosteroid can be injected. Before withdrawal of the needle, the needle tract again should be flushed with a small amount of anesthetic.

The lateral approach to the knee is also simple. With the patient supine, the knee is fully extended or placed in slight flexion. The patella is slightly displaced laterally to increase the gap between the patella and femur laterally. The skin may then be anesthetized with 1% lidocaine. The needle is introduced halfway between the superior pole of the patella and the midline of the patella lateral and inferior to the patella. As the needle is introduced, aspiration is performed until the needle is into the joint. The joint can then be aspirated or injected.

If a large effusion is present, the suprapatellar approach may be used. This does not have any specific advantage over the lateral approach unless the

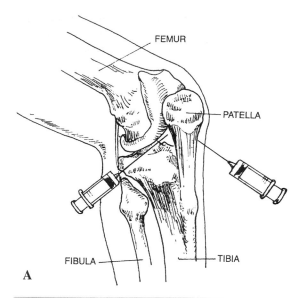

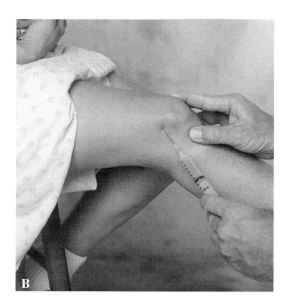

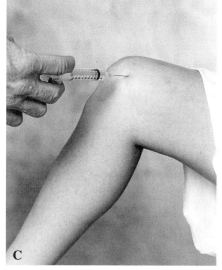

FIGURE 15-14. Internal anatomic (*A*) and approximate surface anatomic (*B,C*) sites for injection of the knee.

effusion is expanding the suprapatellar bursa. The needle is introduced at the point of maximal expansion of the effusion, and the joint is then aspirated. This approach is usually not as good as the lateral approach if the knee is to be injected only and not aspirated. It is much easier to enter the joint space with the medial or lateral approach.

On occasion, an anterior approach to the knee may be desired if a patient cannot fully extend the knee. In these cases, the patient may be sitting or supine with the knee flexed to 90°. The needle is inserted just inferior to the inferior patellar pole from either the lateral or medial side of the patellar tendon. The needle is then advanced parallel to the tibial plateau until the joint space is entered. It is more difficult to aspirate a knee effusion when using this approach.[23] Moreover, the risk of puncturing

the articular cartilage is much higher, as is the risk to the infrapatellar fat pad. Occasionally, the knee is approached anteriorly by inserting the needle directly through the patellar tendon. This approach has no merit because it increases discomfort to the patient and may cause bleeding in the patellar ligament.

Other conditions affecting the knee that may warrant injection of corticosteroid include prepatellar bursitis, iliotibial band syndrome, anserine bursitis, and others. These injections are not intra-articular and will therefore be discussed elsewhere.

Ankle Mortise

The ankle joint is not commonly injected; however, it may be subject to osteoarthritis, rheumatoid arthritis, or chronic pain resulting from instability.

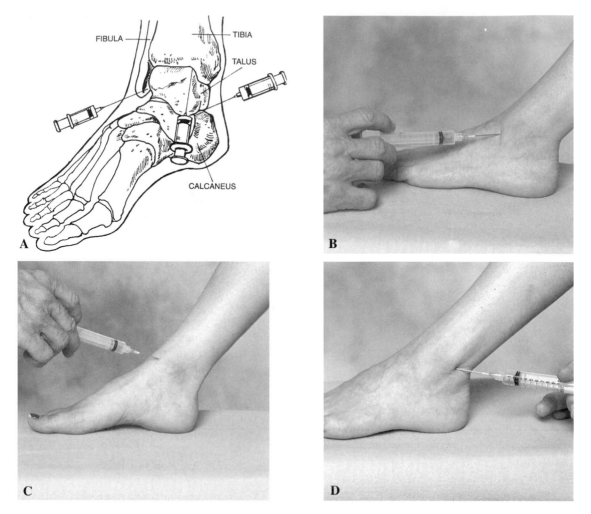

FIGURE 15-15.   Internal anatomic (*A*) and approximate surface anatomic (*B*, medial; *C*, lateral; *D*, posterior) sites for injection of the ankle.

An anterior medial or anterior lateral approach may be used, depending on the location of pain or pathologic process (Fig. 15-15). For the medial approach, a slight depression is felt between the extensor hallucis longus tendon laterally and tibialis anterior tendon medially on the inferior border of the tibia superiorly and the talus inferiorly. The needle is then directed slightly laterally and perpendicular to the tibial joint surface. The talus has a superior curve, and the needle may need to be angled slightly superiorly to avoid contact with the talar joint surface.

The lateral approach is useful in situations in which pathologic processes in the ankle appear to be most prominent either at the talofibular joint or the tibiotalar joint. Here, the foot is placed in moderate plantar flexion. The area enclosed by the tibia superiorly, the talus inferiorly, and the fibular head laterally is palpated. The extensor tendons of the toes should be medial to the injection site. The needle is

then inserted from an anterolateral position and is directed toward the posterior edge of the medial malleolus. If the joint surface is encountered, the physician should direct the needle slightly upward, remembering that the talar dome arches superiorly.

Subtalar Joint

Occasionally, the subtalar joint is the site of a pathologic process. The easiest approach to this joint is to have the patient lie prone with his or her feet extending over the end of the examination table. This allows the ankle to be in the neutral position. The posterior and lateral portions of the ankle are then prepared aseptically. The site of entry for the injection is along a line drawn from the most prominent portion of the distal fibula posterior to the Achilles tendon. This line should be parallel to the plantar aspect of the foot with the foot in neutral

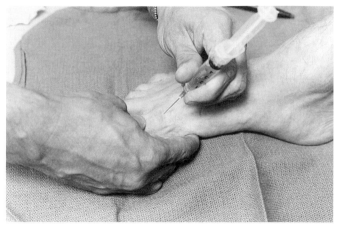

FIGURE 15-16. Dorsal approach to the first metatarsophalangeal joint.

position; halfway between the prominent aspect of the lateral malleolus and the Achilles tendon, the needle is inserted and directed toward a point inferior and medial to the medial malleolus.

Intertarsal Joints

Injection of the tarsal joints may be accomplished similarly to injection of the carpal joints. Palpation of the bony landmarks is obtained, the needle is inserted between the tarsal bones to the desired depth,[32] and aspiration is accomplished if necessary. Fluoroscopic needle guidance simplifies this procedure and ascertains precise needle placement.

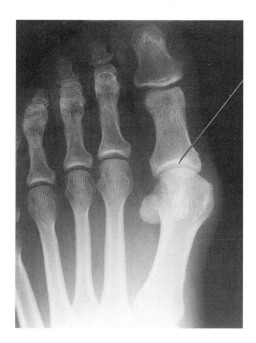

FIGURE 15-17. Anteroposterior x-ray of the foot demonstrating proper needle placement into the first metatarsophalangeal joint.

Metatarsophalangeal Joints

The metatarsophalangeal joints are most frequently infiltrated with a dorsal approach (Figs. 15-16 and 15-17).[31] This approach is carried out by palpating the metatarsophalangeal margins with plantar flexion of the toe in order to facilitate insertion of the needle. The needle is then advanced into the joint. The first metatarsophalangeal joint is frequently affected by arthritic conditions and gout. When a swollen joint is encountered, infiltration and aspiration may be easier with a swollen capsule.

CONCLUSION

The peripheral joints are not difficult to inject. With practice, the clinician can become quite adept at entering these joints with ease, providing an effective addition to the management of peripheral joint problems. After the joints are injected, they should not be subjected to intensive exercise or motion for several days. This period of relative rest helps to promote the retention of the corticosteroid in the joint, allowing longer contact with the joint surface and delaying absorption of the drug systemically.[23]

REFERENCES

1. Adelberg JS, Smith GH: Corticosteroid-induced avascular necrosis of the talus. J Foot Surg 30:66–69, 1991.
2. Alarcon-Segovia D, Ward LE: Marked destructive changes occurring in osteoarthritic finger joints after intra-articular injection of corticosteroids. Arthritis Rheum 9:443–449, 1966.
3. Bain LS, Balch HW, Wetherly JMR, et al: Intra-articular triamcinolone hexacetonide: Double-blind comparison with methylprednisolone. Br J Clin Pract 26:559–561, 1972.
4. Balch HW, Gibson JMC, El Ghobarey AF, et al: Repeated corticosteroid injections into knee joints. Rheumatoid Rehabil 16:137–140, 1977.
5. Behrens F, Shepherd N, Mitchel N: Alterations of rabbit articular cartilage by intra-articular injection of glucocorticoids. J Bone Joint Surg 57A:70–76, 1975.

6. Castles JJ: Clinical pharmacology of glucocorticoids. In McCarty DJ, Hollander JL (eds): Arthritis and Allied Conditions, 12th ed. Philadelphia, Lea & Febiger, 1993, pp 665–682.

7. Doherty M, Hazleman BL, Hutton CW, et al: Rheumatology Examination and Injection Techniques. Philadelphia, W.B. Saunders, 1992.

8. Gordon GV, Schumacher HR: Electron microscopic study for depot corticosteroid crystals with clinical studies after intra-articular injection. J Rheumatol 6:7–14, 1979.

9. Gowans J, Granieri P: Septic arthritis: Its relations to intra-articular injections of hydrocortisone acetate. N Engl J Med 261:502, 1959.

10. Gray RG, Gottlieb NL: Intra-articular corticosteroids: An updated assessment. Clin Orthop 177:235–263, 1983.

11. Gray RG, Gottlieb NL: Rheumatic disorders associated with diabetes mellitus: Literature review. Semin Arthritis Rheum 6:19–34, 1976.

12. Gray RG, Tenenbaum J, Gottlieb NL: Local corticosteroid injection treatment in rheumatic disorders. Semin Arthritis Rheum 10:231–245, 1981.

13. Hardin JG Jr: Controlled study of the long-term effects of "total hand" injection. Arthritis Rheum 22:619, 1979.

14. Hollander JL: Intrasynovial corticosteroid therapy in arthritis. Maryland State Med J 19:62–66, 1972.

15. Hollander JL: Joint problems in the elderly: How to help patients cope. Postgrad Med 21:209–311, 1988.

16. Howard LD, Pratt ER, Punnell S: The use of compound L (hydrocortisone) in operative and nonoperative conditions of the hand. J Bone Joint Surg 35A:994–1002, 1953.

17. Hudson TM: Elbow arthrography. Radiol Clin North Am 19:227–240, 1981.

18. Jalava S: Periarticular calcification after intra-articular triamcinolone hexacetonide. Scand J Rheumatol 9:190–192, 1980.

19. Kothari T, Reyes MP, Brooks N, et al: *Pseudomonas capacia* septic arthritis due to intra-articular injections of methylprednisolone. Can Med Assoc J 116:1230–1235, 1977.

20. Leversee JH: Aspiration of joint and soft tissue injections. Prim Care 13:572–599, 1986.

21. Marks M, Gunther SF: Efficacy of cortisone injection in treatment of trigger fingers and thumbs. J Hand Surg 14A:722–727, 1989.

22. McCarty DJ, McCarthy G, Garrera G: Intra-articular corticosteroids possibly leading to local osteonecrosis and marrow fat-induced synovitis. J Rheumatol 18:1091–1094, 1991.

23. Neustadt DH: Intra-articular corticosteroids and other agents: Aspiration techniques. In Katz W (ed): The Diagnosis and Management of Rheumatic Diseases, 2nd ed. Philadelphia, J.B. Lippincott, 1988, pp 812–825.

24. Neustadt DH: Local corticosteroid injection therapy and soft tissue rheumatic conditions of hand and wrist and rheumatism. J Arthritis Rheum 34:923–926, 1991.

25. Owen DF: Intra-articular and soft tissue aspiration injection. Clin Rheumatol Pract (Mar-May):52–63, 1986.

26. Pavno P, Anderson HJ, Simonson O: A long-term follow up of the effects of repeated corticosteroid injections for stenosing tenosynovitis. J Hand Surg 14B:242–243, 1989.

27. Pfenninger JL: Injections of joints and soft tissue: Part I. General guidelines. Am Fam Physician 44:1196–1202, 1991.

28. Pfenninger JL: Infections of joints and soft tissues: Part II. Guidelines for specific joints. Am Fam Physician 44:1690–1701, 1991.

29. Stanley D, Connolly WB: Iatrogenic injections injuries of the hand and upper limb. J Hand Surg 17B:442–446, 1992.

30. Stefanich RJ: Intra-articular corticosteroids in treatment of osteoarthritis. Orthop Rev 15:65–71, 1986.

31. Steinbrocker O, Neustadt DH: Aspiration Injection Therapy in Arthritis and Musculoskeletal Disorders: Handbook on Technique and Management. Hagerstown, MD, Harper & Row, 1972.

32. Taweepoe P, Frame JD: Acute ischemia of the hand by accidental radial infusion of Depo-Medrol. J Hand Surg 15:118–120, 1990.

33. Wilke WS, Tuggle CJ: Optimal techniques for intra-articular and peri-articular joint injections. Mod Med 56:58–72, 1988.

34. Zuckerman JD, Neislan RJ, Rothberg M: Injections for joint and soft tissue disorders: When and how to use them. Geriatrics 4:45–52, 1990.

16

Soft Tissue Injections

Nicholas K. Olsen, D.O., Joel M. Press, M.D., and Jeffrey L. Young, M.D.

Bursitis accounts for a large number of disorders seen in clinical practices that focus on musculoskeletal dysfunction. Inflamed bursae often respond to conservative treatments offered by the comprehensive rehabilitation team. In patients who fail to respond to conservative rehabilitation, a soft tissue injection into the bursa can serve as a useful diagnostic and therapeutic adjunct to therapy.

Bursae are purse-like sacs that are filled with fluid and function to reduce microtrauma to friction-prone areas. They are positioned between two muscles or between a muscle and its tendon or bone. Inflammation may occur during repetitive activities involving poor body mechanics or following direct trauma. An accurate diagnosis can be made by taking a thorough history, investigating the occupational and recreational activities of the patient. Correction of improper biomechanics is essential to avoid chronic irritation to the involved bursa.

After the history is obtained, a positive physical examination will reveal focal tenderness during palpation of the area overlying the bursa. If the injury is due to acute trauma, a fracture or ligamentous instability of the joint should be ruled out. However, most patients present with bursal irritation from repetitive microtrauma. The physical examination should include a survey of other joints to rule out a systemic process. Skin overlying the area of tenderness should be inspected for evidence of penetrating trauma. The patient may have intense pain upon palpation of the affected area, and an increase in skin temperature may be appreciated. In fact, skin warmth at the bursa may be the most sensitive indicator differentiating between a septic and nonseptic bursa.[16] Aspiration of a septic bursa and identification of a bacterial pathogen are necessary for appropriate antibiotic treatment. Laboratory studies of the serum should include an erythrocyte sedimentation rate, complete blood cell count, and microscopic examination to screen for leukocytosis, bacteria on Gram stain, or crystals. Operative incision and

drainage of a septic bursa may be required for effective treatment.[7,21] Contraindications to bursal injection with corticosteroids include cellulitis, generalized infection, and coagulation disorders.

Bursal injections serve both a diagnostic and a therapeutic role. An initial bursal injection with local anesthetic alone can provide important information that will lead to the correct diagnosis. The patient should be examined before and after administration of an anesthetic. When a septic bursa has been ruled out, a small amount of corticosteroid is introduced into the inflamed bursa to provide long-term relief and promote patient participation in a comprehensive rehabilitation program. Following the injection, the patient should be given instructions to avoid aggravating the condition. A physical therapist may be consulted for soft tissue mobilization and instruction in a stretching and strengthening program, or the clinician may prefer to provide a well-directed home program during the initial visit. Ice may be a useful adjunct during the initial phases of treatment, and nonsteroidal anti-inflammatory drugs (NSAIDs) may provide additional relief. Each of these options should be individualized for the clinical situation, and none of these, especially bursal injections, is to be used as the primary form of therapy. Follow-up should be scheduled within the first few weeks, and the program should be tailored to the patient as symptoms subside.

This chapter describes the basic approach to injection of many of the bursae encountered in clinical practice. Although the rehabilitation program for each bursae has not been detailed in order to allow for closer attention to procedural techniques, it is essential to employ a comprehensive rehabilitation program for each patient.

SUBACROMIAL (SUBDELTOID) BURSITIS

The subacromial bursa rests on the supraspinatus and is covered by the acromion, the coracoacromial ligament, and the deltoid. This is the most common site of bursitis of the shoulder, with inflammation usually occurring secondary to rotator cuff tendinitis or shoulder impingement syndrome. In a pure subacromial bursitis, the impingement signs may be absent, and the inflamed bursa may limit full passive abduction due to compression at the near end range of shoulder motion.[9] However, subacromial bursitis frequently coexists with impingement syndrome or rotator cuff syndrome. Determining the etiology of shoulder pain may be difficult, and a diagnostic injection into the bursa can narrow the field of possibilities. A diagnostic injection may help distinguish weakness and loss of range of motion secondary to a painful bursitis from a full-thickness rotator cuff tear. The patient should be thoroughly examined prior to the administration of local anesthetic and then reexamined 5–10 minutes after injection. Postinjection, the patient may be less guarded and more cooperative during the physical exam, yielding further diagnostic information.

Although an anterior, posterior, or lateral approach may be used, the posterolateral approach is preferred. Following sterile technique, the skin is cleansed with povidone-iodine, and the patient is directed to retract the shoulder to a neutral posture. The posterolateral angle of the acromion is identified by palpation, and the needle is advanced in an anteromedial and slightly inferior direction (Figs. 16-1 and 16-2).[20] If the soft tissues resist needle insertion, a small volume can be injected to expand the bursa so that the needle can be advanced further, resulting in optimal needle position. A mixture of 2–4 ml of 1% or 2% lidocaine hydrochloride and 2–4 ml of 0.5% bupivacaine hydrochloride is injected into the bursa after a 25-gauge, 1.5-inch needle is introduced approximately 1 inch.[1] In the authors' experience, an inflamed subacromial bursa accepts 4–6 ml of total volume. Following the injection, a reduction of pain with improved strength supports the diagnoses of shoulder impingement, supraspinatus tendinitis, and subdeltoid bursitis. Patients who respond with greater than 50% relief are good candidates for an immediate follow-up injection with 1 ml of betamethasone sodium phosphate.[1] Subacromial bursography is helpful when the initial blind injection is unsuccessful or in a patient whose diagnosis is unclear. A normal bursogram casts doubt on a diagnosis of subacromial impingement.[10]

The rehabilitation program should not progress too rapidly after corticosteroid injection, because the patient may be at risk for bicipital tendon rupture.

OLECRANON BURSITIS (DRAFTSMEN'S ELBOW)

The olecranon bursa is located subcutaneously and protects the proximal ulna where the olecranon is often subjected to trauma. Inflammation of this bursa is commonly seen in rheumatologic disorders. Aspiration of the bursa should always precede injection and may be helpful to ensure proper location of the needle, because the wall of the bursa is often thickened and fibrotic from chronic irritation. Gout may be seen at the olecranon, and any bursal fluid aspirated should undergo microscopic examination for crystals. Aspiration of the bursa is more successful using a larger bore needle (18-gauge), because the fluid is likely gelatinous. The needle enters the skin perpendicular to the central swelling while the clinician withdraws on the syringe (Fig. 16-3).[20] The procedure is followed with the application of a compressive dressing, and the patient is instructed to protect the elbow from further trauma. Persistent

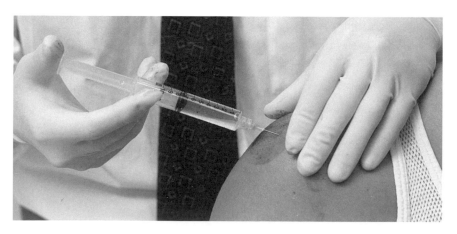

FIGURE 16-1.   The subacromial bursa is approached from posterolateral attitude.

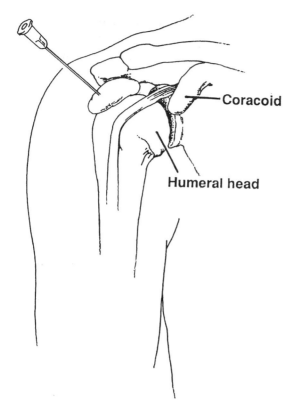

FIGURE 16-2. Schematic of subacromial bursa injection. (Adapted from Vander Slam TJ: Atlas of Bedside Procedures. Boston, Little Brown, 1988, with permission.)

cases may benefit from a low-dose corticosteroid injection. Rarely, surgical excision or an arthroscopic bursectomy is warranted after failure of conservative measures.[7]

TROCHANTERIC BURSITIS

Several bursae may be implicated in trochanteric bursitis. The subgluteus maximus bursa lies lateral to the greater trochanter and the insertion of the gluteus medius and minimus. The subgluteus medius bursa is situated superior and posterior to the trochanter. The gluteus minimus bursa lies anterior to the trochanter. All three bursae may be part of a greater trochanteric pain syndrome.

Trochanteric bursitis is commonly seen in an elderly population and manifests as pain in the lateral thigh during ambulation. Patients may describe a pseudoradicular pattern with the pain extending down the lateral aspect of the lower extremity and into the buttock. The symptoms can be elicited by placing the lower extremity in external rotation and abduction. Direct palpation or deep pressure applied posterior and superior to the trochanter will reproduce the pain.[14] The patient should be examined for limitations in flexibility involving the gluteus maximus, medius, and minimus and the tensor fasciae latae. Hip abduction weakness may contribute to irritation of the bursa. If the history and physical exam are consistent with bursitis, a corticosteroid combined with anesthetic agent is delivered via a 3.5-inch, 22-gauge needle directed at the point of maximal tenderness overlying the greater trochanter (Fig. 16-4).[11,20] Persistent hip pain despite injection therapy and comprehensive rehabilitation should alert the physician to alternate sources of pain including the lumbar spine, hip joint, and distal lower extremity joints.[2,19]

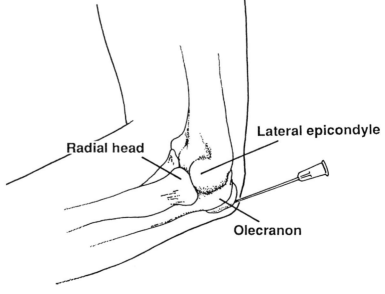

FIGURE 16-3. Approach for olecranon aspiration and injection. (Adapted from Vander Slam TJ: Atlas of Bedside Procedures. Boston, Little Brown, 1988, with permission.)

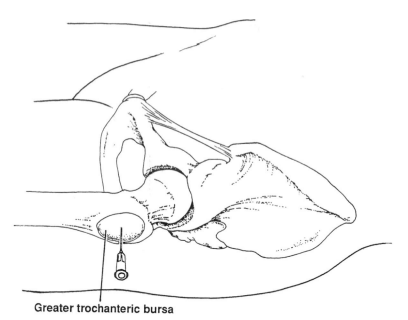

FIGURE 16-4. Greater trochanteric bursal injection. (Adapted from Vander Slam TJ: Atlas of Bedside Procedures. Boston, Little Brown, 1988, with permission.)

Greater trochanteric bursa

ILIOPECTINEAL (ILIOPSOAS) BURSA

The iliopectineal bursa, the largest bursa near the hip joint, is located anterior to the hip capsule and is covered by the iliopsoas. Inflammation of the bursa is not particularly common but may be functionally limiting because it causes the patient to avoid extension of the lower extremity during the gait cycle. Patients hold the lower extremity in external rotation with the hip in flexion to relieve pressure on the inflamed bursa. Referral pain following the femoral nerve distribution may be seen in cases of iliopectineal bursitis. The examiner may elicit symptoms by passively extending the hip in either a supine or prone position. Injection under fluoroscopic guidance is recommended because the bursa may communicate with the hip capsule and correct needle placement is essential.[14,15] Once placement is confirmed by a bursogram, a mixture of anesthetic and corticosteroid is injected through the 3.5-inch spinal needle.

ISCHIAL BURSITIS (TAILOR'S OR WEAVER'S BOTTOM)

The ischial bursa lies between the ischial tuberosity and the gluteus maximus. The examiner's index of suspicion must be high because ischial bursitis—so-called tailor's or weaver's bottom—is not common. Classically, ischial bursitis occurs from friction and the trauma of prolonged sitting on a hard surface. It may occur in adolescent runners, often in conjunction with ischial apophysitis. Pain is aggravated during uphill running.[12] The pain is distributed down the posterior aspect of the thigh and occurs with activation of the hamstring muscles. Initial treatment approaches should address modification of the patient's activity, including a decrease in the duration and frequency of running. If an alternative to running includes cycling, the patient should be advised to avoid the use of toe clips, which increase activation of the hamstrings. When the etiology is due to prolonged sitting, the patient's work station should be modified to allow activities to be conducted in a standing position, and a cushion should be used during sitting. Ice and NSAIDs are helpful in controlling symptoms. Adolescent athletes may require a radiologic series to screen for callus formation secondary to ischial apophysitis if the pain does not resolve with conservative measures. Persistent pain may benefit from injection as an adjunct to rest, ice, and NSAIDs. To perform this, the patient lies on his or her side with the knees fully flexed to relax the hamstrings. A 3-inch, 22-gauge needle is held in a horizontal position and directed toward the point of maximal tenderness overlying the ischial tuberosity. The injection of contrast dye into the bursa under fluoroscopy may be necessary to verify needle placement.

ANSERINE BURSITIS

The anserine bursa separates the three conjoined tendons of the pes anserinus, or goose's foot (semitendinosus, sartorius, and gracilis muscles), from the medial collateral ligament and the tibia. It is one

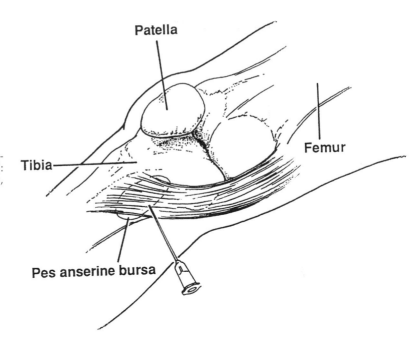

FIGURE 16-5. Anserine bursal injection. (Adapted from Vander Slam TJ: Atlas of Bedside Procedures. Boston, Little Brown, 1988, with permission.)

of the most commonly inflamed bursae in the lower extremity. Anserine bursitis is commonly seen in women with heavy thighs and osteoarthritis of the knees. The bursa may also become inflamed as the result of direct trauma in athletes, especially soccer players.[12] Patients report pain inferior to the anteromedial surface of the knee with ascension of stairs. Moving the patient's knee in flexion and extension while internally rotating the leg will reproduce the symptoms. The palpatory exam will localize the pain to the anserine bursa. The injection is easy and quite effective in reducing inflammatory symptoms. After sterile preparation, the knee is fully extended and a 1.0- to 1.5-inch, 22-gauge needle is directed at the point of maximal tenderness (Fig. 16-5)[20] to deliver a 1- to 3-ml combination of anesthetic and corticosteroid. The patient should enter a rehabilitation program emphasizing flexibility, and the athlete at risk for repetitive trauma may benefit from padded knee protection.

TIBIAL COLLATERAL LIGAMENT BURSITIS

The tibial collateral ligament (TCL) bursa, referred to as the "no name, no fame" bursa,[17] is located between the deep and superficial aspects of the tibial collateral ligament. The bursa does not adhere to the medial meniscus, and it appears to reduce friction between the superficial layer of the TCL and the medial meniscus. TCL bursitis should be considered in any patient with medial joint line

tenderness. During a 3-year study, Kerlan found that 5% of orthopedic patients presenting with medial knee pain suffered from TCL bursitis.[6] Physical examination will not show evidence of new ligamentous or capsular instability. Treatment consists of a local injection of lidocaine and 1 ml of triamcinolone (40 mg/ml)[6] directed perpendicular to the medial joint line at the point of maximal tenderness (Fig. 16-6).

PREPATELLAR BURSITIS

Prepatellar bursitis, often called "housemaid's knee," is the result of frequent kneeling that produces swelling and effusion of the subcutaneous bursa at the anterior surface of the patella. The patient rarely complains of pain unless direct pressure is applied to the bursa. The area is easily entered with a needle at the middle to superior pole of the patella. Repeat injections may be required because the bursa is often multiloculated. Occupational adjustments should include patient education, avoidance of kneeling, and the use of knee pads when pressure must be applied to the patella.

RETROCALCANEAL (SUBTENDINOUS) BURSITIS

The retrocalcaneal bursa lies between the posterior surface of the calcaneus and the tendon of the triceps surae. Inflammation of the bursa may occur from overtraining, such as too early assumption of

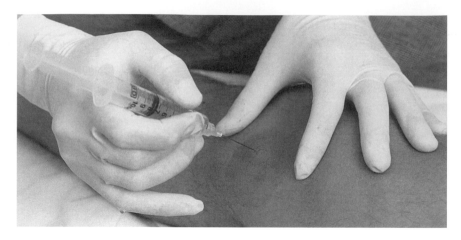

FIGURE 16-6.   Approach for tibial collateral bursa.

increased mileage in a runner, or an ill-fitting shoe resulting in pressure from a restricting heel counter. A positive indicator is discomfort when the examiner places the thumb and index finger on the anterior edges of the Achilles tendon and applies pressure. Modification of the footwear is an important first step to alleviating pain, and symptoms should be controlled with ice and NSAIDs. As the pain is controlled, the patient should stretch the triceps surae complex daily to avoid recurrence. Injections into the bursa are considered only after the above measures have been pursued. A 20- to 22-gauge needle should be inserted where the bursa demonstrates the greatest distention, often on the lateral aspect of the heel. The needle is advanced with an anterior angle of 15–20° to avoid instilling corticosteroid into the Achilles tendon, which weakens the structure and increases the risk of tendon rupture.

SUBCUTANEOUS (ACHILLES) BURSITIS

Subcutaneous bursitis, also known as Achilles bursitis or achillobursitis, affects the bursa that lies subcutaneous to the posterior surface of the tendon. Midline swelling develops where the upper edge of the heel counter comes in contact with the heel cord. Subcutaneous bursitis is common in patients who wear high-heeled shoes that apply direct pressure on the bursa. The mainstay of treatment is to have the patient change the shoes. Ice and anti-inflammatory medications help provide symptomatic relief. Injection of the bursa is usually not necessary, but if the symptoms persist, an injection should be considered. Care should be given to avoid the Achilles.

CALCANEAL BURSITIS

Calcaneal bursitis often develops in elderly patients from a calcified spur that subjects the bursa to trauma after prolonged walking or running. Evaluation of the footwear may reveal poor shock-absorbing capacity. Injection into the point of maximum tenderness may have both diagnostic and therapeutic value. Selection of an appropriate walking or running shoe and the use of a heel cup are beneficial. Athletes should be encouraged to change running shoes every 200–300 miles because midsole breakdown occurs after this amount of wear.[22]

PHARMACOLOGIC AGENTS FOR BURSAL INJECTION

A number of local anesthetics are available for bursal injections, and clinicians should be familiar with their pharmacologic properties. Concentrations of 0.5–1.0% lidocaine or 0.25–0.5% bupivacaine are appropriate for bursal injection. The onset and duration of the anesthetic effect is related to the volume and concentration injected. Lidocaine has an onset of action within 5–15 minutes and may last 3–4 hours, while bupivacaine begins to work in 10–20 minutes, but the anesthetic effect can last 4–6 hours.[3] Bach describes the benefits of using a combination of lidocaine hydrochloride and bupivacaine hydrochloride in subacromial space injections to obtain an early onset of action with prolonged anesthesia.[1]

Corticosteroids are widely available and very effective in alleviating bursal inflammation. Corticosteroids of intermediate or long duration are suitable for treatment of bursitis. Triamcinolone

TABLE 16-1. Guidelines for Bursal Injections

Bursae[a]	Anesthetic Volume[b] (ml)	Corticosteroid Volume (ml)	Needle Length (20–22 gauge)[c]
Subacromial	4.0–6.0	0.5–1.0	1.5″
Trochanteric	4.5–9.0	1.5–1.0	1.5–3.5″
Iliopectineal	4.0–4.5	0.5–1.0	3.5″
Ischial	2.5–4.0	0.5–1.0	3.5″
Anserine	2.5–4.5	0.25–0.5	1.5″
Prepatellar[d]		0.5–1.0	1.5″

[a] Fluoroscopic guidance may be necessary to increase accuracy of bursa injection. A bursogram may be a useful tool, increasing the diagnostic and therapeutic value of injections.

[b] The volume refers to the capacity of the bursa, and the clinician should select a corticosteroid concentration appropriate for the bursal volume.

[c] The clinician may prefer an 18-gauge needle initially for aspiration if gelatinous fluid is anticipated and then change to a finer gauge for instillation of pharmacologic agents.

[d] The prepatellar bursa is often multiloculated, and its capacity may vary.

acetonide (10 mg/ml and 40 mg/ml) is a commonly used intermediate-acting agent with a half-life of 24–36 hours. Betamethasone is a longer acting corticosteroid with a half-life of 36–72 hours and a relative anti-inflammatory potency five times greater than triamcinolone.[3] The dosage is adjusted to the size of the bursa, and the lowest effective dose should be delivered to the bursa. Clinicians may want to avoid corticosteroid injection acutely (the first 7 days after an initial injury) because corticosteroids theoretically inhibit the healing process.[13] About 14–21 days after injury, glucocorticoids can control the inflammation and edema of the proliferative phase. The Achilles and patellar tendons should be avoided because direct injection into the tendon can place the patient at risk for rupture.[13]

The clinician must be careful to select a combination of medications within the recommended volumes to avoid further injury to the bursae. Table 16-1 may be used as a guideline for selecting the type and volume of corticosteroid and anesthetic to be administered.

CONCLUSION

Bursal injections provide a useful diagnostic and therapeutic approach within a comprehensive rehabilitation program. The clinician should have a strong foundation in anatomy and must be familiar with the pharmacologic agents. Diagnosing bursitis can be difficult with only a physical exam, and injection therapy is a useful diagnostic tool. Strong palpatory skills can aid in the injection process, verifying placement of medication into a superficial bursa such as the pes anserine. Fluoroscopic guidance can further ensure accurate delivery of medications to deep lying bursae, avoiding unnecessary repeat injections due to an inaccurately placed needle. Injection therapy is neither a beginning nor an end point of a comprehensive rehabilitation program. Underlying biomechanical deficits of muscle weakness and tightness must be aggressively sought and corrected for an optimal result.

REFERENCES

1. Bach BR, Bush-Joseph C: Subacromial space injections: A tool for evaluating shoulder pain. Physician Sportsmed 2:93–98, 1992.
2. Collée G, Dijkmans BA, Vandenbroucke JD, Cats A: Greater trochanteric pain syndrome (trochanteric bursitis) in low back pain. Scand J Rheumatol 20:262–266, 1991.
3. Covino BG, Scott DB: Handbook of Epidural Anesthesia and Analgesia. Orlando, Grune & Stratton, 1985, pp 58–74.
4. Hemler DE, Ward WK, Karstetter KW, Bryant PM: Saphenous nerve entrapment caused by pes anserine bursitis mimicking stress fracture of the tibia. Arch Phys Med Rehabil 72:336–337, 1991.
5. Kelley WN, Harris ED, Ruddy S, Sledge CB: Textbook of Rheumatology. Philadelphia, W.B. Saunders, 1993, pp 545–560.
6. Kerlan RK, Glousman RE: Tibial collateral ligament bursitis. Am J Sports Med 16:344–346, 1988.
7. Kerr BR: Prepatellar and olecranon arthroscopic bursectomy. Clin Sports Med 12:137–142, 1993.
8. Lee JK, Yao L: Tibial collateral ligament bursa: MR imaging. Radiology 178:855–857, 1991.
9. Magee DJ: Orthopedic Physical Assessment. Philadelphia, W.B. Saunders, 1992, p 102.
10. Nicholas JA, Hershman EB: The Upper Extremity in Sports Medicine. St. Louis, Mosby, 1990, pp 124–125.
11. Rasmussen KJ, Farro N: Trochanteric bursitis: Treatment by corticosteroid injection. Scand J Rheumatol 14:417–420, 1985.
12. Reid DC: Sports Injury Assessment and Rehabilitation. New York, Churchill Livingstone, 1992, pp 631, 1564, 1625–1626, 1636.
13. Saal JA: General principles and guidelines for rehabilitation of the injured athlete. Phys Med Rehabil State Art Rev 1:523–536, 1987.
14. Schumacher RH: Primer on the Rheumatic Diseases. Atlanta, Arthritis Foundation, 1988, pp 263–274.
15. Sheeb MI, Matteson EL: Trochanteric bursitis (greater trochanter pain syndrome). Mayo Clin Proc 71:565–569, 1996.

16. Smith DL, McAfee JH, Lucas LM, et al: Septic and non-septic olecranon bursitis: Utilization of the surface temperature probe in the early differentiation of septic and nonseptic cases. Arch Intern Med 149:1581–1585, 1989.
17. Stuttle FL: The no-name, no-fame bursa. Clin Orthop 15:197–199, 1959.
18. Swezey RL: Pseudo-radiculopathy in subacute trochanteric bursitis of the subgluteus maximus bursa. Arch Phys Med Rehabil 57:387–390, 1976.
19. Traycoff RB: "Pseudotrochanteric bursitis": The differential diagnosis of lateral hip pain. J Rheumatol 18:1810–1812, 1991.
20. Vander Slam TJ: Atlas of Bedside Procedures. Boston, Little Brown, 1988, pp 455, 459, 461.
21. Waters D, Kasser J: Infection of the infrapatellar bursa. J Bone Joint Surg 72A:1095–1096, 1990.
22. Young JL, Press JM: Rehabilitation of running injuries. In Buschbacher RH, Braddom RL (eds): Sports Medicine and Rehabilitation: A Sport-Specific Approach. Philadelphia, Hanley & Belfus, 1994, pp 123–134.

17

Tendon Sheath and Insertion Injections

Steve R. Geiringer, M.D.

ANATOMY AND PHYSIOLOGY

Tendons are impressively strong structures that link muscles to bone. They function to transmit the force of muscular contraction to a bone, thereby moving a joint or helping to immobilize a body part (as in making a fist). Their microscopic organization is thoroughly described elsewhere.[8,24,32]

The organizational unit in a tendon is the collagen fibril, which collectively form fascicles, which as a group compose the tendon itself.[35] Some tendons, especially long ones, are guided and lubricated along their paths by sheaths (Fig. 17-1) (e.g., biceps brachii, extensor pollicis brevis, and abductor pollicis longus).

A prototypical muscle consists of the muscle belly centrally, two musculotendinous junctions, and tendinous insertions into bone at the points of anatomic origin and insertion. Some muscles, such as the extensor carpi radialis longus and brevis at the elbow, attach directly into bone, an arrangement that may be more susceptible to injury.[7]

Much is known about a tendon's response to laceration and operative repair,[24] although this clinical situation is not frequently encountered. Less is understood about the more common and clinically relevant overuse tendinitis. A tendon and its sheath (if present) will undergo a typical inflammatory response to either acute or chronic overuse injury, followed by a regenerative repair process.[4,24] The distinction between an overload type of acute injury and a chronic overuse mechanism will aid in successful rehabilitation of tendinitis.[14]

CORTICOSTEROID INJECTIONS

Cortisone and its derivatives are known to reduce or prevent inflammation. Numerous corticosteroid preparations are available for local injection.[19] The injectable corticosteroids are suspensions of insoluble particles, and therefore, the anti-inflammatory effect is profound only where the material is deposited.[9] It is the ability of corticosteroids to control inflammation that makes them a valuable adjunct in treating tendon injuries, because they do not alter the underlying process that leads to inflammation.[19]

Efficacy

As with many other physical medicine treatment modalities, well-designed scientific studies into the usefulness of corticosteroid injections are rare. These injections should therefore be considered when, in the practitioner's judgment, the recognized anti-inflammatory effect of local corticosteroid placement may be beneficial for the conditions of tendinitis, enthesitis, or tenosynovitis, and no harm will likely result.

McWhorter et al. injected hydrocortisone acetate into rat Achilles peritendons that had been previously injured.[26] There were no deleterious effects of one, three, or even five injections, measured biomechanically (tension to failure) or histologically (light microscopy), compared to controls. This finding should reassure physicians that they are not doing harm with properly placed steroid injections. A recent 30-year literature review identified eight prospective, placebo-controlled studies of steroid injection treatment for sports-related tendinitis.[2] Three of these showed beneficial effects of injections at clinical follow-up. A meta-analysis of properly designed investigations of steroid injection for Achilles tendinitis found no beneficial effects,[37] although very few studies qualified as rigorous. Adverse side effects occurred with a 1% incidence. No "proof" of the usefulness or uselessness of this treatment modality exists.

Contraindications, Complications, and Side Effects

The lack of a specific diagnosis is the single largest contraindication to a local corticosteroid injection. If

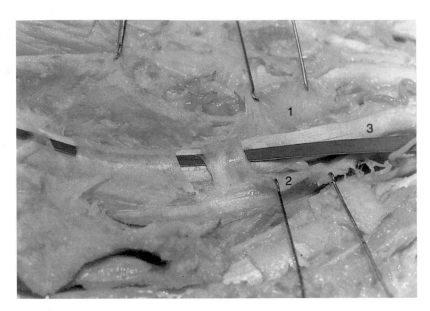

FIGURE 17-1.   Gross specimen demonstrating a flexor tendon (3) within its sheath (metal rod inserted). Ulnar vertical para-tendinous septum (1) and everted radial vertical paratendinous septum (2). (From Zancolli EA, Cozzi EP (eds): Atlas of Surgical Anatomy of the Hand. New York, Churchill Livingstone, 1992, p 357; with permission.)

the diagnosis is clear and the anti-inflammatory effect of a corticosteroid may facilitate the rehabilitation process, injection can be considered.[19]

Repeated injections to the same area are to be avoided, particularly into joints. Alterations in articular cartilage have been documented with repeated administration,[25] possibly resulting in joint damage and weakened ligaments.[31] A widely recognized complication of steroid injection is tendon rupture, a negative outcome that appears to be decreasing in frequency because it is now well understood. Achilles and other tendon ruptures have been reported,[15,18,20,36,39,41,43] and deposition of injected material directly into any tendon substance is contraindicated. One report links the effect of repeated steroid injections to rupture of the plantar fascia.[23]

Some experimental findings have suggested that corticosteroid administration led to smaller, weaker tendons as a side effect.[17] A more common side effect is subcutaneous atrophy, especially at the knee and lateral elbow and more frequently with the use of triamcinolone.[19] Theoretically, atrophy of the specialized fat pads of the heel following steroid injection for plantar fasciitis may lead to a significant disability in an athlete due to the loss of cushioning effect.

Methods of Injection

Cyriax[9] has provided detailed descriptions of soft tissue injection techniques; therefore, these descriptions will not be repeated here.

Tendon and tendon sheath injections are office procedures, typically performed under clean or sterile conditions. The corticosteroid of choice is often combined with a local anesthetic, the latter helping to confirm the proper location of the deposited material. Diagnostic ultrasound has been advocated to guide injections near the heel when guidance by palpation alone fails.[6]

Immobilization of the treated structure usually is not needed following injection, although vigorous use of weight-bearing tendons (Achilles, patellar) should be avoided for 48 hours. Ice application may help when the local anesthesia fades, along with other physical medicine modalities as indicated by the particular condition present, usually starting 48 hours afterwards.

If an initial corticosteroid injection proves useful, one or two repeat injections separated by a few weeks or more may be considered. Numerous injections over time should not be considered the sole or primary treatment.

Indications

Diagnosis

Corticosteroid or local anesthetic injections should not be used routinely to arrive at diagnoses pertinent to the musculoskeletal system. The range of physical examination techniques used by the physician is described elsewhere[13] and, in most cases, will suffice at pinpointing the specific cause of

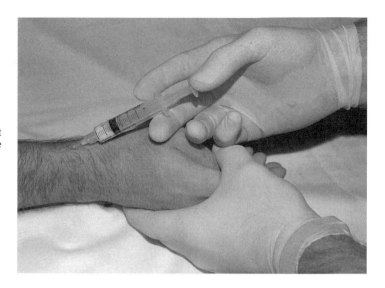

FIGURE 17-2. Injection technique for first dorsal compartment stenosing tenosynovitis (de Quervain syndrome).

pain. The distinction between the conditions of subacromial bursitis and rotator cuff tendinitis can be clarified with injection,[19] but even in this case the physical examination and subsequent rehabilitation program deservedly receive most of the attention.

Treatment

In most instances, the literature supports an adjunctive, not primary, role for injections in the treatment of tendon and tendon sheath injuries.[19,36] When the doctor and patient decide to proceed with injection, the control of inflammation that is obtained should be used to facilitate the prescribed rehabilitation program, rather than being the only treatment. The area of exception to this generalization is the wrist and hand (to be discussed in detail later).

Typically, because of the documented side effects and complications, a limit of about three corticosteroid injections in a given area is considered judicious for an injury. This limit is particularly important for intra-articular injections—as mentioned previously, corticosteroid should not be injected directly into the substance of a tendon.

Upper Extremity Injections

The literature supports the use of corticosteroid injections as a primary treatment for stenosing flexor tenosynovitis in the hand, known as trigger thumb or trigger digit.[3,12,21,22,27,29,33] In this setting, injection has been shown to be as effective as operative release of the tendon sheath and to have fewer complications.[21] Injection has been employed successfully into the hands of patients with diabetes

mellitus and trigger digit.[38] Instillation of the material directly into the tendon sheath has no apparent benefit over subcutaneous placement.[40] As with other soft tissue injections, a physician treating trigger finger with instillation of corticosteroid needs to maintain expertise by performing this procedure at least several times yearly.

Stenosing tenosynovitis of the first dorsal wrist compartment also is known as de Quervain syndrome. This compartment typically transmits the tendons of both the abductor pollicis longus (APL) and extensor pollicis brevis (EPB). However, anatomic studies have demonstrated that multiple APL slips are common, as are two subcompartments.[28] Interestingly, although one or more injections are usually successful in treating de Quervain syndrome nonoperatively,[4,16,45] patients requiring subsequent operative release have been found to have two subcompartments in greater than expected frequency.[16,45] Trigger digit and de Quervain syndrome, therefore, are usually treated successfully nonoperatively, and corticosteroid injection is the primary component of the management (Fig. 17-2).

The use of corticosteroid injection for lateral epicondylitis (tennis elbow) appears widespread (Fig. 17-3), although carefully controlled studies to confirm its efficacy are absent from the literature. One prospective investigation found that corticosteroid injection was more effective in controlling symptoms 8 weeks after injury than anesthetic alone, but the benefit disappeared by 24 weeks.[34] This may be explained by the finding that the histology of tennis elbow is noninflammatory.[30] A prospective chart review found that injection alone was effective in 91% of patients within one week, but was associated

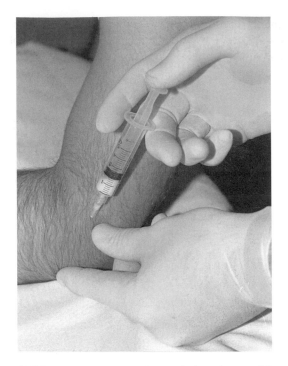

FIGURE 17-3. Injection technique for lateral epicondylitis.

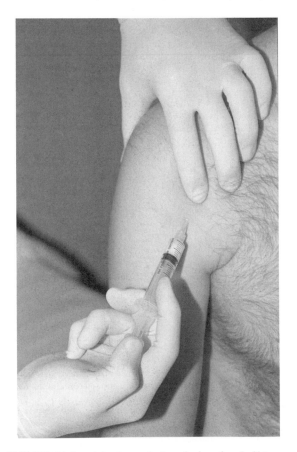

FIGURE 17-4. Injection technique for long head of biceps brachii.

with a 51% recurrence after 3 months. Initially, a standard physical therapy regimen led to improvement in only 74%, but the recurrence rate dropped to 5%.[11] In the typical clinical setting, of course, injection(s) and physical therapy are often combined with careful consideration of the intrinsic and extrinsic biomechanical factors that may be contributing.[14]

No recent studies have examined the use of corticosteroid injections in the treatment of biceps brachii tendinitis. In this area, care should be taken to deposit the suspension to bathe the tendon sheath rather than to deposit it into the body of the tendon itself (Fig. 17-4). Additionally, heavy lifting or vigorous exercise of the arm should be restricted for 48–72 hours following injection.

Corticosteroid injection has been found to be effective for rotator cuff tendinitis, at least for the first several weeks. In one study, injection was superior to placebo and to oral anti-inflammatory medication over the course of 4 weeks.[1] No more than three injections are recommended.[19] The technique itself is detailed elsewhere.[9] After corticosteroid injection for treatment of rotator cuff tendinitis, heavy lifting and excessive overhead work are to be avoided for at least 2 days.

Lower Extremity Injections

The literature contains relatively few references to corticosteroid injections of the lower limb for tendon or tendon sheath injuries. In this arena, as in much of musculoskeletal medicine, the practitioner must rely on anecdotal evidence, clinical experience and judgment, and trial and error when choosing a course of treatment.

Although it is not a true tendinitis, plantar fasciitis is commonly treated with steroid injection(s) (Fig. 17-5). If used, they must be considered complementary to a complete rehabilitation program that includes flexibility training and correction of any contributing intrinsic or extrinsic biomechanical factors.[19] If lipoatrophy occurs in the fat pad of the heel secondary to corticosteroid deposition, true disability in the active individual may result. Cosmesis is less of a problem because of the location.

Most physicians are aware of possible tendon rupture if corticosteroid is injected directly into the Achilles tendon.[13] On the other hand, the Achilles sheath can be injected,[9] often with a good therapeutic result. One double-blind, randomized, controlled study found no advantage of Achilles tendon sheath injections when compared with standard physical therapy measures.[10]

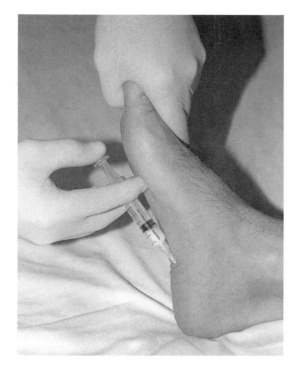

FIGURE 17-5. Injection technique for plantar fasciitis.

Iliotibial band tendinitis, refractory to other measures, sometimes responds to corticosteroid injection. The material is placed around the insertion of the iliotibial band at the proximal, lateral tibia, or, depending on the site of symptoms, where it passes over the prominence of the lateral femoral condyle.[19] Iliopsoas tendinitis has been similarly treated[42] with up to 2 years of symptomatic relief.

The quadriceps (infrapatellar) tendon can be injected for cases of tendinitis,[9] but because this is a weight-bearing structure, many practitioners avoid this procedure for fear of rupture.

CONCLUSION

In most cases of tendinitis or tenosynovitis of the upper or lower limb, corticosteroid injection for control of inflammation should be considered as a supplement to an individualized, well-designed, rehabilitation program. Notable exceptions are trigger digit or thumb, in which corticosteroids are a successful primary intervention, and, to a lesser extent, de Quervain syndrome. The physician using corticosteroid injections must perform them often enough to maintain technical expertise. Three injections for any given injured area is considered a conservative maximum. Subcutaneous atrophy is a common side effect, and the known complication of

tendon rupture strongly recommends against injections of corticosteroid directly into the substance of tendons.

REFERENCES

1. Adebajo AO, Nash P, Haxleman BL: A prospective double blind dummy placebo controlled study comparing triamcinolone hexacetonide injection with oral diclofenac 50 mg tds in patients with rotator cuff tendinitis. J Rheumatol 17:1207–1210, 1990.
2. Almekinders LC, Temple JD: Etiology, diagnosis, and treatment of tendonitis: An analysis of the literature. Med Sci Sports Exerc 30:1183–1190, 1998.
3. Anderson B, Kaye S: Treatment of flexor tenosynovitis of the hand ("trigger finger") with corticosteroids: A prospective study of the response to local injection. Arch Intern Med 151:153–156, 1991.
4. Anderson BC, Manthey R, Brouns MC: Treatment of de Quervain's tenosynovitis with corticosteroids: A prospective study of the response to local injection. Arthritis Rheum 34:793–798, 1991.
5. Badalamente MA, Sampson SP, Dowd A: The cellular pathobiology of cumulative trauma disorders/entrapment syndromes: Trigger finger, de Quervain's disease and carpal tunnel syndrome. Trans Orthop Res Soc 17:677, 1992.
6. Brophy DP, Cunnane G, Fitzgerald Q, Gibney RG: Technical report: Ultrasound guidance for injection of soft tissue lesions around the heel in chronic inflammatory arthritis. Clin Radiol 50:120–122, 1995.
7. Cooper RR, Misol S: Tendons and ligament insertion. J Bone Joint Surg 52A:1–20, 1970.
8. Curwin S, Stanish WD: Tendinitis: Its Etiology and Treatment. Lexington, Collamore Press, 1984.
9. Cyriax J: Textbook of Orthopaedic Medicine: Vol. 2. Treatment by Manipulation Massage and Injection. London, Baillière Tindall, 1980.
10. DaCruz DJ, Geeson M, Allen MJ, Phair I: Achilles paratendonitis: An evaluation of steroid injection. Br J Sports Med 22:64–65, 1988.
11. Dijs H, Mortier G, Driessens M, et al: A retrospective study of the conservative treatment of tennis elbow. Acta Belg Med Phys 13:73–77, 1990.
12. Fauno P, Anderson HJ, Simonsen O: A long-term follow-up of the effect of repeated corticosteroid injections for stenosing tenovaginitis. J Hand Surg 14A:242–243, 1989.
13. Galloway MT, Jokl P, Dayton OW: Achilles tendon overuse injuries. Clin Sports Med 11:771–782, 1992.
14. Geiringer SR, Bowyer BL, Press JM: Sports medicine. The physiatric approach. Arch Phys Med Rehabil 74:S428–S432, 1993.
15. Halpern AA, Horowitz BG, Nagel DA: Tendon ruptures associated with corticosteroid therapy. West J Med 127:378–432, 1993.
16. Harvey FJ, Harvey PM, Horsley MV: deQuervain's disease: Surgical or nonsurgical treatment. J Hand Surg 15A:83–87, 1990.
17. Kapetanos J: The effects of the local corticosteroids on the healing and biomechanical properties of the partially injured tendon. Clin Orthop 163:160–179, 1982.
18. Kennedy JC, Baxter-Willis R: The effects of local steroid injections on tendons: A biochemical and microscopic correlative study. Am J Sports Med 4:11–18, 1976.
19. Kerlan RK, Glousman RE: Injections and techniques in athletic medicine. Clin Sports Med 8:541–560, 1989.
20. Kleinman M, Gross A: Achilles tendon rupture following steroid injection. J Bone Joint Surg 65A:1345–1347, 1983.
21. Kraemer BA, Young VL, Arfken C: Stenosing flexor tenosynovitis. South Med J 83:806–811, 1990.

22. Lambert MA, Morton RJ, Sloan JP: Controlled study of the use of local steroid injection in the treatment of trigger finger and thumb. J Hand Surg 17A:69–70, 1992.

23. Leach R, Jones R, Silva T: Rupture of the plantar fascia in athletes. J Bone Joint Surg 60A:537–559, 1978.

24. Leadbetter WB: Cell-matrix response in tendon injury. Clin Sports Med 11:533–578, 1992.

25. Mankin H, Conger K: The acute effects of intra-articular hydrocortisone on articular cartilage in rabbits. J Bone Joint Surg 48A:1383–1388, 1966.

26. McWhorter JW, Francis RS, Heckmann RA: Influence of local steroid injections on traumatized tendon properties. A biomechanical and histological study. Am J Sports Med 19:435–439, 1991.

27. Marks MR, Gunther SF: Efficacy of cortisone injection in treatment of trigger fingers and thumbs. J Hand Surg 14A:722–727, 1989.

28. Minamikawa Y, Peimer CA, Cox WL, et al: deQuervain's syndrome: Surgical and anatomical studies of the fibro-osseous canal. Orthopedics 14:545–549, 1991.

29. Newport ML, Lane LB, Stuchin SA: Treatment of trigger by steroid injection. J Hand Surg 15A:748–750, 1990.

30. Nirschl RP: Elbow tendinosis/tennis elbow. Clin Sports Med 11:851–870, 1992.

31. Noyes F, Grood E, Nussbaum N: Effect of intra-articular corticosteroids on ligament properties. Clin Orthop 123:197–209, 1977.

32. O'Brien M: Functional anatomy and physiology of tendons. Clin Sports Med 11:505–520, 1992.

33. Panaytopoulos E, Fortis AP, Armoni A, et al: Trigger digit: The needle or the knife? J Hand Surg 17A:239–240, 1992.

34. Price R, Sinclair H, Heinrich I, et al: Local injection treatment of tennis elbow—hydrocortisone, trimacinolone and lignocaine compared. Br J Rheumatol 30:39–44, 1991.

35. Reid DC: Connective tissue healing and classification of ligament and tendon pathology. In Reid DC (ed): Sports Injury Assessment and Rehabilitation. New York, Churchill Livingstone, 1992, pp 65–83.

36. Saal JA: General principles and guidelines for rehabilitation of the injured athlete. Phys Med Rehabil State Art Rev 1:527–528, 1987.

37. Shrier I, Matheson GO, Kohl HW: Achilles tendonitis: Are corticosteroid injections useful or harmful? Clin J Sports Med 6:245–250, 1996.

38. Sibbitt WL, Eaton RP: Corticosteroid responsive tenosynovitis is a common pathway for limited joint mobility in the diabetic hand. J Rheumatol 24:931–936, 1997.

39. Sweetham R: Corticosteroid arthropathy and tendon rupture. J Bone Joint Surg 51B:397–398, 1969.

40. Taras JS, Raphael JS, Pan WT, et al: Corticosteroid injections for trigger digits: Is intrasheath injection necessary? J Hand Surg 23A:717–722, 1998.

41. Tonkin MA, Stern HS: Spontaneous rupture of the flexor carpi radialis tendon. J Hand Surg 16B:72–74, 1991.

42. Vaccaro JP, Sauser DD, Beals RK: Iliopsoas bursa imaging: Efficacy in depicting abnormal iliopsoas tendon motion in patients with internal snapping hip syndrome. Radiology 197:853–856, 1995.

43. Velan GJ, Hendle D: Degenerative tear of the tibialis anterior tendon after corticosteroid injection—augmentation with the extensor hallucis longus tendon. Acta Orthop Scand 68:308–309, 1997.

44. Warwick R, Williams PL: Gray's Anatomy, 36th ed. Edinburgh, Churchill Livingstone, 1980.

45. Witt J, Pess G, Gelberman RH: Treatment of de Quervain tenosynovitis: A prospective study of the results of injection of steroids and immobilization in a splint. J Bone Joint Surg 73A:219–222, 1991.

18

Trigger Point Injection

Andrew A. Fischer, M.D., Ph.D.

TRIGGER POINTS AND TENDER SPOTS: A FREQUENT CAUSE OF PAIN IN MANY CONDITIONS

Trigger points (TrPs) are small, exquisitely tender areas in various soft tissues, including muscles, ligaments, periosteum, tendons, and pericapsular areas. These points may radiate pain into a specific distant area called a "reference pain zone."[1,10–13,15–18] The referred pain may be present at rest. The pain may occur only on activation of the TrP by local pressure, piercing by an injection needle, or activity of the involved muscle (particularly its overuse). TrPs located in muscles are called myofascial because they also may involve the fascia. In addition to the focal tenderness, they are characterized by the presence of a taut band[15,17,18] that is sensitive to pressure, which indicates sensitization of the nerve endings within. The hard resistance to palpation and needle penetration is interpreted as evidence that a group of the affected muscle fibers is constantly contracted. Later, approximately 6–8 weeks after an injury, the resistance to the needle usually becomes very hard. This is characteristic of fibrotic (scar) tissues that fail to respond to conservative therapy. Because there are no definitive histologic studies of TrPs at different stages, it may be assumed that the damaged tissue has healed by a scar.

Trigger point injections (TIs) represent specific techniques used for alleviation of pain caused by the trigger area. Optimally, TIs are aimed at mechanically breaking up the entire abnormal tissue that causes pain. The most frequent findings related to pain are tender spots (TSs), a term reserved for point tenderness without radiating pain. TSs are frequently located within taut bands that have identical characteristics as TrPs. TIs have the same effect, indications, and limitations in both TSs and TrPs. Therefore, the rest of this chapter uses the expression "TrPs" for both tender spots and TrPs, because the technique of injection in both cases is identical:

directed at the point of maximum tenderness and taut bands.

Commonly, tender spots and some TrPs represent local tissue damage that causes inflammation and irritation that can be diagnosed by increased sensitivity to pressure. Figures 18-1 and 18-2 illustrate a possible concept of pathologic changes following local tissue damage. This hypothesis may explain clinical findings in acute and chronic injury and the effect of needling. Conceptually, the TSs or TrP at the chronic stage can be thought of as a pocket of fibrotic tissue that contains sensitizing agents that are the products of tissue damage. These substances cause sensitization of the entrapped nerve fibers. This sensitization increases the nerve's reactivity so that a lower pressure produces pain. The sensitivity of the nerve ending can be quantified by measurement of "pressure pain threshold" (tenderness) using a dolorimeter (algometer).[4–7,12]

Even without infiltration by anesthetic the needling instantaneously abolishes the pain, tenderness, and fibrotic type of resistance. Such effect of dry needling can be best explained by breaking up a fibrotic pocket that has entrapped the nerve endings along with sensitizing substances. This allows the entering blood flow to wash away the sensitizing substances. This concept may explain the effect of TIs but has not been substantiated by histologic studies. Needling also may interrupt neuromuscular mechanisms involved in TrP activity.

Figure 18-2 and Table 18-1 illustrate physical findings over TrPs and taut bands before, during, and after injection combined with needling.

TrPs and TSs are the immediate cause of pain in a variety of conditions. These include sports or work-related injuries, sprains, strains, nerve compression, disc disease, arthritis, or muscle tension related to nonphysiologic posture or stress. Headaches also are frequently caused by TrPs. Certain hormonal disorders such as thyroid or estrogen deficiencies are frequent causes and perpetuators of widespread TrPs.

1. ACUTE STAGE

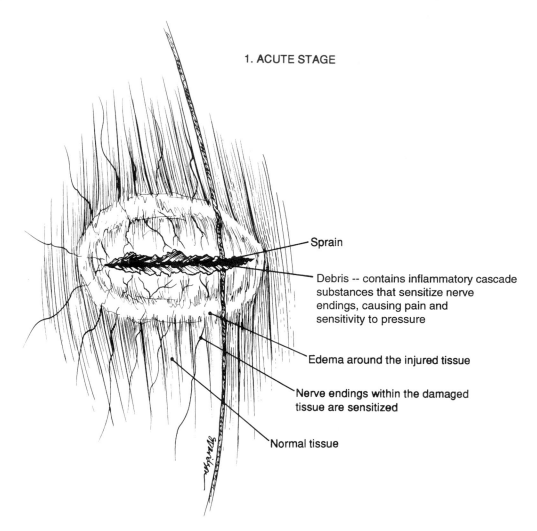

Sprain

Debris -- contains inflammatory cascade substances that sensitize nerve endings, causing pain and sensitivity to pressure

Edema around the injured tissue

Nerve endings within the damaged tissue are sensitized

Normal tissue

FIGURE 18-1. Conceptual illustration of pathologic changes in acute tissue injury that causes focal tenderness with pain. *(Figure continued on following page.)*

TRIGGER POINT INJECTIONS: THE MOST EFFECTIVE TREATMENT

Needling represents the most effective treatment of trigger points, TSs, and acute or chronic soft tissue injuries. Injecting a local anesthetic (usually lidocaine) is combined with a special needling technique to break up the abnormal tissue that causes the pain. The critical factor in TIs is not the injected substance but rather the mechanical disruption of the abnormal tissue and interruption of the TrP mechanism if one has developed.[8,9] Intensive stimulation also may contribute to the prolonged relief of pain by TrP injections.[14] The fact that the symptoms originated in the treated TrP is confirmed by observing whether the pain is reproduced by pressure upon the trigger area and relieved after the TrP injection.[2] The injections are followed by a specific

program of physical therapy and exercises. After fibrotic tissue (scar) has formed in the damaged tissue, the most effective way to break it up is through needling: the repetitive insertion and withdrawal of the injection needle in the affected area.

Local anesthetics, such as 1% lidocaine or 0.5% procaine, provide temporary relief, lasting about 45 minutes. Long-term relief from pain is achieved by the needling, which mechanically breaks up the abnormal tissue. The number of injections needed depends on the number of TrPs present.

One or two areas are usually injected during each treatment visit. Injections may be given two or three times a week for acute pain; once per week or once every 2 weeks is usually adequate as pain relief is being achieved. Each trigger point requires at least one injection. However, in large TrPs, injection may be limited to one segment per visit, depending on

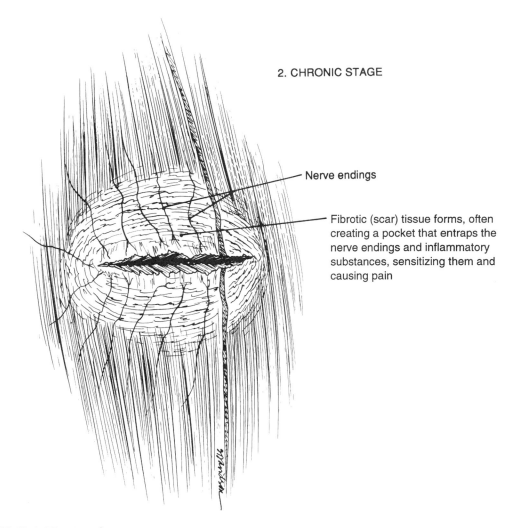

2. CHRONIC STAGE

Nerve endings

Fibrotic (scar) tissue forms, often
creating a pocket that entraps the
nerve endings and inflammatory
substances, sensitizing them and
causing pain

FIGURE 18-1 *(Continued).*   Conceptual illustration of pathologic changes in chronic tissue injury that causes focal tenderness with pain.   *(Figure continued on following page.)*

the patient's tolerance. Sufficient tissue must be left around the needled areas for proper healing. Without proper treatment, TrPs tend to spread to additional muscles, causing flare-up of pain.

The injection technique used for TrPs (combination of needling with infiltration) is effective in alleviating pain and restoring function in focal tenderness. The procedure is effective regardless of the underlying pathology and whether or not the pain is referred or limited to the tender area. Sprains and strains of muscles, ligaments, soft tissue injuries, inflammation, injuries of pericapsular tissues, and bursitis are the most common conditions that improve dramatically after needling combined with injection of local anesthetic. In osteoarthritis, a ligament tear is frequently the main cause of pain. These conditions also respond well to injections combining mechanical needling without the use of corticosteroids. TrPs caused by endocrine dysfunction (especially thyroid or estrogen deficiency), fibromyalgia, psychological tension, or ischemia caused by muscle spasm also may be treated effectively by TIs. Often psychological tension and muscle spasm may not be alleviated without eliminating TrPs, which prevent relaxation of the muscle. Inability to relax tight muscles produces more TrPs, and a vicious cycle ensues. All of the above conditions are called "TIs," because the technique is identical.

The main contraindications for TIs include bleeding disorders, local infection, anticoagulant therapy, certain psychiatric conditions (anxiety, paranoia, schizophrenia), and inability to rest the injured body part following the procedure. Depression is not a contraindication for TIs. On the contrary, relief from chronic pain frequently improves

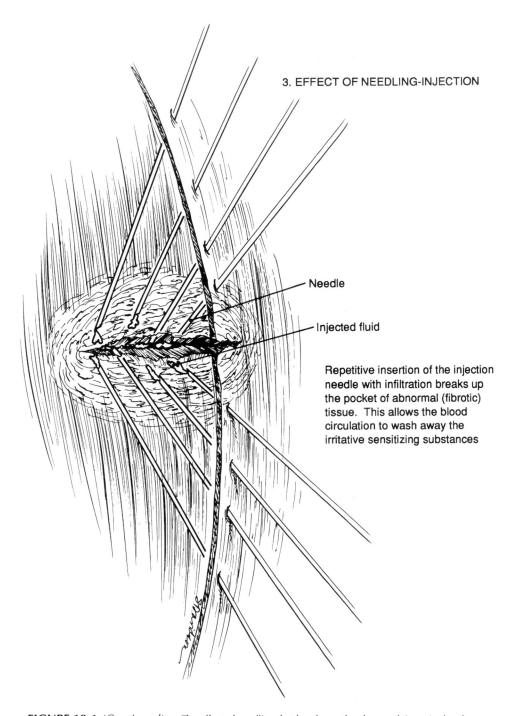

3. EFFECT OF NEEDLING-INJECTION

Needle

Injected fluid

Repetitive insertion of the injection
needle with infiltration breaks up
the pocket of abnormal (fibrotic)
tissue. This allows the blood
circulation to wash away the
irritative sensitizing substances

FIGURE 18-1 *(Continued)*. The effect of needling that breaks up the abnormal tissue is also shown.

depression profoundly. Unless the conditions that caused the TrPs and perpetuating factors are diagnosed and treated, the TrPs will recur.

Three commonly employed trigger point techniques include needling combined with infiltration of the entire taut band, technique of Travell and Simons, and injection of corticosteroids.

1. **Needling combined with infiltration of the entire taut band** is the most effective technique of TI in the author's experience. Infiltration with a local anesthetic such as 1% lidocaine or 0.5% procaine is combined with needling. After withdrawal of the needle to the subcutaneous level, repetitive insertion and redirection of the needle is required to

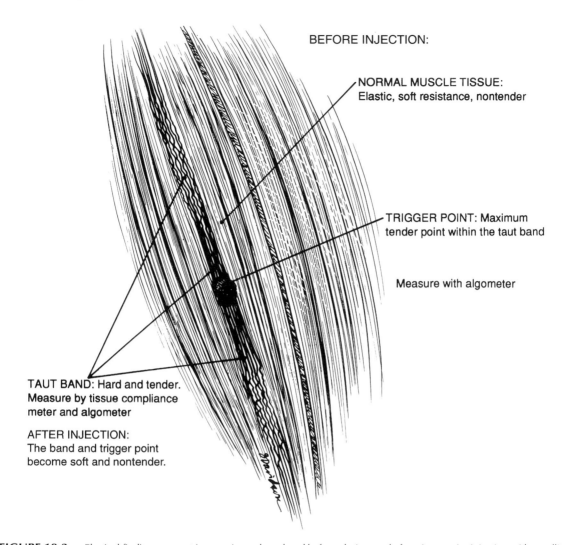

BEFORE INJECTION:

NORMAL MUSCLE TISSUE:
Elastic, soft resistance, nontender

TRIGGER POINT: Maximum
tender point within the taut band

Measure with algometer

TAUT BAND: Hard and tender.
Measure by tissue compliance
meter and algometer

AFTER INJECTION:
The band and trigger point
become soft and nontender.

FIGURE 18-2.   Physical findings over a trigger point and taut band before, during, and after trigger point injection with needling.

cover the entire abnormal (painful) area with as few skin penetrations as possible. The needling and infiltration is extended over the entire taut band, which harbors the TrP/TSs, including its attachment to the bones (enthesopathy).

2. **Technique of J. Travell and D.G. Simons.**[17,18] A small amount of 0.5% procaine is injected into the TrP in order to desensitize the most tender spot. This approach limits the needling and injection of 0.5% procaine to the most tender foci. The goal is to inactivate the neuromuscular TrP mechanism. The needling progresses in millimeters rather than centimeters, as described later.

3. **Steroid injection**. A 1.5-inch needle, usually 25-gauge, is used. Corticosteroids are combined with a small amount (1–3 ml) of local anesthetic, usually lidocaine. Corticosteroids are not necessary for myofascial TrP treatment. Precise needling,

which breaks up the abnormal tissue, is more effective. In fact, corticosteroids may induce local myopathy. However, corticosteroids may be useful in the treatment of conditions involving passive tissues such as bursitis, tendinitis, epicondylitis, or ligament sprain. The disadvantages of corticosteroid injections into ligaments and tendons include loosening and incomplete healing. This may make the injected structures more susceptible to reinjury. Also, the number of corticosteroid injections is limited to 3–5, leaving numerous TrPs untreated.

TECHNIQUE

The purpose of the injection is to mechanically break up the abnormal and sensitized, tender tissue by needling. Injection of any fluid adds to the mechanical effect of the procedure. Usually 1%

TABLE 18-1.   Physical Findings Before, During, and After Trigger Point Injections

Before Injection	During Injection	After Injection
Normal muscle tissue Elastic soft resistance; nontender	Minimal resistance to needle progression; no pain	Normal tissue findings
Taut band Hard and tender. Measure tissue compliance and algometry. Local twitch response can be elicited on snapping.	Penetration of the needle causes pain and encounters hard resistance as in fibrotic tissue (particularly in chronic TrP). Local twitch response occurs when the needle enters the hyperirritable fibers.	The hard and tender areas on palpation become nontender. Pressure pain sensitivity (algometry) becomes normal immediately. Soreness from injection resolves in 3–5 days. Local twitch response can no longer be elicited. Hyperirritability resolves.
Trigger point Maximum tender point within the taut band.	Maximum pain on needle penetration with hard resistance as in the taut band.	Trigger point sensitivity to pressure disappears. Hard consistency becomes normal, similar to improvement in taut bands.
Measure with algometer.		Confirm decreased tenderness with algometry.

lidocaine is optimal. However, in case of allergy to the "-caine" group, saline is satisfactory. The anesthetic also blocks pain and the irritation resulting from tissue damaged by the needle.

The needle should be sufficiently long to be able to reach deeper than the trigger point. The diameter of the needle should be large enough to facilitate mechanical disruption of the abnormal tissue areas. A 22- to 25-gauge needle is usually sufficient. The total amount of 1% lidocaine injected ranges from 1–12 ml. Commonly, an extensive area has to be infiltrated that ranges from 3–25 cm in length and 2–10 cm in width. The size of the infiltration depends on the extent of the trigger point and on the length of the affected muscle fibers. At each stop of the needle's penetration, no more than 0.1 or 0.2 ml

should be injected. Larger volumes can damage the muscle, negating any benefit.

PROCEDURE

1. Ask the patient to point out with one finger the area of most intense pain. If this pain is diffuse and corresponds to a trigger point's reference zone(s), locate the TrP causing the symptoms.[10,15,17,18] Palpate the muscle or ligament[10] that has a corresponding reference zone. Position the patient so that you have proper access to the painful area.

2. Palpate the point of maximum tenderness. Mark it by impression of a fingernail. Palpate around to find the entire taut and tender band, which may reach from the origin to the insertion of the muscle, and mark it by fingernail impressions. Presence of abnormal tenderness (pressure pain sensitivity) can be confirmed quantitatively by a pressure algometer.[4–7,12] Figure 18-3 shows the pressure algometer measuring pressure pain sensitivity (tenderness) of a trigger point.

3. Explain the procedure to the patient.

4. Measure the pressure pain threshold with the algometer (dolorimeter).

5. Clean the skin with Betadine or alcohol. Use surgical gloves.

6. Spray with ethyl chloride to frost. If patient does not like the vapocoolant, pinch the skin in the area of injection and immediately insert the needle. Because the pinching distracts and occupies the sensory pathways, the patient does not feel the needle.

7. Needle the entire area where increased fibrotic type of resistance is present, including the

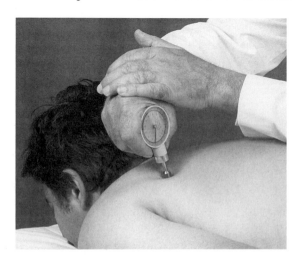

FIGURE 18-3.   A dolorimeter is used for quantification of pressure pain sensitivity. Diagnosis of abnormal tenderness can be confirmed and treatment results quantified.

entire taut band. Explore with the needle beyond the border of the trigger point and the taut band. Inject only a small amount (0.1–0.3 ml) each time you stop the needle penetration. It is of great importance to always aspirate at each needle stop before the injection, especially when the neck or upper body is treated. Terminate the injection if blood is aspirated.

Proceed with the needle insertions through the taut band. Stop in 1–2 cm increments and again deposit only a small amount of anesthetic (0.1–0.2 ml) at each stop. When you reach the normal muscle below the taut band, the pain and hard resistance to the needle cease. Deposit a smaller amount in the normal tissue and then withdraw the needle to the subcutaneous level. Make sure that the needle is out of the muscle when you change the direction of the needle; otherwise, you will cut the tissue. Redirect the needle tip within the subcutaneous tissue along the plane of the taut band. Enter the band in distances 1–3 cm from the previous infiltration. The distance to the next insertion depends on the size of the muscle and the taut band. Proceed similarly until you needle and infiltrate the entire taut band. Depending on the patient's tolerance, about 10 local infiltrations can be performed in one session, covering one large TrP and its taut band. If the patient becomes annoyed or the planned amount of anesthetic has been exhausted, the injection is terminated. If necessary, the remaining parts of the taut band can be injected in the following session, usually 1 week later.

Immediately following an effective injection, the tenderness of the TrP and taut band, as well as the associated harder consistency of the surrounding tissue, disappears or diminishes substantially. Results can be documented by dolorimeter and tissue compliance meter. Figure 18-4 shows the tissue compliance meter, its rubber tip being pressed into the examined tissue. The depth of penetration per unit of force expresses compliance. Taut bands, muscle spasm, and tension, and their reaction to treatment, can be documented objectively and quantitatively.

Special attention should be directed to injecting the myotendon junction as well as the origin and the insertion of the involved muscle(s). Injection is usually particularly painful at these sites. Technique of injection to specific muscles has been described,[12,17,18] and it is highly recommended that these textbooks are consulted before a novice starts TIs.

8. Compress the injected site for about 2 minutes to prevent bleeding. Cover with a Band-Aid.

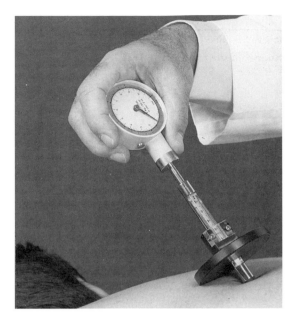

FIGURE 18-4.   A tissue compliance meter measures soft tissue consistency.

9. If the needling was effective, the pressure threshold increases by 3 kg/cm^2.

POSTINJECTION CARE

Postinjection care includes the following steps:
1. Promote hemostasis by pressure.
2. Encourage active slow movement of the injected muscle to its full range; repeat three times.
3. Heat locally.
4. Use physiotherapy consisting of hot packs and electric stimulation using sinusoid surging current (adjust volume to induce strong contractions that are not too painful). Use vapocoolant spray to inactivate remaining painful areas. This is followed by limbering and stretching exercises. Three such sessions of physiotherapy are necessary after each injection for best results, preferably on the days following the procedure.
5. If soreness is excessive, give acetaminophen or celecoxib.
6. Limbering exercises and/or passive stretching should be performed by the patient every 2 hours. Limbering exercises have been proven effective in preventing the recurrence of low back pain.[3] Experience shows that this applies to all types of muscle pain.
7. Advise the patient to avoid heavy use of the injected muscle such as walking or driving long distances after lower body injections and to avoid sports after upper body injections.

Pressure algometers and tissue compliance meters are distributed by Pain Diagnostics and Treatment Inc., 233 East Shore Road, Suite 108, Great Neck, New York 11023.

REFERENCES

1. Bonica JJ: The Management of Pain. Philadelphia, Lea & Febiger, 1990.
2. Bonica JJ: Management of myofascial pain syndromes in general practice. JAMA 164:732–738, 1957.
3. Deyo RA: Conservative therapy for low back pain. JAMA 250:1057–1062, 1983.
4. Fischer AA: Diagnosis and management of chronic pain in physical medicine and rehabilitation. In Ruskin AP (ed): Current Therapy in Physiatry. Philadelphia, W.B. Saunders, 1984.
5. Fischer AA: Pressure threshold measurement for diagnosis of myofascial pain and evaluation of treatment results. Clin J Pain 2:207–214, 1987.
6. Fischer AA: Documentation of myofascial trigger points. Arch Phys Med Rehabil 69:286–291, 1988.
7. Fischer AA: Application of pressure algometry in manual medicine. J Manual Med 5:145–150, 1990.
8. Frost FA, Jessen B, Siggaard-Andersen J: A control, double-blind comparison of mepivacaine injection versus saline injection for myofascial pain. Lancet i:499–500, 1980.
9. Garvey TA, Marks MR, Wiesel SW: A prospective, randomized, double-blind evaluation of trigger-point injection therapy for low-back pain. Spine 14:962–964, 1989.
10. Hackett GS: Ligament and Tendon Relaxation Treated by Prolotherapy, 3rd ed. Springfield, IL, Charles C Thomas, 1958.
11. Kraus H: Clinical Treatment of Back and Neck Pain. New York, McGraw-Hill, 1970.
12. Kraus H: Diagnosis and Treatment of Muscle Pain. Chicago, Quintessence Publishing, 1988.
13. Kraus H, Fischer AA: Diagnosis and treatment of myofascial pain. Mount Sinai J Med 58:235–239, 1991.
14. Melzack R: Prolonged relief of pain by brief, intense transcutaneous somatic stimulation. Pain 1:357–373, 1975.
15. Simons DG: Myofascial pain syndromes due to trigger points. In Goodgold J (ed): Rehabilitation Medicine. St. Louis, Mosby, 1988.
16. Simons DG: Muscular pain syndromes. In Fricton JR, Awad EA (eds): Advances in Pain Research and Therapy. New York, Raven Press, 1990.
17. Travell JG, Simons DG: Myofascial Pain and Dysfunction: The Trigger Point Manual, Vol. I. Baltimore, Williams & Wilkins, 1983.
18. Travell JG, Simons DG: Myofascial Pain and Dysfunction: The Trigger Point Manual. The Lower Extremities, Vol. II. Baltimore, Williams & Wilkins, 1992.

ADDENDUM

Since the first edition of this book progress has been made in several aspects of the diagnosis and management of musculoskeletal pain (see also chapter 23).[1] The reader may consult previous publications for detailed descriptions of technical aspects[2–9] and newer developments.[10–12]

Currently, trigger point injections may be combined with the newer injection techniques such as **preinjection blocks** and **paraspinous blocks**. The cumulative evidence and experience of several dozen physicians who used the recently described injection techniques demonstrate that a combination of three procedures yields the best results:

1. **Paraspinous block**, which desensitizes the irritated spinal segment, is the first in sequence if spinal segmental sensitization is present. This is usually part of a pentad (vicious circle) consisting of discopathy, radiculopathy, and paraspinal muscle spasm.[1] The paraspinous block consists of two steps: (1) the spreading of the anesthetic (1% lidocaine) along the sprained (tender) supra/interspinous ligaments in order to achieve long-term healing and relief of spinal segmental sensitization; and (2) needling and infiltration of the sprained supra/interspinous ligaments.[1]

2. **Preinjection block** spreads anesthetic to prevent nociceptive impulses from the tender area to be injected.[1,5,8] Preinjection block is administered before the injection of the tender area. The purpose is to block the pain sensation from the sensitive structure about to be injected. Preinjection block prevents central sensitization caused by injecting the irritative focus (a tender area) and also relaxes the neurogenic component of the taut band associated with the trigger point or tender spot.[5] This makes the trigger point injection easier to perform and renders needling and infiltration more effective.[5,8] Therefore, preinjection blocks should be used before any trigger point injection or other injections to tender spots, tender areas, and inflamed tissues.

3. Unlike other methods of trigger point injections that also use needling and infiltration, **needling and infiltration of the taut band** is not confined to the trigger point or tender spot. On the contrary, the procedure extends over the entire taut band, which also includes its attachment to the bones on both sides (origin and insertion of the muscle). Needling and infiltration has been proven to achieve long-term pain relief and restoration of function.[1]

REFERENCES

1. Fischer AA, Imamura M: New concepts in diagnosis and management of musculoskeletal pain. In Lennard TA (ed): Pain Procedures in Clinical Practice, 2nd ed. Philadelphia, Hanley & Belfus, 2000.
2. Fischer AA: Local injections in pain management. Trigger point needling with infiltration and somatic blocks. Phys Med Rehabil Clin North Am 6:851–870, 1995.
3. Fischer AA: Injection techniques in the management of local pain. J Back Musculoskeletal Rehabil 7:107–117, 1996.
4. Fischer AA: Quantitative and objective compliance recording. In Nordhoff LS (ed): Motor Vehicle Collision Injuries. Gaithersburg, MD, Aspen, 1996, pp 142–148.

5. Fischer AA: New approaches in treatment of myofascial pain. Phys Med Rehabil Clin North Am 8:153–169, 1997.
6. Fischer AA: New developments in diagnosis of myofascial pain and fibromyalgia. Phys Med Rehabil Clin North Am 8:1–21, 1997.
7. Fischer AA: Algometry in diagnosis of musculoskeletal pain and evaluation of treatment outcome: An update. In Fischer AA (ed): Muscle Pain Syndromes and Fibromyalgia. New York, The Haworth Medical Press, 1998, pp 5–32.
8. Fischer AA: Myofascial pain. In Windsor RE, Lox DM (eds): Soft Tissue Injuries: Diagnosis and Treatment. Philadelphia, Hanley & Belfus, 1998, pp 85–100.
9. Fischer AA: Treatment of myofascial pain. J Musculoskeletal Pain 7:131–142, 1999.
10. Fischer AA, Imamura ST, Imamura M: Myofascial trigger points are most frequently a manifestation of segmental spinal sensitization. J Musculoskeletal Pain 6(Suppl 2):20, 1998.
11. Fischer AA, Imamura ST, Imamura M: New injection techniques and concepts for treatment of myofascial pain. J Musculoskeletal Pain 6(Suppl 2):51, 1998.
12. Fischer AA, Imamura ST, Kaziyama HS, Imamura M: Trigger point injections and "paraspinous blocks" which relieve segmental spinal sensitization are effective treatment for chronic pain. J Musculoskeletal Pain 6(Suppl 2):52, 1998.

19

Basic Principles of Medical Acupuncture

Joseph M. Helms, M.D.

Medical acupuncture is acupuncture that has been successfully incorporated into medical or allied health practices in Western countries. It is derived from Asian and European sources and is practiced in both pure and hybrid forms. Therapeutic insertion of solid needles in various combinations and patterns is the foundation of medical acupuncture. The choice of needle patterns can be based on traditional principles such as encouraging the flow of *qi* (pronounced *chee*), a subtle vivifying energy, through classically described acupuncture channels; modern concepts such as recruiting neuroanatomic activities in segmental distributions; or a combination of these two principles. The adaptability of classical and hybrid acupuncture approaches in Western medical environments is the key to their clinical success and popular appeal.

HISTORICAL PERSPECTIVES

In the United States, acupuncture has been increasingly embraced by practitioners and patients since the appearance of James Reston's landmark article describing his experience with successful postappendectomy pain management using acupuncture needles.[5] Before that time, acupuncture had been practiced only in urban Asian communities, discreetly and primarily by and for Asians. In the early 1970s, widespread enthusiasm for acupuncture was fueled by reports from physician visitors to China, who witnessed surgical analgesia using only acupuncture needles. Respect for the technique grew in the medical and scientific communities in the late 1970s, when it was shown that acupuncture analgesia was linked to the central nervous system activities of endogenous opioid peptides and biogenic amines. Since the 1970s, guidelines for education, practice, and regulation in acupuncture have been established and implemented. State, regional, national, and international societies have evolved to represent the interests of affinity groups of practitioners.

Acupuncture is one discipline extracted from a complex heritage of Chinese medicine—a tradition that also includes massage and manipulation, stretching and breathing exercises, and herbal formulas, as well as exorcism of demons and magical correspondences. The earliest major source of acupuncture's theory is the *Huang Di Nei Jing* (*Yellow Emperor's Inner Classic*), whose oldest portions date from the Han dynasty in the 2nd century B.C. The *Nei Jing* authors regarded the human body as a microcosmic reflection of the universe and considered the physician's role that of maintaining the body's harmonious balance, both internally and in relation to the external environment.

The *Nan Jing* (*Classic of Difficult Issues*) was written in the 1st and 2nd centuries A.D., also during the Han dynasty. This text presented a unified and comprehensive system that advanced the theories of points and channels and addressed the etiology of illness, diagnosis, and therapeutic needling. The *Zhen Jiu Jia Yi Jing* (*Comprehensive Manual of Acupuncture and Moxibustion*), attributed to Huang-Fu Mi in 282 A.D. and based on the previous texts, is the oldest existing classical text devoted entirely to acupuncture and moxibustion (heating the acupuncture points and needles with smoldering mugwort, a dried herb).

Between the Han dynasty (206 B.C.–200 A.D.) and the Ming Dynasty (1368–1644 A.D.), acupuncture practice was refined and its literature underwent continued exegesis. Research, education, clinical refinement, and collation and commentary on previous classics flourished in the Ming dynasty. The *Zhen Jiu Da Cheng* (*Great Compendium of Acupuncture and Moxibustion*) of Yang Ji-Zhou, published in 1601, synthesized many classical texts as well as unwritten traditions of practice and became the most influential medical text for later generations in Asia and Europe. The *Da Cheng* was the source of acupuncture information transmitted to Europe in the 17th through the 19th centuries via

Latin translations by Portuguese, French, Dutch, and Danish missionaries, traders, and physicians traveling and working in China and Japan. It was also the primary source translated into French in the 20th century.

There was a flurry of primitive acupuncture experimentation by physicians in France, England, Germany, Italy, Sweden, and the United States in the first three decades of the 19th century; this experimentation did not renew itself in Europe until a century later and in the United States until the 1970s. The most influential impact on the development of 20th-century European acupuncture was the work of George Soulié de Morant, a scholar-diplomat engaged in the French diplomatic service in China between 1901 and 1917. Soulié de Morant published articles and French translations of Chinese and Japanese medical texts, and on his return to France, he taught clinical applications of acupuncture to French physicians. He systematically introduced acupuncture theory from the classical texts to the French and European medical community. The commonly used terms *meridian* and *energy* both originated in his texts as translations for the two fundamental tenets of acupuncture: anatomy and physiology. In 20th-century France and throughout much of Europe since the 1950s, clinical acupuncture has codeveloped with biomedical science. Europe has thus served as another influence for acupuncture approaches that integrate into the practice of conventional Western medicine.[2]

CLASSICAL CONCEPTS

Acupuncture has evolved over two millennia, both through refinements based on treatment responses and through adaptations to changing social situations. The language in classical Chinese medicine texts reflects nature and agrarian village metaphors and describes a philosophy of man functioning harmoniously within an orderly universe. The models of health, disease, and treatment are presented in terms of patients' harmony or disharmony within this larger order and involve their responses to external extremes of wind, heat, damp, dryness, and cold, as well as to internal extremes of anger, excitement, worry, sadness, and fear. Illnesses likewise are described and defined poetically, by divisions of the yin and yang polar opposites (interior or exterior, cold or hot, deficient or excessive), by descriptors attached to elemental qualities (wood, fire, earth, metal, and water), and by the functional

influences traditionally associated with each of the internal organs.

The classic anatomy of acupuncture consists of energy channels traversing the body. The principal energy pathways are named for organs whose realms of influence are expanded from their conventional biomedical physiology to include functional, energetic, and metaphorical qualities (e.g., Kidney supervises bones, marrow, joints, hearing, head hair, will, and motivation; Spleen oversees digestion, blood production, blood-related functions such as menstruation, and nurturing and introspection). Acupuncture anatomy is a multilayered, interconnecting network of channels that establishes an interface between an individual's internal and external environments, permitting energy to move through the muscles and the various organs.

The most superficial of these pathways are the tendinomuscular meridians, which serve as an interface between the organism and its external environment. They provide the first defense for the body's response to climatic conditions and external traumas. The principal meridians travel through the muscles and provide nourishment to all tissues and vitality for animation and physical activity. The distinct meridians go directly from the surface of the body deep to the organs and allow the nourishment and the energy produced by the organs to circulate throughout the body. Finally, a system of pathways called the curious meridians create connections among the principal acupuncture channels and serve as energy reservoirs for extreme conditions of emptiness or fullness. The network of energy circulation is organized into three bilaterally symmetrical plates that divide the body into six sagittal territories of influence. Each plate manifests the energy derived from four organs as it circulates in their anatomic territory of influence.

Figure 19-1 represents the schematic organization of one plate in the acupuncture energy circulation. The core rectangle is the principal meridian subcircuit, from which the subdivisions of energy circulation are derived: tendinomuscular meridians on the surface, distinct meridians going to the organs, and curious meridians creating connections among several principal meridian subcircuits. Figure 19-2 shows the deep pathways of the distinct meridians for the kidney and bladder.

The classical physiology of acupuncture involves a dozen internal organs that interact to produce basic energy and blood from ingested solid and liquid nourishment, then mix in the energy from inspired air and propel the transformed energy and blood

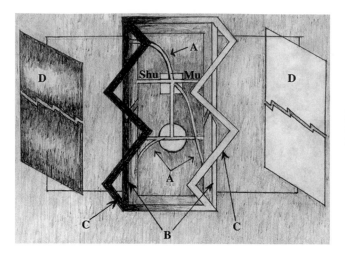

FIGURE 19-1. Acupuncture energy circulation: *A*, distinct meridian; *B*, principal meridians; *C*, curious meridians; *D*, tendinomuscular meridians.

through all the body's organs and tissues. The organs are divided into six parenchymal, energy-producing organs (solid, yin), and six visceral, substance-transporting organs (hollow, yang). These organs are coupled into groups (one yin and one yang) to make up the three symmetrical energy circulation plates. Pathology in acupuncture involves an early manifestation of disharmony associated with the subtle influences of an organ, a disruption of the qi flow in one of the subdivisions of the circulation network associated with an organ, or a frank disturbance in an organ's metabolic or transport function.

Diagnosis in acupuncture involves recognizing the level of manifestation of a disturbance. Premorbid symptomatology is organized according to the organs' subtle spheres of influence, where early energetic and functional symptoms are linked to the organ that supervises the disturbed anatomic region or physiologic function (e.g., Kidney energy supervises head hair; premature graying or balding reflects a deficient Kidney vitality). Obstruction of the flow of energy or blood through the principal meridians manifests as musculoskeletal pain in the territory of the channel (e.g., the Bladder principal meridian passes through the lower back; lumbar pain reflects an obstruction of qi and blood flow through that channel). Organ pathology is identified either in conventional biomedical terms or as a disturbance in the organ's physiological activities according to acupuncture terms (e.g., nephrolithiasis is a disturbance in both Kidney and Bladder organs and spheres of influence). Treatment in acupuncture involves the insertion of needles along the channels of the involved organs to stimulate energy circulation that can influence the problem at its level of manifestation, thus restoring energetic balance and organ function in the organism.

MODERN CONCEPTS

Since the late 1970s, acupuncture analgesia has been demonstrated to activate the endogenous opioid peptide system and thereby influence the body's pain regulatory system by changing the processing and perception of noxious information at various levels of the central nervous system. Two model systems of acupuncture analgesia have been advanced: (1) an endorphin-dependent system involving low-frequency, high-intensity electrical stimulation of acupuncture needles (2–4 Hz) that is

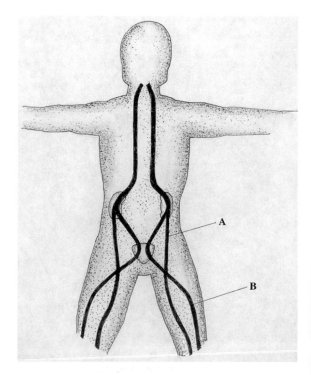

FIGURE 19-2. Kidney (*A*) and bladder (*B*) distinct meridians.

slow in onset, generalized through the body, and cumulative on subsequent stimulation and (2) a monoamine-dependent system involving high-frequency, low-intensity electrical stimulation of acupuncture needles (70 Hz or greater) that is rapid in onset, segmental, and not cumulative.[6]

By combining the neurohumoral models with other observations and speculations about the mechanism of acupuncture's impact, a model is created of an acupuncture needle simultaneously activating multiple systems in the body's physiology:

- the nervous system, which includes peripheral afferent transmission, perivascular sympathetic fiber conduction, and the central neurohumoral and neuropeptide mechanisms
- the blood circulation system, which transmits the biomolecular elements locally and centrally, along with the biochemical and cellular changes stimulated by acupuncture
- the lymphatic system, which serves as a medium for ionic flow along fascial planes and perivascular interstitial fluid circulation
- the electromagnetic bio-information system, which consists of static electricity on the surface, ionic migration in the interstitial fluid between the needles and as currents of injury at the needled site, and fascial and perineural semiconduction throughout the body.[2]

The above hybrid assemblage of descriptions creates a contemporary working model of a multisystem information network that obliges the medical acupuncture practitioner not only to consider classical paradigms to arrive at diagnostic and therapeutic decisions, but also to take into account neuroanatomic and neurophysiologic parameters. These considerations are of special importance in acupuncture's application in pain management, where knowledge of dermatomal, myotomal, sclerotomal, and autonomic innervation patterns is indispensable.

HISTORY AND PHYSICAL EXAMINATION

In an acupuncture evaluation, the initial encounter with the patient is similar to that of a conventional allopathic medical interview and examination. The patient is encouraged to speak candidly and thoroughly about the presenting problems and background. In addition to a conventional assessment and differential diagnosis, the practitioner explores the characteristics and behaviors of the problems in an effort to link them with the gross or subtle spheres of influence of one or several of the internal organs. In the case of musculoskeletal pain problems, the location of the pain is identified neuroanatomically and according to the acupuncture channel in whose territory it lies. The goal of the interview is to identify the organs and energy circulation divisions involved in the patient's disorder, whether the association be with the subtle symptoms linked to the traditional sphere of influence of the organs, with the trajectory of a meridian through a painful region, with a dense organ lesion, or with a combination of these factors.

The patient's past medical history, childhood illnesses, family history, and review of systems are elicited during the interview, and all information is tagged with the organ or meridian under whose supervision it falls. During this period the acupuncturist poses questions of particular importance: possible cyclicity in the appearance of the symptoms, seasonal exacerbations, general seasonal preferences or dislikes, positive or negative flavor affinities and color affinities, response of symptoms to external climatic environments, and the lesion's response to pressure, movement, heat, or cold.

A standard physical examination appropriate for the patient and the problem is undertaken, with several additional acupuncture inspections included. The musculoskeletal evaluation includes identification of painful muscle knots and trigger points as well as subcutaneous nodules and bands overlying contracted muscles. Specific reflex points on the front and back of the trunk (*mu* points and *shu* points) correspond to the organs associated with them. If any mu or shu points are sensitive to palpation during the physical examination, those findings also are recorded.

In acupuncture, several diagnostic somatotopic systems that microcosmically reflect the internal organs are routinely used to evaluate the balance of relative strengths and weaknesses within the organs. Those most commonly employed are the external ear, reflex systems of the tongue, and radial pulse, inspections of which are undertaken as part of the routine physical evaluation.

Evaluation of the external ear confirms findings from the physical exam or other reflex systems and may indicate new directions for exploration during the interview and examination. The diagnostic examination includes visual inspection, palpation with a probe, or scanning with a battery-powered electrical resistance detector. The external ear also can be used as a treatment system in isolation or as an adjunct to body acupuncture points.

The tongue reflects the basic condition and underlying problem of the patient at the time of examination by way of its color, body, coating, and surface irregularities. Changes in tongue qualities are easily noted from week to week and often day to day. The tongue serves as an indicator of change in the patients as they evolve through illness and respond to medical interventions.

The diagnostic microsystem of the radial pulse provides another means of evaluating the patient's overall condition and of comparing the relative strengths of energetic activity in the organs and their meridians. The pulse changes from minute to minute and therefore can be used to verify whether an input has had its intended effect before one continues or concludes the treatment. The pulses also serve as a subjective measurement from visit to visit, revealing the stability of the changes made through the acupuncture treatments.

DIFFERENTIAL DIAGNOSIS AND TREATMENT PLANNING

Before concluding the diagnostic process, a review of past medical records, radiographs, and laboratory studies is undertaken, and appropriate new studies are requested to confirm and specify mechanical and organic disorders. From all available information, subtle and gross symptoms and characteristics are organized into affinity clusters, and patterns of disharmony are identified. The organ or organ's influence that is most disturbed is then defined as is the level of manifestation of this greatest disturbance. The energy-functional level of disturbance involves the balance of energetic and metabolic activities of the organs and their spheres of influence, including, especially, their psychoemotional expressions; the channel-structural level involves skin, fascia, muscles, and bones; and the organ level involves the metabolic or transport functions of the organs themselves. A decision is then made as to which division of the energy circulation network gives best access to the level of greatest disturbance.

The initial interview affords an understanding of the manifestations and course of the disorder as well as the patient's constitutional strengths and weaknesses. The ideal diagnostic conclusion is a clear perception of the patient's health course: the presenting problems and their origins as well as the likely future health events. An algorithm of treatment approaches should be constructed. The goal of the overall treatment strategy must be kept in mind while working with the various tactics at each session. For example, the immediate treatment plan may address only relief of the most urgent symptoms, and long-standing problems can be addressed after change in the presenting symptoms.

PATIENT SELECTION AND TREATMENT DESIGN

The first steps in treatment design involve identifying the levels of manifestation of the patient's complaints and establishing an order of treating the problems. Treatment strategy involves activating the appropriate layers of the energy circulation network to address each problem on its own level of manifestation. A simple strain or sprain may need nothing more than dispersion with needles surrounding the local lesion and an activation of the appropriate tendinomuscular meridian. Musculoskeletal pain of long-standing duration will need placement of needles around one of the principal meridian subcircuits to encourage energy flow in addition to local needles to focus on the site of the problem. Such a treatment may involve electrical stimulation of the points needled to move the energy through the subcircuit as well as the local points. Psychosomatic or premorbid problems may respond to the needling of several front or back mu or shu points, to a rarefied equilibration treatment based on more arcane models of organ and energy interactions, or perhaps to an activation of energy flow through the disturbed principal meridian subcircuit.

It is important to aim treatment at the level of manifestation of the problem being addressed. The circulation levels being activated may be changed during a series of treatments to better address the presenting problem or to introduce treatment for secondary problems. It is better to proceed slowly than with vigor, so that the patient's response to the treatment can be properly evaluated. As with any other medical intervention, factors influencing the outcome of a treatment include the patient's age; the duration and complexity of the presenting problem; the presence of concurrent acute or chronic illness, medications, history of surgical interventions, lifestyle, and personal health factors; and the patient's emotional state and basic vitality. The patient's attitude toward acupuncture usually does not affect the result, as it is not necessary to believe in acupuncture for it to be effective.

TREATMENT

Treatment Options

Along with the majority of physician acupuncturists in the United States, the author uses the hybrid model of combining energy movement through the channels with local or focusing treatment. This model, known as "acupuncture energetics," is derived from European interpretations of the Chinese classics and blended with neuromuscular anatomy of trigger points and segmental innervation for pain treatments. Traditional Japanese meridian acupuncture is akin to the linear energy movement programs represented in the following section, although Japanese practitioners commonly needle more superficially than do Europeans or Americans.

Of the acupuncture systems currently practiced in the United States, the traditional Chinese medicine that is taught at the training colleges in China is the most widespread. This approach to acupuncture is linked with traditional herbal prescribing as the core of the discipline, which can be an effective approach for internal medicine problems. The acupuncture points are selected for their traditional functions to reinforce the goals of herbal therapy, rather than to move energy through the circulation network.

Five elements acupuncture is another widely practiced discipline. Imported from England, five elements acupuncture reflects French and other European interpretations of classical information. The greatest value of this approach lies in its potential to assist in the repair of problems that originate in the psychoemotional sphere.

Three somatotopic systems have established themselves as valuable disciplines, used either as exclusive approaches to acupuncture or as adjuncts to body acupuncture. Auricular acupuncture, developed in France, offers a homuncular reflex organization of all body parts on the external ear. Korean hand acupuncture identifies a microsystem on the hand of the complete meridian circulation. Scalp acupuncture is another recent development, several systems of which divide cranial territories into neurologic regions corresponding to cerebrocortical influences on the body structures. These somatotopic systems appear to be effective for modifying neurologic problems that can be elusive to body acupuncture.

Description of Treatment

The acupuncture treatment consists of inserting fine needles into the body in patterns designed to influence the flow of qi in one of the subdivisions of the energy circulation network. Usually only one energy subdivision is selected to stimulate energy movement, along with a collection of local points to focus the attention of the energy movement. Each subdivision of the circulation has a unique therapeutic point combination necessary for activation. The combinations involve the insertion of at least three needles—the energy moving needles—that are usually in the extremities and usually inserted bilaterally. The focusing needles are inserted at trunk points that influence the organs being stimulated or at muscular points tender to palpation in the region of the pain.

Needles are inserted to the depth necessary to elicit the patient's sensation of *de qi*, or needle grab, a dull ache that radiates from the point. This can be 0.5–8.0 cm, depending on the location. The patient is positioned comfortably, usually lying supine or prone. The acupuncture needles are left in place for 5–20 minutes. It is crucial to protect the patient from energy depletion during an acupuncture treatment. The older or more fatigued the patient, the shorter the duration of treatment must be. The energy-moving needles may be stimulated when an additional activation of the acupuncture system is desired, such as when the problem is one of deficiency according to acupuncture principles or when the patient has low vitality. This additional activation is accomplished through manual manipulation, by heating the needle with burning mugwort (moxibustion), or by connecting the needles to an electrical stimulating device.

Focusing needles can likewise be stimulated through manual, thermal, or electrical means. It is common to treat the patient using front, back, and extremity points during the course of a single treatment session. This means that the treatment is typically divided into two sections: the energy movement section using extremity points to activate flow through the meridians and the section to focus the energy on one or several organs or to influence a pain problem.

An example of preventive intervention that makes use of the traditional influences of the organs would be that of a 35-year-old man who complains of a general diminution of energy, including decreased sexual interest, increased sensitivity to cold weather, mild generalized joint aches, and a new affinity for salt. He is wearing a black T-shirt and black underpants and has significantly graying in his temples (such symptoms and presentation are features of Kidney influence). This man's medical evaluation and laboratory tests are negative. His case is a premorbid manifestation of weakness in the Kidney sphere of influence. An appropriate treatment would be to activate Kidney energy with needles and moxibustion at the shu points for Kidney on the back, bilaterally, as the first section of the treatment. The second section could consist of creating an energy flow through the *shao yin* (Kidney–Heart) and *tai yang* (Small Intestine–Bladder) principal meridian subcircuit by placing one needle in the Kidney meridian, one in the Heart meridian, and one in the Bladder meridian, bilaterally in the extremities, and manually stimulating them in addition to moxibustion. Each section would last 5–10 minutes and would take place in one session.

The local treatments for pain problems can be quite complex because, in addition to honoring the classical directive of encouraging the flow of qi and blood through the channels that traverse the painful area, neuromuscular anatomy must be considered. Deliberately searching for and deactivating intramuscular trigger points in the region of the pain and along the myotomal distribution of the spinal segments involved in the pain is a necessary component of the local treatment. Likewise, recruiting the neurologic activity of the spinal origins of the dermatomal, myotomal, sclerotomal, and sympathetic innervation of the pain problem is a common local treatment for chronic pain. In these cases, electrical stimulation is commonly used, with the frequencies ranging between 2 Hz and 150 Hz.

If the above 35-year-old man also has chronic lumbar pain with an occasional L5 radicular component, the acupuncture treatment will consist of an initial energy moving section involving two needles bilaterally in the extremities in the Kidney meridian, one in the Heart meridian, one in Small Intestine, and one in Bladder. The two needles in the Kidney meridian to enhance the energetic activity in the subcircuit as well as moxibustion can be applied to the other points. This section of the treatment lasts approximately 10 minutes. The second section is the local treatment for the lumbar pain and involves needles placed on the Bladder meridian, for example, at the L2 level (somatic sympathetics for lower extremities), L4 and L5 levels (myotomal and dermatomal levels of pain), and the S2 level (parasympathetics for lower extremities) to recruit the spinal segments involved in his pain. Electrical stimulation at 4 Hz or 15 Hz can be connected among these needles. This second section lasts for 20 minutes.

Treatment Duration

Patient visits are usually scheduled once weekly, although two or three visits each week are not uncommon especially during the initial stages of an acute problem. When a favorable response lasts for the full week between visits, the interval is opened to 2 weeks. As the response stabilizes for a 2-week period, the interval is opened again to 3 weeks, then 4 weeks. When the symptoms are stable for 4 weeks, a decision is made as to whether the patient should return for a maintenance treatment in another month or 6 weeks or call for an appointment only if the condition returns. Chronic pain problems typically require maintenance treatments at 1-month, 6-week, or 2-month intervals. Medical problems of lesser severity and chronicity can often be resolved adequately and do not require maintenance treatments, although chronic medical problems — even when they respond well to acupuncture — typically call for quarterly maintenance treatments.

Treatment Response

During initial treatments, any change, even a transient exacerbation of symptoms, is considered a favorable response. No response to the initial treatment can mean that the therapeutic input was not strong enough, that the problem is deep seated and requires several treatments to influence, that the treatment design is inappropriate, or that the problem is not accessible to acupuncture intervention. An exacerbation of symptoms after the initial treatment usually means that the treatment decision is accurate but that the manipulation or the duration of the needles was too extensive. An examination of the diagnostic microsystems such as the radial pulse and the tongue gives another means for the practitioner to subjectively evaluate change in the patient's condition from visit to visit and thereby decide whether a change in treatment is indicated.

With the cumulative effect of the treatments, enduring improvement is the desired goal. Enduring improvement may mean a thorough resolution of the presenting problem, or it may mean enabling the patient to function on a plateau of discomfort that is less incapacitating or requires less medication than at the time of initial presentation. Ideally, a dozen visits are scheduled to follow the course of the disorder and its response to acupuncture. Usually, the extent of response can be approximated by six or eight visits, but an enduring response often requires the full schedule of visits. After the first dozen treatments, the problem and its response to acupuncture are reevaluated and the acupuncturist and patient decide whether to continue intensive treatments, maintain treatments, or abandon the acupuncture intervention.

Acupuncture treatments are as individual as the patients and their responses to acupuncture. It is common to stay with an initial treatment approach for at least three or four visits before modifying the approach. It is common for the patient to report changes in general well-being and vitality, or a reduction in medication, before a clear change in the presenting symptoms occurs. If no progress has been made by the sixth visit, it is reasonable to consider including additional modalities to complement the acupuncture. It is best not to abandon a case that shows reasonable hope for response to acupuncture before a full trial of 12 visits has been completed.

USES IN MUSCULOSKELETAL PAIN

In the United States, acupuncture has found its greatest acceptance and success in the management of musculoskeletal pain. Acute musculoskeletal lesions such as soft tissue contusions, acute muscle spasms, musculotendinous sprains and strains, and the pain of acute nerve entrapments are among the problems most frequently and successfully addressed with acupuncture. In such cases, acupuncture can legitimately serve as the initiating therapy.

Chronic musculoskeletal pain problems are also commonly and appropriately treated with acupuncture, although not usually as the only approach. Those problems likely to be responsive to acupuncture intervention include repetitive strain disorders (e.g., carpal tunnel syndrome, tennis elbow, plantar fasciitis), myofascial pain patterns (e.g., temporomandibular joint pain, muscle tension headaches, cervical and thoracic soft tissue pain, regional shoulder pain), arthralgias (particularly osteoarthritic in nature), degenerative disc disease with or without radicular pain, and pain following surgical intervention (both musculoskeletal and visceral). In the management of chronic musculoskeletal pain, acupuncture offers a broad range of potential value between the conventional therapy poles of pharmaceuticals and invasive procedures. Other chronic pain problems commonly responsive to acupuncture include postherpetic neuralgia,

peripheral neuropathic pain, and headaches from other causes.

USES AND LIMITATIONS IN PRIMARY CARE

Although acupuncture has been established as an effective tool to treat many forms of musculoskeletal pain, its limitations must be recognized in dealing with the consequences of spinal cord injuries and cerebrovascular accidents. In these conditions, acupuncture's effectiveness is diminished, and the frequency of treatments is increased and protracted over a longer time. Furthermore, acupuncture is usually not useful for thalamically mediated pain and, apart from symptom management and general vivifying effects, is not of great value in the treatment of chronic neurodegenerative diseases.

Perhaps the most fertile ground for acupuncture intervention is for disorders in their premorbid state, problems commonly encountered by primary care providers but rarely associated with positive laboratory findings, definitive medical diagnoses, or successful therapies. Such states often can be described within the acupuncture diagnostic paradigms and then modified through activation of the appropriate level of energy circulation. These disorders can be loosely categorized into three groups: aesthenic states, autonomic dysregulation disorders, and immune dysregulation disorders.

Aesthenic states include ill-defined fatigue (e.g., "tired all the time," "low energy"), mild depression, stress-related myofascial symptoms (e.g., upper thoracic and cervical myofascial pain, muscle tension headache), and early functional disturbances (e.g., diminished libido). Autonomic dysregulation disorders may manifest as anxiety, sleep disturbances, and bowel dysfunction. Immune dysregulation disorders include recurrent infectious and inflammatory states without underlying frank immunodeficiency: sinusitis, pharyngitis, bronchitis, gastroenteritis, and viral illnesses.

In addition to the treatment of acute and chronic musculoskeletal pain and premorbid or functional problems, medical acupuncture can be used successfully to address many diagnosable medical conditions, although it may need to be used in collaboration with other therapies, whether conventional or unconventional. The four divisions of medicine that appear to be most responsive to acupuncture intervention in this country are respiratory, gastrointestinal, gynecologic, and genitourinary.

Respiratory ailments potentially accessible to acupuncture intervention include allergic rhinitis, sinusitis, and bronchitis. Gastrointestinal ailments include gastritis, irritable bowel syndrome, hepatitis, and hemorrhoids. Gynecologic problems include dysmenorrhea and infertility. Genitourinary problems include irritable bladder, prostatitis, male infertility, and some forms of impotence.

Acupuncture, particularly when applied to the external ear, has proven valuable for managing substance abuse problems and reducing prescription narcotic analgesics. One of the most socially visible for acupuncture, this application has gained the respect of rehabilitation programs internationally.[1]

For mental and emotional disturbances, acupuncture can be useful as a transient aid in early and acute emotional states such as anxiety, excitability, worry, early stages of depression, and fearful states. Acupuncture should not be considered as a primary or ongoing therapy for deep-seated or chronic psychoemotional illness, because its effect on these conditions is not enduring.

Acupuncture as a sole therapy has not shown itself to be of substantial value in severe and chronic inflammatory and immune-mediated disorders such as ulcerative colitis, asthma, rheumatoid arthritis, and collagen-vascular diseases, especially if those conditions have advanced to require systemic corticosteroid medication. Likewise, acupuncture is not appropriate as the primary intervention for chronic fatigue states or HIV disease. There can be general value, however, for the symptom control and vitality-promoting effects of acupuncture in all of these conditions. In malignancies, acupuncture can be considered as an additional therapy to combat the secondary effects of conventional therapy and as an adjunct in pain management.

COMPLICATIONS

In the hands of a medically trained practitioner, acupuncture is a fairly safe and forgiving discipline. It is difficult to introduce new and lasting problems with an acupuncture treatment, even if the treatment is not designed as skillfully as an experienced provider would desire. Many patients report a sensation of well-being or relaxation following an acupuncture treatment, especially if electrical stimulation has been used. That sense of relaxation, however, sometimes evolves into a feeling of fatigue or depression that lasts for several days. Other transient psychophysiological responses can be light-headedness, anxiety, agitation, and tearfulness.

The possible risks and complications of an acupuncture treatment are undesirable consequences of penetrating the body with a sharp instrument: syncope, puncture of an organ, infection, and a retained needle. These risks can be reduced by scrupulous sterilizing of needles, acquiring good clinical skills, understanding surface and internal anatomy, and executing responsible clinical judgment. Pneumothorax is the most frequently reported and the most easily produced visceral complication of acupuncture needling. Pneumoperitoneum, hemothorax, cardiac tamponade, and penetrating of the kidney, bladder, and spinal medulla have been reported, although infrequently.

Contact dermatitis to stainless steel needles, local inflammation, and bacterial abscesses can occur, as can chondritis from needling points on the ear. Outbreaks of hepatitis B documented in Europe and America have been traced to single practitioners reusing unsterilized needles.[4] There have been no epidemiologically responsible reports of HIV transmission through the use of acupuncture.

CONCLUSION

Medical acupuncture is a highly adaptable discipline, and is of potential therapeutic value in many pain and general medical conditions. Whether it is introduced as the primary or the complementary therapy depends on the nature and severity of the presenting problem as well as the training, orientation, and practice environment of the provider. The physician trained in medical acupuncture who sees patients early in the course of their disturbances can initiate treatment of a pain or medical problem with acupuncture and introduce additional therapies if acupuncture proves insufficient as the sole treatment. The physician who receives cases later in their evolution and after conventional treatments have been initiated can add acupuncture to assist, or possibly replace, conventional treatments.

Many patients seeking attention from acupuncture providers demand acupuncture or other unconventional interventions as the starting treatment, agreeing to conventional methods only later in their management. Other patients and many physicians wait until conventional therapies have been exhausted and then resort to acupuncture intervention. Acupuncture therapy is not miraculous. It has its appropriate range of applications, and, like any other medical intervention, yields good results in well-selected early problems and less successful results when chronicity and complexity of the presenting problems increase. Usually the best moment to initiate acupuncture therapy is early in the evolution of a problem; however, the flexibility and adaptability of acupuncture allow it to be integrated at almost any stage of treatment.

The potential for medical acupuncture is just beginning to be understood. Future clinical research and utilization evaluations should clarify how best to integrate acupuncture into the conventional health care system. Medical acupuncture offers the opportunity to expand contemporary medicine to treat conditions for which current interventions either are ineffective or have undesirable secondary effects. Because of its usefulness and adaptability to so many aspects of allopathic medicine, medical acupuncture will likely be integrated with increasing frequency into private and institutional practices.

This chapter has been modified from Helms JM: An overview of medical acupuncture. Altern Ther 4:35–45, 1998, with permission.

REFERENCES

1. Culliton PD, Kiresuk TJ: Overview of substance abuse acupuncture treatment research. J Altern Complement Med 2:149–159, 1996.
2. Helms JM: Acupuncture Energetics: A Clinical Approach for Physicians. Berkeley, CA, Medical Acupuncture Publishers, 1995.
3. Helms JM: Report on WHO consultation on acupuncture. Med Acupunct 7(1), 1997.
4. Norheim AJ: Adverse effects of acupuncture: A study of the literature for the years 1981–1994. J Altern Complement Med 2:291–297, 1996.
5. Reston J: Now, about my operation in Peking. New York Times, July 26, 1971, pp 1, 6.
6. Stux G, Pomeranz B: Acupuncture: Textbook and Atlas. Berlin, Springer-Verlag, 1987, pp 1–26.

20

Prolotherapy: Basic Science, Clinical Studies, and Technique

K. Dean Reeves, M.D.

Prolotherapy (growth factor or growth factor stimulation injection) raises growth factor levels or effectiveness to promote tissue repair or growth. Growth factors are complex proteins (polypeptides), and their beneficial effects on human ligament, tendon, cartilage, and bone are under intense investigation. Prolotherapy may utilize inflammatory or noninflammatory mechanisms.

NORMAL TENDON AND LIGAMENT HEALING

To understand prolotherapy, a knowledge of the pathology of sprain or strain and the normal healing process is necessary. Sprains (ligaments) and strains (tendons) become chronic when healing does not result in sufficient tensile strength or tightness.[14,50] This condition also is termed *connective tissue insufficiency* (CTI), in which the structure is either too loose or has insufficient tensile strength.[33] Load bearing in CTI stimulates pain mechanoreceptors.[33] Biedert et al. reported that "as long as connective tissue remains functionally insufficient, the pain mechanoreceptors can continue to malfunction."[4] Recent studies show that in chronic pain of soft-tissue origin the pathologic lesion is degenerative rather than inflammatory.[3,33] Therefore, *tendinosis* is a more appropriate description of this tissue state than *tendinitis*.[3,33]

Abnormal ligaments and tendons relate directly to myofascial pain because mechanoreceptors also trigger twitch contractions,[4] which may explain the taut bands observed in myofascial pain. Individual fiber bundles correspond to tight portions of the muscle belly.

Significant sprain or strain results in cell damage, which in turn triggers an inflammatory healing cascade and the appearance of monocytes within hours, fibroblast proliferation and migration within

48 hours, procollagen deposition within one week, and maturation of procollagen to collagen by 8 weeks.[6] In the maturation phase water is lost, causing constriction of the tendon and tightening and allowing for both thickening and tightening of weak or loose ligament, tendon, or joint capsules. After injury, growth factors are elevated enough to stimulate growth only for a matter of days. Thereafter, healing is dependent on maturation of immature repair tissue.

If laxity or tensile strength deficit is not corrected sufficiently to stop pain mechanoreceptor stimulation, a chronic sprain or strain results. Without further stimulation by growth factors, sufficient repair cannot take place. In repetitive trauma, each individual trauma may be insufficient to provide a proliferation stimulus, so that even minor injury may be enough to accumulate damage to the point of initiating chronic pain. Prolotherapy raises the level of growth factors to resume or initiate a repair sequence that has prematurely aborted or never started. Cells in the area of exposure, such as chondrocytes or osteocytes in osteoarthritis (OA), also can be expected to respond if the growth factors are those that proliferate such cells.

The Role of Growth Factors

Growth factors are powerful, hormone-like proteins produced by peripheral cells. Examples include insulin-like growth factor (IGF), platelet-derived growth factor (PDGF), epidermal growth factor (EGF), fibroblast growth factor (FGF), transforming growth factor (TGF), bone morphogenetic proteins (BMPs), nerve growth factor (NGF), and hepatocyte growth factor (HGF).[60] Normal cells require growth factors (mitogens) for proliferation; in their absence they withdraw from the cell cycle and stop developing.[62] In order for a growth factor to work, it needs to be produced, approach the target cell, avoid binding factors, and attach to its receptor. Disrepair factors such as interleukin 1 (IL-1) can interfere with these processes.

SUMMARY OF BASIC SCIENCE AND CLINICAL STUDIES

Chronic sprain and strain pathology consists of decreased tensile strength and often laxity in ligaments and tendons[3,33] (changes are primarily degenerative rather than inflammatory). Osteoarthritis similarly involves primarily degenerative changes in cartilage and cortical and subcortical bone. Polypeptides are growth factors produced in peripheral cells that powerfully initiate growth and repair in connective tissue (fibroblasts) and cartilage (chondrocytes).[60] Direct exposure of fibroblasts to growth factors causes new cell growth and collagen deposition.[9,28,34,36,40,57] Inflammation creates secondary growth factor elevation. Studies of injection of inflammatory proliferant solutions have demonstrated ligament thickening, enlargement of the tendinoosseous junction, and strengthening of tendon or ligament in animal studies.[19,35,44] In humans, inflammatory proliferant injection in two prospective, randomized, double-blind studies of chronic low back pain has resulted in clinically and statistically significant improvement in pain and disability measures.[31,43] Cartilage effects of polypeptide growth factors are considerable: healing of full-thickness cartilage defects in animals has been shown in several injection studies.[45,56,59,61]

Simple dextrose or hyper- or hypoosmolarity exposure causes cells to proliferate and produce a number of growth factors.[2,8,10,32,41,42,47,51,52,58] A recently completed prospective, randomized, double-blind study by this author indicates the ability of simple dextrose injection interarticularly to tighten human ACL ligament.[50a] Two recently completed prospective, randomized, double-blind studies on osteoarthritis (knees and fingers) indicate substantial and statistically significant clinical benefit from dextrose injection as compared with control solution.[50a,50b]

EFFECTS OF PROLOTHERAPY ON LIGAMENTS AND TENDONS

Injection of Growth Factors

Studies involving exposure of fibroblasts from ligaments and tendons have exposed cells to various growth factors, primarily in vitro. Responses to growth factors differ between animal species[9,28,57] and between different tendons and ligaments within the same animal or human.[36,57] Transforming growth factor beta 1 (TGF-β1), erythrocyte growth factor (EGF), PDGF, and basic fibroblast growth factor (bFGF) appear to be particularly important growth factors for either new cell growth or collagen growth in animals and humans.[28,34,36] Application of this information to growth factor injection studies has only been reported in one animal study to date, in which direct injection of injured patellar ligament in rats was performed. The injected material contained a virus altered to produce a key growth factor (PDGF), which resulted in a substantial increase in collagen deposition compared to noninjected controls.[40]

Growth Factor Stimulators

Inflammatory Solutions

The injection of inflammatory solution briefly stimulates the inflammatory cascade to simulate an injury without actually stretching or deforming tissue.[1] Such an approach causes a complex cascade of chemical events, and measurement of individual growth factors and disrepair factors to determine the exact mechanism is not feasible. Dextrose > 10% concentration partially works by this mechanism, as do phenol and sodium morrhuate. *Sclerotherapy* is an older term for inflammatory prolotherapy. It is recommended only in varicose vein injection; sclerosis implies scar induction for therapeutic effect. Biopsy studies have not demonstrated scar formation with mechanical, inflammatory, or growth factor prolotherapy with the agents and concentrations currently in use.

Clinical research on inflammatory prolotherapy has demonstrated an increase in tendon diameter and tendinoosseous junction in animals (Figs. 20-1 and 20-2). Strengthening of knee medial collateral ligament has been demonstrated in a double-blind study in rabbits,[35] and reduction of knee laxity has been suggested by an initial study in humans using an electroarthrometer.[44] Nonblinded studies in whiplash, chronic headache, chronic cervical and low back pain, and temporomandibular joint syndrome have indicated improvement in 70–85% of cases using dextrose-glycerine-phenol, sodium morrhuate, or hypertonic dextrose ($\geq 12.5\%$).[16,29,38,38,49,55]

Two double-blind studies of inflammatory proliferant injection with 6-month follow-up have

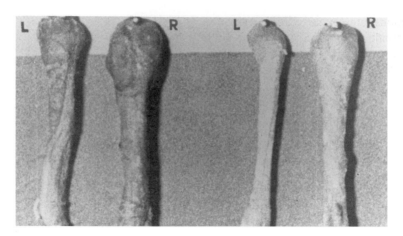

FIGURE 20-1.   Rabbit tendons 9 and 12 months after injection of proliferant; controls (L), treated (R). (From Hackett GS, Hemwall GA, Montgomery GA: Ligament and Tendon Relaxation by Prolotherapy, 5th ed. Oak Park, IL, Gustav A. Hemwall, 1992, p 96, with permission.)

been performed on patients with low back pain. The first study was on 82 patients with chronic back pain for more than 1 year who had failed to respond to conservative treatment.[43] Patients in the active treatment arm received extensive injection throughout the sacroiliac (SI) ligament and lower lumbar attachments with a solution containing 12.5% dextrose + 12.5% glycerine + 1.25% phenol + 0.25% lidocaine. Control patients received injection of saline solution in the same locations. All patients were injected weekly for 6 weeks. Only 1 patient dropped out. Between 0 and 6 months the Visual Analogue Scale pain score improved 60% in the active group and 23%

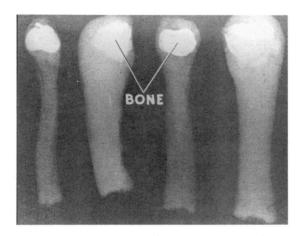

FIGURE 20-2.   Paired radiographs of tendon-to-bone attachment of rabbit tendons 1 and 3 months after injection of proliferant. Controls are on the left side of each pair, treated tendons on the right. (From Hackett GS, Hemwall GA, Montgomery GA: Ligament and Tendon Relaxation by Prolotherapy, 5th ed. Oak Park, IL, Gustav A. Hemwall, 1992, p 96, with permission.)

in the control group with p value for an intergroup difference of < 0.001. A hybrid disability score improved 70% in the active group and 30% in the control group (p < 0.001 for intergroup difference).

The second study involved 80 patients with more than 6 months of low back pain and failure to respond to conservative methods.[31] Patients were treated with a solution containing 12.5% dextrose + 12.5% glycerine + 1.25% phenol + 0.25% lidocaine versus a 1-to-1 mixture of 0.5% lidocaine and normal saline. Injections again were given weekly for 6 weeks. Between 0 and 6 months the Visual Analogue Scale pain score improved 53% in the active group and 37% in the control group with p value for intergroup difference of 0.056. The hybrid disability score improved 57% in the active group and 47% in the control group with a p value of 0.068. Therefore, despite similar improvements in the active treatment group in study 2 compared to study 1, the control group in study 2 improved to the point at which the differences between groups were only marginally significant. An examination of the osmolarity of the solutions indicates that in the second study the control solution was hypotonic (which may not be a placebo solution).

Weaknesses of these studies include the use of phenol (whose inflammatory properties may impair blinding), multiple treatment methods applied simultaneously (i.e., all patients also performed back exercises), and a treatment technique that is difficult to duplicate, and the second study included a control group that may have been an active treatment group. On the other hand, the first study did demonstrate a statistically impressive advantage of proliferant injection versus true placebo solution as well as a substantial and comparable percentage improvement in pain and disability in both studies.

Glucose

A variety of cells, including human gingival ligament cells, promptly produce growth factors or facilitators such as IGF-1, TGFβ, platelet-derived growth factor beta receptor beta (PDGFR-B), TGFα visual analogue scale, and bFGF with resultant proliferation[10,41,47,51] when exposed to elevation of glucose levels to as little as 0.5%.

Gale Borden, M.D., performed a large number of biopsies in the white rat after injection of a variety of dextrose concentrations (unpublished observations). His slides show inflammation with ≥ 12.5% concentration of dextrose (Fig. 20-3), but no inflammation with up to 10% dextrose in 0.5% Xylocaine. This is consistent with the common hospital practice of limiting peripheral venous dextrose concentrations to about the 10% range.

It is not fully understood how elevation of glucose raises growth factor levels. However, even transport of glucose into the cell requires a rise in growth factor(s).[13,47] Two studies have used dextrose injection as a single agent for proliferation.[39,49] The first study used 25% dextrose (D form of glucose in water) injected into the iliolumbar (IL) ligament versus a control of 1% Xylocaine.[39] This study showed a superior outcome in the dextrose-treated patients but had insufficient patient numbers to reach statistical significance. The dextrose concentration was likely in the inflammatory range with potential effect from stimulation of the inflammatory healing cascade. A second study involved 40 patients with severe fibromyalgia injected with 12.5% dextrose solution and demonstrated the ability to inject dextrose solution extensively in patients with severe pain with no significant side effects.[49] That study was consecutive patient-controlled rather than placebo-controlled.

The most recent study involving dextrose as a single agent for treating ligament/tendon was a prospective study of knees with anterior cruciate ligament (ACL) laxity.[50a] An electroarthrometer was used as an objective measure of ACL laxity with anterior displacement difference (ADD), which is the difference in anterior excursion measurement between knees in the same patient. To qualify for the study, patients had to have an ADD

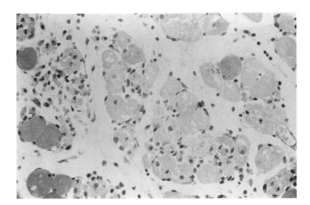

FIGURE 20-3. Photograph of a cross-section of rat muscle 48 hours after injection of proliferant (12.5% dextrose in 0.5% lidocaine) and stained with hemotoxylin and eosin. (Courtesy of Gale Borden, M.D.)

level that was 85% sensitive and 85% specific for ACL laxity. Individual, paired t tests indicated that blinded measurement of goniometric knee flexion range improved by 12.8° (p = 0.005), and ADD improved by 57% (p = 0.025). Eight out of 13 dextrose-treated knees with ACL laxity were no longer lax at the conclusion of 1 year. The rationale for tightening of connective tissue structures is the normal loss of end-to-end length of immature collagen as it dehydrates during the maturation process.

Solutions with Altered Osmolarity

Although hypertonic glucose solution is more effective than equivalently hypertonic mannitol solution, in studies comparing their growth factor stimulation effects, elevation of osmolarity about a cell clearly causes release of growth factors.[47] Osmoregulation, the cellular response to environmental changes of osmolarity and ionic strength, is important for the survival of living organisms. Elevation of osmolarity by as little as 50 mOsm has been found to activate multiple growth factors.[2,8,32,42,52,58] PDGF is among the growth factors activated.[42] Several investigators have demonstrated that hypotonicity also stimulates growth factor release,[8,53] and Sadoshima et al. demonstrated that hypotonicity stimulates a rise in DNA for growth factor production within seconds of cellular exposure.[53] Preventing a cell from shrinking or expanding with changes in osmolarity appears to prevent growth factor release, and stretching a cell without changing osmolarity leads to release of growth factors.[32] These findings imply that cells detect alterations in cell size but not changes in osmolarity or ionic strength.

PROLOTHERAPY EFFECTS ON CARTILAGE OR OSTEOARTHRITIS

Effects of Direct Injection of Growth Factors on Cartilage

Studies on effects of growth factors on human chondrocytes have so far been in vitro.[7,12,25,36] However, in animal studies, results of application of growth factors by infusion or injection have been encouraging. Van Beuningen et al. demonstrated chondrogenesis with single injection of TGF-β1 or BMP-2; TGF-β1 in particular increased proteoglycan synthesis for 3 weeks after injection.[59] Single injection of bFGF into 4-week-old rat knees induced chondrocyte growth and caused a thicker cartilage to develop.[56] Continuous infusion of FGF-2 (fibroblast growth factor-2) and injection of hepatocyte growth factor have both been shown to heal full-thickness lesions (3–4 mm induced injuries) in articular cartilage in rabbit knee and rat knee respectively.[45,61]

Growth Factor Stimulators

Inflammatory Solutions

The injection of inflammatory solutions as a growth factor stimulator has not been studied formally or in a measurable way in terms of effect on cartilage.

Glucose

Two randomized, prospective, placebo-controlled, double-blind clinical trials of dextrose injection of osteoarthritic joints have been conducted.[50a,50b] The first was on 77 patients with 111 knees meeting radiographically confirmed symptomatic knee osteoarthritis.[50a] These patients had an average weight of 193 pounds and pain for more than 10 years in qualifying knees. This study included 38 knees with no cartilage remaining in at least one compartment. Multivariate analysis indicated superior benefit from the dextrose solution over control by 6 months (p =

0.015). Data from 1 year (6 bimonthly injections of 9 ml of 10% dextrose) revealed pain improvement of 44%, swelling improvement of 63%, knee buckling improvement of 85%, and a range of motion improvement in flexion of 14°. X-rays at 1 year showed no progression of osteoarthritis and are being followed for 3 years to further confirm this.

The second study was on 27 patients with finger osteoarthritis and an average age of 64 years.[50b] One hundred fifty joints met the radiographic criteria and the symptom-duration criteria of more than 6 months of pain (average pain duration was more than 4 years). After three injections of 0.5 ml of 10% dextrose on either side of each symptomatic joint, pain with movement of fingers improved significantly in the dextrose group (with a p value of 0.027). Flexion range of motion improved more in the dextrose group (p = 0.003) than in the control group. After six injections of 10% dextrose, pain improvement averaged 53%, and there was a range of motion gain of 8°. X-rays at 1 year again showed no progression of osteoarthritis and are being followed.

Disrepair Factor Blockers

Blocking disrepair factors can promote growth by disinhibiting growth factors. Pelletier et al. demonstrated virus-altered fibroblasts can be made to produce antagonists to IL-1, a key disrepair factor that prevented osteoarthritic changes after the ACL ligament in dogs was cut.[46]

APPROACHES TO PROLOTHERAPY

There are two general approaches to proliferation therapy (Table 20-1). Physicians tend to combine aspects of both methods. The first, known as the Hackett method, is based on the approach of George Hackett with subsequent refinements made primarily by Drs. Gustaff Hemwall and Gerald Montgomery.[17–23] The West Coast method,

TABLE 20-1. Comparison of Prolotherapy Approaches

	Hackett Method	West Coast Method
Proliferant used	Predominantly dextrose	Predominantly phenol/dextrose/glycerine or sodium morrhuate
Manipulation	Rarely or not used	Used more often
Needle size	Smaller bore	Larger bore
Sedation	Anesthetic gel/blebs + IV sedation	IV sedation less often
Frequency of treatment	Every 6–12 weeks	Weekly
Exercise recommendations	Gentle activity	Fast resumption

popularized by physicians in this region, was promoted by Dorman, Ongley, and others.[11] The comparisons in Table 20-1 result from direct observation of techniques used by Hemwall, Montgomery, and Ongley and the author's personal experience.

In the Hackett method, dextrose is used as the proliferant in the vast majority of cases. Cellular disruption is minimal and nerve damage has not been reported. This method is slower to perform, but is easier to teach and is uniform in distribution of solution. In contrast, the West Coast approach utilizes phenol 1.25%, glycerine 12.5%, and dextrose (D-glucose in water) 12.5%. The needles are generally larger, and needle movements are more rapid and difficult to learn.

PRE- AND POSTPROCEDURE TREATMENT AND SEDATION

In addition to needle insertion and injection method, other considerations include proper patient selection, timing, proliferant solution choice and preparation, identification of injection sites, sedation, positioning and anesthesia issues, postprocedure care, and complications.

Patient Selection

Patients with peripheral joint laxity such as shoulder, knee, metacarpophalangeal joint, and ankle usually will not show clinical laxity on examination. Symptoms related to reflex muscular dysfunction include clicking, popping, or stiffness with reduced range of motion. Symptoms related to more significant soft tissue abnormality with secondary muscle inhibition include feeling a need to self-manipulate the area or benefitting only briefly from manipulation. A feeling of weakness or very easy fatiguability, such as the head feeling too heavy for the neck or immediate pull in the low back when bending over, can occur from either inhibition or laxity origin. Insufficient tautness in cervical ligaments or ankle ligaments can cause a feeling of being off balance from reduced cervical proprioceptive information or repetitive ankle giveway that is resistant to strengthening alone.

Symptoms related to referral from tendons and ligaments include pseudoradicular pain or pseudoradicular or whole extremity numbness. Pseudoradicular referral patterns for selected cervical ligaments are shown in Figure 20-4 and for selected sacroiliac region ligaments in Figure 20-5. In patients with segmental sensitization such as complex regional pain syndrome or fibromyalgia, the pains may be interpreted as burning and hyperalgesia is common. In such cases the normal pulling sensations felt in the lax patient may sometimes be felt as "tearing" sensations.

When prolotherapy is widely practiced, it will be an early choice to alleviate pain from sprain and strain that has lasted more than 2 months and to repair peripheral nociceptors in chronic pain. Basic science clearly points to the entheses as the source of peripheral pathology in chronic sprain and strain. Early treatment may obviate the need for prolonged therapy by providing direct treatment. If treatment does not result in improvement in two

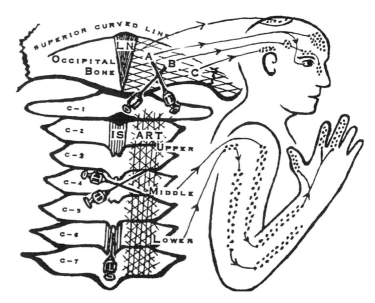

FIGURE 20-4. Common referral patterns of cervical structures. Forehead, eye (*A*); temple, eyebrow, nose (*B*); above ear (*C*); interspinous ligaments (*IS*); and articular ligaments (*ART*). (From Hackett GS, Hemwall GA, Montgomery GA: Ligament and Tendon Relaxation by Prolotherapy, 5th ed. Oak Park, IL, Gustav A. Hemwall, 1992, p 70, with permission.)

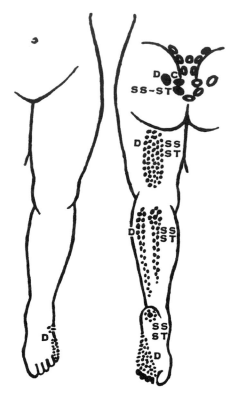

FIGURE 20-5. Common referral patterns of the sacroiliac, sacrospinous, and sacrotuberous ligaments. (From Hackett GS, Hemwall GA, Montgomery GA: Ligament and Tendon Relaxation by Prolotherapy, 5th ed. Oak Park, IL, Gustav A. Hemwall, 1992, p 32, with permission.)

sessions or if symptoms worsen, the diagnosis should be reconsidered.

Timing

In the case of focal pain over the subacromial region, the superior trochanteric bursa, or de Quervain's area, steroid trial may be advisable before initiating proliferant injection because secondary inflammation in these conditions is more prominent.

An 8-week delay after injury is recommended to allow the body to self-repair. If the patient is severely affected after sprain or strain, the pain cycle should be stopped before secondary fibromyalgia syndrome develops. The effectiveness of prolotherapy in aborting conversion of acute pain to chronic pain syndrome is an important topic to research. Reasons for intervening earlier than 8 weeks may include previous chronic sprain and strain in a region in which spontaneous healing is not expected to be efficacious or the patient's inability to work. The success of early intervention depends on a well-educated patient who understands the extent of the damage; typically this situation arises in a patient previously treated who has another accident.

Pregnant patients generally are not treated during the first trimester (except for focal peripheral joint problems) or the last trimester due to positioning issues.

If inflammatory prolotherapy methods are to be performed, it is preferable to discontinue all non-steroidal anti-inflammatory drugs (NSAIDs) three days before treatment and 10 days after. The use of anti-inflammatories does not preclude treatment, however; clinical benefit occurs in patients on regular prednisone.

Proliferant Solution Choice and Preparation

Syringes or bags can be prepared using ¼ volume of 50% dextrose (i.e., 3 ml in a 12-ml syringe) to make 12.5% soft tissue solution, or ½ volume for 25% joint injection solution. Xylocaine percentage varies between 0.4 and 0.075%, depending on the size of the area to be injected. Bacteriostatic water is recommended for the diluent. Single-use containers should be discarded at the end of each day. Solution made in advance should be refrigerated. Benzyl alcohol can be obtained from the manufacturer for large-volume solution preparation if other than bacteriostatic water is used as diluent.

Bottled phenol is obtainable from the manufacturer, allowing for small amounts to be added to ≥ 250 ml of 12.5% dextrose to convert solution to phenol-dextrose. Concentrations of 0.5–0.75 are alternatives to the 1.25% phenol concentration in the Ongley solution; remember to keep the volume of injection low. The glycerine component function has not clearly been determined or studied individually.

Sodium morrhuate is available as a 5% solution. One to 2 ml per 10-ml syringe makes a 0.5–1% concentration. Again, low volumes should be used. Its advantages over phenol are not established.

For the first treatment, using dextrose is advisable in any patient before using phenol, but particularly in patients with central sensitivity who misinterpret postinjection discomfort as more painful than it should be. Phenol has not been found to create scarring in the maximum prolo concentrations (1.25%), and permanent dysesthesia has not been reported, even with concentrations up to 6% used for nerve block.[48] However, postinjection stiffness and discomfort are more significant; phenol is best reserved for more local treatment in patients well-known to the treating physician. Small amounts for each injection site should be used. Be especially careful to avoid the spinal canal.

Identifying Injection Sites

Potential pain referral sources for the patient's clinical complaints are palpated with the prolotherapist's fingertip. A knowledge of ligament and tendon referral patterns is essential to determine the sites of injection. Common sites of injection for regions of pain in the upper and lower body are shown in Tables 20-2 and 20-3 respectively. The objective presence of twitch contractions can often be elicited with crossfiber palpation over the tendon or ligament in question and reproduce the patient's pain pattern. After these specific areas are identified, the skin is marked. Trigger points from muscle usually are not marked because the primary pathology in chronic sprain and strain is in connective tissue, and reflex twitch contractions to muscle stimulation are likely a secondary phenomenon.[4] Consistent with this hypothesis, large numbers of twitch contractions in muscle occur during injection of the entheses.

Sedation, Positioning, and Anesthesia

Anesthetic gel (a simple preparation containing benzocaine or an alternative) is applied to diminish skin sensation. Anesthetic blebs are an alternative, especially if IV sedation is not used.

Immediately prior to treatment, prophylactic antinausea medication such as hydroxyzine may be given. The length of the procedure and the patient being treated on his or her stomach create special concerns for sedation hypoventilation. Standard precautions with any sedation include no eating for 6–8 hours and not drinking for 1 hour before treatment. If more than 25 mg of meperidine is given, constant oximetry is recommended with a nasal cannula in place with oxygen ready to initiate. Single-agent sedation is recommended. Midazolam is not recommended for the nonhospital setting unless the patient is constantly monitored by the staff and an alarmed oximeter and the physician is highly familiar with intubation. The physician should routinely inquire if patients have taken any anxiolytics or narcotics before the procedure. Intravenous diazepam may be administered before giving low-dose meperidine, but it should not be given during a treatment to a patient who has already been given IV meperidine, because the tendency for

TABLE 20-2. Common Sites of Injection for the Upper Body (Regions of Pain)

Referral Source Examples	Head	Head and Neck	Neck	Top of Shoulder	Shoulder	Elbow	Arm	Upper Back
Semispinalis capitis	■	■						
Splenius capitis	■	■						
Rectus capitis	■	■						
TMJ capsule/ligaments	■	■						
Cervical intertransverse ligaments		■	■	■	■		■	
Cervical facet ligaments		■	■	■	■		■	
Anterior/posterior tubercles		■	■	■	■		■	■
Posterior superior trapezius		■	■	■	■			
Costotransverse ligaments			■	■	■		■	■
Longissimus thoracis			■	■	■		■	■
Iliocostalis thoracis			■	■	■		■	■
Shoulder capsule				■	■		■	
Biceps					■		■	
Subscapularis					■		■	
Pectoralis					■		■	
Deltoid					■		■	
Infraspinatus					■		■	
Teres major					■		■	
Teres minor					■		■	
Common extensors						■	■	
Common flexors						■	■	

TABLE 20-3. Common Sites of Injection for the Lower Body (Regions of Pain)

Referral Source Examples	Back	Back and Leg	Buttock	Thigh	Knee	Calf/Shin	Ankles	Heel	Arch	Toes
Facet ligaments	■	■	■	■		■				
Lumbar intertransverse ligaments	■	■	■	■		■				
Sacroiliac ligament/joint	■	■	■	■		■	■	■	■	■
Iliolumbar ligament	■	■	■	■						
Gluteal insertions			■	■		■				
Sacrospinous ligament			■	■		■	■			
Deep articular ligaments, hip			■	■		■	■	■	■	■
External rotators, hip			■	■						
Distal knee adductors				■	■					
Distal hamstrings				■	■	■				
Knee capsule				■						
Distal vastus medialis			■	■						
Anterior tibialis					■					
Peronei					■					
Talofibular ligament						■				
Calcaneofibular ligament						■				
Tibionavicular ligament						■				
Tibiotalar ligament						■				
Tibiocalcaneal ligament						■				
Achilles tendon							■			
Calcaneonavicular ligament								■		
Calcaneocuboid ligament								■		
Long plantar ligament								■		
Tarsometatarsal ligaments									■	

hypoventilation is substantial. Because both lidocaine and meperidine in the solution cause hypotension and because nausea is related to postural hypotension during and after the procedure, ephedrine, 50 mg intramuscular, and low-dose epinephrine in solutions (0.25 mg per 500–1000 ml) can be quite helpful in limiting hypotension after treatment. Before doing so, blood pressure check or monitoring is advised to confirm that hypertension is not present, and each patient's cardiac status should be known. Oxygen saturation values in the 90s should be maintained, and predrawn naloxone hydrochloride should be available. When a patient falls asleep, this is equivalent to his or her receiving another 50 mg of intravenous meperidine, so keeping the patient in the conscious sedation range is important.

Postprocedure Care

After the procedure, patients generally can be discharged to the care of a responsible driver when they can walk without dizziness. Analgesics are provided for pain, but NSAIDs should be avoided. The inflammatory cascade stimulation of fibroblast migration occurs in the first few days, so three days is a reasonable minimum period to wait. If glucose/osmotic or growth factor proliferation is used, avoidance of NSAIDs may not be necessary. Application of ice or heat in combination with slow, gentle stretching is recommended, and activities should be light for 2–4 days. Resumption of activities that were tolerated before injection should be tolerated after injection, but the patient who has received phenol should be warned that reactions are variable in terms of work tolerance after injection.

Complications

Proliferation therapy is quite safe when used judiciously. The most common complication is an exacerbation of pain that lasts 2–7 days after the injection session. If pain persists beyond this time, residual ligament or tendon trigger points may be present, excess volume injection may have occurred, or a stronger proliferant may have resulted in a central hypersensitivity overreaction. A superimposed inflammatory process also may be present.

Avoiding anaphylaxis is imperative. With sodium morrhuate the risk is real; incidence of anaphylaxis with this solution does not necessarily correspond to a coexisting shellfish intolerance. Preservative-free Xylocaine, bacteriostatic water without methylparabens, and latex-free rubber gloves are recommended. Using chlorhexidine gluconate 2% solution for skin preparation is well tolerated. Nevertheless, epinephrine should be readily available in case of emergency.

Other complications are specific to the injected body part and usually are a result of improper needle placement. Injections around the thorax can lead to pneumothorax, although with proper technique this is rare. Injection into a vertebral artery is rare and safe if ≤ 0.5 ml of standard solution is used.[5] Five cases of substantial neurologic impairment from spinal cord irritation caused by subdural injection above the sacrum have been reported since 1955[26,30,54] and were attributed to strongly inflammatory proliferants that are not in current use.

PROCEDURE PERFORMANCE

Positioning and Volume of Injection

In whole body treatment, the patient begins on his or her stomach with 2–3 pillows under the stomach, with the head above the pillows enough to not have to stretch for the table, and with the mouth and nose clear for breathing. Because gastroesophageal reflux is not uncommon and may increase with length of sedation, performing the back injections first is preferable. Tapping of the bone surface is recommended when the bone is palpated by needle tip, injecting very small amounts of fluid until 0.5–1 ml is injected into the area.

Posterior Neck and Upper Back Injection Techniques

Neck and upper extremity pain often is treated with proliferation therapy. Although understanding common trigger point referral patterns is helpful, as with muscular trigger point, chronic pain often is associated with atypical referral patterns with spread of stimuli from lowered interneuron thresholds. Many cases of upper extremity pain resembling thoracic outlet syndrome or pseudo–reflex sympathetic dystrophy may result from cervical or thoracic nociceptors. This disruption also may affect the posterior cervical sympathetic outflow, resulting in organ dysfunction with chronic sinus

drainage problems, ringing in the ears or intermittent hearing loss, swallowing dysfunction, blurry vision, off balance sensation, and nausea (Barré-Lieou syndrome).[15,24] In addition, many tension and migraine headaches unresponsive to medication and other traditional treatments may be treated with injection into the cervical structures.

A nonindenting, reangulation technique is recommended for costotransverse ligament injection because it allows injection of ribs up to 3 inches in depth (patients ≥ 350 lbs) with safety. The nonindenting technique is preferred by the author because it allows the treating physician to know exactly how far from the skin surface the needle is traveling, which is useful for ribs that cannot accurately be palpated. This method begins at about T5–T6 where the ribs are most superficial. Use of a short (i.e., ½ to 1-inch needle) is recommended, palpating, inserting, and searching at ½-inch depth with 5–10° angulation changes of the needle. Redirection is performed by coming out nearly fully to avoid bending of the needle and then reinserting at a different angle. If the rib is not found, re-palpate if the rib is palpable, and then reinsert and search again with a ⅛-inch to ¼-inch increase in depth. Repeat the process until the rib is found. Because of the many reangulations attempted at each depth, passing the rib will seem highly difficult. Nonpublished observations suggest frequency of pneumothorax at 1 per 2,500 to 10,000 needle insertions over the ribs.

After the most superficial costotransverse ligament (CTL) is found, mark that rib and use the depth to find the other levels, inserting at a right angle to the skin surface. Marking as ribs are found is more accurate than premarking. Figure 20-6 demonstrates the row of CTL injection sites on the left about 1½ to 1¾ inches from the midline. Using the superficial rib as a template, inject up and down from that level. Note that depth increases about ¼ inch traveling up to T1 and about ¼ inch traveling down to T12, depending on the size of the patient and varying with the distance from the midline. Slowly increasing the length of the needle may be helpful to the physician. At each level, insert to a level known to be safe from the previous rib, and if the rib is not touched, search in a similar manner to that described previously. This method is used for both CTLs and iliocostalis thoracis, commonly involved in upper back pain and with referral pain as far as the hand or up into the head.

Because the depth for T1 approximates the depth for injection of the posterior cervical vertebral body (cervical intertransversarii), needle insertions

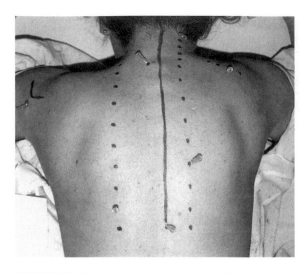

FIGURE 20-6.   Injection of posterior neck, upper back, posterior superior trapezius, and shoulder capsule.

for injection along that row are often the most convenient. At cervical levels the needle is directed about 10–20° inferiorly to avoid any possibility of passing between vertebral bodies. The top level injected is C2. This is recognized by palpating the posterior spinous process of C2 about 1 cm below the base of the skull. Note that for C2 injection the same angulation may not be feasible; in this case a shorter and more vertically oriented needle may be used for this level.

Thoracic facet ligament injection depth is usually about ½ inch deeper with the needle directed slightly medially. Figure 20-6 demonstrates marks for a row of facet ligament injections on the right with a point of entry about 1 inch from the midline and needle angulation 10–20° medially and 10–20° inferiorly for safety. Although the distance of the facet articulation from midline varies, spread of solution is satisfactory to achieve the necessary result and uniformity of injection. For each injection a finger is on the spinous process to ensure that the distance from the midline remains about one inch and to rule out or compensate for scoliosis. Carrying the injections up into the cervical region to C2 is again recommended to complete the row of treatments. Note that, with the vertebra prominens varying, it may be difficult to distinguish C7 from T1 level. However, because the depths are constant and an entire row is being injected, this is irrelevant.

Although patients with chronic pain often complain of weakness in the back and the erector spinae, injection of the costotransverse and facet ligaments usually is enough to correct this. However, if the patient continues to complain of weakness or if the

sides of the spinous processes or the interspinous ligament are painful, he or she may be injected in the painful regions. Figure 20-6 shows multifidi injection at vertebra prominens level on the L and insertion into the interspinous ligament at approximately the T9–10 level. The insertion point for multifidi injection is typically ½ inch from the midline. It is not clearly established how critical it is with interspinous ligament to tap bone. The author prefers to inject into the central portion with a 1-inch needle. The injection is done vertically to avoid any chance of entering the spinal canal, which may occur with the use of a 1½ inch-needle in thin patients.

After completing the thoracic and cervical posterior injections, the base of the skull is injected, addressing multiple entheses such as rectus capitis, semispinalis, and splenius capitis. Marks for insertion are made on a line across the width of the neck about 1 fingerbreadth inferior to the base of the skull (about C2 spinous process level) with 4 insertion points along each side, beginning about ½ inch from midline. For safety the midline is again palpated and confirmed visually. Insertion of the needle medially is no closer than ½ inch to the midline. Typically a 2-inch, 25-gauge needle is used. Insertion is at the C2 spinous process level to reach the rectus capitis row (see Fig. 20-6). Insertion is best done aiming slightly laterally and superiorly to be sure the skull is touched and the midline is avoided. After the skull is touched, the needle is redirected inferiorly several times until the depth increases slightly, indicating that the base of the skull has been reached. The first row of injection sites is then complete. Note that an injection here may inadvertently reach the vertebral artery, so aspiration is recommended. The next two rows are located superior to the first at about ½ to ⅔-inch intervals to touch the semispinalis and splenius capitis insertions using a 1-inch needle.

Injection of the posterior superior trapezius is facilitated by bringing the arm up such that the elbow is even with the shoulder (R trapezius area in Fig. 20-6), which elevates the clavicle so that the posterior superior trapezius insertion can be injected posteriorly. If preferred, insertion may be at 90° to the table surface, but because the clavicle travels anteriorly from lateral to medial, angling the needle laterally will find the clavicle with the least distance traveled. Typical insertion points are shown in Figure 20-6.

For the rhomboid and levator scapulae injection, the patient's arm rests either on his or her back or on the leg of the examiner to elevate the scapula so that distance to the ribs is increased (see right scapulae in Fig. 20-7). Levator scapulae injections travel up to the superior extent of attachment, with depth about ½ inch deeper than that for the rhomboid injection. For teres major and minor and infraspinatus injection (see left scapulae in Fig. 20-7), the arm usually is down at the patient's side. The scapula outline is shown with needle insertion along the lateral border for teres major and minor and in the mid portion of the scapula for the infraspinatus origin.

Low Back and Buttock Injections

Acute and chronic back, hip, buttock, and lower extremity pain often may be attributable to referred pain from trigger points within ligaments or tendon structures around the sacrum or lumbar spine. Failed back syndrome from surgery may be due to instability of ligament and tendon structures. Chronic pain from osteoporotic fractures can be due to traumatic laxity of spinal ligaments with pain from the facet and CTLs or longissimus muscle attachments. Selected ligament referral patterns for the lower back and leg are illustrated previously in Figure 20-5. Sacroiliac (SI) joint referral is similar to the SI ligament pattern depicted.

As in other locations, before performing injections in the lumbar spine, gluteal region, and hips, thorough palpation is necessary to identify abnormal ligaments that appear painful, but the patient with minimally painful palpation may still have SI ligament involvement due to the ligament's depth. Although the posterior superior iliac spine (PSIS) is at the S2 level and the iliac crest corresponds to the L4 level, while palpating it is not uncommon to misjudge the top of the iliac crest as much as 2 cm: thus insertion of a needle vertically is helpful in accurately marking the peak of the iliac crest and potentially in several locations in large individuals.

After the top of the crest is marked, two rows of injection sites can be marked paralleling the top of the crest as shown on the left side of Figure 20-8. The superficial portions of the iliolumbar (IL) and SI ligament are injected from the first row of sites and the deeper portions from the superior row. The medial sites on the top row often will access the SI joint, but this is seldom necessary as long as adequate tapping and instillation is carried out in the ligament. Each insertion site indicated is usually injected with 1.5 ml total volume, for a total volume approximating 20 ml for each IL-SI ligament region.

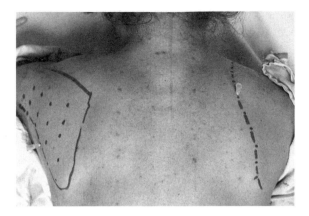

FIGURE 20-7. Injection of the right posterior thromboids/levator and left infraspinatus/teres.

Insertion sites for intertransverse ligaments and facet ligaments are shown in Figure 20-8 on the R. L5 is just below the level of the crest, so usually it is easily approached by inserting a 2–3-inch needle about 2 inches lateral to the midline, about ¼ inch above the top of the crest, touching the top of the crest, and then redirecting medially and inferiorly to slip off the top and down onto L5. The exact tip of L5 may not be touched but spread of solution occurs. Then, L4–L2 are injected, with L4 injection shown in Figure 20-8. The author prefers to inject fairly vertically for L4 and L3 to effectively gauge the distance from midline and then enter on the

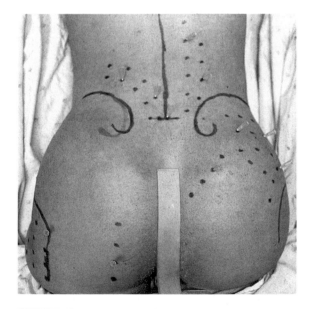

FIGURE 20-8. Injection of the iliolumbar (*IL*) and sacroiliac (*SI*) ligaments, intertransverse and facet ligaments, lumbosacral junction, gluteal attachments, deep hip articular ligament, sacrospinous and sacrotuberous ligaments, and multiple insertions on the posterior femur.

same vertical line for L2 and L1 with the needle angled medially to optimize safety. Note that L1 transverse process level is not marked, because novices frequently misjudge the top of the crest. It may be wiser to depend on solution spread to travel from L2–L1 to avoid risk of pneumothorax. The facet ligaments are similarly injected in the thoracic and cervical regions with a slight inferior and medial direction of needle. Note the L5–S1 facet articulation is about ¾ inch above the top of the sacrum. After facet ligament injection, the top of the sacrum usually is injected with a needle short enough (1½ inch) to avoid entering epidural space. The top of the sacrum is injected laterally as well but with inferior direction to avoid inadvertent spinal headache.

In the posterior gluteal region, multiple ligaments and muscular attachments are potential pain generators. Groin or inferior abdominal pain often originates in the IL ligament, pain to the great toe is often from the hip articular ligament, and SI ligament and gluteal attachments can refer pain in a variety of directions into the leg. Figure 20-8 shows needle insertion for gluteal insertions medial to the PSIS, insertions in the mid portion of the gluteus, and insertions for the deep hip articular ligament. Injection volumes in the medial gluteal insertions and hip articular ligament are about 1.5 ml for each site due to redirections with the needle to cover the gluteal insertion and hip ligament region.

The inferior borders of the sacrum are injected for sacrospinous and sacrotuberous insertions that typically radiate posteriorly down the leg. It is important to start on the sacrum and then "walk off" with the needle to avoid excessively deep entry.

Attachments of the gemelli, obturator internus, piriformis, and gluteal muscles at the posterolateral femoral trochanter also can be injected (Fig. 20-8, left side). These attachments are injected in three rows, with the most medial row located ¾ inch off the midline of the posterior thigh. Lateral trochanteric pain usually resolves with this approach if steroids for bursitis are unsuccessful or as an alternative to steroid injection. The gemelli origin shown above the ischial tuberosity can radiate pain down the back of the leg, and sometimes into the groin and testicular area causing pseudo–tailor's bottom. It is approached directly vertically, finding it first just above the ischial tuberosity and then reinserting vertically, noting that depth typically increases about ¾ of an inch from the first insertion location. Injections are stopped about even with the top of the trochanter to avoid touching the sciatic nerve.

Figure 20-9 shows marks down the lateral thigh with the patient in a side-lying position. At times, injection down the leg appears to address the many slips of the tensor fascia lata as it travels to insert below the knee in patients with resistant lateral thigh pain with weight bearing or persistent difficulty with pain upon side lying. Twitch contractions are particularly large with this injection, especially in distal thigh portion, so sedation may need to be increased.

Foot Injections

Due to substantial pain sensitivity, injections into the feet usually precede knee injections. Medial injection site examples are shown in Figure 20-10. Metatarsophalangeal joints are most comfortably injected from the top of the foot for metatarsalgia; response to this method appears to approximate that of injection directly over the head from the plantar aspect. The needle insertion is lateral to the top of the metatarsal head, which is felt by flexing the toe down or approximated from the metatarsal head through the bottom of the foot, and the needle is directed distally and medially. Entering the joint is not critical—injection under the joint capsule appears to have an equivalent result.

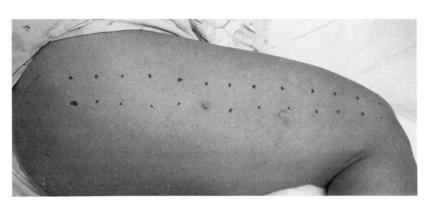

FIGURE 20-9. Injection of the tensor fascia lata.

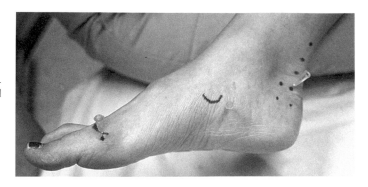

FIGURE 20-10. Injection of the metatarsophalangeal (MTP) joints, plantar fascia, and Achilles tendon.

Plantar area insertion point for plantar fasciosis is shown just posterior to the navicular bone and even with its tip. Insertion of a 30-gauge needle in that location to 1-inch depth and injecting 3 ml of lidocaine at the same level and along the needle track is recommended for anesthesia. Wait a few minutes before inserting a 2-inch, 25-gauge needle. A 2-inch needle is required to reach the plantar ligament origins and insertions from one injection site.

If a steroid injection is elected for the first approach to this problem, a similar insertion method can be used to find the origin of the plantar ligament.

Achilles tendonosis (not usually a true "-itis") can be injected over its insertion as shown in Figure 20-10. Usually this is performed on both the medial and lateral aspect. Other insertion points along the tendon for about 2 inches can be injected using a 27-gauge needle, inserting gently through the skin and advancing until slight resistance is met to inject about the peritendinous area. Rupture of the Achilles tendon is not a concern with this as it is with Achilles steroid injection.

Injection of the calcaneofibular and talofibular ligaments (Fig. 20-11) is performed by palpating about the lateral malleolus anteriorly and inferiorly and injecting at tender origins. It is helpful in chronic ankle sprain with inadequate proprioceptive

feedback and repetitive sprain tendency. The needle location shown enters the subtalar joint. Filling the subtalar joint with 3–4 ml of 25% dextrose solution has particular merit in chronic ankle strain because it can affect articulations chronically affected about the talus. The lateral talocalcaneal ligament or intercarpal ligaments may be painful to palpation and require injection. Injection of the medial ankle is similar with palpation revealing tenderness in the tibionavicular, tibiotalar, and tibiocalcaneal portion.

Knee Injections

The thigh adductor insertions and vastus medialis insertions are injected from a semicircle about the medial condyle of the femur and the hamstring insertions from several rows oriented vertically below the knee articular line (Fig. 20-12). This is most easily done with the knee bent and the leg in external rotation resting on the examiner's bent leg. The collateral ligament origin and insertion are injected when painful. In addition, the knee capsule often is injected inferomedially with 6 ml of 25% dextrose. Due to tibiotalar-patellofemoral communication, injection of the infrapatellar joint does not appear necessary when 25% dextrose is used.

FIGURE 20-11. Injection of the calcaneofibular and talofibular ligaments and subtalar joint.

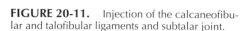

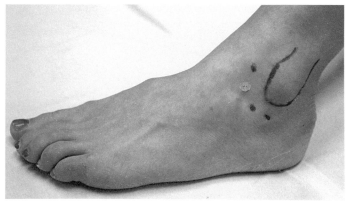

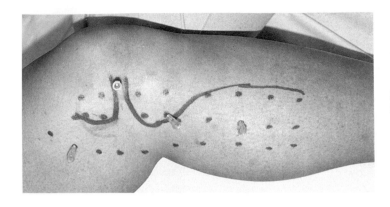

FIGURE 20-12. Injection of hamstring insertions, collateral ligament, and joint capsule.

Forearm, Wrist, and Finger Injection Techniques

Proliferation treatment of medial and lateral epicondylosis is preferable to use of steroids and is best performed before the development of prominent disorientation of tissue. Abundant tapping and low volume (4–6 ml total) proliferant are recommended to avoid excess inflammatory effect, particularly with the first treatment. In lateral epicondylosis, the common extensors are injected starting at the supracondylar ridge, with injections also over the radial head ligament, medial to the condyle, and directly on the lateral condyle (Fig. 20-13). The forearm should be fully supinated to make all attachment sites needle-accessible. Similar spread of fluid about the medial epicondyle is recommended for medial epicondylosis (Fig. 20-14).

Wrist injection is typically in the region of the radial collateral ligament (Fig. 20-13). This is particularly helpful in resistant cases of de Quervain's disease not resolved completely with a single steroid injection (radial wrist strain will mimic this disorder). In cases of marked pain over the first dorsal compartment, initially a steroid injection followed by proliferant injection for connective tissue repair is reasonable. Other common injection sites about the wrist include intercarpal ligaments in cases of wrist hyperextension.

Metacarpophalangeal (MCP) injection for painful function is performed by entering over the palpable joint line with the MCP in flexion, with a 5–10° distal inclination from vertical (Fig. 20-13). PIP and DIP injection is performed from a lateral approach with sufficient capsule infiltration and injection slightly above midline to minimize contact with digital nerves.

Anterior Shoulder and Anterior Chest Injections

The subscapularis, coracobrachialis, and pectoral insertions often are sources of anterior shoulder pain that mimic bicipital tendinitis. The subscapularis and pectoralis major insertion sites are injected with the shoulder in external rotation to expose the anterior insertions (Fig. 20-14). Injection is given in two to three rows over the proximal 3–4 inches of the anterior humerus. Coracobrachialis and pectoralis minor insertions are injected vertically. A chondrosternal ligament row often is helpful for patients with chest pain and pain with palpation of this row.

Scalene Region Injections

Because whiplash and other cervical sprain or strain often affect anterior structures, a safe and effective strengthening of these structures is important.

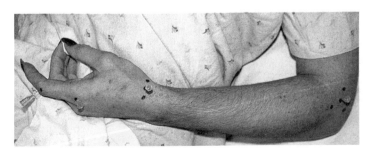

FIGURE 20-13. Injection of common extensor origin at elbow, radial collateral ligament at wrist, and metacarpophalangeal (MCP) and proximal interphalangeal (PIP) joints.

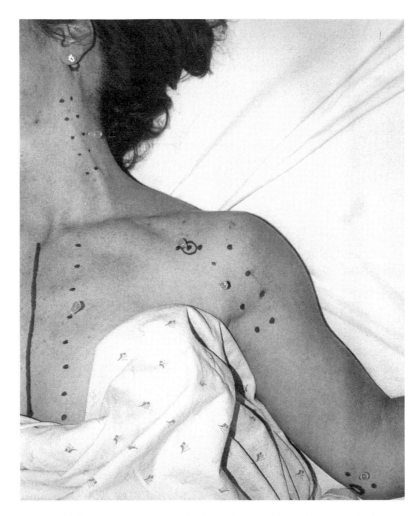

FIGURE 20-14.   Injection of subscapularis, coracobrachialis, and pectoralis attachments on the humerus, chondrosternal ligaments, and scalene origins.

Palpation of anterior and posterior tubercles to inject tender areas may be used, but these structures are normally somewhat tender and palpation may not be sufficiently tolerated for exact determination, especially because the tubercles are often just a few millimeters wide. The author prefers to inject in two rows. The patient's head is rotated 45°–60° away from the side of injection. The first row of injection sites is even with the anterior line of the ear and the second ⅓ inch anterior to the first. The second cervical tubercles are located 1½ finger-breadths (FB) below the mastoid process. The C6 tubercles correspond to a point three FB above the clavicle (see Fig. 20-7). The needle used usually is a 1¼-inch, 27-gauge with a depth of ⅝ inch, or more, depending on patient size. Injection on bone is again the rule. Note that the C2 level in the anterior row is not injected because there is no C2 anterior tubercle. This is an area in which touching a bone

does not guarantee avoiding a vessel, so aspiration and caution are strongly suggested. Complications from injections into the deep cervical structures may include cervical nerve irritation with temporary paresthesia or vertebral artery injection.

Temporomandibular Joint Injection Techniques

Treatment of temporomandibular joint (TMJ) pain with proliferation therapy is directed at the joint capsule and supportive tendons and ligaments internal to the joint. The objective is to strengthen these structures by thickening and tightening the ligaments, thereby providing joint stability and less pain. With the patient's mouth closed and teeth unclenched (closed-mouth approach), the physician palpates the zygomatic arch adjacent to the condylar process of the mandible

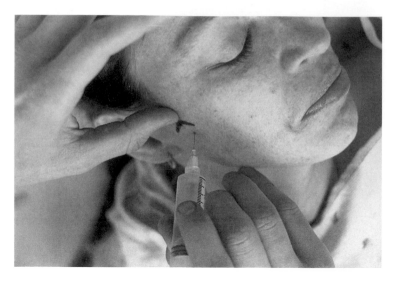

FIGURE 20-15.   Needle placement for the closed-mouth approach when injecting for temporomandibular (TMJ) joint disorders.

with a finger of the injecting hand. A 1-inch, 30-gauge needle or 1¼ inch-, 27-gauge needle is inserted ¼ inch inferior to the apex of this palpable structure, felt as a semicircle (Fig. 20-15). The needle is advanced about 1 inch, and 0.75 ml of 25% dextrose solution is injected.

CONCLUSION

Prolotherapy involves placement by needle of a solution that raises growth factor activity enough to stimulate cell growth or cell production of collagen or matrix. Although inflammatory prolotherapy has been used for many years, noninflammatory prolotherapy methods are rapidly expanding. Two impressive but difficult to reproduce inflammatory prolotherapy studies on low back pain have been performed. Three double-blind studies with simple dextrose are underway in knee, finger arthritis, and knee ACL laxity; one-year data shows statistically and clinically significant results. Future studies on growth factor use should include low-cost options (e.g., growth factor stimulator) as well as more expensive alternatives (e.g., primary growth factor application) to determine cost efficacy factors.

Whole-body treatment of a patient in pain can be tedious and technically difficult. Considerable experience and personal instruction from an experienced prolotherapist is recommended before administering such treatment.

REFERENCES

1. Banks A: A rationale for prolotherapy. J Orthop Med (UK) 13:54–59, 1991.
2. Berl T, Siriwardana G, Ao L, et al: Multiple mitogen-activated protein kinases are regulated by hyperosmolality in mouse IMCD cells. Am J Physiol 272:305–311, 1997.
3. Best T: Basic science of soft tissue. In DeLee JC, Drez D Jr (eds): Orthopaedic Sports Medicine Principles and Practice, Vol 1. Philadelphia, W.B. Saunders, 1994, p 3.
4. Biedert R, Stauffer E, Freiderich N: Occurrence of free nerve endings in the soft tissue of the knee joint. Am J Sports Med 20:430–433, 1993.
5. Bonica J: Anatomic and physiologic basis of nociception and pain. In Bonica JJ (ed): The Management of Pain, 2nd ed. Philadelphia, Lea & Febiger, 1990, pp 28–94.
6. Buckwalter J, Cruess R: Healing of musculoskeletal tissues. In Rockwood CA, Green DP (eds): Fractures. Philadelphia, J.B. Lippincott, 1991.
7. Bujia J, Pitzke P, Kastenbauer E, et al: Effect of growth factors on matrix synthesis by human nasal chondrocytes cultured in monolayer and in agar. Eur Arch Otorhinolaryngol (Germany) 253:336–340, 1996.
8. Caruccio L, Bae S, Liu A, et al: The heat-shock transcription factor HSF1 is rapidly activated by either hyper- or hypo-osmotic stress in mammalian cells. Biochem J 327:341–347, 1997.
9. Des Rosiers E, Yahia L, Rivard C: Proliferative and matrix synthesis response of canine anterior cruciate ligament fibroblasts submitted to combined growth factors. J Orthop Res 14:200–208, 1996.
10. Di Paolo S, Gesualdo L, Ranieri E, et al: High glucose concentration induces the overexpression of transforming growth factor-beta through the activation of a platelet-derived growth factor loop in human mesangial cells. Am J Pathol 149:2095–2106, 1996.
11. Dorman T, Ravin T: Diagnosis and Injection Techniques in Orthopedic Medicine. Baltimore, Williams & Wilkins, 1991.
12. Dunham B, Koch R: Basic fibroblast growth factor and insulin like growth factor I support the growth of human septal chondrocytes in a serum-free environment. Arch Otolaryngol Head Neck Surg 124:325–330, 1998.
13. Fladeby C, Bjonness B, Serck-Hanssen G: GLUT1-mediated glucose transport and its regulation by IGF-I in cultured bovine chromaffin cells J Cell Physiol 169:242–247, 1996.
14. Frank C, Amiel D, Woo SL-Y, et al: Normal ligament properties and ligament healing. Clin Orthop Res 196:15–25, 1985.

15. Gayral L, Neuwirth E: Oto-neuro-ophthalmologic manifestations of cervical origin: Posterior cervical sympathetic syndrome of Barré-Lieou. N Y State J Med 54:1920–1926, 1954.
16. Grieve E: Mechanical dysfunction of the sacroiliac joint. Int Rehabil Med 5:46–52, 1983.
17. Hackett G: Joint stabilization through induced ligament sclerosis. Ohio St Med J 49:877–884, 1953.
18. Hackett G: Shearing injury to the sacroiliac joint. J Int Coll Surg 22:631–642, 1954.
19. Hackett GS: Ligament and Tendon Relaxation Treated by Prolotherapy, 3rd ed. Springfield, IL, Charles C Thomas, 1956.
20. Hackett G: Prolotherapy in whiplash and low back pain. Postgrad Med 27:214–219, 1960.
21. Hackett G: Prolotherapy for sciatica from weak pelvic ligaments and bone dystrophy. Clin Med 8:2301–2316, 1961.
22. Hackett G, Huang T, Raftery A: Prolotherapy for headache. Headache 2:20–28, 1962.
23. Hackett G, Hemwall G, Montgomery G: Ligament and Tendon Relaxation Treated by Prolotherapy, 5th ed. Oak Park, IL, Gustav A. Hemwall, 1992.
24. Hemwall G: Barre-Lieou syndrome. J Orthop Med 11:79–81, 1989.
25. Horner A, Kemp P, Summers C, et al: Expression and distribution of transforming growth factor-beta isoforms and their signaling receptors in growing human bone. Bone 23:95–102, 1998.
26. Hunt W, Baird W: Complications following injections of sclerosing agent to precipitate fibro-osseous proliferation. J Neurosurg 18:461–465, 1961.
27. Johnson LL: Arthroscopic abrasion arthroplasty. In Mcginty JB (ed): Operative Arthroscopy. New York, Raven Press, 1991, pp 341–360.
28. Kang H, Kang ES: Ideal concentration of growth factors in rabbit's flexor tendon culture. Yonsei Med J 40:26–29, 1999.
29. Kayfetz D, Blumenthal L, Hackett G, et al: Whiplash injury and other ligamentous headache—Its management with prolotherapy. Headache 3:1–8, 1963.
30. Keplinger J, Bucy P: Paraplegia from treatment with sclerosing agents. JAMA 173:113–115, 1960.
31. Klein R, Bjorn C, DeLong B, et al: A randomized double-blind trial of dextrose-glycerine-phenol injections for chronic low back pain. J Spinal Disord 6:23–33, 1993.
32. Krump E, Nikitas K, Grinstein S: Induction of tyrosine phosphorylation and Na+/H+ exchanger activation during shrinkage of human neutrophils. J Biol Chem 272:17303–17311, 1997.
33. Leadbetter W: Soft tissue athletic injuries. In Fu FH (ed): Sports Injuries: Mechanisms, Prevention, Treatment. Baltimore, Williams & Wilkins, 1994, pp 736–737.
34. Lee J, Harwood F, Akeson W, et al: Growth factor expression in healing rabbit medial collateral and anterior cruciate ligaments. Iowa Orthop J 18:19–25, 1998.
35. Liu Y, Tipton C, Matthes R, et al: An in-situ study of the influence of a sclerosing solution in rabbit medial collateral ligaments and its junction strength. Connect Tissue Res 11:95–102, 1983.
36. Marui T, Niyibizi C, Georgescu HI, et al: Effect of growth factors on matrix synthesis by ligament fibroblasts. J Orthop Res 15:18–23, 1997.
37. Mitchell N, Shephard N: The resurfacing of adult rabbit articular cartilage by multiple perforations through the subchondral bone. J Bone Joint Surg 58A:230–233, 1976.
38. Myers A: Prolotherapy treatment of low back pain and sciatica. Bull Hosp Joint Dis 22:48–55, 1961.
39. Naeim F, Froetscher L, Hirschberg GG: Treatment of the chronic iliolumbar syndrome by infiltration of the iliolumbar ligament. West J Med 136:372–374, 1982.
40. Nakamura N, Shino K, Natsuume T, et al: Early biological effect of in vivo gene transfer of platelet-derived growth factor (PDGF)-B into healing patellar ligament. Gene Ther 5:1165–1170, 1998.
41. Ohgi S, Johnson P: Glucose modulates growth of gingival fibroblasts and periodontal ligament cells: Correlation with expression of basic fibroblast growth factor. J Periodontal Res 31:579–588, 1996.
42. Okuda Y, Adrogue H, Nakajima T, et al: Increased production of PDGF by angiotensin and high glucose in human vascular endothelium. Life Sci 59:455–461, 1996.
43. Ongley M, Klein R, Dorman T, et al: A new approach to the treatment of chronic low back pain. Lancet 2:143–146, 1987.
44. Ongley M, Dorman T, Eck B, et al: Ligament instability of knees: A new approach to treatment. Manual Med 3:152–154, 1988.
45. Otsuka Y, Mizuta H, Takagi K, et al: Requirement of fibroblast growth factor signaling for regeneration of epiphyseal morphology in rabbit full-thickness defects of articular cartilage. Dev Growth Differ 39:143–156, 1997.
46. Pelletier J, Caron J, Evans C, et al: In vivo suppression of early experimental osteoarthritis by interleukin-1 receptor antagonist using gene therapy. Arthritis Rheum 40:1012–1019, 1997.
47. Pugliese G, Pricci F, Locuratolo N, et al: Increased activity of the insulin-like growth factor system in mesangial cells cultured in high glucose conditions: Relation to glucose-enhanced extracellular matrix production. Diabetologia 39:775–784, 1996.
48. Reeves KD: Mixed somatic peripheral nerve block for painful or intractable spasticity: A review of 30 years of use. Am J Pain Mgmt 2:205–210, 1992.
49. Reeves KD: Treatment of consecutive severe fibromyalgia patients with prolotherapy. J Orthop Med 16:84–89, 1994.
50. Reeves KD: Prolotherapy: Present and future applications in soft tissue pain and disability. Phys Med Rehabil Clin North Am 6:917–926, 1995.
50a. Reeves KD, Hassanein K: Randomized, prospective double-blind, placebo-controlled study of dextrose prolotherapy for knee osteoarthritis with or without ACL laxity. Evidence of pain improvement, range of motion increase, reduction of ACL laxity, and early evidence for radiographic stabilization. Altern Ther Health Med [in press].
50b. Reeves KD, Hassanein K: Randomized, prospective, double-blind, placebo-controlled study of dextrose prolotherapy for osteoarthritic thumb and finger (DIP, PIP, and trapeziometacarpal) joints: Evidence of clinical efficacy. J Altern Complement Med [in press].
51. Roos MD, Han IO, Paterson AJ, et al: Role of glucosamine synthesis in the stimulation of TGF-alpha gene transcription by glucose and EGF. Am J Physiol 270:803–811, 1996.
52. Ruis H, Schuller C: Stress signaling in yeast. Bioessays 17:959–965, 1995.
53. Sadoshima J, Izumo S: Cell swelling rapidly activates Src tyrosine kinase, a potential transducer of mechanical stress in cardiac myocytes [abstract]. Circulation 1(Suppl 1):409, 1996.
54. Schneider RC, Liss L: Fatality after injection of sclerosing agent to precipitate fibro-osseous proliferation. JAMA 170:1768–1772, 1959.
55. Schultz LW: Twenty years experience in treating hypermobility of the temporomandibular joints. Am J Surg 92:925–928, 1956.
56. Shida J, Jingusih S, Izumi T, et al: Basic fibroblast growth factor stimulates articular cartilage enlargement in young rats in vivo. J Orthop Res 14:265–272, 1996.
57. Spindler KP, Imro AK, Mayes CE: Patellar tendon and anterior cruciate ligament have different mitogenic responses to platelet-derived growth factor and transforming growth factor beta. J Orthop Res 14:542–546, 1996.
58. Szaszi K, Buday L, Kapus A: Shrinkage-induced protein tyrosine phosphorylation in Chinese hamster ovary cells. J Biol Chem 272:16670–16678, 1997.

59. van Beuningen H, Glansbeek H, van der Kraan P, et al: Differential effects of local application of BMP-2 or TGF-beta 1 on both articular cartilage composition and osteophyte formation. Osteoarthritis Cartilage 6:306–317, 1998.

60. Ward CW, Gough KH, Rashke M: Growth factors in surgery. Plast Reconstr Surg 97:469–476, 1996.

61. Wakitani S, Imoto K, Kimura T, et al: Hepatocyte growth factor facilitates cartilage repair much better than saline control. Full thickness articular cartilage defect studied in rabbit knees. Acta Orthop Scand 68:474–480, 1997.

62. Zubay G: Integration of metabolism in vertebrates. In Zubay G (ed): Biochemistry, 4th ed. Dubuque, IA, Wm. C. Brown, 1998, p 691.

21

Botulinum Toxin Use in Myofascial Pain Syndromes

Martin K. Childers, D.O., and David G. Simons, M.D.

This chapter will outline potential uses of botulinum toxin type A (Botox) for pain management in putative conditions best described as myofascial pain syndromes. Although the uses for botulinum toxin type A that are licensed by the Food and Drug Administration (FDA) do not include pain management, this product currently is being used by a range of medical specialists to address pain control of various etiologies. However, there is a dearth of empiric clinical data that directly addresses these issues. The purpose of this chapter, therefore, is to provide some clinical insight for physicians regarding the use of botulinum toxin in myofascial pain syndromes, based on the authors' experience and similar applications in a variety of neuromuscular disorders. As with all medications and procedures, one should obtain the necessary training and knowledge to achieve the most effective outcome. Accordingly, one should know some essential features about this product before treating patients for pain. These vital elements include:
- Mechanism of action (MOA)[17,31]
- Concept of median lethal dose (LD$_{50}$)
- Dosing and administration[57]
- Basic neuromuscular physiology
- Treatment(s) that might be helpful in conjunction with botulinum toxin therapy[13,33]
- Contraindications

Because it is beyond the scope of this chapter to address all of the topics listed above, the authors urge the reader to visit other informational sources listed at the end of this chapter. However, a few words regarding some physiologic aspects of botulinum toxin type A (herein referred to simply as botulinum toxin) are worthwhile mentioning here. First, clinical effects of botulinum toxin injections are delayed a day or two with the maximal effects of functional muscular weakness peaking at about 2 weeks.[14,31] Second, effects last for approximately 12 weeks due to sprouting at the neuromuscular junction.[19] Third, the anatomic location of the neuromuscular junction varies among muscles and depends on the type of structural arrangement of myofibers; some studies suggest that the methods of localizing neuromuscular junctions potentiate the effects of botulinum toxin.[14,71] Finally, putative mechanisms by which botulinum toxin achieves pain relief are at best incompletely understood and may be complex. Additional clinical research is required not only to gain insight into the pathophysiology of painful conditions of muscle, but also to identify and explore potential agents that might be effective, such as botulinum toxin.

CLINICAL USES OF BOTULINUM TOXIN TYPE A

In 1989, the FDA licensed Botox in the United States for treatment of the following inpatients over the age of 12 years:
- Strabismus (a condition in which one or both eyes do not move together in tandem)
- Essential blepharospasm (involuntary blinking)
- Hemifacial spasm (involuntary facial muscle spasms)

In addition to the approved uses in the U.S., there are other published uses of botulinum toxin,[12] which include painful or potentially painful conditions such as:

Achalasia
Anismus (painful)
Cervical dystonia (sometimes painful)
Detrusor-sphincter dysinergia
Essential blepharospasm
Essential tremor
Facial wrinkles

Hemifacial spasm (sometimes painful)
Hyperhydrosis
Myofascial pain syndrome (painful)
Occupational dystonia (sometimes painful)
Muscle spasm (often painful)
Piriformis muscle syndrome (painful)
Spasmodic dysphonia
Spasticity (sometimes painful)
Strabismus
Whiplash (painful)

Outside of publications, noteworthy medical organizations have commented on the effectiveness and safety of botulinum toxin. The National Institutes of Health (NIH) Consensus Development Conference published a statement in 1990 that summarized the indications and contraindications of botulinum toxin usage for the treatment of a variety of conditions.[60] The NIH conference endorsed the use of the neurotoxin as safe and effective for the symptomatic treatment of adductor spasmodic dysphonia, blepharospasm, cervical dystonia, hemifacial spasm, jaw-closing oromandibular dystonia, and strabismus. The same year, the Therapeutics and Technology Assessment Subcommittee of the American Academy of Neurology further endorsed the use of this product for the symptomatic treatment of these conditions.[84]

BOTULINUM TOXIN TYPE A USE IN PAINFUL CONDITIONS: REPORTS IN THE LITERATURE

A Medline search conducted in 1997 for the headings "botulinum toxin," "myofascial pain," and "pain" for the period 1966 to September 1997 resulted in 18 references that included 463 subjects. Of these, 7 studies included "pain" or "myofascial pain" within the article title.[1,3,5,8,26–28,30,46,58,59,62,64,68,69,72,73,85] The remaining references reported pain response within the context of treatment for underlying spasticity, cervical dystonia, fibromyalgia, focal dystonia and hemifacial spasm, masseteric hypertrophy, painful dystonia in Parkinson's disease, pain of chronic pancreatitis, and writer's cramp. Variables in these studies include dosing, concentration and injection techniques, use of concurrent therapeutic modalities, varying diagnoses, and chronicity of neurologic dysfunction. Some patients treated for disorders of involuntary muscle contraction (e.g., dystonia) also reported benefits in pain reduction (Table 21-1) in muscles injected with botulinum toxin.

WHEN TO CONSIDER BOTULINUM TOXIN THERAPY

A few words of caution before considering using botulinum toxin in the treatment of a patient with myofascial pain. Recall that the approved indications for use of botulinum toxin in the U.S. are for three conditions: strabismus, blepharospasm, and hemifacial spasm.[44] Use of botulinum toxin for myofascial pain, therefore, is off-label and accordingly should be considered only for patients with conditions that remain unsatisfactory or for patients judged inappropriate for more conservative treatment. Before considering specific examples, however, first consider some fundamental properties of skeletal muscle and also one of the hallmarks of muscle associated pain, the myofascial trigger point (MTrP).[80]

In general, botulinum toxin therapy for pain management may be specifically appropriate (and probably only appropriate) when the pain is determined by the clinician to be dependent on uncontrolled contractile activity of skeletal muscle.[12] Because all skeletal muscle contraction depends on release of acetylcholine (ACh) from nerve terminals at motor end plates, treatments that prevent ACh release accordingly will inhibit contraction of muscle and thus benefit the patient troubled by muscle-associated pain. For example, when spasticity is sufficiently intense that it causes pain or that MTrPs cause pain,[77–79] treatment with botulinum toxin should be helpful.

Injection of botulinum toxin should be considered for treatment of pain caused by MTrPs when noninvasive manual treatments[80] are not effective or not available or when less destructive analgesic medications are ineffective *after mechanical and systemic perpetuating factors have been corrected.* Based on the mechanism of action of botulinum toxin, injections should be made into the end-plate zone of the muscle as much as possible. When MTrPs are determined to be the etiology of pain, one way of achieving accurate placement of the toxin is to inject under electromyographic (EMG) guidance at sites exhibiting end-plate potentials (end-plate noise and spikes).[14] Injection of botulinum toxin should be directed into the end-plate zone because that is the only part of the muscle where the susceptible nerve terminals are found. One example of a painful condition amenable to such an approach is the painful shoulder in the hemiplegic stroke patient. The combination of spasticity and MTrPs that may be found in such a patient is, in the authors' opinion, a double

TABLE 21-1. Summary of References Generated by Medline Search of "Botulinum Toxin," "Myofascial Pain," and "Pain" for the Period 1966 to September 1997

Reference	N	Diagnosis	Pain Outcome Measures	Mean Dose of BTX-A	Results/Conclusions
Odergren 1994[62]	20	CD	VAS	149 units	↓ VAS (p < 0.01)
Greene 1990[30]	55	CD	Numeric	118 units	"Statistically significant improvement in pain" (p = 0.003)
Jedynak 1990[46]	36	CD	Descriptive	Varied	"20 of 22 positive results . . . duration over 4 weeks" (French transl.)
Gelb 1989[26]	20	CD	Numeric	Varied	16 of 20 patients ↓ pain
Tsui 1987[85]	56	CD	Numeric	50–70 units	Pain scores ↓ 2.1 to 0.9 (p < 0.001)
Paulson 1996[68]	5	Fibromyalgia	Descriptive	100 units	"Ineffective for pain"
Sherman 1995[73]	7	Chronic pancreatitis	Descriptive	1.5–2.5 U/kg	"Ineffective for pain"
Sheean 1995[72]	2	Writer's cramp	Descriptive	Varied	Occurrence of shoulder pain in 2
Pacchetti 1995[64]	30	Parkinson's foot dystonia	McGill pain questionnaire	80 units	Improved in all (p = 0.001)
Cheshire 1994[8]	6	Myofascial pain	VAS, descriptive	50 units	↓ VAS and most pain descriptors weeks 2–4 (p < 0.05)
Pierson 1996[69]	39	Spasticity	Not specified	180 units	Improvement in 10 of 13
Monsivais 1996[58]	68	Thoracic outlet syndrome	VAS	Not specified	↓ VAS (p = 0.011)
Brin 1988[5]	97	Focal dystonia and hemifacial spasm	Not specified	Varied	Moderate/marked benefit in 16 of 19 specified
Acquadro 1994[1]	2	Myofascial pain	Descriptive	50, 150 units	Improved
Girdler 1994[28]	1	Facial pain in temporomandibular joint (TMJ) dysfunction	Descriptive	250 units (Dysport®)	Improved
Girdler 1997[27]	1	Chronic muscle spasm of facial arthromyalgia	Descriptive	250 units (Dysport®)	"48 hours later . . . complete cessation of facial pain"
Moore 1994[59]	1	Masseteric hypertrophy	NA	100	NA

BTX-A = botulinum toxin type A; CD = cervical dystonia; VAS = Visual Analogue Scale; NA = not applicable; ↓ = decrease

indication for injection of botulinum toxin using EMG guidance.

BOTULINUM TOXIN USE IN MYOFASCIAL PAIN CAUSED BY TRIGGER POINTS

Injection of muscles with botulinum toxin can be appropriate therapy for myofascial pain caused by trigger points (TrPs) but is likely to be inappropriate for treatment of myofascial pain of unspecified origin, when that term is used in the general sense.[74] Myofascial pain that is diagnosed only as muscle tenderness in a patient with a regional pain syndrome without having identified the specific TrPs responsible for the clinical pain is an ambiguous diagnosis. The tender spots may be due to fibromyalgia, bursitis, or one of many other diagnoses the causes for which do not justify injection with this product.

A myofascial pain syndrome caused by TrPs characteristically results from either an acute episode of muscle overload or a chronic and/or repetitive muscle overload.[80] Active MTrPs that cause a pain complaint exhibit marked localized tenderness and often refer the pain to a distant location, disturb motor function, and may produce autonomic changes.

MTrPs are identified on physical examination by palpating a localized tender spot in a nodular portion of a taut rope-like band of muscle fibers. Pressure (usually with the examiner's fingertip) over a trigger point elicits pain at that area and may also elicit pain at a distance from the point under the fingertip. This is known as *referred pain*. Another important feature of the trigger point is that the elicited pain mirrors the patient's experience. Applied pressure often garners the response: "That's my pain!" Insertion of a needle, snapping palpation, or even a brisk tap with the fingertip directly over the trigger point may elicit a brief muscle contraction detectable by the examiner. This brisk contraction of muscle fibers of the ropy taut band is termed a *local twitch response*.[80] In muscles that move a relatively small mass or in those that are large and superficial (e.g., the finger extensors or the gluteus maximus), the response is easily seen and may cause the limb to "jump" when the examiner introduces a needle into the trigger point. Localized abnormal response from the autonomic nervous system may cause piloerection, localized sweating, or even regional temperature changes in the skin because of altered blood flow.

The local twitch response is a transient contraction of taut myofibers that occurs in response to snapping palpation of the MTrP or in response to rapid insertion of a needle into the MTrP. Animal studies[38–40] and a human study[35] have shown that this response is propagated as a spinal reflex that is not dependent on a supraspinal component. This response is a valuable indicator that the needle being injected into an MTrP has effectively reached at least one necessary target in the MTrP. Demonstration of a local twitch is additional confirmation of the diagnosis. In addition, passive stretch range of motion of the muscle is limited by pain, and both maximal contraction in the shortened position and maximum voluntary contraction are likely to be inhibited or to be associated with pain.

At present, no routine laboratory test or routine imaging test is available to confirm the presence of MTrPs, but the newly developed tissue impedance imaging shows much promise. In addition, two objective tests can be used to confirm the presence of MTrPs. One requires electrodiagnostic technique and the other uses ultrasound imaging. Both animal and human research studies have shown that MTrPs are characterized by electrically active loci that exhibit end-plate noise and often spikes.[37] Electromyographers generally recognize these end-plate potentials as normal.[36,37] However, physiologists have distinguished these potentials from normal miniature end-plate potentials and have shown that they represent a pathologic increase in spontaneous release of ACh.[42,55] Studies to date indicate that these abnormal end-plate potentials can always be found in an active MTrP, but the physiology studies suggest that they can also be present for other reasons. Contraction knots (hypercontracted myofibers) to account for the nodule at the TrP and the taut band that causes increased muscle tension were demonstrated histologically in MTrPs of dogs.[76]

Myofascial TrPs are known to be a clinical condition in dogs as well as in humans.[45]

Injection of MTrPs with botulinum toxin is usually performed on patients with chronic pain symptoms. It is important to remember that the commonly occurring, acute, single-muscle MTrP syndromes often revert from active to latent TrPs without specific treatment if the individual simply avoids the muscle overload situation that activated the MTrPs and proceeds with daily activities within limits that are not painful. This activity tends to actively stretch the involved muscle gently but repeatedly, which is an effective treatment. The recovery from acute MTrP syndromes is expedited and the likelihood of lasting relief greatly improved if the patient learns to perform slow, gentle, active, full range-of-motion exercises specifically for the involved muscles at least once daily. Following injection of chronic MTrPs, the authors consider these exercises essential for optimum results.

The chronic myofascial pain syndromes may become chronic because the initial acute TrP pain was not properly diagnosed or not treated effectively. Characteristically, chronic MTrPs are chronic because of unresolved perpetuating factors that may be mechanical or systemic.[80] Simply injecting these chronic MTrPs with botulinum toxin (or anything else) can be expected to provide relief only for a limited time if perpetuating factors are not identified and resolved. Completely eliminating the MTrPs in a muscle with a neurotoxin without eliminating or correcting the muscle overload situation that activated the MTrPs in the first place may result in that muscle stress activating another TrP in the same muscle. In any case, because recovery occurs in the injected end plates in a few months,[19] persistence of the stress that activated the TrP in the first place will very likely again activate it. When dealing with chronic or recurrent MTrPs, resolving perpetuating factors is often an essential step to lasting relief.

NATURE OF MYOFASCIAL TRIGGER POINTS

Research studies indicate that the clinical characteristics of an MTrP can be explained by hypercontracted muscle fibers located at and produced by a region of muscle with multiple dysfunctional motor end plates (neuromuscular junctions). The dysfunction is a markedly excessive continuous release of the normal synaptic transmitter, acetylcholine. The noise-like potentials and spikes that are strongly associated with MTrPs[40,41,75] were first interpreted as coming from muscle spindles.[41] However, EMG studies clearly identify these noise-like and spike potentials as motor end-plate potentials of skeletal muscle fibers.[89] Although the EMG literature often refers to these end-plate potentials as representing normal end-plate activity,[51,89] the physiology literature shows that the noise-like potentials result from a greatly increased release of ACh,[18,34] which means those potentials are abnormal. The end-plate noise component can result from mechanical strain of the neuromuscular junction caused by stresses applied to the nerve terminal[55] or produced by muscle overload. The end-plate noise component of end-plate potentials appears to be present before the needle examination and is commonly caused by stressful activity of the muscle, especially in latent TrPs that cause no clinical pain complaint. The end-plate spikes, however, are often induced by the presence of the needle[21] and are more likely to appear in more active MTrPs.

Histologically, MTrPs show large, darkly staining, round myofibers in cross section in canine[76] and in human[90] studies. Sections of myofibers several hundred microns in length of longitudinal sections of canine muscle show hypercontracted fibers (also called *contraction knots*). The integrated hypothesis for the pathophysiology of MTrPs attributes these contraction knots to the observed depolarization of the postjunctional membrane that continuously releases calcium from the sarcoplasmic reticulum. This hypothesis identifies contraction knots as limiting circulation because the strong contraction of the sarcomeres is sustained within the hypercontracted fiber while local energy consumption is increased. The resulting energy crisis should exhibit severe local hypoxia, demonstrated in the German equivalent to MTrPs, nodules of myogelosis.[6] The increased tension of involved muscle fibers accounts for the palpable taut band consistently associated with an MTrP. The energy crisis and local hypoxia that was observed to extend for several millimeters could account for the release of substances that sensitize local nociceptors, causing the local and referred pain characteristic of MTrPs.[80]

An interesting study examined rabbit muscle after a marker (iron deposit) was placed at precisely the location where an active trigger point was identified by twitch response, taut band, and spontaneous electrical activity. Small C nerve fibers (most likely nerves that carry pain information) were found in the immediate vicinity.[37] Taken together, these data support the idea that MTrPs are related to abnormal motor end-plate activity and subsequent hypercontraction of the associated myofibers.[7]

RATIONALE FOR USE OF NEUROMUSCULAR BLOCKING AGENTS

If abnormal end-plate activity is responsible for MTrPs, then a powerful rationale exists for the use of neuromuscular blocking agents, such as botulinum toxin, in the treatment of myofascial pain syndromes and trigger points.[16] The increased tension of muscles caused by MTrPs is clearly not due to involuntary motor unit activity (spasticity) but apparently is caused by the localized contracture of sarcomeres due to endogenous end-plate dysfunction. When involuntary muscle contraction (spasticity) is associated with muscle hypoxia, it characteristically is painful. Based on this understanding, it seems likely that any intervention that (at least temporarily) relieves pain by preventing or reducing muscle contractions might predict how a patient responds to botulinum toxin. However, while TrP injections or intramuscular compartment blocks by anesthetic agents may predict future response to treatment with botulinum toxin, an eventual problem arises in differentiating the beneficial effects caused by blocking sensory nerves (with anesthetic agents) from the effects produced by a sensory nerve-sparing neurotoxin. However, the effect of blocking sensory nerves by injected anesthetic agents lasts no longer than the duration of the anesthetic action. On the other hand, needling a TrP (dry or with anesthetic) can treat the TrP definitively. Ambiguity arises when a good result occurs because of effective TrP treatment by needling with anesthetic injection and also arises when a poor result occurs because serious unidentified perpetuating factors promptly reactivate an effectively treated TrP.

TRIGGER POINT INJECTIONS WITH BOTULINUM TOXIN IN THE LITERATURE

Studies to evaluate the effectiveness of injections of botulinum toxin into MTrPs are prone to several errors of design and execution that can lead to misleading results. A study that includes placebo injections should use a placebo injection that is not considered by many to be an effective treatment for MTrPs. If the placebo injection is effective treatment then the study is not placebo controlled but rather is a comparison of different kinds of treatment without placebo control. There is serious question about whether injection of TrPs with normal saline is a placebo treatment. Injection into an adjacent non-tender site in the muscle should be a more valid placebo control. Another error that can obscure the effectiveness of any injection treatment of MTrPs is to inject only one or some of the multiple muscles with MTrPs that are contributing to the patient's pain. If only some of the muscles with pain-producing MTrPs are treated, then one could expect that the patient would experience at most only partial pain relief. Frequently in this case, the patient feels little total pain relief and instead feels only that less of his body is hurting. Poor results reported could just as well be the result of experimental design rather than ineffectiveness of the treatment being tested. Another similar error is the injection of only one of several MTrPs in a muscle so that the untreated MTrP(s) continue to cause pain that obscures the relief obtained by the treatment.

Another comparable study design error is to fail to identify the presence of several different sources of the subject's pain. For example, if the patient has a bursitis or joint dysfunction (such as facet joint problem) that is generating a pain pattern similar to an active TrP pattern[4] and only the MTrP source of pain is eliminated, the subject will report only partial relief at best. Focal tenderness can be (and often is) produced at two different kinds of locations in a muscle. The central MTrP in the end-plate zone is tender because of the local end-plate dysfunction. Attachment TrPs where the muscle fibers attach to the aponeurosis or bone can also exhibit similar focal tenderness that can also refer pain. However, this tenderness is usually secondary to the tension of the taut band produced by the central MTrP. Thus, injection of botulinum toxin into an attachment site rather than in the end-plate zone does not have a rational physiologic basis. Accordingly, effective treatment by injection in the attachment region of the muscle is likely to occur only by permeating at least half of the muscle with botulinum toxin. Moreover, the location of the end-plate zone depends strongly on the architecture of the muscle, and there can be two attachment MTrPs for every central MTrP.[80] Because studies appear to depend strongly on muscle tenderness to identify the site for injection without fully considering the location of the end-plate zone, this error in injection location could be a major source of conflicting findings.

Cheshire et al. described patient responses to trigger point injections with botulinum toxin in 6 individuals with chronic myofascial pain in a randomized, double-blind, placebo-controlled study.[8] Cervical paraspinal or shoulder girdle trigger points

in 6 patients received either saline or 50 units of botulinum toxin reconstituted in 4 ml of saline injected equally in two or three sites. Responses were measured over 8 weeks by verbal pain descriptors, Visual Analogue Scale (VAS), pressure algometer, and palpable muscle spasm or firmness. A reduction of more than 30% from baseline was considered a positive response.

Four of 6 subjects experienced reduction in pain and spasm following botulinum toxin, but not saline, injections. One subject experienced no change by any variables following either treatment, and another subject responded favorably in all variables after both placebo and botulinum toxin injections. Onset of responses occurred within the first week following neurotoxin injections, with a mean duration of 5–6 weeks. The authors concluded that beneficial effects of botulinum toxin in myofascial pain occurred through the interruption of muscle contraction and that a larger study was needed to confirm these preliminary findings before treatment could be recommended unequivocally.

In comparison, Wheeler et al. conducted a randomized, double-blinded, controlled study comparing injections of normal saline versus injections of 50 and 100 units of botulinum toxin at the most tender trigger points in 23 patients with myofascial pain syndrome.[88] The authors found no significant difference in VAS pain or disability scores, patients' global assessment of symptoms, or pressure algometer readings throughout 4 months of follow-up. There was a statistical trend toward significant improvement in scores among a small cohort, 39% of the original participants, who were originally treated with botulinum toxin and then chose to receive a second 100-unit injection. Authors speculate that there may be a dose-related effect of the neurotoxin that was not evident in this study, and therefore further study may be warranted. It is worth mentioning, however, that the group receiving second injections contained significantly fewer patients with work-related injuries than the control group.

In a report of 4 revealing case studies, the same investigator injected botulinum toxin in patients who had refractory headaches associated with pericranial muscle tension.[87] These cases illustrate the importance of identifying all of the sources of pain. Three patients had true tension-type headache due to uncontrolled contraction of facial muscles; 1 patient responded to botulinum toxin in the corrugator supercillii and frontalis, 1 patient responded to botulinum toxin in contracted glabellar and supraorbital muscles, and the third in the orbicularis oculi, corrugator, and frontalis muscles. One of the 3 patients with MTrPs required injections in four sites in the splenius capitis muscle; another required treatment of the splenius capitis, splenius cervicis, and middle trapezius muscles; and the third was injected in the temporalis, right cervical paraspinals, middle scalene, right upper thoracic paraspinal, and trapezius muscles. One patient experienced relief following MTrP injections except at the time of her menses. This was managed with medication.

IDENTIFYING MYOFASCIAL PAIN SYNDROMES FOR BOTULINUM TOXIN THERAPY

Any of the approximately 500 muscles in the body can develop myofascial pain caused by TrPs and therefore could, when indicated, benefit from accurately placed injection with botulinum toxin. However, only a limited number have been reported in the literature to date. Factors that might identify a pain syndrome of any myofascial origin as potentially responding favorably to botulinum toxin injections include muscle hypertrophy, neurogenic or vascular compression, anatomic localization that isolates the target muscle from other structures, and more than one outcome measure to determine efficacy of treatment.[16] Under these criteria, piriformis muscle syndrome and thoracic outlet syndrome appear to qualify.

Piriformis Muscle Syndrome

Piriformis muscle syndrome is a myofascial pain condition that presents with seemingly bizarre symptoms.[32,79,81] Patients are typically female with a recent history of trauma to the buttocks or pelvis (usually from a fall) who complain of a deep-seated pain in the buttocks and hip, with radiation into the thigh or even into the leg and foot. These characteristic signs and symptoms are sometimes caused by pain referred from piriformis MTrPs[67,77–79] and sometimes caused by compression of the sciatic nerve between the bony rim of the foramen and a hypertrophied piriformis muscle.[10] The nodular MTrP and its taut band can provide the increased muscle bulk and tension. Pain in these patients may come from both the nerve entrapment and the referred pain from the piriformis MTrPs. An additional source of pain in these patients is the tendency for compression of motor nerves to activate MTrPs in the muscles supplied by that nerve. Although some clinicians feel that this diagnosis is

controversial, numerous peer-reviewed articles clearly define clinical, anatomic, and electrophysiologic evidence for this distinct condition causing low back and leg pain.[22,32,43,48,61,79,81,82]

On clinical examination, deep pressure over the buttocks at a point midway between the sacrum and greater trochanter of the hip will reproduce the patient's pain complaint. Full stretch range of motion of the piriformis muscle is limited by pain. Since the piriformis muscle is so deep, palpation of this trigger point can only be properly performed by rectal or vaginal examination and requires unusually long fingers. Deep along the posterolateral portion of the rectal (or vaginal) vault, cephalad to the levator ani muscle, palpation of the intrapelvic attachment area of the taut band of the trigger point elicits pain at the site of compression and refers pain either into the thigh or down the leg. However, the intrapelvic examination alone can only barely reach the attachment region of the piriformis and may therefore be palpating first nerve root tenderness and then piriformis attachment TrP tenderness. The attachment of the muscle at the greater trochanter is prone to be equally involved and tender and is readily available for palpation. It is very useful to identify both the central TrP tenderness in the region of the midbelly and also the attachment tenderness at both ends. This strengthens the MTrP diagnosis considerably.

Beatty's maneuver has been described to elicit pain in this condition as well.[2] It requires the patient to lie on the nonpainful side, and the thigh is abducted by moving the painful leg off the table. This maneuver effectively contracts the piriformis muscle and should reproduce the patient's pain in the buttocks. However, contraction of muscles with TrPs appears to be most painful when the muscle is voluntarily contracted in the shortened position. If the enthesopathy is sensitive enough, the muscle hurts when forcefully loaded in any position but particularly in the shortened position.

Alternatively, to stretch the piriformis muscle one must internally rotate and adduct the thigh at the hip. The most effective way to put this muscle on stretch is to have the patient lie on the nonpainful side, flex the hip to 90°, and adduct it by allowing it to drop over the edge of the table. This is also a very effective treatment position for contract-relax manual therapy.[20,80,82]

However, because the syndrome commonly includes sciatic nerve compression at the level of the hip, other causes of sciatica should be ruled out (such as a herniated lumbar disc). One helpful diagnostic aid is EMG. In the case of sciatic neuropathy at the level of the nerve root in the back, the EMG exam may reveal abnormal spontaneous electrical activity in the extensor muscles of the back, while in piriformis syndrome no such abnormal electrical activity should be seen in the lumbar paraspinal muscles.[54] Since the site of nerve compression is distal to the nerve root,[66] other investigators have reported that H-wave studies are delayed when comparing the patient's extended painful leg to the same leg in a position of adduction, internal rotation, and flexion.[22] Conduction may be delayed when the muscle is at its thickest in the shortened position.

Diagnosis of Piriformis Muscle Syndrome

The syndrome described above may be caused by two distinct etiologies: piriformis MTrP syndrome and that syndrome complicated by sciatic nerve entrapment. Accordingly, the clinician should evaluate patients with this putative diagnosis for other causes of sciatic neuropathy from compression at the level of the spine (e.g., a herniated disc or space-occupying lesion). Imaging studies, such as computed tomography (CT) or magnetic resonance imaging (MRI) may also be considered to rule out other potential sources of compression at or near the sciatic notch, such as intrapelvic abscess, occult tumor, or hematoma.[9,52,53] Additionally, all the criteria described above should be met to accurately identify and determine the location of the MTrP. Taken together, these clinical findings, electrodiagnostic data, and imaging studies should enable the clinician to reach an accurate diagnosis.

When to Consider Botulinum Toxin

In some cases, conservative treatment of piriformis syndrome fails, and local injections of anesthetics or steroids may be considered. Surgical resection of the piriformis muscle is an additional option.[49,56,70] However, some patients may gain short-term benefits from local TrP injections into the muscle but remain refractory to other treatment for long-term pain control. This subset of patients might benefit from botulinum toxin treatment, especially if the piriformis muscle shows EMG evidence of involuntary muscle contraction. When injecting MTrPs in the piriformis muscle, they are hard to localize accurately in such a deep muscle and are located in the end-plate zone in the midbelly region of the muscle (Fig. 21-1). In this case, use of EMG guidance to inject the neurotoxin specifically where end-plate potentials are observed will insure

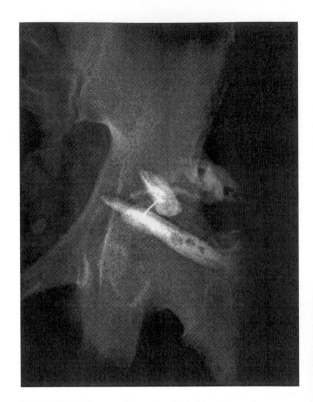

FIGURE 21-1. Radiograph of left hip with radiocontrast material injected into the piriformis muscle. Note the needle placement inferior to contrast material above (placed superior to the piriformis muscle). Special imaging techniques, such as fluoroscopy, CT, or ultrasound, may facilitate accurate localization of deep muscles of the pelvis and back.

optimal placement of the product.[14] Since all or part of the sciatic nerve may occasionally traverse this part of the muscle, this use of EMG guidance is of additional importance.

To examine the effectiveness of intramuscular botulinum toxin injections as a treatment for piriformis muscle syndrome, one author (MKC) examined a convenience sample of 3 consecutive patients.[24] All patients presented with findings consistent with a diagnosis of piriformis syndrome and all had failed a trial of conservative management including nonsteroidal anti-inflammatory agents (NSAIDs), stretching, ultrasound, and piriformis TrP injections. H-reflexes and segmental nerve conduction studies in all patients confirmed conduction block along the sciatic nerve above the gluteal fold, consistent with the diagnosis.[22,67]

The involved piriformis muscle in each patient was injected under fluoroscopic guidance with 100 units of botulinum toxin reconstituted in 5 ml of preservative-free saline. Pain reduction was assessed through pretreatment to post-treatment differences on a patient self-reporting instrument that recorded

VAS of pain intensity, psychological distress from pain, spasm frequency, and interference with daily activities. Results of this open label case series demonstrated that the average pain scores decreased from 6.1 to 3.4 and were 3.6 two weeks later. Twelve weeks later, 2 out of 3 patients had returned to their previous pain levels, whereas 1 patient sustained longer lasting benefit. The same author is currently conducting a double-blind, placebo-controlled crossover study of the effectiveness of botulinum toxin injections for refractory piriformis syndrome. As of yet, there are no definitive answers for dose, injection location, or dilution, but anecdotal evidence and this small case series suggest injections of botulinum toxin may be beneficial in some chronic, refractory cases.

Thoracic Outlet Syndrome

Thoracic outlet syndrome is a myofascial pain syndrome involving compression of the nerves of the brachial plexus or the vessels (subclavian artery and vein) of the upper limb.[23,83] Compression occurs as the vulnerable structures pass over or adjacent to the first rib as they exit the thoracic cavity or neck region, because the thoracic outlet is bounded by the anterior and middle scalene muscles, the first rib, the clavicle, and (inferiorly) the tendon of the pectoralis minor muscle (Table 21-2). Increased tension of these two scalene muscles elevates the first rib, and hypertrophy (enlargement) of these muscles can cause or contribute to signs and symptoms of this syndrome.[80]

Signs and Symptoms

Signs and symptoms of thoracic outlet syndrome include painful sensations in the shoulder and ulnar nerve distribution of the hand. In a clinical maneuver, Adson's test, the patient turns his head to the involved side and holds a beep breath while raising the chin.[20,65,83] The examiner palpates the radial pulse. A positive test is determined in the individual if his

TABLE 21-2. Scalene Muscles

Scalene anterior muscle:
Elevates the first rib in breathing
Bends the neck laterally and forward
Rotates the neck to the opposite side

Scalene medius muscle:
Same as scalene anterior

Scalene posterior muscle:
Raises the second rib in breathing
Bends the neck laterally
May slightly rotate the neck

pulse diminishes and pain is reproduced during this maneuver.

A similar clinical maneuver, known as Roos' test, requires the patient to abduct the shoulders 90°, flex the elbows 90°, and open and close his hands slowly for 3 minutes.[65,86] The examiner observes the patient for hand pallor, diminished pulses, and ulnar dysesthesias, all of which are positive for thoracic outlet syndrome.

Scalene MTrPs are found by examining the head and neck for painful restriction of side bending of the head to the opposite side. Also, one should examine the digitations of the anterior and middle scalene muscles for tender spots in taut bands. Other causes of compression (besides muscle hypertrophy) in the thoracic outlet should be considered because the thoracic outlet is an enclosed, relatively small space. Anything that might narrow the space or cause swelling and edema of any of the associated structures should be considered, including:

- Fractured clavicle
- Cervical rib
- Tumor within the thoracic outlet
- Movements that compress the thoracic outlet (shoulder hyperabduction)
- Paradoxical or chest breathing (vs. coordinated diaphragm breathing, an aggravating factor for scalene MTrPs)[80]

Treatment Options

Traditional treatment options[83] include:
- Weight loss, postural reeducation, shoulder muscle exercises
- Physical modalities for pain relief (heat, cold, electrical stimulation, ultrasound)
- Spinal manipulation
- Manual release and/or injection of scalene MTrPs
- Surgical removal of first rib
- Surgical removal of one of the scalene muscles

Similar to piriformis syndrome, it is reasonable to consider botulinum toxin treatment for thoracic outlet syndrome due to scalene muscle tension or enlargement caused by MTrPs. However, special precautions should be considered when injecting the scalene muscles because of the possibility of weakening accessory muscle(s) of respiration, the potential for pneumothorax, and the close proximity to vascular or nerve structures. For these reasons, special imaging techniques (CT, fluoroscopy, ultrasound) most likely are warranted.[11,12] Effective and safe injection of these muscles takes considerable skill and a thorough working knowledge of the anatomy of that region.

REPORTED EFFICACY FOR PAIN

Pain associated with spasticity was reported to respond to botulinum toxin type A injections in 21 of 27 patients in the studies cited in Table 21-1. Shoulder pain was reported by 6 patients.[3,69] Five patients reported wrist pain, and the remainder of patient injection sites were not specified.[3,69]

In 187 individuals with pain associated with cervical dystonia, most reported pain relief associated with reduction in dystonia,[26,30,46,62,85] although the percentage of patients with pain reduction was not specified in every study.

Not all studies reported positive results. Botulinum toxin was reported to be ineffective in pain attributed to fibromyalgia[68] and pain attributed to chronic pancreatitis.[73] In two cases, a syndrome resembling neuralgic amyotrophy (a painful condition associated with intense sharp or throbbing pain around the shoulder) was reported following botulinum toxin injections for writer's cramp.[72]

Perhaps the most compelling description of pain relief from botulinum toxin injections is seen in a report of 30 patients with the painful dystonia of Parkinson's disease known as "off painful dystonia" (OPD).[29,64] The authors hypothesized that pain of OPD was due to sustained muscle contraction, which is by definition a prolonged muscle spasm. In 30 cases of OPD treated with botulinum toxin, pain improved in all cases within 10 days, and in 21 cases, patients' pain completely abated for 4 months.

REMAINING QUESTIONS

Variables in studies previously discussed include the presence or absence of concurrent therapy, variable diagnoses, length of time since onset of pain, dosing and concentration, and outcome measurement. Further studies that control for each of these variables are needed to rigorously measure the putative analgesic effects of botulinum toxin in the treatment of muscular pain. For example, there is no clear indication in human spasticity research that injection localization of botulinum toxin is clinically important,[15] yet animal data show superior paralytic effects by injecting botulinum toxin at motor end-plate zones.[14,63,71] Future clinical trials might investigate similar responses in MTrP pain by relating the precision of end-plate zone and TrP location to the amount and concentration of neurotoxin injected. To be valid, such studies must assure accurate and complete localization of the end-plate zone.

CONCLUSION

An existing body of literature in related conditions of muscular hyperactivity provides a rationale for using botulinum toxin in painful muscular syndromes.[8,12,25,28,47,50,58] A rational basis has now been proposed for the injection of botulinum toxin to relieve myofascial pain that is caused by TrPs. Although there is evidence to suggest that botulinum toxin effectively reduces painful muscular contractions associated with a variety of neurologic disorders, further research is needed to define conditions in which injections might be most effective. Any of the readily available head, neck, and shoulder or lower extremity muscles could serve as targets for injection with botulinum toxin. However, a formidable problem in designing future prospective multicenter studies may be in finding clinicians who have developed the considerable skills required to accurately locate the TrPs by palpation (or by EMG guidance) and who can then inject exactly the spot that was localized. Unless there is another TrP mechanism that has not yet been identified, the results obtained injecting MTrPs with botulinum toxin may more accurately reflect the adequacy of the technique that was used rather than the effectiveness of the study medication. Research instruments that incorporate physical measures to quantify the effects of pain and meet criteria similar to self-reported pain scales and that are physiologically relevant should be applied to rigorously examine effects of botulinum toxin in the treatment of painful muscular conditions.

REFERENCES

1. Acquadro MA, Borodic GE: Treatment of myofascial pain with botulinum A toxin [letter]. Anesthesiology 80:705–706, 1994.
2. Beatty RA: The piriformis muscle syndrome: A simple diagnostic maneuver [see comments]. Neurosurgery 34:512–514, 1994.
3. Bhakta BB, Cozens JA, Bamford JM, et al: Use of botulinum toxin in stroke patients with severe upper limb spasticity. J Neurol Neurosurg Psychiatry 61:30–35, 1996.
4. Bogduk N, Simons DG: Neck pain: Joint pain or trigger points? In Vakakis N, Merveille O (eds): Progress in Fibromyalgia, 6th ed. Amsterdam, Elsevier, 1993, pp 267–273.
5. Brin MF, Fahn S, Moskowitz C, et al: Localized injections of botulinum toxin for the treatment of focal dystonia and hemifacial spasm. Adv Neurol 50:599–608, 1988.
6. Bruckle W, Suckfull M, Fleckenstein W, et al: [Tissue pO_2 measurement in taut back musculature (m. erector spinae)]. [German]. Z Rheumatol 49:208–216, 1990.
7. Cazzato G, Walton JN: The pathology of the muscle spindle. A study of biopsy material in various muscular and neuromuscular diseases. J Neurol Sci 7:15–70, 1968.
8. Cheshire WP, Abashian SW, Mann JD: Botulinum toxin in the treatment of myofascial pain syndrome [see comments]. Pain 59:65–69, 1994.

9. Chen WS: Sciatica due to piriformis pyomyositis. Report of a case. J Bone Joint Surg 74A:1546–1548, 1992.

10. Chen WS, Wan YL: Sciatica caused by piriformis muscle syndrome: Report of two cases. J Formos Med Assoc 91:647–650, 1992.

11. Childers MK: Rationale for injection procedures for botulinum toxin type A in skeletal limb muscles. Eur J Neurol 4(Suppl 2):37–40, 1997.

12. Childers MK: Use of Botulinum Toxin Type A in Pain Management. Columbia, MO, AIS, Inc., 1999.

13. Childers MK, Biswas SS, Petroski G, et al: Inhibitory casting decreases a vibratory inhibition index of the H-reflex in the spastic upper limb. Arch Phys Med Rehabil 80:714–716, 1999.

14. Childers MK, Kornegay JN, Aoki R, et al: Evaluating motor end-plate–targeted injections of botulinum toxin type A in a canine model. Muscle Nerve 21:653–655, 1998.

15. Childers MK, Stacy M, Cooke DL, et al: Comparison of two injection techniques using botulinum toxin in spastic hemiplegia. Am J Phys Med Rehabil 75:462–469, 1996.

16. Childers MK, Wilson DJ, Galate JF, et al: Treatment of painful muscle syndromes with botulinum toxin. J Back Musc Rehab 10:89–96, 1998.

17. Coffield JA, Considine RB, Simpson LL: The site and mechanism of action of botulinum neurotoxin. In Jankovic J, Hallett M (eds): Therapy with Botulinum Toxin. New York, Marcel Dekker, 1994, pp 3–14.

18. DeBassio WA, Schnitzler RM, Parsons RL: Influence of lanthanum on transmitter release at the neuromuscular junction. J Neurobiol 2:263–278, 1971.

19. de Paiva A, Meunier FA, Molgo J, et al: Functional repair of motor endplates after botulinum neurotoxin type A poisoning: Biphasic switch of synaptic activity between nerve sprouts and their parent terminals. Proc Natl Acad Sci U S A 96:3200–3205, 1999.

20. Dobrusin R: An osteopathic approach to conservative management of thoracic outlet syndromes. J Am Osteopath Assoc 89:1046–1050, 1989.

21. Dumitru D, King JC, McCarter RJ: Single muscle fiber discharge transformations: Fibrillation potential to positive sharp wave. Muscle Nerve 21:1759–1768, 1998.

22. Fishman LM, Zybert PA: Electrophysiologic evidence of piriformis syndrome. Arch Phys Med Rehabil 73:359–364, 1992.

23. Fricton JR: Myofascial pain syndrome. Neurol Clin 7:413–427, 1989.

24. Galate JF, Childers MK, Gnatz S: Effectiveness of botulinum toxin in refractory piriformis muscle syndrome [abstract]. Arch Phys Med Rehabil 78:1041, 1997.

25. Gandhavadi B: Bilateral piriformis syndrome associated with dystonia musculorum deformans. Orthopedics 13:350–351, 1990.

26. Gelb DJ, Lowenstein DH, Aminoff MJ: Controlled trial of botulinum toxin injections in the treatment of spasmodic torticollis [see comments]. Neurology 39:80–84, 1989.

27. Girdler NM: Uses of botulinum toxin [letter; comment]. Lancet 349:953, 1997.

28. Girdler NM: Use of botulinum toxin to alleviate facial pain [letter]. Br J Hosp Med 52:363, 1994.

29. Grazko MA, Polo KB, Jabbari B: Botulinum toxin A for spasticity, muscle spasms, and rigidity. Neurology 45:712–717, 1995.

30. Greene P, Kang U, Fahn S, et al: Double-blind, placebo-controlled trial of botulinum toxin injections for the treatment of spasmodic torticollis. Neurology 40:1213–1218, 1990.

31. Hallett M: One man's poison—clinical applications of botulinum toxin [editorial; comment]. N Engl J Med 341:118–120, 1999.

32. Hallin RP: Sciatic pain and the piriformis muscle. Postgrad Med 74:69–72, 1983.

33. Hesse S, Jahnke MT, Luecke D, et al: Short-term electrical stimulation enhances the effectiveness of botulinum toxin in the treatment of lower limb spasticity in hemiparetic patients. Neurosci Letters 201:37–40, 1995.

34. Heuser J, Miledi R: Effects of lanthanum ions on function and structure of frog neuromuscular junctions. Proc R Soc Lond B Biol Sci 179:247–260, 1971.

35. Hong CZ: Persistence of local twitch response with loss of conduction to and from the spinal cord. Arch Phys Med Rehabil 75:12–16, 1994.

36. Hong CZ, Simons DG: Histological findings of responsive loci in a myofascial trigger spot of rabbit skeletal muscle from where localized twitch responses could be elicited [abstract]. Arch Phys Med Rehabil 77:962, 1996.

37. Hong CZ, Simons DG: Pathophysiologic and electrophysiologic mechanisms of myofascial trigger points. Arch Phys Med Rehabil 79:863–872, 1998.

38. Hong CZ, Torigoe Y: Electrophysiological characteristics of localized twitch responses in responsive taut bands of rabbit skeletal muscle. J Musculoskel Pain 1:15–34, 1995.

39. Hong CZ, Torigoe Y: Electrophysiological characteristics of localized twitch responses in responsive taut bands of rabbit skeletal muscle. J Musculoskel Pain 2:17–43, 1994.

40. Hong CZ, Yu J: Spontaneous electrical activity of rabbit trigger spot after transection of spinal cord and peripheral nerve. J Musculoskel Pain 6:45–58, 1998.

41. Hubbard DR, Berkoff GM: Myofascial trigger points show spontaneous needle EMG activity. Spine 18:1803–1807, 1993.

42. Ito Y, Miledi R, Vincent A: Transmitter release induced by a "factor" in rabbit serum. Proc R Soc Lond B Biol Sci 187:235–241, 1974.

43. Jankiewicz JJ, Hennrikus WL, Houkom JA: The appearance of the piriformis muscle syndrome in computed tomography and magnetic resonance imaging. A case report and review of the literature. Clin Orthop Rel Res 262:205–209, 1991.

44. Jankovic J, Brin MF: Therapeutic uses of botulinum toxin. N Engl J Med 324:1186–1194, 1991.

45. Janssens LA: Trigger points in 48 dogs with myofascial pain syndromes [see comments]. Vet Surg 20:274–278, 1991.

46. Jedynak CP, de Saint Victor JF: [Treatment of spasmodic torticollis by local injections of botulinum toxin]. [French]. Rev Neurol (Paris) 146:440–443, 1990.

47. Johnstone SJ, Adler CH: Headache and facial pain responsive to botulinum toxin: An unusual presentation of blepharospasm. Headache 38:366–368, 1998.

48. Julsrud ME: Piriformis syndrome. J Am Podiatr Med Assoc 79:128–131, 1989.

49. Kao JT, Woolson ST: Piriformis tendon repair failure after total hip replacement. Orthop Rev 21:171–174, 1992.

50. Kaufman DM: Use of botulinum toxin injections for spasmodic torticollis of tardive dystonia. J Neuropsychiatry Clin Neurosci 6:50–53, 1994.

51. Kimura J: Electrodiagnosis in Diseases of Nerve and Muscle: Principles and Practice, 2nd ed. Philadelphia, F.A. Davis, 1989, p 631.

52. Kinahan AM, Douglas MJ: Piriformis pyomyositis mimicking epidural abscess in a parturient. Can J Anaesth 42:240–245, 1995.

53. Ku A, Kern H, Lachman E, et al: Sciatic nerve impingement from piriformis hematoma due to prolonged labor [letter]. Muscle Nerve 18:789–790, 1995.

54. LaBan MM, Meerschaert JR, Taylor RS: Electromyographic evidence of inferior gluteal nerve compromise: An early representation of recurrent colorectal carcinoma. Arch Phys Med Rehabil 63:33–35, 1982.

55. Liley AW: An investigation of spontaneous activity at the neuromuscular junction of the rat. J Physiol (London) 132:650–666, 1956.

56. Lu MY, Dong BJ, Ma XY: [Piriformis syndrome and its operative treatment: An analysis of sixty cases]. [Chinese]. Chung-Hua Wai Ko Tsa Chih 23:483–484, 510, 1985.

57. Mellanby J: Comparative activities of tetanus and botulinum toxins. Neuroscience 11:29–34, 1984.

58. Monsivais JJ, Monsivais DB: Botulinum toxin in painful syndromes. Hand Clin 12:787–789, 1996.

59. Moore AP, Wood GD: The medical management of masseteric hypertrophy with botulinum toxin type A. Br J Oral Maxillofac Surg 32:26–28, 1994.

60. National Institutes of Health: Consensus conference. Clinical use of botulinum toxin. Conn Med 55:471–477, 1991.

61. Noftal F: The piriformis syndrome. Can J Surg 31:210, 1988.

62. Odergren T, Tollback A, Borg J: Efficacy of botulinum toxin for cervical dystonia. A comparison of methods for evaluation. Scand J Rehabil Med 26:191–195, 1994.

63. Ottaviani L, Childers MK, Kornegay J: Identification of motor endplates in the dog to guide botulinum toxin injections [unpublished]. 1997.

64. Pacchetti C, Albani G, Martignoni E, et al: "Off" painful dystonia in Parkinson's disease treated with botulinum toxin. Mov Disord 10:333–336, 1995.

65. Pang D, Wessel HB: Thoracic outlet syndrome. Neurosurgery 22:105–121, 1988.

66. Papadopoulos SM, McGillicuddy JE, Albers JW: Unusual cause of "piriformis muscle syndrome." Arch Neurol 47:1144–1146, 1990.

67. Parziale JR, Hudgins TH, Fishman LM: The piriformis syndrome. Am J Orthop 25:819–823, 1996.

68. Paulson GW, Gill W: Botulinum toxin is unsatisfactory therapy for fibromyalgia. Mov Disord 11:459, 1996.

69. Pierson SH, Katz DI, Tarsy D: Botulinum toxin A in the treatment of spasticity: Functional implications and patient selection. Arch Phys Med Rehabil 77:717–721, 1996.

70. Sayson SC, Ducey JP, Maybrey JB, et al: Sciatic entrapment neuropathy associated with an anomalous piriformis muscle. Pain 59:149–152, 1994.

71. Shaari CM, Sanders I: Quantifying how location and dose of botulinum toxin injections affect muscle paralysis. Muscle Nerve 16:964–969, 1993.

72. Sheean GL, Murray NM, Marsden CD: Pain and remote weakness in limbs injected with botulinum toxin A for writer's cramp. Lancet 346:154–156, 1995.

73. Sherman S, Kopecky KK, Brashear A, et al: Percutaneous celiac plexus block with botulinum toxin A did not help the pain of chronic pancreatitis. J Clin Gastroenterol 20:343–344, 1995.

74. Simons DG: Myofascial pain syndrome: One term but two concepts: A new understanding [editorial]. J Musculoskel Pain 3:7–13, 1995.

75. Simons DG, Hong CZ, Simons LS: Nature of myofascial trigger points, active loci [abstract]. J Musculoskel Pain 3(Suppl 1):62, 1995.

76. Simons DG, Stolov WC: Microscopic features and transient contraction of palpable bands in canine muscle. Am J Phys Med 55:65–88, 1976.

77. Simons DG, Travell JG: Myofascial origins of low back pain. 1. Principles of diagnosis and treatment. Postgrad Med 73:66–70, 1983.

78. Simons DG, Travell JG: Myofascial origins of low back pain. 2. Torso muscles. Postgrad Med 73:81–92, 1983.

79. Simons DG, Travell JG: Myofascial origins of low back pain. 3. Pelvic and lower extremity muscles. Postgrad Med 73:99–105, 1983.

80. Simons DG, Travell JG, Simons LS: Travell & Simons' Myofascial Pain and Dysfunction: The Trigger Point Manual, 2nd ed. Baltimore, Williams & Wilkins, 1999.

81. Solheim LF, Siewers P, Paus B: The piriformis muscle syndrome. Sciatic nerve entrapment treated with section of the piriformis muscle. Acta Orthop Scand 52:73–75, 1981.

82. Steiner C, Staubs C, Ganon M, et al: Piriformis syndrome: Pathogenesis, diagnosis, and treatment. J Am Osteopath Assoc 87:318–323, 1987.

83. Sucher BM: Thoracic outlet syndrome—a myofascial variant: Part 2. Treatment. J Am Osteopath Assoc 90:810–812, 1990.

84. Therapeutics and Technology Assessment Subcommittee of the American Academy of Neurology: Training guidelines for the use of botulinum toxin for the treatment of neurologic disorders. Report of the Therapeutics and Technology Assessment Subcommittee of the American Academy of Neurology. Neurology 44:2401–2403, 1994.

85. Tsui JK, Fross RD, Calne S, et al: Local treatment of spasmodic torticollis with botulinum toxin. Can J Neurol Sci 14:533–535, 1987.

86. Urschel HCJ: Management of the thoracic-outlet syndrome. N Engl J Med 286:1140–1143, 1972.

87. Wheeler AH: Botulinum toxin A, adjunctive therapy for refractory headaches associated with pericranial muscle tension. Headache 38:468–471, 1998.

88. Wheeler AH, Goolkasian P, Gretz SS: A randomized, double-blind, prospective pilot study of botulinum toxin injection for refractory, unilateral, cervicothoracic, paraspinal, myofascial pain syndrome. Spine 23:1662–1666, 1998.

89. Wiederholt WC: "End-plate noise" in electromyography. Neurology 20:214–224, 1970.

90. Windisch A, Reitinger A, Traxler H, et al: Morphology and histochemistry of myogelosis. Clin Anat 12:266–271, 1999.

22

Botulinum Toxin Injections for Neurologic Conditions

Robert G. Schwartz, M.D.

The popularity of botulinum toxin injections has evolved partly due to botulinum's unique properties as well as its proven efficacy, especially in difficult medical conditions involving neuromuscular abnormalities. This chapter discusses the properties of botulinum, its mechanisms of action, and clinical uses. A comparison of botulinum injections to traditional phenol motor point blocks is also provided, along with a description of the actual technique of botulinum toxin injections.

Botulinum, a toxin produced by *Clostridium botulinum*, an anaerobic organism responsible for food poisoning (botulism), was first discovered in 1897. Since that time, seven immunologically distinct toxins have been identified (types A–G). Only types A, B, and E have been linked to cases of botulism in humans, and an antitoxin is available for each of these types. In the United States, type A is found primarily west of the Mississippi River; type B, east of the Mississippi River; and type E is usually found in shellfish. Types C, D, F, and G are less prevalent.

PROPERTIES OF BOTULINUM TOXIN TYPE A

Botulinum toxin type A (botulinum toxin) is one of the most lethal biologic toxins. Its neurotoxic component has a molecular weight of 150,000. However, the toxin forms a complex with nontoxic proteins and hemagglutinin, creating a much larger molecule.

Cultures of *Clostridium botulinum* are established in a fermenter, grown and harvested by acidification and centrifugation, and further purified and processed for commercial use. Currently, in the United States, botulinum toxin type A is marketed by Allergan Pharmaceuticals in a freeze-dried form known as Botox. Dissolved in normal saline, Botox is clear and odorless. It is harvested from broth culture

and purified and microfiltered, resulting in a crystallized toxin that is complexed with nontoxic proteins.[6,12,18,26]

Botulinum toxin for clinical use is supplied in a highly purified freeze-dried and lyophilized state. It must be stored at $-5°C$ and diluted with normal cellulin without preservative before its use. Once reconstituted, it remains effective for about 4 hours at room temperature. Studies are in progress to determine whether reconstituted toxin may be refrozen for later use. It is an expensive agent (about \$285 a vial, and two vials are needed for standard treatment of torticollis), and the ability to save unused reconstituted toxin for future use would result in significant cost savings.

The standard method of measuring the potency of commercially available toxin in the United States is derived from a mouse assay. In this assay, one unit of botulinum toxin (mouse unit) is the amount that kills 50% of a 18–20 female Swiss-Webster mice (average weight, 400 gm) (lethal dose [LD_{50}]). The toxin available in the United Kingdom (Dysport) is much more potent than what is available in the United States. One nanogram of the British toxin contains 40 mouse units, whereas 1 nanogram of the American toxin contains 2.5 mouse units. The lethal dose for humans, projected from primate experiments, is approximately 2700 mouse units.

The dosages used in human therapeutic applications are roughly proportional to the mass of the muscle being injected and are much lower than the estimated LD_{50}. Clinical resistance to the effect of subsequent injections of botulinum toxin has been demonstrated in some patients after repeat treatment. This resistance also has been correlated with the presence of antibodies to botulinum toxin detected with bioassays. A cumbersome in vivo mouse neutralization assay has been used to detect serum antibodies to botulinum toxin. The presence of neutralizing (blocking) antibodies is suggested if the mice remain healthy after the injection of both serum and botulinum toxin. When unprotected mice die, a negative assay results. Enzyme-linked immunosorbent assays for the detection of antibodies have been developed, but the specificity and clinical correlation with resistance to treatment of botulinum toxin have not been demonstrated.[22]

In human studies of adult patients injected with 250–400 units of toxin, no systemic side effects have been reported. Single doses of greater than 500 units have produced mild, transient systemic symptoms. No cumulative effects of repeated botulinum injections have been noted locally or in distant muscles. Motor function and electromyographic measurements returned to preinjection levels 12–24 weeks after injection. No evidence seems to suggest chronic denervation following repeat Botox injections. After Botox has altered the neuromuscular junctions, sprouting of the motor axons occurs, reinnervating the muscle fiber. Clinically significant muscular weakness is noted 1–3 days after intramuscular botulinum injections. The localized weakness usually lasts 6–28 weeks and varies with the site of botulinum toxin injection. Terminal neural axon sprouting occurs with reinnervation of the muscle fibers and return of muscular contractions in 6–12 weeks. It is believed that botulinum toxin does not cross the normal blood-brain barrier. Radionuclide labeling has shown that toxin diffuses approximately 4 cm per injection site. The advantage of such a large diffusion area is that the medication does not have to be placed exactly at the neuromuscular junction. Electromyographic guidance is preferred in order to ascertain that the proper muscle is being injected. However, crisp, clean motor units generated by this muscle demonstrate that needle placement is close enough to obtain the desired effect. As a result of this feature, the desired neurolytic effect can be achieved much more rapidly than with the use of other materials such as phenol or alcohol.

MECHANISM OF ACTION

Botulinum toxin exerts its paralytic action by rapidly and strongly binding to presynaptic cholinergic nerve terminals. It becomes internalized and ultimately inhibits the exocytosis of the acetylcholine by decreasing the frequency of acetylcholine release (Figs. 22-1 and 22-2). The treatment of muscle with botulinum toxin results in an accelerated loss of junctional acetylcholine receptors. The speed of axon destruction depends on the volume of toxin exposure, but generally occurs within 72 hours. This results in a blockade of neural transmission at the motor end plate, caused by inhibition of acetylcholine release from nerve endings and by interference of the uptake of cytoplasmic acetylcholine. A reduction in miniature end-plate potentials occurs within a few hours after the injection of botulinum toxin. The muscle becomes functionally denervated, atrophies, and develops extrajunctional acetylcholine receptors. The effects of botulinum injection are not immediate but depend on the supply of acetylcholine from the presynaptic nerve terminal being exhausted via spontaneous release of acetylcholine. Within 2 days

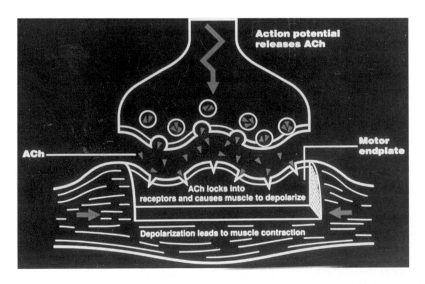

FIGURE 22-1.   Normal neuromuscular transmission. (Courtesy of Allergan, Inc., Irvine, CA.)

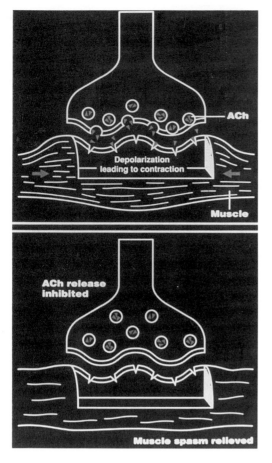

FIGURE 22-2. Action of Botox on the neuromuscular junction. Botox inhibits the release of acetylcholine (ACh) from nerve endings and interferes with the uptake of cytoplasmic ACh. (Courtesy of Allergan, Inc., Irvine, CA.)

after muscle exposure to the toxin, the axon terminal begins to sprout, and the proliferating branches form contacts on the adjacent muscle fibers.

Although it is likely that the clinical effect of botulinum toxin primarily is due to its action at the neuromuscular junction, the toxin can enter into the central nervous system after peripheral administration. It is believed to be transported to the spinal cord by retrograde axonal transport and later can be detected in the appropriate segment of the spinal cord. Intraspinal transfers evidenced by the subsequent appearance of botulinum toxin in the contralateral half segment are believed to occur. In the cord, the toxin appears to block recurrent inhibition mediated by the Renshaw cells.

Other data confirm distant effects of botulinum toxin on neuromuscular transmission and autonomic function. Botulinum toxin injection was found to induce and increase the mean jitter values above normal limits in patients who underwent two sessions of treatment. The onset of these changes has been reported by Garner et al. to occur 3–13 days after injection.[14] In the second session, the dosage of botulinum injection was doubled from that of the usual dosage. An increase of fiber density was recorded on single fiber studies 6 weeks after the treatment. In addition, cardiovascular reflexes showed mild abnormalities in 4 of 5 patients, although they remained asymptomatic. However, in one individual, borderline postural hypotension was indicated by a fall of 20 mmHg in systolic blood pressure during standing. In the autonomic nervous system, botulinum toxin blocks ganglionic nerve endings, preganglionic sympathetic nerve endings, and postganglionic sympathetic nerve endings in which acetylcholine has been transmitted. A partial antagonistic action and motor response has also been demonstrated in some adrenergic and nonadrenergic atropine-resistant autonomic neuromuscular sites. The effect of botulinum toxin on distant sites is dose-dependent. An additional mechanism of spread to distant sites is presumed to be vascular after local administration.[14,16]

BOTULINUM INJECTIONS VERSUS PHENOL MOTOR POINT BLOCKS

When phenol motor point blocks are used to control a spastic muscle, an electrical stimulator is used as a constant current generator, working at a frequency of approximately 2 pulses per second (see chapter 4). The intensity of current is set at approximately 1 mA, and the duration is varied from 0.1–0.2 ms. Typically, a 5% aqueous phenol solution is injected. However, 2% and 3% solutions also have been advocated. In most centers, it is easy to obtain phenol in its clinically useful form.[4,13,25] The amount of phenol solution required for an effective motor point block ranges from 0.5–5 ml per site. Typically, one to three sites per muscle group are injected.

With phenol blocks, a direct current stimulator and a 22-gauge, 2- or 3-inch insulated spinal needle are used to accurately locate the nerve fiber neuromuscular junction. The technique used with a phenol motor point block causes it to become a time-consuming and often painful procedure. Precise localization of motor points with a surface stimulator is commonly performed but is often difficult. Also, because of the cost of phenol, judicious selection of injection sites is important. Because of practicalities involving this procedure, its frequency of use has diminished in the clinical setting.

Botulinum toxin injections have been received favorably by physicians over phenol motor point blocks. The procedure can be carried out with a typical electromyography machine and does not require exact needle placement in the neuromuscular junction. In fact, rather than targeting the nerve in the neuromuscular junction, as with phenol motor point blocks, botulinum injection is directed toward the muscle belly as the target itself.

As in the case of phenol motor point blocks, the Teflon-coated monopolar cannula is used for botulinum injection. A surface electrode is sufficient for a reference and ground. With botulinum toxin, depending on the site that is to be injected, the size of the cannula varies. In small ocular muscles, a 25-gauge, 1-inch cannula is used; for larger muscles such as the trapezius, a 26-gauge, 1- or 1½-inch cannula is used.

Although patients may complain of pain after botulinum injection—as they do with phenol—the amount of pain experienced with botulinum injection is no different than that from standard electromyographic examinations.

CLINICAL USES

Botulinum toxin has been found to have value in the treatment of various neurologic and ophthalmologic disorders. It is approved by the Food and Drug Administration (FDA) as a therapeutic agent in patients with strabismus, blepharospasm, hemifacial spasm, and other facial nerve disorders. It has been endorsed by the National Institutes of Health, American Academy of Neurology, and American Medical Association's Department of Drug Divisions in Toxicology for peripheral and central nervous system disorders where hypertonic spastic conditions exist (Fig. 22-3).[23]

SPECIFIC INDICATIONS

Extraocular Disorders

Botulinum toxin was first used to weaken extraocular muscles. The toxin was later introduced for the treatment of strabismus as an alternative to conventional incisional surgery. Follow-up studies up to 5 years after the injection revealed that 85% of the patients available for reassessment had satisfactory improvement of their condition. Side effects, including presbyopia and secondary vertical deviations, are usually transient and do not result in concomitant amblyopia. Strabismus, lateral rectus palsy, and nystagmus have all been treated with botulinum toxin injections.

Dysphonia

The American Academy of Otolaryngology-Head and Neck Surgery has made a statement of the clinical usefulness of botulinum toxin for the treatment of spasmodic dysphonia. In this condition, patients present with a choked and constrained voice pattern with a break in vocalization. The original dystonia has been characterized as a slowly developing voice disorder with increasing vocal fatigue, spastic constriction of the throat muscles, and pain around the larynx. Patients sound as if they are trying to talk while being choked. The voice strain and voice arrest are believed to derive from hyperadduction of the true and false vocal cords; however, 10% of patients will present with the abductor form. In this form of phonation, the cord will have spasmodic motion of the posterior cricoarytenoid muscles as well as several other of the original muscles.

Botulinum injection also represents an alternative to recurrent laryngeal nerve resection when return of dysphonia from continued vocal cord paralysis occurs despite previous nerve resection.

Facial Disorders

Other disorders that have been treated in the cranial region with botulinum toxin include oral mandibular dystonia, Meige's syndrome, and hemifacial spasm. These conditions involve various muscles in the face, either alone or in association with ocular findings.

In the treatment of blepharospasm (Fig. 22-4), hemifacial spasm, Meige's syndrome and the oral mandibular dystonias, various studies have documented relief of spasm ranging from 85–94%. The duration of a spasm-free interval as well as the incidence of ptosis, diplopia, or facial weakness is dose-dependent. When an additional 20–25 units are injected into each muscle, there is a marked increase in the incidence of side effects but only a small increase in the duration of spasm-free intervals. Spasm-free intervals range from 3–5 months, and the effect is reproducible with reinjection. For patients with oral mandibular findings alone, the success rate has been lower (47%); however, this technique remains the best treatment for this condition. Generally, spasms diminish only as long as the muscles are clinically weak, because uninjected muscles remain strong and exhibit spasms.[2,5,15,20,24,29]

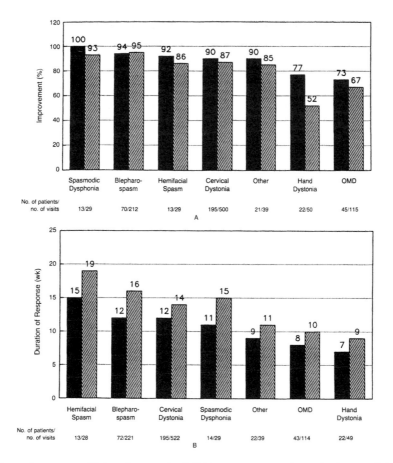

FIGURE 22-3.   Effects of treatment with botulinum toxin. Solid bars represent patients who improved; hatched bars represent percentage of treatment sessions at which improvement was made. (From Jankovic J, Brin MF: Therapeutic uses of botulinum toxin. N Engl J Med 324:1192, 1991, with permission.)

Cervical Dystonia

Botulinum injection is frequently used in patients with cervical dystonia (spasmodic torticollis). In this condition, the involved neck muscles cause a pattern of repetitive, clonic (spasmodic), and tonic (sustained) head movement. Abnormal posture of the head as a result of twisting (torticollis), tilting one's shoulder (lateral collis), flexing (anterocollis), or extending (retrocollis) the neck is usually present (Table 22-1). The majority of patients with cervical dystonia have a combination of these abnormal postures. Approximately one-third of patients with cervical dystonia have involvement of a contiguous body part, such as the oral mandibular region, shoulder, and arm.

The efficacy and safety of botulinum toxin in the treatment of cervical dystonia have been demonstrated in several controlled and open studies. A total of 61–92% of patients have reported improvement after the injection of botulinum toxin.

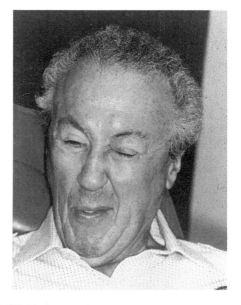

FIGURE 22-4.   Blepharospasm involving lower facial and neck contractions. (Courtesy of David R. Jordan, M.D., Ottawa, Ontario, Canada.)

TABLE 22-1. Muscles Involved in Cervical Dystonia*

Torticollis	Ipsilateral splenius, contralateral SCM
Head tilt	Ipsilateral SCM, splenius capitis, scalene complex, levator scapulae, posterior vertebrals
Shoulder elevation	Ipsilateral trapezius and levator scapulae
Retrocollis	Splenius capitis, upper trapezius, deep postvertebrals
Anterocollis	SCM, both sets scalene, submental muscles, longus capitis, longus colli

* Special thanks to Mitchell F. Brin, M.D., and Judith Blazer at WE MOVE (Worldwide Education and Awareness for Movement Disorders) for providing this information.

Furthermore, 93% had marked relief of neck pain. The average length between the injection and onset of improvement (and muscle atrophy) was 1 week, and the average duration of maximal improvement was $3\frac{1}{2}$ months. The total duration of improvement, however, was about 6 weeks longer. Most patients required injection every 3 months. Some patients received benefit for only weeks and others for as many as 4–5 months.

Complications with injections for cervical dystonia include dysphagia, neck weakness, nausea, generalized malaise, and pain. The pain is the most frequent side effect secondary to the local injection. The pain is more severe in individuals in whom botulinum toxin is injected directly into or around a peripheral nerve.

The use of electromyographic assistance during the injections has minimized the likelihood of these side effects (with the exception of weakness). At least one study also has demonstrated that a lower total dosage of botulinum toxin is required and a better clinical effect occurs as a result of an improved ability to effectively identify and treat the deep muscles electromyographically.[10]

Abnormal excessive weakness following injection begins to occur within 3 days. Patients usually report immediate change in strength as well as dystonia after injection. Usually, weakness is maximal 2–3 weeks after injection. Appropriate supportive measures are required for the muscle groups that become weak. Cervical collars are frequently used when the neck musculature is involved, and minor changes in daily diet to prevent aspiration may be required if too high a dosage of toxin is injected in the area of the anterior strap muscles. Typically, these side effects are temporary and resolve over a period of weeks, leaving the desired clinical effect to last for months.[11,20,23]

Focal Dystonias

One of the most rewarding changes associated with botulinum injections can be observed when treating focal dystonias. Focal dystonias, either fixed or task-specific, are often disabling and usually unresponsive to medical therapy. Several groups have noted the efficacy of botulinum toxin in the treatment of occupational cramps and limited task-specific dystonias. Affected muscles are identified clinically and by recording with electromyography (EMG) from needle electrodes at rest and during performance of tasks that precipitate these abnormal postures. Subjective improvement lasting for 1–4 months has been reported in 82% of patients. The major side effect is transient focal weakness; it has been noted in 53% of patients injected with the toxin.

Writer's cramp is the most common form of focal dystonia in the general population and frequently involves the flexor pollicis longus, flexor digitorum profundus, extensor indicis, extensor hallucis longus, extensor carpi ulnaris, and flexor carpi radialis muscles. The first dorsal interosseous and abductor digiti minimi are other muscles that are frequently involved (Fig. 22-5).

Focal dystonia of the limbs has been reported in reflex sympathetic dystrophy, in musicians with movement disorders, and in overuse syndromes. Equinovarus changes in the foot and involvement in other distal lower extremity muscles also may present as focal dystonias.[7,8,27,30,33,34]

Tremors

Another indication for botulinum toxin injections is tremors (Fig. 22-6). In a study in which 51 treatments were given to patients with disabling tremors classified as dystonic, essential, a combination of dystonic and essential, parkinsonian, peripherally induced, and midbrain, 67% of patients improved with the injection of botulinum. EMG recordings showed decreased amplitude of motor units after treatment with botulinum toxin. The most common side effects were weakness and dysphagia.[22]

Additional Uses

Additional indications for botulinum injections include stroke-related hemiplegia, spinal cord injury, multiple sclerosis, cerebral palsy, and detrusor sphincter dyssynergia. In contrast to focal and segmental dystonias, which are usually idiopathic,

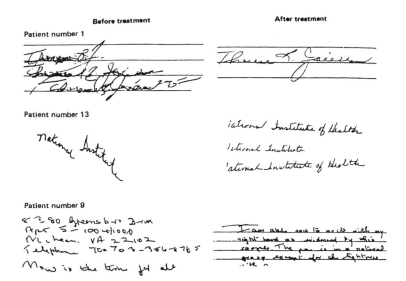

FIGURE 22-5. Handwriting before and after treatment with botulinum toxin injections for dystonic writer's cramp in three patients. (From Cohen L: Treatment of focal dystonias of the hand with botulinum toxin injection. Neurol Neurosurg Psychiatry 52:360, 1989, with permission.)

the majority of patients with hemidystonia have an identifiable etiology such as head trauma, stroke, arteriovenous malformation, tumor, encephalitis, or other pathology affecting the contralateral basal ganglia.[1,3,28,32]

New uses of botulinum toxin injections include the treatment of painful conditions that result from prolonged muscle spasm and contractures. Other indications are chronic pain, especially in the postoperative back, and myofascial pain. Thoracic outlet syndrome associated with spasm of the scalene musculature can be relieved with botulinum injection, which results in significant improvement in peripheral blood flow. Botulinum toxin should be used as a last resort in these patients and requires careful patient selection.[19]

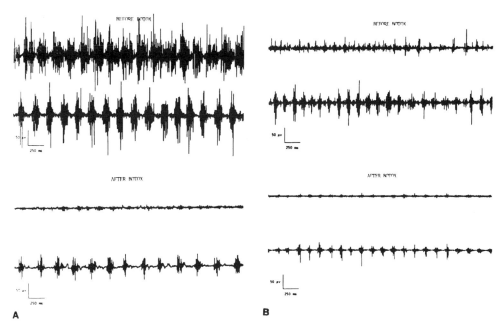

FIGURE 22-6. Reduction in tremor amplitude after Botox injections into (A) forearm muscles in a patient with postural hand tremor and (B) splenius capitis muscles in a patient with lateral head oscillation. (From Jankovic J, Schwartz K: Botulinum toxin treatment of tremors. Neurology 41:1187, 1991, with permission.)

Botulinum toxin has been used in children even though the FDA's statement of efficacy applies to individuals no younger than 12 years. Abnormal tone as a result of cerebral palsy is the most common condition treated. A generalized form of dystonia can occur with childhood onset, as in dystonia musculorum deformans, which also may be treated with botulinum injections.[3,9,17,21,28]

CONTRAINDICATIONS

Botulinum toxin injection is contraindicated in patients receiving aminoglycoside or spectinomycin antibiotics or with known sensitivity to botulinum, myasthenic syndrome, myasthenia gravis, motor neuron disease, upper eyelid apraxia, and ptosis. A paucity of data exists regarding the use of botulinum toxin during pregnancy.[1] In one report of 9 patients treated during pregnancy (dose unspecified), 1 gave birth prematurely, but this complication was not thought to be related to the botulinum.

PROCEDURAL DETAILS

Prior to injection with botulinum toxin, patients should be notified of all potential complications. Although these complications may not occur, it is always best to cover every potential side effect that could occur, especially weakness. Many clinicians find it useful to photograph or videotape patients before, during, and after treatment with botulinum toxin in order to have a pictorial history of improved function as a result of the treatment. It is also helpful for patients to evaluate their pre- and post-treatment outcomes. Most patients who receive botulinum injections are told beforehand that outcomes are variable. On a statistical basis, an average of 85% of individuals are pleased with the results. As long as patients are notified of potential weakness prior to the injection, they are not particularly disturbed if weakness occurs. Most patients are appreciative of any benefit that results from the botulinum injection therapy. The only true concern becomes how long the effect will last.

While superficial muscles are accessible for injection with a tuberculosis syringe with a 25-gauge, 5/8-inch needle, most practitioners prefer to inject with a monopolar Teflon-coated cannula and identify the muscle electromyographically prior to injection. With standard reference and ground electrodes, the clinician can use electrodiagnostic equipment that is readily available on the market today. For the smaller facial muscles, a 30-gauge, 1-inch cannula is preferred; for larger muscles, a 26-gauge, 1½-inch cannula is used. All injections are intramuscular. If alcohol is used to cleanse the skin, it should be allowed to dry because it can deactivate the toxin.

Once the needle is inserted into the muscle, the practitioner looks for the classic dystonic firing of the muscle group involved on EMG. In cases of spastic dystonia associated with hemiplegia or other central nervous system pathology, excessive firing of motor unit action potentials helps to identify the muscle groups involved.

Exact dosages of botulinum toxin for specific diagnoses have not been well established, but general guidelines do exist. It is preferable to underdose an individual with botulinum toxin during the first treatment and repeat the treatment within 30 days should the desired effect not occur. The dosage may be increased proportionally until the desired clinical effect is obtained.

In the eye, 25 units injected into the orbicularis oculi and corrugator muscles is an appropriate starting point. This may be increased up to 75 units per eye, as required, in order to achieve the desired clinical effect. It may take two or three office visits to achieve this effect. A dilution of 5.0 units per 0.1 ml is preferred. To achieve this dose, 2 ml of preservative-free saline is injected into the 100-unit vial of botulinum. Complications with these ocular injections may include tearing, irritation, paralysis, eye opening, and ptosis.

For hemifacial spasms, a 30-gauge needle is used. However, 4 ml of preservative-free saline is added to the 100-unit vial of botulinum to achieve a concentration of 2.5 units per 0.1 ml. Facial weakness can occur with just a few more units over the therapeutic dose, which may be as little as 20 or 25 units. As with all botulinum toxin injections, titrate upward until the clinical effect is achieved is advised.

When larger muscles are to be injected, as in cervical dystonia (spasmodic torticollis), a 26-gauge, 1½-inch cannula is used and 2 ml of preservative-free saline is added to a 100-unit vial of botulinum to achieve a 5-unit per 0.1 ml concentration. These muscles typically require a minimum of 35–40 units and as much as 300 units in order to achieve the desired effect. It is not uncommon to use 50–75 units per muscle to achieve a therapeutic response; however, this depends entirely on the patient (Table 22-2). Typically, 200 units per session is the starting therapeutic dose. If the desired effect is not achieved, an additional 100 units is given in 30 days. The FDA does not approve the use of more than 300 units

TABLE 22-2. Common Doses of Botox When Injected into Neck Muscles for Cervical Dystonia*

Muscle	Units (U)	Range (U)
SCM	50	15–75
Trapezius	75	50–100
Splenius capitis	75	50–150
Levator scapulae	50	25–100
Semispinalis capitis	75	50–150
Longissimus capitis	75	50–150

SCM = sternocleidomastoid
* Special thanks to Mitchell F. Brin, M.D., and Judith Blazer at WE MOVE (Worldwide Education and Awareness for Movement Disorders) for providing this information.

per month. However, 500 units have been given in the clinical setting without ill effect in individual cases.

Important cervical structures to avoid during botulinum injection into the cervical muscles include the brachial plexus, carotid sheath, and greater occipital nerve. The pharynx, esophagus, pleura and apex of the lung also should be avoided. Depending on the site that is being injected, knowledge of regional anatomy that may be affected by such needle placement should be carefully considered.[15,19,20,31]

If individual muscles are being treated that have spastic dystonia, 200 units per muscle may be required to achieve a therapeutic response. It would not be uncommon to begin at 100 units, for example, with the gastrocnemius soleus muscle and increase the dose as needed. In cases of generalized spasticity, it becomes clear that treatment with botulinum toxin injection is difficult, if not impossible. If, however, focal muscle groups can be identified as the primary generator of a diffuse spastic reaction or for cases in which individual muscle groups are explicitly involved in function and hygiene, botulinum injections may be helpful.

Treatments are repeated as necessary and should be individualized among patients. Usually 3 months of clinical benefit can be expected from the botulinum toxin. The duration of benefit is variable, lasting only weeks in some individuals and as long as 5 or 6 months in others. Periodic assessment of function and response should be done for each patient as medically necessary.

It is essential that patients be as relaxed as possible for their injections. This requires proper positioning so that the practitioner can be certain that the muscles that are contracting are not doing so in a normal postural response to their current positioning. This is especially true if one is having difficulty

obtaining the classic burst of rhythmic firing pattern seen with dystonia. If individuals do not demonstrate dystonic firing of individual muscles during needle placement, tricks that initiate their dystonia may be sought. Patients frequently can diminish their dystonia through tricks, but they also can initiate dystonia through different body movements or postures. This procedure is always patient-specific and requires explicit knowledge of the patient and his or her particular characteristics.

The presence of family members is not required during the procedure. However, many patients feel more comfortable knowing that someone will drive them home, especially if it is a patient's first botulinum injection.

In patients who have taken nonsteroidal drugs or are taking anticoagulants, the possibility of increased bruising at the injection site should be considered but is not a contraindication to the procedure. It is quite helpful to needle muscles that are not obviously involved from the clinical examination alone. Frequently, the muscles will be firing in a dystonic fashion and should be injected. Although some individuals achieve an excellent response when the entire dosage is injected at one site, spreading the dosage among three sites is widely believed to provide a more effective response.

Due to the high cost of the medication, it is useful to schedule more than one patient at a time for botulinum injections. Any medication left over from one patient can be given to the next. Once the medication has been prepared, it must be used within 4 hours. The vial should not be agitated, and the vacuum-sealed valve should draw the preservative-free saline into it from the prefilled syringe. If this does not occur, the vial should be returned to the manufacturer and not used.

POSTPROCEDURE CARE

Muscle relaxants or acetaminophen may be given to patients after treatment if any discomfort occurs over the ensuing 24–48 hours. Patients rarely require stronger analgesics.

A follow-up appointment in 2–3 weeks after the first time that an individual receives botulinum injection therapy is quite helpful to determine if an adequate dosage was given. A telephone call to the patient 3–4 days after the injection also will help determine if the desired response is likely to occur or if there are adverse side effects as a result of the injection. This approach also results in patient reassurance, which is usually appreciated.

CONCLUSION

Botulinum injection therapy offers the clinician a powerful tool in the treatment of individuals with movement disorders and painful conditions associated with dystonia and hyperactive muscle tone. These injections can dramatically improve patient function and enhance the rehabilitation program for individuals with disabling impairments. When the injections are properly used, the side effects can be minimized and the desired effect achieved in a most gratifying manner for both patient and practitioner.

REFERENCES

1. American Academy of Neurology: Assessment: The clinical usefulness of botulinum toxin A in treating neurologic disorders. Report of the Therapeutics and Technology Assessment Subcommittee. Neurology 40:1332–1336, 1990.
2. American Academy of Otolaryngology–Head and Neck Surgery: Physician's Statement on the Clinical Usefulness of Botulinum Toxin and Treatment of Monosphonia. Alexandria, VA, AAOHN, 1990.
3. American Medical Association Drug Evaluations and Subscription, Vol. 3. Chicago, AMA, 1990.
4. Awad E: Phenol block for control of hip flexor and adductors spasticity. Arch Phys Med Rehabil 53:554–557, 1972.
5. Blitzer A: Botulinum toxin injection for the treatment of oral mandibular dystonia. Rhinolaryngology 98:93–97, 1989.
6. Chesleff S: Motive action of botulinum toxin and the effect of drug antagonist. Adv Psychopharmacol 3:35–43, 1979.
7. Cohen L: Treatment of focal dystonias of the hand with botulinum toxin injection. J Neurol Neurosurg Psychiatry 52:355–363, 1989.
8. Cole RA, Cohen LG, Hallett M: Treatment of musician's cramp with botulinum toxin. Med Probl Perform Art 6:137–143, 1991.
9. Cooper IS, Riklan RM: Dystonia musculorum deformans. Arch Phys Med Rehabil 43:607, 1962.
10. Comella C, Buchman AS, Tanner CM, et al: Botulinum toxin injection for spasmodic torticollis: Increased magnitude of benefit with electromyographic assistance. Neurology 42:878–882, 1992.
11. Comella C, Tanner CM, DeFoor-Hill L, Smith C: Dysphagia after botulinum toxin injections for spasmodic torticollis: Clinical and radiologic findings. Neurology 42:1307–1310, 1992.
12. Drachman DB: Effect of botulinum toxin on speed of skeletal muscle contraction. Am J Physiol 216:1453–1455, 1982.
13. Felsenthal G: Pharmacology of phenol in peripheral nerve blocks: A review. Arch Phys Med Rehabil 55:1, 1974.
14. Garner CG: Time course of distant effects of local injection of botulinum toxin. Mov Disord 8:33–37, 1993.
15. Geller B: Botulinum toxin therapy in hemifacial spasms: Clinical and electrophysiologic studies. Muscle Nerve 12:716–722, 1989.
16. Girlamda P: Botulinum toxin therapy: Effects of neuromuscular transmission and autonomic nervous systems. J Neurol Neurosurg Psychiatry 55:844–845, 1992.
17. Gormley M: Botulinum toxin disease in children. Presented at the 55th Annual Meeting of the American Academy of Physical Medicine and Rehabilitation, Miami, October 31–November 4, 1993.
18. Holland R: Nerve growth in botulinum toxin poisoned muscles. Neuroscience 6:1167–1179, 1981.
19. Hughes HF: Botulinum toxin in the treatment of posttraumatic thoracic outlet syndrome [poster]. Annual Meeting of the American Academy of Electrodiagnostic Medicine, Ralston, SC, October 1992.
20. Jankovic J: Botulinum toxin for cranial cervical dystonia. Neurology 37:616–663, 1989.
21. Jankovic J: Botulinum toxin therapy for focal dystonia. Med Probl Perform Art 6:122–124, 1991.
22. Jankovic J: Botulinum toxic treatment of tremors. Neurology 41:1185–1188, 1991.
23. Jankovic J: Therapeutic uses of botulinum toxin. N Engl J Med 324:1186–1194, 1991.
24. Jordan DR, Anderson RL: Essential Blepharospasm: Focal Points 1988: Clinical Modules for Ophthalmologists. Vol. 6, Module 6, 1988.
25. Khalili AA, Betts HB: Peripheral nerve block with phenol in the management of spasticity. JAMA 200:1155–1157, 1967.
26. Lange DJ: Distant effects of local injection of botulinum toxin. Muscle Nerve 10:552–555, 1987.
27. Lockwood E: Reflex sympathetic dystrophy after overuse: The possible relationship with focal dystonia. Med Probl Perform Art 4:114–117, 1989.
28. National Institutes of Health: Botulinum Toxin. Consens Statement 8(8):1–20, 1990.
29. Ophthalmic Procedures Assessment Committee of the American Academy of Ophthalmology: Botulinum Toxin Therapy of Eye Muscle Disorders: Safety and Effectiveness. San Francisco, American Academy of Ophthalmology, 1989.
30. Rivest J, Lees AJ, Marsden CJ: Writer's cramp: Treatment with botulinum toxin injections. Mov Disord 6:55–59, 1991.
31. Rivner M: Botulinum injection in training sessions [course materials]. Department of Neurology, Medical College of Georgia, Augusta, GA.
32. Rome S: Use of botulinum toxin in the treatment of spasticity in large muscles [poster]. Presented at the 54th Annual Meeting of the American Academy of Physical Medicine and Rehabilitation, San Francisco, November 13–17, 1992.
33. Schwartzman R: The movement disorder of reflex sympathetic dystrophy. Neurology 40:57–61, 1990.
34. Yoshimura DM, Aminoff MJ, Olney RK: Botulinum toxin therapy for limb dystonias. Neurology 42:627–630, 1992.

23

New Concepts in the Diagnosis and Management of Musculoskeletal Pain

Andrew A. Fischer, M.D., Ph.D., and Marta Imamura, M.D., Ph.D.

The purpose of this chapter is fourfold: (1) to describe improved neurologic sensory examination techniques and relation of results to pain; (2) to describe a new pentad of discopathy and radiculopathy, paraspinal muscle spasm and supra/interspinous ligament sprain and its treatment by a new injection technique; (3) to describe three new injection techniques that produced documented, long-term relief of musculoskeletal pain (MSkP); and (4) to present a new concept of myofascial pain syndrome (MPS). Overlapping of referred pain zones of trigger points with corresponding dermatomes and other findings leads to the conclusion that MPS is frequently a manifestation of spinal segment sensitization. Treatment results of MPS improved when the spinal segment sensitization was treated along with trigger points.

This chapter reviews the clinical observations and experience of the authors and many of their trainees in the use of new diagnostic and therapeutic approaches for pain management, which includes a study of 120 patients with low back, neck, and extremities pain conducted by the authors. The successful use of new diagnostic methods extends over more than two decades and has even yielded good results in patients who failed to respond to other therapies.[15–17,19,20,23] The results and conclusions have been validated by independent observers who witnessed the injections and their immediate effects—the relief of pain and restoration of function. Long-term effects lasting several months and sometimes years have been documented by independent observers on follow-up examinations.[41,43–44] In addition, residents of the Mt. Sinai Physical Medicine and Rehabilitation program and other physicians working with the authors were able to reproduce the results by performing the injections independently or under the authors' supervision.

INTRODUCTION TO TERMS

Trigger points (TrPs) are small, exquisitely tender areas that spontaneously or on compression needle penetration cause pain in a distant region (a referred pain zone [RPZ]).[39,60,64] Treatment should focus on the TrP causing the symptoms, which is identified from maps of referred pain zones.[39,60,64]

In contrast to TrPs, **tender spots** (TSs) induce pain locally. When patients indicate the area of the most intense pain with a finger, the TS manifested by a point of maximum tenderness is located exactly underneath said finger. Treatment should thus concentrate on this spot.

Taut band (TB) is a consistent finding associated with muscle pain and damage and TSs and TrPs. TBs consist of a group of muscle fibers that are tender and have a hard consistency on palpation.

Muscle spasm (MSp) also is diagnosed by tenderness and a hard consistency; however, these findings extend over the entire muscle and are not limited to selected fibers as in TBs. MSp has been defined as a usually painful involuntary muscle contraction that cannot voluntarily be relieved completely: during sleep electromyographic activity was present over the spasmodic muscles.[25]

Table 23-1 summarizes commonly used terms and abbreviations.

PALPATION TECHNIQUES

POSTAIRE is a system of palpation that renders substantially improved results by reducing diagnostic error.[22] The first letter of each pair of letters in this acronym expresses an *action*, and the following letter indicates the *goal* of the previous action (Table 23-2).

TABLE 23-1. Terms and Abbreviations

ESC	electric skin conductance
MPS	myofascial pain syndrome
MSkP	musculoskeletal pain
MSp	muscle spasm
NandI	needling and infiltration of taut band
PandR	pinch and roll
PIB	preinjection block
PSB	paraspinous block
RPZ	referred pain zone
SSS	spinal segmental sensitization
TB	taut band associated with trigger points and tender spots
TrP	trigger point
TS	tender spot
VAS	Visual Analogue Scale

INJECTION TECHNIQUES FOR LONG-TERM RELIEF OF MUSCULOSKELETAL PAIN[24,28,29]

The new procedures consist mainly of three injection techniques. **Paraspinous blocks** (PSBs) spread local anesthetic along the spinous processes and frequently desensitize the irritated spinal segment.[19,29] **Preinjection blocks** (PIBs) prevent nociceptive impulses generated by painful areas from reaching the spinal cord. The sensitive points can then be injected without pain and irritation.[17,19,23] The third procedure, **needling and infiltration** of taut bands (NandI), is an improvement upon trigger point injections, because it is not limited to the trigger point itself but extends to its attachments to the

TABLE 23-2. POSTAIRE

Position patient in order to
Open access to the examined area.

Stretch in order to induce
Tension in the examined muscle.

Activate in order to
Identify the muscle. While palpating the examined muscle, ask the patient to contract it.

Relax the target muscle in order to
Examine it. Ask patient to contract minimally the antagonist of the examined muscle, a maneuver that relaxes the examined muscle and makes it possible to "palpate through" the relaxed muscle so that the taut bands and the most tender point within them can be diagnosed.

Example: Examination of the right quadratus lumborum muscle.

1. Patient lies on opposite (left) side, stretches elbow above head, and drops upper (right) knee behind the left knee.
2. Pull down right iliac crest and identify the quadratus lumborum by palpation.
3. While palpating the muscle, ask patient to lift right shoulder. Bending to right activates the quadratus lumborum.
4. Ask patient to push left shoulder into examination table to relax the right quadratus lumborum (relaxation by activation of antagonist).

bones.[15–17,19,23,24] These techniques, particularly the combination of NandI with PSB, brought instantaneous as well as long-lasting relief of pain with restoration of function in the vast majority of patients who had failed to respond to other treatments such as physical therapy, anti-inflammatory drugs and painkillers, acupuncture, and chiropractic techniques. The results were validated by several independent observers.

PATHOPHYSIOLOGIC BASIS OF MUSCULOSKELETAL PAIN AND TREATMENT

Effects of Needling and Infiltration

The pathophysiologic basis of musculoskeletal pain originating in the periphery is the sensitization of the nerve fibers.[2,5,10,57,58] This sensitization is the reaction of the nerve fibers to inflammatory and irritative substances, products of the local cell injury. Any damage to the cell membrane initiates the arachidonic acid cascade of inflammation, which sensitizes the nerve fibers and causes spontaneous pain as well as sensitivity to mechanical compression.[10] The degree of pressure pain sensitivity, which can be quantified by a pressure algometer,[14] expresses the degree of nerve fiber sensitization.[14,22,40] In the acute stage of tissue damage, vasoactive substances such as histamine and bradykinin that cause edema are released along with prostaglandins, causing sensitization of the nerve fiber.[10] The edema formed around the damaged cells entraps and seals the sensitizing substances with the nerve fibers and causes gradual augmentation of pain and inflammation. The edematous pocket that entraps the nerve endings with the inflammatory sensitizing substances[15,17] can be disrupted mechanically by NandI using local anesthetic.[15–17,19] The efficacy of needling itself has been proven previously by several double-blind studies.[31,33,35,53] The result is an immediate relief of the pain caused by the mechanical break-up of the edema entrapping the nerve endings.[15,17] NandI by local anesthetic has better results.[38] In the chronic stage the local edema around the damaged tissue becomes fibrotic, sometimes creating a pocket that entraps the nerve endings with the sensitizing, inflammatory substances. Palpatory findings can identify fibrotic (scar) tissue about 3 weeks after an injury. Fibrotic tissue becomes the cause of protracted pain and disability, and its mechanical breakdown is the only long-term effective treatment.[15–17,19,23,41,43,44] This conclusion is based upon clinical observations as well as widely recognized studies of wound healing.

Sensitization of nerve fibers manifests clinically by two characteristic findings: (1) tenderness (i.e., mechanical allodynia[10,57,58]), in which stimuli such as pressure that under normal circumstances fail to cause pain become painful, and (2) hyperalgesia, whereby normally painful stimuli such as a pinprick or scratch generate a much more painful reaction than under normal circumstances. The degree of sensitization will determine whether the pain is present spontaneously or is elicited only by mild or strenuous activity.

The Pentad

The pentad consists of the following:
1. Narrowed disc space
2a. Narrowed neural foramen
  b. Narrowed space between spinous processes
3. Sprain of supraspinous ligament
4. Paraspinal muscle spasm, causing #5, below
5. Nerve root compression by the narrowed foramen causes radicular dysfunction that induces spinal segmental sensitization

Spinal Segmental Sensitization

Spinal segmental sensitization (SSS)[5,34,48,54] occurs in reaction to a peripheral irritative focus formed by sensitized nerve fibers.[6,7,58,70] SSS represents a state of hyperactivity that spreads from the sensory component of the spinal segment to the anterior horn cells that control the myotome and also to the sympathetic centers located in the involved spinal level. Injection of local anesthetic into the spasmodic paraspinal muscle relieves the signs and symptoms of the radiculopathy.[13] It was therefore concluded that SSS secondary to radicular compression is frequently caused by paraspinal spasm that narrows the neural foramen at the level of discopathy.

The supra/interspinous ligament sprain component of the pentad acts as an irritative focus, causing SSS (including paraspinal MSp) or contributing to its occurrence. This conclusion is based upon the effects of PSBs, which relieved the paraspinal MSp as well as the signs and symptoms of SSS by blocking nociceptive impulses from the supra/interspinous ligaments.

Treatment of SSS

Paraspinous block (PSB) has been established as an effective treatment of SSS.[19,28,29] It is a new technique that spreads a local anesthetic along the sprained supra/interspinous ligaments. Desensitization of SSS results; pain, dermatomal hyperalgesia, and a corresponding increase in ESC frequently revert to normal, paraspinal MSp is relieved, and TrPs/TSs in the myotome are inactivated. This effect of PSB can be explained by the fact that sprain of the interspinous ligament[36] or its irritation by injected hypertonic saline[47] causes segmental pain and sensitization. Infiltration of the irritated ligament by anesthetic relieved segmental symptoms and signs of sensitization.[47]

Positive results have advanced new concepts in the pathophysiology of MSkP and related disorders, specifically the pentad and the causal relations between its components. These ideas became the basis of treatment for several conditions that were previously resistant to conventional therapies.

NEW DIAGNOSTIC AND THERAPEUTIC APPROACHES FOR PAIN MANAGEMENT

Material and Methods

The authors' study included 120 consecutive patients (62 males and 38 females, age range 22–92 years) with MSkP who were evaluated in physiatric practices specializing in pain management. Twenty-six physicians-in-training alternated in witnessing examinations and treatment results as independent observers. The testing and treatments were performed by the senior author (AAF) in the Department of Physical Medicine and Rehabilitation of the Veterans Affairs Medical Center in Bronx, New York, and in his private practice in Great Neck, New York. Several follow-up examinations confirmed the original findings in all patients.

All subjects complained of pain and had visited the physiatrists for pain management. Causes of pain included recent sports injuries, injuries at the work place, motor vehicle accidents, acute and chronic discopathy, radiculopathy, myofascial pain syndrome, postoperative pain, bursitis, osteoarthritis, sacroiliac joint sprain, and fibromyalgia.

Patients filled out a questionnaire. They indicated on a body chart the areas of tingling, pins and needles, numbness, as well as the intensity and distribution of pain. Areas of pain were compared with location of paresthesia. In selected representative patients, photographs were taken in order to document the patterns of altered skin sensitivity and for use in further analysis.

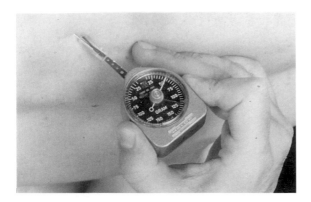

FIGURE 23-1. Quantified nociceptive stimuli produced by scratching of skin. The angle of the opened paper clip is maintained at 45° and the force at 40 g.

Evaluation Techniques

Skin Sensitivity

Sensitivity to painful stimuli (pinprick) was tested by scratching the tip of an open paper clip against the skin as it was slowly dragged across the dermatomal borders. Patients were asked to indicate if the sensation of the paper clip became sharper or duller.

The intensity of stimuli on scratching can be quantified as recommended by Vechiett et al.[67,68] by maintaining the angle between the skin and the measuring paper clip at 45° while applying a standard pressure of 40 g (Fig. 23-1). A disposable paper clip helps to prevent infection.

Electric Skin Conductance

Electric skin conductance (ESC) indicates sympathetic dysfunction[3] and was measured by a microampere meter. If skin conductance is measured with an electrode having a relatively sharp tip, sensitivity to pinprick (scratch) can be tested simultaneously with skin conductance. Measurements of pinprick sensitivity to indicate sensory function and ESC representing sympathetic activity do not require more time to evaluate than measurement of sensitivity to pinprick alone. ESC was measured by Point Finder (Joanco Co., Toronto, Canada), an electronic device featuring an analogue microampere meter with a range of 50 microamperes. Any change in the current between the electrodes was indicated by a sound whose pitch was altered by an increase in the current. The neutral electrode was placed in each patient's palm as the exploring electrode was moved across the dermatomes. The device was calibrated before each measurement. ESC measurements were performed in 32 consecutive patients with different MSkP and disorders by M. Imamura. Her observations were performed independently and the results were marked on the skin along with the patients' indication of change in feeling of sharpness.

Sensitivity of Subcutaneous Tissue

Sensitivity of subcutaneous tissue was tested by the pinch and roll (PandR) method,[54,55] which is performed by picking up the skin between the thumb and forefinger and rolling the tissue beneath. PandR can be quantified by a pressure algometer, a pocket-sized, mechanical force gauge fitted with a standard 1 cm² rubber disc.[14,22] After executing the pinch with the fingers, the tip of the algometer is applied to the side of the skinfold to measure its pressure sensitivity[22] (Figs. 23-2 and 23-3).

Muscle Tenderness

Deep tissue (muscle) tenderness was assessed by digital pressure. In selected cases the test was

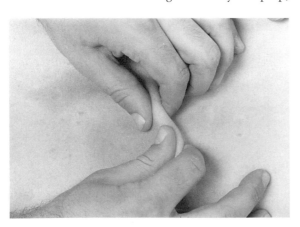

FIGURE 23-2. Pinch and roll (PandR) tests the pressure pain sensitivity of the subcutaneous tissue. PandR is more sensitive than pinprick for diagnosis of radicular dysfunction.

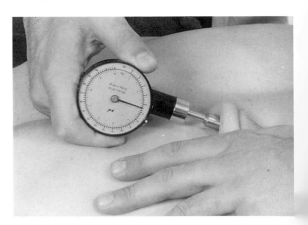

FIGURE 23-3. The technique of quantified pinch uses a pressure threshold meter (algometer) to test the sensitivity of subcutaneous tissue.

quantified with a pressure algometer (Fig. 23-4.) Pressure pain threshold (i.e., the minimum pressure to induce pain) is considered abnormal if it is lower by 2 kg/cm^2 relative to a normosensitive control point. The pressure pain threshold is usually measured over the opposite side.[22]

Muscle Tone

Muscle tone was assessed by manual palpation and confirmed in selected cases by a tissue compliance meter,[12] a hand-held, mechanical instrument that measures soft-tissue consistency objectively and quantitatively. Increased muscle tone manifests as decreased compliance (i.e., the same force pressing a rubber tip into the examined tissue causes less penetration than in soft, normal tissue). Depth of penetration was monitored by a scale attached to the shaft of the algometer. The advantage of tissue compliance measurement is that this method is completely objective (i.e., independent of the patient's reaction) and also quantitative.[12,18] Excellent validity of compliance measurements was reported.[69] Algometers and tissue compliance meters are distributed by Pain Diagnostics and Treatment, Inc., Great Neck, New York.

Trophoedema

Quantitative evaluation of trophoedema (microedema) is performed with a pressure algometer. It is diagnosed by a pitting indentation that lasts several minutes, which is a sign of increased sympathetic activity (Fig. 23-5). Such edema is constantly present in the area of any local tissue damage. After a PSB or PIB, the trophoedema immediately decreases or normalizes completely. This reaction probably indicates that the spasm of venules caused by sympathetic overactivity plays a role in inducing trophoedema.

NEW APPROACHES IN TREATMENT

Special Injection Techniques

Preinjection Block

The preinjection block (PIB) was introduced by the senior author 2 years ago and represented substantial improvement of the treatment for TSs, TrPs, MSp, local inflammation, acute and chronic stage injuries, and arthritis.[16,17,19,23]

PIB (Fig. 23-6) consists of infiltration of the sensory nerve supply to the painful area later to undergo NandI. Pressure algometry demonstrated that, as in PIB,[19] preoperative local infiltration with anesthetic accelerated healing after hernia repair.[65] PIB and PSB

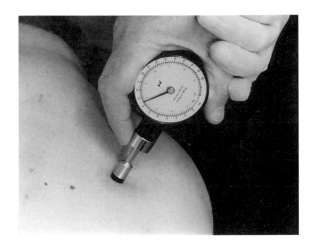

FIGURE 23-4. Pressure threshold meter (algometer) measuring pressure pain sensitivity of deep (muscle) tissues.

correspond to the concept of preemptive analgesia and demonstrate the same positive effects.

Needling and Infiltration of Taut Bands

Needling and infiltration of taut bands (NandI) is a special injection technique unlike other methods of trigger point injections. NandI is used in the treatment of regional pain caused by TSs, TrPs, TBs, and inflamed or scar tissue. Of all modalities used in the study, this injection technique was the most effective. Essentially this technique differs from the usual TrP injections[39,60,64] because it involves a relatively thicker and sufficiently long needle (up to 22 gauge and 10 cm) for deep muscles such as quadratus lumborum, piriformis, or large thigh muscles. The needling consists of repetitive insertion and withdrawal of the injection needle while slowly infiltrating a small amount of 1% lidocaine (Fig. 23-7).

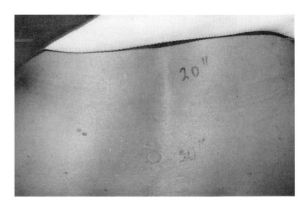

FIGURE 23-5. Trophoedema (microedema) very precisely and objectively localizes the site of dysfunction. It may be caused by extravasation secondary to constriction of venules due to increased sympathetic tone.

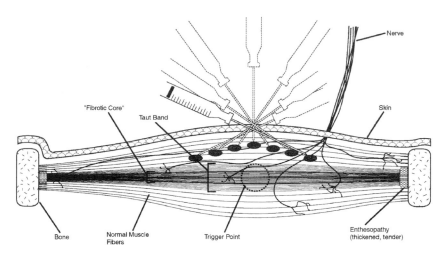

FIGURE 23-6. Preinjection block (PIB) consists of spreading the anesthetic along the taut band to prevent pain and sensitization when injection of the sensitive area is to follow.

The goal is to disrupt and mechanically break up the entire area of abnormal tissue that is causing pain. Emphasis is placed on covering not only the trigger point itself as in conventional techniques,[39,64] but also the entire TB,[17,19,23] including its attachment to the bone at the origin and insertion of the muscle, where tenderness and edema of a mushy consistency indicate enthesopathy.

After NandI, instantaneous relief of pain and substantial restoration of previously limited function occurs.[15–17,19,23] Successful NandI results in long-term relief of pain,[17,19,23,41,43,44] whereas inactivation of the trigger point itself without mechanical disruption of the entire underlying pathology often has only a temporary effect. Usually only 1–2 trigger areas or points are injected in one session.

Paraspinous Block

Paraspinous block (PSB) was introduced about 2 years ago as a preinjection block for NandI of supra/interspinous ligaments. PSB alone relieved the segmental sensitization and radicular pain. Therefore, it became the standard first step in the management of SSS. A 25-gauge needle, 38 mm or longer, is inserted next to the spinous processes at the affected level where the space between them is narrowed and the supra/interspinous ligaments are sprained (Fig. 23-8). These findings are a component of the pentad, which also includes SSS.

Lidocaine (1%) is infiltrated slowly proximally and distally along the spinous processes into the loose connective tissue, which offers no resistance. Penetration of muscles is avoided. The amount of 1% lidocaine injected for PSB depends on the treated region and the patient's size. In the cervical area about 1.5 ml is spread over one segment. This amount includes the NandI of supra/interspinous ligaments. Usually 1 or 2 levels are injected per session. If severe pain of other, unattended levels persists, the additional level is injected after about

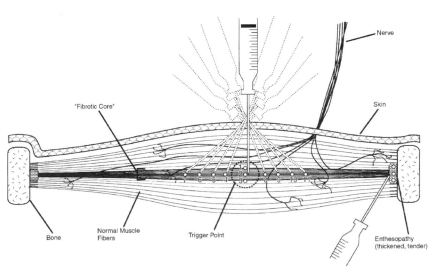

FIGURE 23-7. Needling and infiltration (NandI) of the taut band extends over its attachment to the bones.

45–60 minutes, during which time the patient can receive a physical therapy session. The maximum amount of anesthetic injected in the neck per one session should not exceed 3 ml. At the thoracic level, 2 or 3 segments requiring about 2 ml/segment usually may be injected. More anesthetic is required in the lumbosacral area, and about 3–5 ml/segment and 2–3 segments can be attended per session. In addition, peripheral painful areas (TSs/TrPs) should be injected after PSB. The PIB usually requires 3–8 ml and NandI of TB of a similar amount depending on the size of muscle and size of pathology. The total amount of 1% lidocaine should not exceed 15 maximum 20 ml per session over the entire body or a total of 5 ml in the neck area.

Diffuse infiltration of spasmodic muscle[16,17,19] instantaneously alleviates pain and breaks the pain-spasm-pain vicious circle. A needle of adequate length (38 mm–10.5 cm) is used, and the lidocaine is spread within the spasmodic muscle. Spasm is caused by an irritative focus that must be identified and eliminated for best immediate and long-term results.[19]

Physical Therapy Modalities

Each injection is followed by at least three sessions of physical therapy to promote healing of the injected areas in the muscle as well as to prevent recurrence of pain.[19,52]

Electrical Stimulation

Application of a moist heating pad for 20 minutes is followed by electrical stimulation using sinusoid surging current for 15 minutes, which induces strong periodic contractions and relaxation of the treated muscles. The contractions squeeze out the edema formed at the injection site and prevent inflammation caused by the injury. If a spasmodic component is present, tetanizing current is applied and followed by sinusoid surging current to induce periodic contractions for 10 minutes each.[19,52]

Exercise

Double-blind studies prove that active limbering and relaxation exercises are effective in the treatment of low back pain and its prevention as long as the patient does them systematically.[8] Postisometric relaxation also has been proven effective in a double-blind study.[1] However, the authors' experience demonstrates that the most effective treatment consists of inhibition of painful muscles when a patient voluntarily contracts the antagonists.[16,19] A

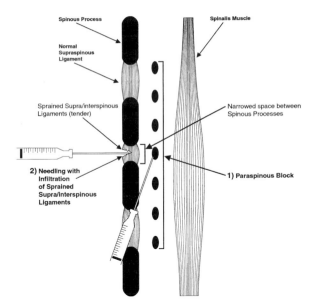

Technique of 1) Paraspinous Block and
2) Needling with Infiltration of Sprained
Supra/interspinous Ligaments.

FIGURE 23-8. Paraspinous block (PSB) for treatment of the pentad. At the levels of discopathy-radiculopathy the distance between the spinous processes is narrowed due to palpable spasm in paraspinal muscles. The injecting needle progresses a few millimeters laterally from the spinous process into the loose connective tissue and is moved proximally and distally to cover several tender levels of sprained supra/interspinous ligaments.

spray of vapocoolant inactivates the TrPs/TSs and renders relaxation exercises[52] and passive stretching of the involved muscle[64] more effective.

Removal of Pain-Causing Factors

The etiologic and perpetuating factors that caused the TPs, TSs, MSp, or other painful dysfunction must be identified and eliminated to prevent recurrence of pain. Treatment of pain has short-lived and limited effects unless its causes can be removed.[19,23,52,60,64]

The pentad of discopathy, radiculopathy, and paraspinal spasm was the cause of pain in 82% of patients (Figs. 23-9 and 23-10).

CLINICAL FINDINGS

Efficacy of Paraspinous Block

Paraspinous block relieved pain and normalized segmental sensitization in 87% of treatments. The sprained supra/interspinous ligaments act as an irritative focus that causes SSS, part of which is the

The Pentad of Vicious Cycle:
Discopathy - Radiculopathy - Paraspinal Spasm

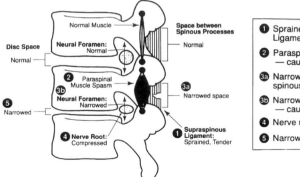

1. Sprained Supraspinous Ligament — causing →
2. Paraspinal muscle spasm — causing →
3a. Narrowed space between spinous processes and
3b. Narrowed Neural Foramina — causing →
4. Nerve root compression
5. Narrowed disc space

FIGURE 23-9. The pentad of vicious circle in discopathy-radiculopathy with paraspinal spasm.

paraspinous MSp. Relaxation of spasm immediately after the PSB is palpable. Evidently, the relief of signs and symptoms of radiculopathy is related to the relaxation of paraspinal spasm. Simultaneously, hyperalgesia and increased ESC, which are manifestations of segmental sensory sensitization, also were reversed to normal. Substantial reduction of activity (pain and tenderness) in TBs, TSs, TrPs, and MSp within the treated myotome was noted regularly. Long-term results were observed when patients returned for treatment of other areas that were not the subject of the initial therapy. In the majority of cases, treatment results persisted for several months, particularly if the patient was regularly adhering to the exercise program. In some cases, the sprain of supra/interspinous ligaments and paraspinal spasm recurred with radicular irritation. The recurrence, however, always had much milder symptoms than were present before the initial treatment. A possible cause of recurrence is respraining of the supra/interspinous ligaments. Statistical data on long-term treatment results of the pentad are not yet available.

Neurologic Findings

Dermatomes as described by Keegan and Garrett[46] matched perfectly the zones of pain, hyperalgesia, and increased skin conductance in all patients and in each and every dermatome. Descriptions of dermatomes by other authors[4,30,45] failed to match the hyperalgesic zones and are considered incorrect (Figs. 23-11, 23-12, and 23-13).

Neurologic findings of sensitization and their relation to pain-generating mechanisms have been established. A correlation was found between pain distribution and positive (irritative) neurologic findings consisting of tingling and feelings of pins and needles (subjective). On physical examination, which is more sensitive for diagnosis, sensory changes included hyperalgesia, increased ESC, and deep tissue tenderness. Motor sensitization is manifested by spasm, point tenderness, and TBs in the myotome. The increase in ESC overlapped exactly with hyperalgesic zones and confirmed objectively and quantitatively the segmental sensitization. Negative neurologic findings, which indicate conduction block such as numbness, based on subjective

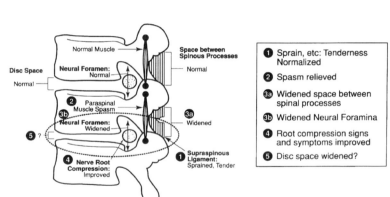

1. Sprain, etc: Tenderness Normalized
2. Spasm relieved
3a. Widened space between spinal processes
3b. Widened Neural Foramina
4. Root compression signs and symptoms improved
5. Disc space widened?

FIGURE 23-10. Changes in the pentad after infiltration of the supra/interspinous ligaments.

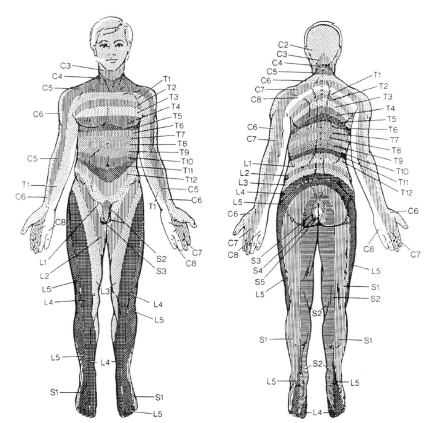

FIGURE 23-11. The dermatomal territories that accurately correlate with pain, hyperalgesia, and increased skin conductance as described by Keegan and Garrett.[46]

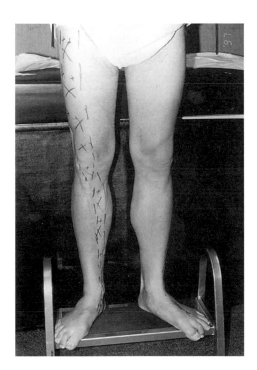

FIGURE 23-12. Hyperalgesic zones marked by "X" corresponding to L4 dermatome. X-ray showed degenerative disc disease with narrowed disc space at the L4–L5 level.

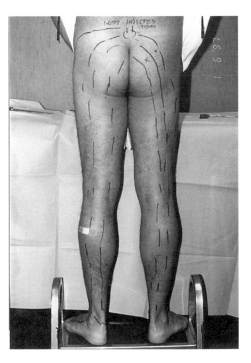

FIGURE 23-13. Hyperalgesic zones corresponding to L5–S1 dermatomes. Blocking of the supra/interspinous ligaments at L5–S1 levels bilaterally decreased sensitivity over the affected dermatomes.

determination and a decreased sensation to pinprick on physical examination do not correlate with pain distribution.

Sometimes only the dorsal primary rami of the roots are involved, sparing the ventral primary rami. The dorsal primary rami supply the skin of the paraspinal area and extensor muscles of the spinal column, which also are located in the paraspinal area. In contrast, the ventral primary rami supply the rest of the trunk and extremities in terms of both sensory and motor innervation. Both sensory and motor fibers of the dorsal primary rami usually are involved.

Relation between Location of Pain and Its Cause

TSs were the most frequent immediate cause of pain, whereas trigger points were relatively infrequent. TSs were the causative factor of MSkP in 93% of point tenderness, yet TrPs were the cause of pain in not more than 7% of subjects. As a rule, TSs or TrPs were not isolated but part of SSS. SSS was manifested by sensitization of the entire myotome (TSs or/and TrPs in the remaining muscles of the segment) and hyperalgesia was detected in the corresponding dermatome.

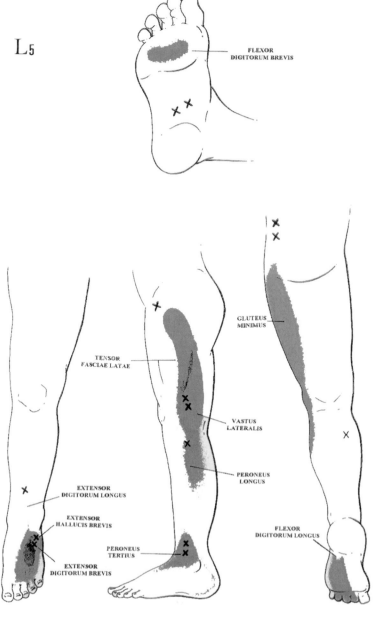

L5

FLEXOR DIGITORUM BREVIS

GLUTEUS MINIMUS

TENSOR FASCIAE LATAE

VASTUS LATERALIS

PERONEUS LONGUS

EXTENSOR DIGITORUM LONGUS

EXTENSOR HALLUCIS BREVIS

PERONEUS TERTIUS

EXTENSOR DIGITORUM BREVIS

FLEXOR DIGITORUM LONGUS

FIGURE 23-14. Referred pain zones (RPZs) of trigger points located in muscles supplied by the fifth lumbar spinal segment. The RPZs overlap with the corresponding L5 dermatome shown in Fig. 23-11.

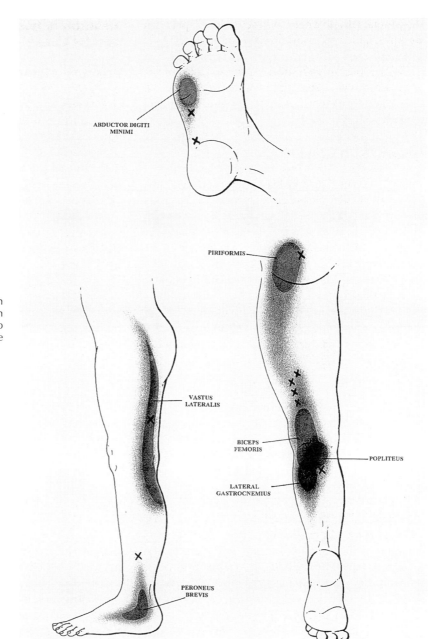

FIGURE 23-15.   Referred pain zones of trigger points located in S1 myotome. The RPZs overlap with parts of the S1 dermatome shown in Fig. 23-11.

There is perfect overlapping of dermatomes with the referred pain zones (RPZs) of TrPs located in muscles belonging to the identical spinal segment. For example, the RPZs of TrPs located in muscles are supplied by the 5th lumbar spinal segment (Fig. 23-14).

The RPZs overlap perfectly with the corresponding L5 dermatome (see Fig. 23-11). Similar correlations were found in all other dermatomes and RPZs of TrPs situated in corresponding myotomes. RPZs are generated by TrPs located within the first sacral segment. Note that each RPZ corresponds to a part of the identical S1 dermatome as presented in Figure 23-11 (Fig. 23-15).

EVALUATION OF NEUROLOGIC EXAMINATION TECHNIQUES

Scratch

Scratching with the tip of an open paper clip is preferable to the pinprick: it shows the borders of dermatomes within millimeters and requires little time, a fraction of that required by the pinprick method.

Pinch and Roll

PandR tests subcutaneous tissue sensitivity. It is particularly valuable in the detection of hyperalgesia within the dermatome or peripheral nerve distribution because the test has a higher diagnostic sensitivity than pinprick.

Electric Skin Conductance

ESC can confirm hyperalgesia objectively and quantitatively. In the authors' experience, ESC has proven highly valuable in the diagnosis of sensory radiculopathy because it is more sensitive than pinprick or scratch and its results are quantitative and independent of the patients' subjective reaction. Such objective measurement is helpful in clinical practice because patients often are unable to provide reliable and repeatable information on the sharpness of a pinprick. Objective and quantitative tests of sensory dysfunction also are necessary for accurate medicolegal documentation.

ESC also reflects quantitatively the severity of the sensitization.[56] In addition, reversal of sensitization (desensitization) can be documented by ESC.[56] Desensitization can usually be achieved instantaneously in case of a radicular dysfunction by PSB. The effect of injection is monitored readily by the reversal of increased skin conduction to normal values. The authors' results confirm those in previous publications about ESC,[56] but the former applied ESC in the daily routine of pain diagnosis, whereas previous studies were done under experimental conditions. Also, the combination of scratching and ESC allowed us to perform both tests simultaneously. Results of both tests can be correlated instantaneously for clinical diagnosis. Increased ESC is caused by augmented sympathetic activity, which induces sweating.[3,63] Radiculopathy induced increased ESC corresponding exactly to the sensory radicular innervation territory, but not to the "sympathetic dermatome" that features a different shape and localization.[32,63] Such a distribution of augmented ESC, which corresponded to the hyperalgesic dermatomal zones, can be explained only by the spreading of the excitatory process through the sensory root fibers antidromically to the periphery. There it is switched over to the axon reflex causing local sympathetic hyperactivity that includes sweating and vasomotor disturbances. Increased ESC related to neural dysfunction and pain[32,56,62,66] has been well documented in segmental, radicular,[62,63] and peripheral

nerve dysfunction[37] as well as local soft tissue damage.[48–51]

Pressure Algometry

Pressure algometry proved to be of great value in the quantified diagnosis of tenderness. The validity and sensitivity of pressure algometry for detection of focal tenderness has been well established.[11,21,22,61] The value of algometry for quantitative evaluation of pain relief by medication and physical modalities also has been proven[59] and was confirmed in our observations.

Relation between Neurologic Findings and Pain

The diagnosis of radiculopathy or SSS by conventional neurologic examination is based mainly on decreased sensitivity to pinprick. Radiculopathy limited to only sensory deficit is not pain-related, a conclusion that is supported by the fact that the conduction deficit cannot produce the irritative, hyperactive phenomena that are associated with pain. Only irritative, positive neurologic findings can be correlated with pain distribution. Irritative phenomena include tingling, buzzing, pins and needles, and hyperalgesia and tenderness found on physical examination.

Sensitivity of Diagnostic Tests

The tests used to diagnose radiculopathy, segmental sensitization, and muscle pain not only demonstrated higher sensitivity but also were quantitative (i.e., pressure algometry for tenderness; scratching for hyperalgesia) and objective (i.e., tissue compliance for muscle spasm and taut bands; ESC for sympathetic dermatomal dysfunction, which confirms the subjective response to pinprick; and surface electromyography for abnormal muscle activity, particularly spasm).

The most sensitive methods for diagnosing segmental or peripheral sensitization are PandR and ESC, which apply whether the sensitization is caused by a local injury, peripheral nerve irritation, or radiculopathy. Point tenderness, muscle spasm, and taut bands are highly constant findings indicating sensitization of the myotome. Parietal structures such as skin and subcutaneous and deep tissues (muscles) in radiculopathy as well as in other conditions demonstrate different degrees of sensitization.[67,68] Subcutaneous tissues are the most sensitive and are examined by the PandR technique.

In summary, for a quick orientation, PandR of the paraspinal area or ESC (if available) and palpation for spasm and taut bands with tenderness in the paraspinal musculature are the most sensitive and reliable tests for diagnosis of radicular involvement.

IMPLICATIONS OF RESULTS FOR MANAGEMENT OF MUSCULOSKELETAL PAIN AND DISORDERS

The management of MSkP consists of two phases[19,20] (Table 23-3). Phase 1 identifies the immediate cause of pain, which usually consists of TSs, TrP, MSp, local injury, or inflammation and has the short-term goal of relieving pain before the patient leaves the office.

In 93% of cases the immediate cause of pain is found exactly underneath the finger pointing to the area of most intense pain. In a much lower percentage of cases (not more than 7%), pain is caused by TrPs, which shoot symptoms into a distant area (RPZ). If a patient is unable to identify a specific point as the location of the most intense pain because the symptoms are dispersed, an RPZ should be sought and identified and its trigger point diagnosed and treated.

Phase 2 in the management of MSkP consists of the identification and removal of factors that had induced the immediate cause(s) of pain, which usually cannot be achieved in a short period.[19] The efficacy of treating MSkP has substantially improved since MPS was discovered to be a frequent manifestation or component of SSS; therapy was extended to also include SSS by PSB.

EFFICACY OF NEEDLING AND INFILTRATION OF TAUT BANDS

Our present results and previous publications[15–17,19,23,41,43,44] demonstrate clearly that for long-term therapeutic results the thorough needling of the entire local pathology (NandI of TBs) is the most effective. For best results, NandI should be followed by physical therapy. Electrical stimulation is particularly important for promoting healing of the tissue damage resulting from the injections.[19] Regular exercise specifically prescribed based on each patient's individual deficiency in range of motion and the weakness and tightness of key postural muscles reduced the risk of pain recurrence.[16,19]

TABLE 23-3. Management of Musculoskeletal Pain

Phase 1: Identify the immediate cause of pain.

1. Ask the patient to point with one finger to the area of most intense pain.
2. Recognition of pain pattern: Identify the point of maximum tenderness by palpation and compress it while asking the patient, "Is this the location of the pain you indicated?"
3. Confirm that abnormal tenderness is present: Measure the pressure pain threshold over the point of maximum tenderness using an algometer. Pressure threshold lower by 2 kg/cm2 relative to a normally sensitive control point (which is usually on the opposite, nonpainful side) is considered abnormal tenderness.
4. Infiltrate the point of maximum tenderness TSs or TrP. If infiltration eliminates symptoms, it confirms that the treated area was the cause of pain. The entire taut band should be needled and infiltrated for best results.

Phase 2: Identify and treat (remove) the causative and perpetuating factors that induced the immediate cause(s) of pain (TSs, TPs, MSp).

The long-term positive results of NandI of TBs also are supported by several recent studies. In the first randomized, controlled study also supported by pressure algometry, M. Imamura showed that treatment of the TSs/TrPs by NandI of TBs shortened recovery and return to work to less than one-third the time (4.88 ± 3.04 weeks as compared to 16.23 ± 7.92 weeks of a control group treated by conventional active physical therapy). The study included 20 control subjects and 13 injected patients. The diagnosis consisted of plantar fasciitis with TrPs in the calf muscles.[42] These TrPs were injected. There were no statistically significant differences between both groups in terms of duration of pain complaint, initial Visual Analogue Scale (VAS), and functional level on a test of the American Orthopedic Foot and Ankle Society (AOFAS). Upon discharge the injected group showed more improvement than the control group, but the difference was not significant. VAS in the injected group dropped from 8.21 ± 1.20 to the final level of 2.92 ± 1.98. The conventionally treated group decreased VAS from 8.46 ± 1.39 to the final 3.73 ± 3.42. Treatment consisted of ultrasound at insertion of the plantar fascia, with electrical stimulation over plantar fascia and gastrocnemius muscle followed by stretching of both structures. Functional improvement on the AOFAS test was significant in both groups, but no significant difference was found between them. The identical level of pain relief and functional improvement allowing return to work has been achieved in the injected group in a substantially shorter time: 4.83 ± 3.04 weeks vs. 16.23 ± 7.92 (p = 0.0002) in control group (U Mann

Whitney test with significance level 5%). Also, the number of treatment sessions were significantly lower in the injected group 3 ± 1.13 vs. 21.77 ± 9.24 (p < 0.0001) (U Mann Whitney test with significance level of 5%).

Using the NandI of TBs, S.T. Imamura statistically documented improvement of pain and function in patients scheduled for total hip replacement.[44] This study focused on treatment of the myofascial component and included 19 patients with hip pathology scheduled for total hip replacement. The follow-up extended to an average of 2 years. Patients were divided into two groups; 9 patients were not operated on and treated only with NandI of TB technique in the involved muscles. Initial VAS in this group was 5.72 ± 2.05 and at follow-up evaluation dropped to 2.39.0 ± 2.85 (p = 0.0023). According to the Wilcoxon test with significance level of 5%, reduction of pain was statistically significant. Ten patients underwent hip replacement. Their initial VAS was 6.71 ± 2.86, which at follow-up dropped to 1.0 ± 1.41 (p = 0.003). The decrease in VAS was statistically significant at the level of 5%. The comparison of VAS values between the two groups was performed by U Mann Whitney test. Neither the initial nor the follow-up VAS values of the groups showed statistically significant differences (p = 1, ns). The improvement of pain and functioning achieved by NandI of TBs associated with TSs/TrPs located in muscles of patients with hip pathology was equal to the outcome of total hip replacement in an average of a 2-year follow-up. These impressive results underscore the importance of diagnosing TSs/TrPs as the immediate cause of pain and illustrate further the high treatment efficacy that can be achieved by NandI of TBs even in patients whose conditions are severe enough to indicate total hip replacement.

MYOFASCIAL PAIN SYNDROME (MPS) MOST FREQUENTLY IS A MANIFESTATION OF SSS[27]

Diagnosis of MPS is based on the presence of TrPs or TSs in muscles. MPS is considered a typical local or regional pain condition. However, several findings and observations indicate that in the vast majority of cases MPS is a clinical manifestation of SSS affecting the myotome. TrPs located in the muscles are usually not isolated: other muscles within the same myotome also demonstrate TBs and point tenderness. Such findings are indicative of sensitization of the entire myotome belonging to

the sensitized spinal segment. In fact, TSs and TrPs, which are located in ligaments, bursitis, tendinitis, epicondylitis, and enthesopathy usually are accompanied by signs and symptoms of SSS affecting the involved level. Careful and correct palpation identifies TrPs and point tenderness only if it is performed after relaxation of the muscle by reciprocal inhibition (contraction of the antagonists), which allows palpation "through" the relaxed muscle. When a patient presented with complaints indicating a TrP, as a rule it was located within a sensitized spinal segment.

In addition to sensitization of the myotome manifested by point tenderness and TrPs, evidence of sensitization affecting the sensory component of the spinal segment or route is found regularly. It is diagnosed by hyperalgesia to pinprick, affecting exactly and circumscriptively the corresponding dermatome. In addition, PandR reveals sensitization of the subcutaneous tissue, which corresponds exactly to the hyperalgesic area and to the area of increased ESC. All three sensory tests, namely the sensitivity to pinprick (scratch), PandR, and ESC, can be quantified for diagnosis.

The referred pain zone (RPZ) of each TrP territorially overlap exactly with the corresponding dermatome.[26] For example, the L5 dermatome overlaps with RPZs of the TrPs located within the L5 myotome (see Figs. 23-14 and 23-15). This finding strongly supports the conclusion that symptoms in RPZs of myofascial pain as well as other TrPs correspond to sensitization of the related dermatome.

Concerning the area to be treated as the cause of pain, it is significant that TrPs shooting pain into a distant region are much less frequent, amounting to only 7% of focal tenderness, whereas TSs, which induce symptoms locally in the area of maximum tenderness, are responsible for the vast majority of local pain.

RELATION BETWEEN SPINAL SEGMENTAL SENSITIZATION AND PAINFUL MUSCULOSKELETAL DISORDERS

Painful MSk disorders include a wide variety of clinical diagnoses with various etiologies, such as muscle pain without defined cause, sprains, and overuse or inflammation of different soft tissues (e.g., muscles, ligaments, bursae, and tendons). Osteoarthritis, neurologic conditions causing muscle pain, and degenerative disc disease with radiculopathy also are classified as MSkP.

Clinical experience proved that when any type of MSkP is present, sensitization of the corresponding spinal segment may be identified by proper examination techniques in the majority of cases. In addition, desensitization of the irritated spinal segment (i.e., normalization of the pathologic findings by PSB) regularly induced considerable relief of local MSkP that was located in the periphery. Usually PSB caused a substantial decrease in pain intensity in the range of approximately 40–60% and sometimes even 100%. Such pain relief after PSB is associated with desensitization of the irritated segment as proven by normalization of hyperalgesia (pinprick), PandR, and partial inactivation of TSs/TrPs within the affected myotome. The amount of pain relief following PSB expresses the component of symptoms caused by the central sensitization, as opposed to the pain generated locally in the periphery by sensitization of nerve fibers due to inflammatory substances (e.g., prostaglandins). The relation between the SSS, which represents a central component of the pain, and the peripheral component is best understood as a vicious circle: the central component makes the periphery more vulnerable. This is the case when TS/TrPs prevent a muscle from relaxing. For example, when the body weight lands on the toes while running or jumping, the gastrocnemius muscle is supposed to relax in order to absorb the shock. If TSs, TrPs, or MSp and tension prevent the sudden relaxation of the muscle, it may develop a tear.

Neurogenic inflammation secondary to SSS may explain the presence of bursitis, tenosynovitis, epicondylitis, and enthesopathy (also induced by muscle tension) within the supply territory of sensitized spinal segment.

Another mechanism that explains the concomitant findings of central, segmental, and peripheral sensitization may develop in the opposite sequence; central sensitization may be induced by an irritative focus in the periphery.[2] The irritative focus may consist of a severe acute injury or even minor chronic pathology, such as injuries, or inflammation (e.g., arthritis, bursitis, tendinitis, epicondylitis, fasciitis). The acute or chronic nociceptive barrage generated by the irritative focus induces the sensitization of the spinal segment that subsequently may spread to higher sections of the central nervous system.[2] Clinical experience shows that treatment of both components, namely the SSS by PSB, combined with the elimination of the peripheral irritative focus renders far superior results as compared to therapy, which is limited to local peripheral problems. This applies regardless of the mechanism of the vicious circle that constitutes the central and peripheral sensitization. Therefore, for practical purposes SSS should be ruled out in any case of MSkP. If SSS is present it should be treated as a separate entity in addition to therapy aimed at the peripheral cause of pain.

CURRENT TREATMENT OF TRPs, TSs, TBs, AND MUSCLE SPASM

Conventional treatment concentrates on local findings because the conditions are considered local or regional pain disorders. The treatment of local pain such as TSs, TrPs, MsP, and other musculoskeletal disorders is much more effective when combined with management of the associated SSS. In this regard the description of the pentad of discopathy/radiculopathy and paraspinal muscle spasm is helpful; it was identified as the cause of pain in 82% of patients suffering from MSkP. Breaking the vicious circle by PSB effectively relieves the symptoms of radicular compression and sensitization in 87% of treatments. It is important to address the irritative focus, specifically the sprain of supra/interspinous ligaments, which plays a prominent role in initiating and inducing the vicious circle of the pentad.

The authors' routine management of TrPs, TSs, MSp, and inflammatory MSkP consists of three injections, administered in the following order:

1. **Paraspinous block** is administered at the level of SSS if this condition is present. The PSB interrupts the nociceptive impulses that originate in the sprained supra/interspinous ligaments and cause sensitization of the spinal segment. PSB is a simple injection without any side effects; no complications were observed over the period of more than two years since the authors started to use it. PSB itself effectively relaxes the paraspinal muscle spasm that is instrumental in inducing the nerve root compression by narrowing the neural foramen.

2. Paraspinous block is followed on the periphery by **preinjection block** of the tender spot or TrP to be needled. PIB not only prevents pain caused by penetration of the injection needle into the sensitive, tender tissue, but also prevents sensitization.

3. **NandI** is essential for breaking up the pathologic and dysfunctional tissue causing the pain. The concept that functional changes are instrumental in causing root compression (particularly paraspinal muscle spasms) is of basic importance for management of radiculopathies and may explain why no

correlation exists between a disc herniation as seen on imaging and pain.[9]

CONCLUSION

New injection techniques can relieve pain and signs caused by radicular compression. Paraspinous block frequently achieves such improvement instantaneously by relieving paraspinal muscle spasm, which causes the root compression. New injection techniques improved success rates and achieved long-term relief of pain caused by trigger points and tender spots.

Acknowledgment

The valuable suggestions of Ruth Frischer, Ph.D., and the assistance of Helen Lax, M.D., in preparation of this manuscript are appreciated.

REFERENCES

1. Aleksiev A: Longitudinal comparative study on the outcome of inpatient treatment of low back pain with manual therapy vs. physical therapy. J Orthop Med 17:10–14, 1995.
2. Bonica JJ : Biochemistry and modulation of nociception and pain. In Bonica JJ: The Management of Pain. Philadelphia, Lea & Febiger, 1990.
3. Carmichael EA, Honeyman WM, Kolb LC, Stewart WK: A physiological study of the skin resistance response in man. J Physiol 99:329–337, 1941.
4. Chusid JG, McDonald JJ: Correlative Neuroanatomy and Functional Neurology, 13th ed. California, Lange Medical Publications, 1967.
5. Coderre TJ, Melzack R: Cutaneous hyperalgesia: Contributions of the peripheral and central nervous systems to the increase in pain sensitivity after injury. Brain 404:95–106, 1987.
6. Devor M: Abnormal excitability in injured axons. In Waxman SL, Kocsis J, Stys PK (eds): The Axon. Oxford, Oxford University Press, 1995.
7. Devor M, Jänig W, Michaelis M: Modulation of activity in dorsal root ganglion neurons by sympathetic activation in nerve injured rats. J Neurophysiol 71:38–47, 1994.
8. Deyo RA, Walsh NE, Martin DC, et al: A controlled trial of transcutaneous electrical stimulation (TENS) and exercise for chronic low back pain. N Engl J Med 322:1627–1634, 1990.
9. Ellenberg MR, Ross ML, Honet JC, et al: Prospective evaluation of the course of disc herniations in patients with proven radiculopathy. Arch Phys Med Rehabil 74:3–8, 1993.
10. Fields HL: Pain. New York, McGraw-Hill, 1987.
11. Fischer AA: Pressure algometry over normal muscles: Standard values, validity and reproducibility of pressure threshold. Pain 30: 115–126, 1987.
12. Fischer AA: Clinical use of tissue compliance meter for documentation of soft tissue pathology. Clin J Pain 3:323–330, 1987.
13. Fischer AA: Relief of nerve root compression by trigger point injection into the quadratus lumborum muscle. Arch Phys Med Rehabil 74:1263, 1993.
14. Fischer AA: Pressure algometry (dolorimetry) in the differential diagnosis of muscle pain. In Rachlin ES (ed): Myofascial Pain and Fibromyalgia, Trigger Point Management. St. Louis, Mosby, 1994.
15. Fischer AA: Trigger point injection. In Lennard TA (ed): Physiatric Procedures in Clinical Practice. Philadelphia, Hanley & Belfus, 1995, pp 28–35.
16. Fischer AA: Local injections in pain management. Trigger point needling with infiltration and somatic blocks. Phys Med Rehabil Clin North Am 6:851–870, 1995.
17. Fischer AA: Injection techniques in the management of local pain. J Back Musculoskelet Rehabil 7:107–117, 1996.
18. Fischer AA: Quantitative and objective documentation of soft tissue abnormality: Pressure algometry and tissue compliance recording. In Nordhoff LS (ed): Motor Vehicle Collision Injuries. Gaithersburg, MD, Aspen, 1996.
19. Fischer AA: New approaches in treatment of myofascial pain. Phys Med Rehabil Clin North Am 8:153–169, 1997.
20. Fischer AA: New developments in diagnosis of myofascial pain and fibromyalgia. Phys Med Rehabil Clin North Am 8:1–21, 1997.
21. Fischer AA: Algometry in the daily practice of pain management. J Back Musculoskelet Rehabil 8:151–163, 1997.
22. Fischer AA: Algometry in diagnosis of musculoskeletal pain and evaluation of treatment outcome: An update. In Fischer AA (ed): Muscle Pain Syndromes and Fibromyalgia. New York, Haworth Medical Press, 1998.
23. Fischer AA: Myofascial pain. In Windsor RE, Lox DM (ed): Soft Tissue Injuries: Diagnosis and Treatment. Philadelphia, Hanley & Belfus, 1998.
24. Fischer AA: Treatment of myofascial pain. J Musculoskeletal Pain 7:131–142, 1999.
25. Fischer AA, Chang CH: Electromyographic evidence of paraspinal muscle spasm during sleep in patients with low Back pain. Clin J Pain 1:147–154, 1985.
26. Fischer AA, Imamura ST, Imamura M: Referred pain zones from trigger points overlap exactly with the dermatomes of the corresponding spinal segment (roots). [Poster.] 4th World Congress on Myofascial Pain and Fibromyalgia, Silvi Marini, Italy, August 1998.
27. Fischer AA, Imamura ST, Imamura M: Myofascial trigger points are most frequently a manifestation of segmental spinal sensitization. J Musculoskeletal Pain 6(Suppl 2):20, 1998.
28. Fischer AA, Imamura ST, Imamura M: New injection techniques and concepts for treatment of myofascial pain [abstract]. J Musculoskeletal Pain 6(Suppl 2):51, 1998.
29. Fischer AA, Imamura ST, Kaziyama HS, Imamura M: Trigger point injections and "paraspinous blocks" which relieve segmental spinal sensitization are effective treatment for chronic pain [abstract]. J Musculoskeletal Pain 6(Suppl 2):52, 1998.
30. Foerster O: The dermatomes in man. Brain 56:1–39, 1933.
31. Frost FA, Jessen B, Siggaard-Andersen J: A controlled, double blind comparison of mepivacaine injection versus saline injection for myofascial pain. Lancet 8:299–500, 1980.
32. Furer M, Hardy JD: The reaction to pain as determined by the galvanic skin response. Proc Assoc Res Nerv Ment Dis 29:72–89, 1949.
33. Garvey TA, Marks MR, Wiesel SW: A prospective, randomized, double blind evaluation of trigger-point injection therapy for low-back pain. Spine 14:962–964, 1989.
34. Gunn CC: The Gunn Approach to the Treatment of Chronic Pain. New York, Churchill Livingstone, 1996.
35. Gunn CC, Milbrandt WE, Little AS, Mason KE: Dry needling of muscle motor points for chronic low-back pain. A randomized clinical trial with long-term follow-up. Spine 5:279–291, 1980.
36. Hackett GS: Ligament and Tendon Relaxation Treated by Prolotherapy, 3rd ed. Springfield, IL, Charles C. Thomas 70:27–36, 1958.
37. Herz E, Glaser GH, Moldover J: Electrical skin resistance test in evaluation of peripheral nerve injuries. Arch Neurol Psychiatry 56:365–380, 1946.

38. Hong C-Z: Lidocaine injection versus dry needling to myofascial trigger point: The importance of the local twitch response. Am J Phys Med Rehabil 73:256–263, 1994.
39. Hong C-Z: Considerations and recommendations regarding myofascial trigger point injection. J Musculoskeletal Pain 2:29–59, 1994.
40. Hong C-Z: Algometry in evaluation of trigger points and referred pain. In Fischer AA (ed): Muscle Pain Syndromes and Fibromyalgia. Pressure Algometry in Quantification of Diagnosis and Treatment Outcome. New York, Haworth Press, 1998.
41. Imamura M, Fischer A, Imamura ST, et al: Treatment of myofascial pain components in plantar fasciitis speeds up recovery. In Fischer AA (ed): Muscle Pain Syndromes and Fibromyalgia. New York, Haworth Press, 1998, pp 91–110.
42. Imamura M, Fischer AA, Imamura ST, et al: Randomized controlled study of the effect of N&I of trigger points [unpublished data]. Presented at the course and workshop "New Approaches in Diagnosis and Management of Musculoskeletal Pain," April 25–26, 1999, Uniondale, New York.
43. Imamura ST, Fischer AA, Imamura M, et al: Pain management using myofascial approach when other treatment failed. Phys Med Rehabil Clin North Am 8:179–196, 1997.
44. Imamura ST, Riberto M, Fischer AA, et al: Successful pain relief by treatment of myofascial components in patients with hip pathology scheduled for total hip replacement. In Fischer AA (ed): Muscle Pain Syndromes and Fbromyalgia. New York, Haworth Press, 1998, pp 73–89.
45. Inman VT, Saunders JB deC: Referred pain from skeletal structures. J Nerv Ment Dis 99:660–667, 1944.
46. Keegan JJ, Garrett FD: The segmental distribution of the cutaneous nerves in the limbs of man. Anat Rec 102:409–437, 1948.
47. Kellgren JH: On the distribution of pain arising from deep somatic structures with charts of segmental pain areas. Clin Sci 4:35–46, 1939–1942.
48. Korr IM: Sustained sympathicotonia as a factor in disease. In The Neurobiologic Mechanisms in Manipulative Therapy. New York, Plenum, 1978, pp 229–268.
49. Korr IM, Thomas PE, Wright HM: Patterns of electrical skin resistance in man. Acta Neurovegetativa 77–96, 1958.
50. Korr IM, Wright HM, Chace JA: Cutaneous patterns of sympathetic activity in clinical abnormalities of the musculoskeletal system. Acta Neurovegetativa 589–606, 1964.
51. Korr IM, Wright HM, Thomas PE: Effects of experimental myofascial insults on cutaneous patterns of sympathetic activity in man. Acta Neurovegetativa 22–355, 1962.
52. Kraus H, Fischer AA: Diagnosis and treatment of myofascial pain. Mt Sinai J Med 58:235–239, 1991.
53. Lewit K: The needle effect in the relief of myofascial pain. Pain 6:83–90, 1979.
54. Maigne R: Diagnosis and Treatment of Pain of Vertebral Origin. Baltimore, Williams & Wilkins, 1996.
55. Maigne R: Pain syndromes of the thoracolumbar junction. A frequent source of misdiagnosis. Phys Med Rehabil Clin North Am 8:87–100, 1997.
56. Mamichev RV: An objective method for observing neuritis of the sciatic nerve. Klin Med 32:47–51, 1954.
57. Mense S: Nociception from skeletal muscle in relation to clinical muscle pain. Pain 54:241–289, 1993.
58. Mense S: Pathophysiologic basis of muscle pain syndromes. Phys Med Rehabil Clin North Am 8:23–53, 1997.
59. Pratzel HG: Application of pressure algometry in balneology for evaluation of physical therapeutic modalities and drug effects. In Fischer AA (ed): Muscle Pain Syndromes and Fibromyalgia. New York, Haworth Press, 1998, pp 111–137.
60. Rachlin ES: Trigger points. In Rachlin ES (ed.): Myofascial Pain and Fibromyalgia. St. Louis, Mosby, 1994, pp 145–157.
61. Reeves JL, Jaeger B, Graff-Radford SB: Reliability of the pressure algometer as a measure of myofascial trigger point sensitivity. Pain 24:313–321, 1986.
62. Richter CP, Woodruff BG: Facial patterns of electrical skin resistance. Their relation to sleep, external temperature, hair distribution, sensory dermatomes and skin disease. Bull Johns Hopkins Hosp 70:442–459, 1942.
63. Richter CP, Woodruff BG: Lumbar sympathetic dermatomes in man determined by the electrical skin resistance method. J Neurophysiol 8:323–338, 1945.
64. Travell JG, Simons DG: Myofascial Pain Dysfunction: The Trigger Point Manual: The Lower Extremities, vol. 1. Baltimore, Williams & Wilkins, 1983.
65. Tverskoy M, Cozacov C, Ayache M, et al: Postoperative pain after inguinal herniorrhaphy with different types of anaesthesia. Anaesth Analg 70:29–35, 1990.
66. Van Metre, Jr: Low electrical skin resistance in the region of pain in painful acute sinusitis. 409–415, 1949.
67. Vecchiet L, Dragani L, De Bigontina P, et al: Experimental referred pain and hyperalgesia from muscles in humans. In Vecchiet L, Albe-Fessard D, Lindblom U (eds): New Trends in Referred Pain and Hyperalgesia. Amsterdam, Elsevier, 1993, pp 239–249.
68. Vecchiet L, Giamberardino MA: Referred pain. Clinical significance, pathophysiology, and treatment. Phys Med Rehabil Clin North Am 8:119–136, 1997.
69. Waldorf T, Devlin L, Nansel DD: The comparative assessment of paraspinal tissue compliance in asymptomatic female and male subjects in both prone and standing positions. J Manipulative Physiol Ther 14:457–461, 1991.

24

Cervical Discography with CT and MRI Correlations

Joseph D. Fortin, D.O.

Learning is not attained by chance. It must be sought with ardor and attended to with diligence.

—Abigail Adams

The Scandinavian reports surrounding lumbar discography in the late 1940s and early 1950s invited an opportunity for comparable explorations in other areas of the spine.[19,28,52] Working independently in the late 1950s, Smith and Cloward developed similar cervical disc injection techniques for evaluating patients with cervicocephalgia and shoulder girdle pain.[5,7,47,48] They found that injection of symptomatic discs could reproduce patients' axial complaints, thereby identifying painful disc or differentiating primary discogenic versus neurogenic pain. To this end, Smith and Cloward used discography to select the proper levels for their cervical fusion techniques, which are still practiced.[6,49]

In the early 1960s, several large studies proclaimed that the contrast roentgenography study of discs was superior to myelography for evaluating patients with internal disc problems.[10,12] However, the prodiscography tide began to turn in 1964. Earl Holt studied 148 cervical discs with sodium diatrizoate (an irritating contrast medium) in 50 penitentiary inmates.[21] Fluoroscopic guidance was not employed, and the injection technique has been described as suspect in mechanical performance, discometric data, and imaging results.[2] Holt concluded that "injections into any cervical disc causes great pain" and "the volume of injectable media is also quite unreliable as an indication of pathology, since 93% of perfectly normal discs allow rapid extravasation."

Although Holt's study discouraged widespread acceptance of cervical discography, many authors have since reported favorable experience with discography in evaluating patients with chronic cervical syndromes.[1,3,9,16,18,24,30,33,36,41,43,51] Several studies clearly define a viable role for diagnostic disc injections in selecting symptomatic or deranged levels for a proposed anterior cervical fusion.[39,46,55]

During Holt's era, the disc was not viewed as the primary putative pain source but only as secondarily capable of causing pain through neurocompression. Many clinicians since have been reluctant to ascribe symptoms to a disc, however internally disrupted, that is not producing direct pressure on a nerve root. One study of cervical discography noted that pain on injection was indicative of disc abnormality but not diagnostic of protrusion.[25,26] The authors therefore discounted discography in general; one later concluded that induced pain, even if similar to the presenting symptoms, was of no diagnostic value.[25,26]

If the cervical annulus is an innervated ligamentous structure,[4,31] is it not capable of generating its own pain response when disrupted or strained?

The indications and preprocedural evaluation for cervical discography are comparable to those for lumbar discography, which is discussed in detail in chapter 25.

TECHNICAL PERFORMANCE OF DISCOGRAPHY

Cervical Diagnostic Disc Injection

Following sedation, as described in chapter 25, the patient is sterilely prepped and draped in the supine position (Fig. 24-1A).

The C-arm fluoroscope can be used alone or in combination with an overhead fluoroscopy unit.[2]

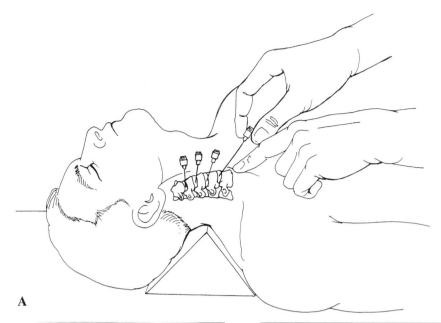

A

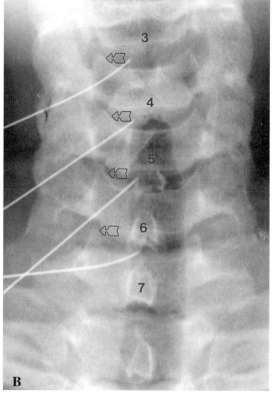

B

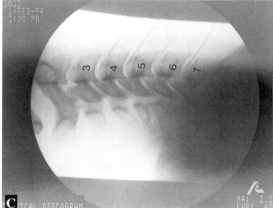

C

FIGURE 24-1. Cervical disc injection technique. *A*, The patient is positioned supine with the head extended over a triangular pillow. A right anterior approach is employed with the index finger applying pressure to move airway and vessels from the needle pathway. *B*, Compare this anteroposterior (AP) preinjection spot film with *A* and *D*. Again, consider the proximity of the needle at each level to its respective uncinate process (*arrows*). There is a gradual progression toward midline, paralleling the sternal head of the sternocleidomastoid muscle, from the C3–4 needle to the C6–7 one. All needles except the C6–7 one will need to be advanced to midline prior to injection. *C*, Preinjection lateral view. The inclination of the needles generally follows the cervical lordosis. *(Figure continued on next page.)*

Under the lateral beam of a C-arm, a segmentation count is taken first. A rule of thumb is to count down from the C2–3 level to at least one disc space below the lowest segment intended for study. Longitudinal, downward traction of the bilateral upper limbs is often necessary to optimally visualize the lower cervical segments because the overlying shoulders cause beam attenuation. This "screening process" allows an estimation of the orientation of each disc space, because the needle must enter at an angle commensurate with the amount of lordosis at the selected level. The posteroanterior beam is used to visualize the appropriate interspace, and the right uncinate process is identified as a landmark (Fig. 24-1B).

The left index finger applies firm pressure to divide the great vessels laterally and the laryngeal

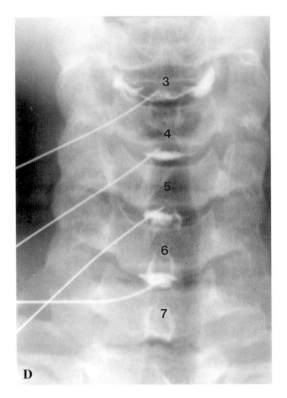

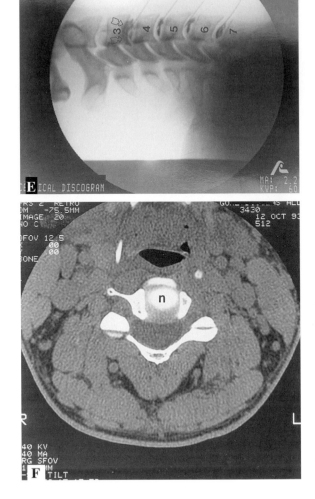

FIGURE 24-1 *(Cont.).* *D,* Postinjection AP projection. All needles have been advanced into the central nuclear zone (compare the needle tip positions with *C* as evidenced by the nucleograms. At C3–4, contrast extends into the bilateral uncinate recesses. *E,* Lateral nucleography spot film. Contrast is contained within the central nuclear region at each level except C3–4, where there is some "blushing" of the C3 inferior end plate secondary to uncinate recess extravasation (*arrows*). *F,* Postdiscography-CT discloses contrast circumscribed in the central nuclear zone (*n*) and substantiates the integrity of the nuclear envelope.

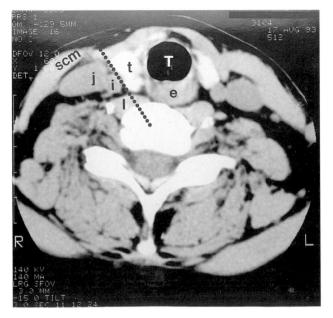

FIGURE 24-2. Axial CT at C6–7 (photographed at soft tissue window and level settings) demonstrates the relationship of soft tissue structures to the needle trajectory. T = trachea, t = thyroid, i = internal carotid artery, j = internal jugular vein, e = esophagus, l = longus colli muscle, scm = sternocleidomastoid muscle.

structures and trachea medially. This maneuver exposes a safe and adequate path for the right anterolateral needle trajectory, providing access to the disc while avoiding the great vessels, larynx, thyroid, and esophagus. The medial border of the sternocleidomastoid muscle is a relative skin surface marker for the needle position at each respective level. At the C2–3 and C3–4 levels, the hypopharynx must be avoided with a lateral entry point, and the apex of the lung must be considered at C7–T1 with medial entry point. A 25-gauge, 3.5-inch spinal needle is directed under the posteroanterior beam of an image intensifier into the selected interspace. Occasionally, the tensile strength of a 22-gauge needle is required to circumvent anterior spondylitic ridges or spurs.

The tip of the left index finger not only applies pressure at the correct site but also serves as a marker for percutaneous entry (see Fig. 24-1A). Once the skin and subcutaneous tissue is penetrated, the needle will course through the platysma muscle, the areolar tissue between the carotid sheath and larynx, the thin strap-like longus colli muscle, and the prevertebral fascia (Fig. 24-2) before purchasing the ligamentous substance of the anterior annulus. If the needle is directed past the medial aspect of the right uncinate process of the subjacent vertebrae toward the center of the interspace, it usually finds its way to the central nuclear zone. For depth confirmation, the novice discographer should learn to strike the end plate of the subjacent vertebrae prior to puncturing the annulus

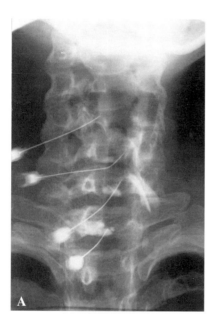

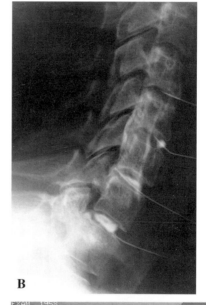

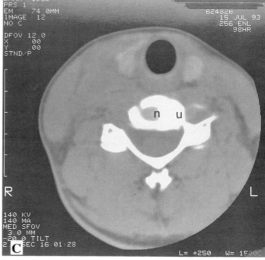

FIGURE 24-3. This 23-year-old college student was given a diagnosis of C4–5, C5–6, and C6–7 internal disc disruption. These films were sent to the author for review. Compare these photos with Figure 24-1. They represent a common misapplication of discography that facilitates its unfounded duplicitous reputation. A, AP view. The C4–5, C5–6, and C6–7 needles are malpositioned, rendering the study nondiagnostic. Based on this investigation, the above diagnosis is unsubstantiated because the only nuclear injection is at C7–T1. B, Lateral film. Note the annular injection at C5–6 and the bend in the needle (likely due to multiple passes). At the C6–7 the needle has been inadvertently advanced beyond the posterior annulus into the epidural space. The C7–T1 injection is nuclear. C, Postdiscography-CT at C5–6 documents a perinuclear-annular injection. The contrast is anterior and to the left lateral side of the central nuclear region.

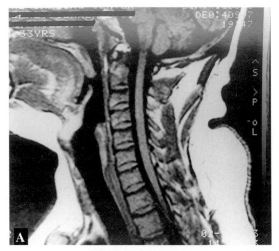

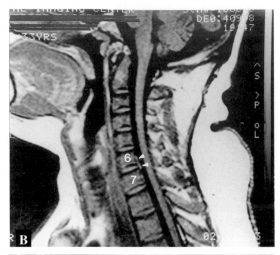

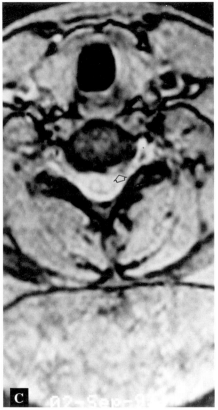

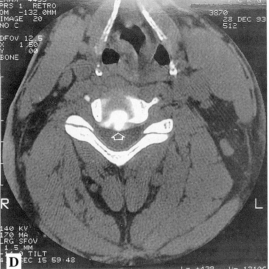

FIGURE 24-4. Imaging studies of a 33-year-old man who was rear-ended in a motor vehicle accident as he was looking at traffic over his left shoulder. *A,* T1-weighted (TR 455, TE 28, RF 90°) midline sagittal MR image is within normal limits. *B,* Left parasagittal T1 image (TR 500, TE 16, RF 90°) discloses a small disc extrusion at C6–7 *(arrows). C,* Same disc lesion *(arrowhead)* seen in *B* on gradient echo axial section (TR 1417, TE 18, RF 30°). *D,* At C4–5, an asymptomatic posterior radial fissure is revealed on postdiscography-CT *(arrowhead). (Figure continued on next page.)*

and then slightly withdraw and direct the needle upward into the disc space. Upon piercing of the annulus, the patient will experience an abrupt, unsustained pang of neck or shoulder girdle pain. Relative to its lumbar counterpart, the cervical annulus is meager and the depth of the disc space narrow; therefore, one must proceed with caution when advancing the needle beyond the annulus (Fig. 24-3). The needle depth and height within the disc space is now examined under the lateral beam (see Fig. 24-1C) and adjusted accordingly.

Discometry

Recording discometric data during operative intervention, Kambin observed that a normal cervical disc held 0.2–0.4 ml of solution while sustaining high intradiscal pressures.[22] Conversely, discs that allowed "posterior escape" of contrast medium accepted greater than 1.5 ml at low, wavering pressures. Herniated or degenerated discs with an intact outer annular capsule held intermediate volumes (0.5–1.5 ml) at sustained, yet intermediate,

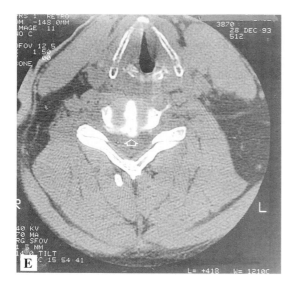 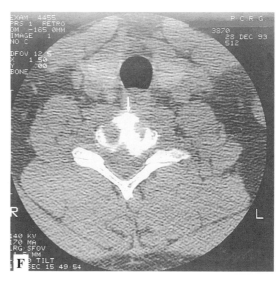

FIGURE 24-4 *(Cont.).* *E,* A radial fissure extends from the central nuclear zone into a concentric outer annular fissure or small prolapse at C5–6. Neither this lesion (which was provocation positive) or the one above were demonstrable on MRI (*arrowhead*). *F,* C6–7 postdiscography-CT (*arrowhead*). Compare with *B.* Also note the anterior circumferential fissuring (*arrow*).

pressures. In a cadaveric investigation, Saternus discovered that cervical discs that accepted more than 0.5 ml most often demonstrated posterolateral extravasation from the uncinate portions of the annulus.[42]

These studies indicate that cervical discometry yields reproducible information concerning discal hydrodynamic competence. Upon injection, the intact cervical disc holds less than 0.5 ml of solution, at which time a firm end point is appreciated. For complete details on discometry, see chapter 25.

Nucleography

Cervical nucleograms vary widely in configuration. They may appear spherical, disc shaped, or tubular. As in lumbar discograms, contrast material extravasating beyond the nuclear region indicates annular disruption; however, extension of contrast from the nucleus to the uncinate recesses is common and may simply reflect disc maturation.[20,37,45] Following adolescence, linear annular clefts develop that allow communication between the nucleus and the uncinate recesses.[20,45] Uncovertebral recesses are present only in adults. Curiously, one study demonstrated a slightly higher rate of provocation with flow of contrast material to the joints of Luschka.[38]

Lumbar postdiscography–computed tomography (CT) has been widely applied, but technical difficulties have hampered the acceptance of cervical postdiscography-CT. Because of the small

amount of contrast material employed and sparse dispersal pattern, transverse imaging of the elusive cervical nucleogram is challenging. High-resolution, thin-section CT may garner novel cervical imaging information.[14] At times, cervical magnetic resonance imaging (MRI) fails to identify annular and nuclear pathology because findings of annular fissures, small protrusions, annular attenuation, and nuclear degradation in subjects with normal MRI have been demonstrated by discography.[44] Obscuration may occur with MRI, because slice thickness (3.0–5.0 mm) is wide relative to the cervical nuclear region, and long acquisition sequences are susceptible to motion artifact and low signal-to-noise ratio.

Gradient echo images are prone to magnetic susceptibility and may erroneously create a pseudomyelographic effect. Cervical discography-CT may be employed to visualize pathology that may be confusing, ill-defined, or absent on MRI or CT (Fig. 24-4). The postdiscography data is obtained in 1.5-mm contiguous sections using a gantry angle commensurate with each interspace (Fig. 24-5).

The author initially employed postdiscography-CT to resolve the dilemma of small prolapse versus pseudoprolapse (i.e., extension of contrast medium into the recesses). If contrast medium extends to the uncinate recesses upon injecting, it may masquerade as a small prolapse on the lateral projection (Fig. 24-6). Orthogonal nucleography rectifies this problem. For further details on nucleography, please see chapter 25.

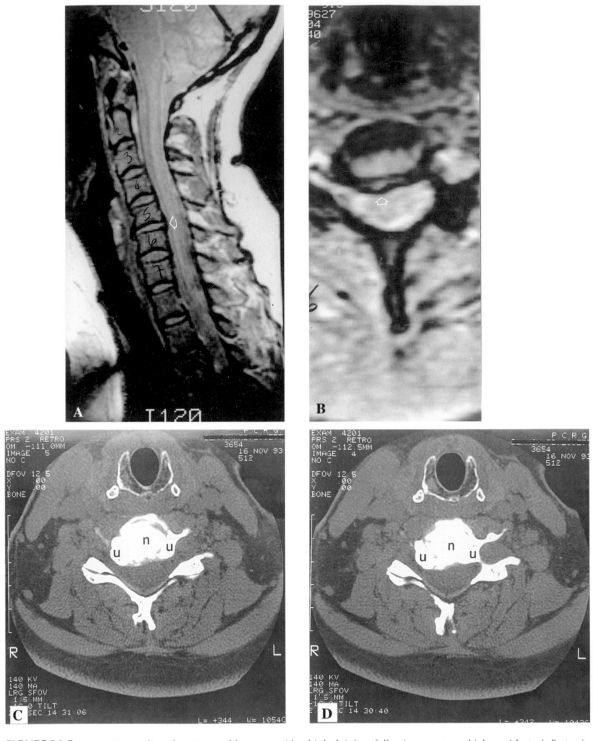

FIGURE 24-5. Imaging studies of a 39-year-old woman with whiplash injury following a motor vehicle accident. *A,* Fast spin echo sagittal MRI with spin density characteristics (TR 3380, TE 17 Ef). A mild, contained prolapse creates a myelographic-like impression at C5–6. *B,* On gradient echo axial section (TR 33, TE 15, RF 5°), a right paracentral herniation effaces the right anterolateral subarachnoid space. No cord compression is visualized. *C* and *D,* Thin section (1.5 mm) postdiscography-CT employing a bone algorithm and an angled gantry minimizes partial volume effect and provides optimal resolution of contrast within the disc space. Compare the contrast resolution and edge enhancement with Figures 24-3C and 24-6C. Cervical postdiscography-CT may provide information regarding the annular integrity that is not apparent on MRI. In addition to the above prolapse, these CT films reveal gross nuclear disarray, anterior outer annular circumferential fissuring, and contrast extending into the bilateral uncinate recesses.

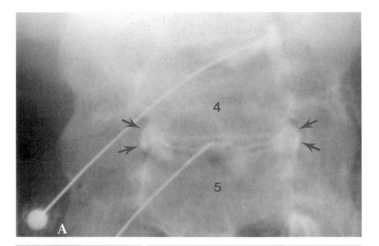

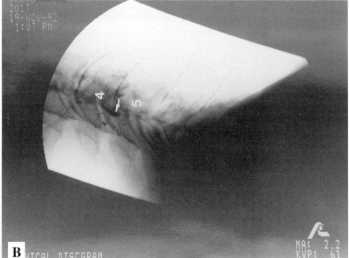

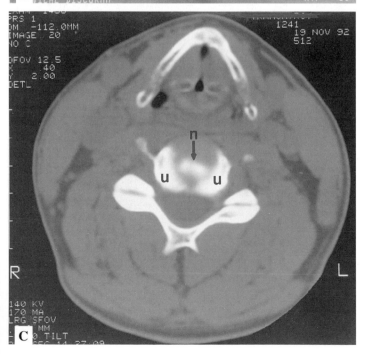

FIGURE 24-6. *"Pseudoprolapse." A,* Contrast in the uncinate recesses creates a bulbous appearance at C4–5 *(arrows)*. Incidentally, the needle tip at C3–4 is left of midline. The needle was repositioned following this photo. *B,* This lateral view suggests a posterior disc prolapse at C4–5 *(arrows)*. *C,* Post discography-CT axial section excludes a posterior prolapse and demonstrates contrast within nucleus *(n)* and uncinate recesses *(u)* only. The "pseudoprolapse" on the lateral view was created by contrast within the posterolateral-oriented recesses.

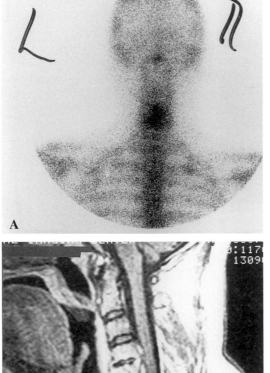

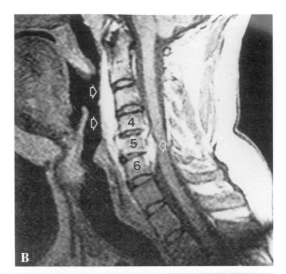

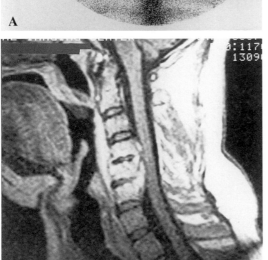

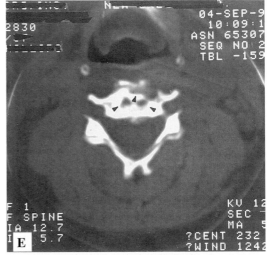

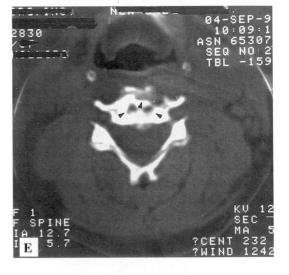

FIGURE 24-7. This patient presented with a history of crescendo neck and shoulder girdle pain and spasm. White blood cell count and sedimentation rate were markedly elevated (14,000 and 47, respectively). He was status post cervical discography at C3–4 through C6–7. *A,* Radionuclide scan demonstrates abnormal tracer uptake in the mid to lower cervical spine (about 2 weeks after the procedure). *B,* Gadolinium-enhanced T1-weighted (TR 500, TE 16, RF 90°) sagittal MRI discloses (1) collapse of C4–5 and C5–6 disc space with nascent end plate destructive changes, (2) vertebral body hyperemia as evidenced by the marrow enhancement (high signal), (3) retropharyngeal and prevertebral abscess, and (4) epidural abscess with cord compression but without intramedullary signal changes. This image was obtained 2 weeks after the procedure. *C,* One week following wide-spectrum IV antibiotic coverage (no organism was identified), a serial gadolinium-enhanced T1 MRI provides further testimony to a virulent organism. Hyperemic and destructive end plate changes have advanced despite the patient's subjective favorable response to treatment. The abscesses appear unchecked but may reflect a common lag between clinical response and imaging findings. *D,* Four weeks following antibiotic therapy (6 weeks postprocedure), both abscesses have dissipated, hyperemia has resolved, and spontaneous arthrodesis of the affected segments is occurring. No further signs of cord compression exist. *E,* Two months after the procedure transaxial CT (bone window and level settings) at C4–5 reveal "moth-eaten" low-density areas in the C4 end plate. An aggressive staphylococcal organism is a likely culprit of these osteolytic remains.

COMPLICATIONS

See chapter 25 for complete details on complications and information on postprocedural care. Although of low incidence, infection of the disc space is the most widely recognized complication associated with the performance of diagnostic disc injections, and once multiplication of bacteria has occurred it can lead to destruction of the vertebral end plates and degradation of the disc despite treatment with intravenous antibiotics (Fig. 24-7).[9–11,15,17,28,34,40,54] In a prospective clinical trial, Osti et al. instilled cefazolin into the discs of 127 patients undergoing discography.[34] None of the 127 patients developed any clinical or radiographic evidence of discitis. A single prophylactic dose of a broad-spectrum antibiotic during discography suffices to prevent disc space infection.[34]

The potential for permanent damage to the disc from puncture or distension is speculative. Oddly, Smith and Kim attributed a herniated cervical disc to the performance of discography.[47] In their case report, Smith and Kim provide gradient echo sagittal MRI images that demonstrate that the patient already had a disc prolapse prior to the procedure. The prolapse was simply enlarged following the procedure. Additionally, the patient's sedimentation rate was 55 mm per hour (normal less than 20), increasing to 70 mm per hour, and the white blood cell count was 12,700. To no surprise, a bone scan obtained within 24 hours of the procedure was normal. Two days following the procedure the patient underwent anterior discectomy/corpectomy with spinal decompression because the patient was experiencing progressive neurologic symptoms. The surgical findings revealed a thickened and edematous posterior longitudinal ligament as well as scattered inflammatory cells and a few white blood cells in the interspace. The clinical presentation and surgical findings are suspicious for an iatrogenically induced chemical or aseptic discitis.[11]

Fernstrom attributed 6 lumbar disc herniations to discography on performing more than 1500 disc injections.[13] He did not have the aid of fluoroscopic guidance nor the ability to validate these findings with transverse imaging. With the exception of Smith and Kim's suspect report, no modern studies have related disc damage to the performance of diagnostic disc injections.

CONTRAINDICATIONS

Cervical discography is potentially life threatening when contraindicated. For example, discography in a patient with evidence of cord compression, such as spasticity, weakness, and paresthesias from a massive disc prolapse, has resulted in frank quadriplegia.[27] Discography is contraindicated in patients with central stenosis,[53] myelopathy, neoplasms, infections, infiltrative processes, and relative (borderline) stenosis[53] combined with bilateral root canal stenosis, especially when multiple levels are involved.

Prima facie imaging studies, which adequately assess spinal stenosis and cord compression, must be examined prior to cervical discography. While MRI is superior in examining the intrinsic substance of the cord, significant annular tears at times escape MRI detection, and cervical internal disc disruption will not be diagnosed unless discography is performed.[35,44] CT affords greater osseous detail and spatial resolution in evaluating stenosis.[23,32] In this setting, MRI is hampered by thicker sections and variable signal intensity in degenerative osseous ridges.[32] With equal or greater accuracy, intrathecal-enhanced CT resolves extradural compression from bone or disc material on neural elements, such as theca, cord, or dural pouches.[32]

CONCLUSION

Cervical discography is an important adjunct for definitively diagnosing primary discogenic pain.[35] It should not be used as a screening imaging modality. In fact, cervical diagnostic disc injection should not be performed, even when clinically warranted, until other imaging studies such as high-resolution CT or MRI have been thoroughly studied. Pain provocation is the sine qua non of discography. Additionally, nucleography in the transverse mode may enhance imaging information garnered by CT or MRI.[14]

REFERENCES

1. Altenstein G: Erfahrungen mit der diskographic anhals und lendenwirbelsaule. Z Orthop 102:358–366, 1967.
2. Aprill CN III: Diagnostic disc injection. In Frymoyer JW (ed): The Adult Spine: Principles and Practice, 2nd ed. Philadelphia, Lippincott-Raven, 1997, pp 523–538.
3. Bettag W, Grote W: Die bedeutung der diskographie fur die behandlung des "zervikalsyndroms." Hippokrates 40:138–141, 1969.
4. Bogduk N, Windsor M, Inglis A: The innervation of the cervical intervertebral discs. Spine 13:2–8, 1988.
5. Cloward RB: Cervical diskography. Technique, indications and use in the diagnosis of ruptured cervical disks. Am J Radiol 79:563–574, 1958.
6. Cloward RB: The anterior approach for removal of ruptured cervical disks. J Neurosurg 15:602–617, 1958.
7. Cloward RB: Cervical diskography. A contribution to the etiology and mechanism of neck, shoulder, and arm pain. Ann Surg 150:1052–1064, 1959.

8. Cloward RB: Cervical diskography. Acta Radiol Suppl (Stockh) 1:675–688, 1963.
9. Cloward RB: Cervical diskography defended [letter]. JAMA 233:862, 1975.
10. Collis JS Jr, Gardner WJ: Lumbar discography. An analysis of 1,000 cases. J Neurosurg 19:452–461, 1962.
11. Crock H: Practice of Spinal Surgery. New York, Springer Verlag, 1983.
12. Feinberg SB: The place of discography in radiology as based on 2,320 cases. AJR Am J Roentgenol 92:1275–1281, 1964.
13. Fernstrom U: A discographical study of ruptured lumbar intervertebral discs. Acta Chir Scand Suppl 258:1–60, 1960.
14. Fortin JD: Cervical nucleography and post discography/CT [unpublished data]. 1991.
15. Fraser RD: Chymopapain for the treatment of intervertebral disc herniation: The final report of a double blind study. Spine 9:815–818, 1984.
16. Grote W, Wappenschmidt J: Uber technik und indikation zur-zervikalen diskographie. Rofo Fortschr Geb Rontgenstr Neuen Bildgeb Verfahr 106:721–727, 1967.
17. Guyer RD, Collier R, Stith WJ, et al: Discitis after discography. Spine 13:1352–1354, 1988.
18. Hatt MU: Hohenlokalisation der cervicalen discushernie in klinil, elektromyographe (EMG) und myelographie. Dtsch Zeitschr Nerveheilk 197:56–65, 1969.
19. Hirsch C: An attempt to diagnose level of disc lesion clinically by disc puncture. Acta Orthop Scand 18:131–140, 1948.
20. Hirsch C, Schajowicz R, Galante J: Structural changes in the cervical spine: A study on autopsy specimens in different age groups. Acta Orthop Scand Suppl 109:7–77, 1967.
21. Holt EP Jr: Fallacy of cervical discography: Report of 50 cases in normal subjects. JAMA 188:799–801, 1964.
22. Kambin P, Abda S, Kurpicki F: Intradiskal pressure and volume recording: Evaluation of normal and abnormal cervical disks. Clin Orthop 146:144–147, 1980.
23. Karnaze MG, Gado MH, Sartor KJ, Hodges FJ III: Comparison of MR and CT myelography in imaging the cervical and thoracic spine. AJR Am J Roentgenol 150:397–403, 1988.
24. Kikuchi S, Macnab I, Moreau P: Localization of the level of symptomatic cervical disc herniation. J Bone Joint Surg 63B:272–277, 1981.
25. Klafta LA Jr, Collis JS Jr: The diagnostic inaccuracy of the pain response in cervical discography. Cleve Clin Q 36:35–39, 1969.
26. Klafta LA Jr, Collis JS Jr: An analysis of cervical discography with surgical verification. J Neurosurg 30:38–41, 1969.
27. Laun A, Lorenz R, Agnoli AL: Complications of cervical discography. J Neurosurg Sci 25:17–22, 1981.
28. Lindblom K: Technique and results of diagnostic disc puncture and injection (discography) in the lumbar region. Acta Orthop Scand 20:315–326, 1951.
29. Lownie SP, Ferguson GG: Spinal subdural empyema complicating cervical discography. Spine 14:1415–1417, 1989.
30. Massare C, Bard M, Tristant H: Cervical discography: Speculation on technique and indications from our own experience. J Radiol 55:395–399, 1974.
31. Mendel T, Wink C, Zimny M: Neural elements in human cervical intervertebral discs. Spine 17:132–135, 1992.
32. Modic MT, Masaryk TJ, Mulopulos GP, et al: Cervical radiculopathy: Prospective evaluation with surface coil MR imaging, CT with metrizamide and metrizamide myelography. Radiology 161:753–759, 1986.
33. North American Spine Society: Position statement on discography. The Executive Committee of the North American Spine Society. Spine 13:1343, 1988.
34. Osti OL, Fraser RD, Vernon-Roberts B: Discitis after discography. The role of prophylactic antibiotics. J Bone Joint Surg 72B:271–274, 1990.
35. Parfenchuck TA, Janssen ME: A correlation of cervical magnetic resonance imaging and discography/computed tomographic discograms. Spine 19:2819–2825, 1994.
36. Pascaud JL, Mailhes F, Pascaud E, et al: The cervical intervertebral disc: Diagnostic value of cervical discography in degenerative and post-traumatic lesions. Ann Radiol (Paris) 23:455–460, 1980.
37. Payne EE, Spillane JD: The cervical spine. Brain 80:572–596, 1957.
38. Poletti SC, Handal JA: Cervical discography: Morphology versus pain response. Presented at the annual meeting of the North American Spine Society, Boston, July 1992.
39. Riley LH Jr, Robinson RA, Johnson KA, Walker AE: The results of anterior interbody fusion of the cervical spine: Review of 93 consecutive cases. J Neurosurg 30:127–133, 1969.
40. Roosen K, Bettag W, Fiebach O: Komplikationen der cervikalen diskographie. Rofo Fortschr Geb Rontgenstr Neuen Bildgeb Verfahr 122:520–527, 1975.
41. Roth DA: Cervical analgesic discography: A new test for the definitive diagnosis of painful-disc syndrome. JAMA 235:1713–1714, 1976.
42. Saternus KS, Bornscheuer HH: [Comparative radiologic and pathologic-anatomic studies on the value of discography in the diagnosis of acute intervertebral disc injuries in the cervical spine]. [German]. Rofo Fortschr Geb Rontgenstr Neuen Bildgeb Verfahr 139:651–657, 1983.
43. Schaerer JP: Anterior cervical disc removal and fusion. Schweiz Arch Neurol Neurochir Psychiatr 102:331–334, 1968.
44. Schellhas KP, Smith MD, Gundry CR, Pollei SR: Cervical discogenic pain. Prospective correlation of magnetic resonance imaging and discography in asymptomatic subjects and pain sufferers. Spine 21:300–311; discussion 311–312, 1996.
45. Sherk H, Parke W: Developmental anatomy. In Bailey RW (ed): The Cervical Spine. Philadelphia, JB Lippincott, 1983, pp 7–8.
46. Simmons EH, Segil CM: An evaluation of discography in the localization of symptomatic levels in discogenic disease of the spine. Clin Orthop 108:57–69, 1975.
47. Smith GW: The normal cervical diskogram with clinical observations. AJR Am J Roentgenol 81:1006–1010, 1959.
48. Smith GW, Nichols P Jr: Technique for cervical discography. Radiology 68:718–720, 1957.
49. Smith GW, Robinson RA: The treatment of certain cervical spine disorders by anterior removal of the intervertebral disc and interbody fusion. J Bone Joint Surg 40A:607–623, 1958.
50. Smith MD, Kim SS: A herniated cervical disc resulting from discography: An unusual complication. J Spinal Disord 3:392–395, 1990.
51. Stuck RM: Cervical discography. AJR Am J Roentgenol 86:975–982, 1961.
52. Unander-Scharin L: Diskografier. Nord Med 57:116, 1957.
53. Verbiest H: Fallacies of the present definition, nomenclature and classification of the stenoses of the lumbar vertebral canal. Spine 1:217–225, 1976.
54. Volgelsang H: Discitis intervertrablis cervicalis nach diskographie. Neurochirurgia 16:80–83, 1973.
55. Whitecloud TS III, Seago RA: Cervical discogenic syndrome: Results of operative intervention in patients with positive discography. Spine 12:313–317, 1987.

25

Lumbar and Thoracic Discography with CT and MRI Correlation

Joseph D. Fortin, D.O., Nalini Sehgal, M.D., and Ricardo A. Nieves, M.D.

There is no sadder or more frequent obituary on the pages of time than "We have always done it this way."

—The English Digest

HISTORICAL PERSPECTIVE

To appreciate the historical controversy surrounding discography is to understand that its inception was a tenuous one, tainted by admonitions, suppositions, and contradictions. Before the description of herniated discs by Mixter and Barr in 1934, posterior disc prolapses were routinely mistaken for chondromas of the disc.[71] Goldthwait (1911) had long before suspected the disc to be the major offender in cases of lumbago and sciatica, but was ignored. Later, Mixter and Barr's work focused attention on the tendency of the disc to prolapse posteriorly into the spinal canal or the neuroforamen, cause cord compression or neurocompromise, and evoke sciatica.[71] The Mixter and Barr precepts not only became the central model of spine pain but also unfortunately fixated the medical community and diverted attention from other possible causes for several years. This neurocompressive model of disc pathology, however, accounted for only a small percentage of all patients presenting with axial complaints.[98,112]

In the early 1930s, low back pain was usually treated with triple arthrodesis, i.e., fusion of lumbosacral articulations and the sacroiliac joints bilaterally. This treatment approach reflected the prevalent shotgun mind-set to a complex problem wherein extensive spine surgeries were performed without defining the actual source of low back pain. The futility of treating without localizing the pain generator prompted Steindler and Luck to utilize procaine hydrochloride injections for allocating the source of pain in low back pain disorders. In order to establish causal connection between local pain and radiation of pain unrelated to direct nerve root compression, they recommended stringent fulfillment of five criteria.[103] These principles of provocation-analgesic response have been integrated into the diagnostic armamentarium of the spinal interventionist and serve to identify pain generators in the spine. Carl Hirsch in 1948 was the first to use this principle in localizing pain to lumbar discs in subjects with back pain. He described pain relief following intradiscal instillation of small volumes of Novocain.[52] This raised the possibility of an intradiscal pain mechanism independent of the neurocompressive model of disc-mediated pain.

A neurogenic substrate for discogenic pain independent of a neurocompressive paradigm was established in 1940 when Roofe reported on the innervation of the annulus fibrosus.[86] Half a century later this basic science information was applied by Vanharanta et al. to demonstrate and explain pain provocation in mid to outer annular fissures.[110] Using sophisticated staining and magnification techniques, the rich innervation of the mid to outer layers of the annulus has since been substantiated independently by other investigators.[15,44,67,117] With the information available today, which includes the awareness of potent inflammatory mediators within the nucleus of disrupted discs[89] and low-pressure, chemical sensitization of annular nociceptors,[32] the need to expand the concept of spine pain beyond a purely mechanical model is obvious.

Four years after Roofe's discovery, Knut Lindblom demonstrated the presence of radial annular fissures by injecting cadaveric discs.[63] He watched with fascination as red lead dye from the injected nucleus leaked into attenuated annular areas. Could disc injections be employed to detect annular pathology in patients with low back pain? Lindblom hesitated for fear of disc damage; case reports in the literature warned of possible disc damage. These admonitions stemmed from iatrogenic discitis that followed inadvertent disc puncture on attempted lumbar thecal puncture in children with purulent meningitis.[24,81] However, the claims of disc damage, secondary to disc puncture, have never been rigidly validated.[40] Encouraged by Carl Hirsch's reports of no secondary disc "damage" on intraoperative disc injections, Lindblom then described the nucleographic patterns of 15 discs in 13 patients and thereby provided the catalyst for future investigations.[64]

At a time when discography was poised to eclipse myelography as the premier disc imaging study in evaluating patients with internal disc pathology,[24,38] Holt published his data on discography.[54] Reports of high false-positive rates of 37% for lumbar disc injections and 100% for cervical disc injections swiftly turned the tide against discography. Holt sought to demonstrate that a disc that is internally disrupted or nondemonstrable on myelography should not be an indication for surgery.

The same year as Holt's lumbar study, Wiley et al. studied 2517 disc injections and reported a viable role for discography in the diagnostic evaluation of patients with axial pain and no definite disc prolapse on myelography.[114] However, Wiley's study was overshadowed by Holt's; the medical community seemed impervious to accepting favorable discography reports. Unfortunately, Holt's work continues to be cited as an authoritative treatise to discount discography.

Critical reviews of Holt's methods have found his data to be flawed by poor selection, technical inadequacies, and fallacious interpretation.[100,111] Employing modern techniques, a well-controlled prospective study refuted Holt's data.[111] Unlike Holt, Walsh et al. considered a provocative discogram positive only if the disc was radiographically abnormal and the patient's pain pattern was reproduced during the administration of the injection.[111] The false-positive rate in the Walsh study was 0% compared to 26% in Holt's study. Walsh and colleagues found discography to be a highly specific and reliable method of distinguishing symptomatic versus asymptomatic discs. Additionally, a host of investigations have disclosed an important application of both cervical and lumbar diagnostic disc injections in prefusion planning.[13,19,33,99,114] Specifically, if the levels selected for fusion are based on discography, the success rate is high.

Holt's studies are a reflection of their time, limited by methodology and technology[4,28,100]; still Holt's work continues to haunt discographers to this day. The medical community remains divided on some of the same fundamental issues of Holt's time such as the existence of internal disc disruption and the value of discography.[16] There are those who feel that this procedure has no demonstrable benefit in improving patient outcomes and in fact leads to inappropriate surgery. Conversely, many proponents consider discography a superior tool that garners vital dynamic information on the disc hitherto unrivaled by any other available spinal diagnostic modality.[46]

WHEN IS DISCOGRAPHY INDICATED?

In 1988 the Executive Committee of the North American Spine Society released its Position Statement on Discography[77] and reaffirmed it subsequently in 1995[46]:

Discography is indicated in the evaluation of patients with unremitting spinal pain, with or without extremity pain, of greater than four months' duration, when the pain has been unresponsive to all appropriate methods of conservative therapy. Before discography, the patients should have undergone investigation with other modalities which have failed to explain the source of pain; such modalities should include, but not be limited to, either CT scanning, MRI scanning and/or myelography. In these circumstances, discography, especially when followed by CT scanning may be the only study capable of providing a diagnosis by permitting a precise description of the internal anatomy of a disc and a detailed determination of the integrity of the disc substructures. Additionally, the anatomic observations may be complimented by the critical physiologic induction of pain which is recognized by the patient as similar to or identical with his/her clinical complaint. By including multiple levels in the study, the patient acts as his/her own control for evaluation of the reliability of the pain response.[77]

Discography is invaluable in ruling out secondary internal disc disruption or recurrent herniation in the postoperative patient, exploring pseudarthrosis, determining the number of levels to include in a spine fusion, and determining the primary symptom-producing level when chemonucleolysis is contemplated.[23] It aids in determining the significance of equivocal or multiple level abnormalities, defining surgical options, and evaluating the previously operated spine.[5,11,50,69] In patients with persistent symptoms, despite a normal or equivocal magnetic resonance imaging (MRI) study, discography is used to establish a diagnosis of internal disc disruption.[18,123]

Predicating treatment on a rapidly established diagnosis is the key to successful treatment and to preventing long-term disability from misdiagnosis or improper treatment and recidivism. If a patient has failed an initial trial of aggressive functional restoration, the use of spinal diagnostic injections (including discography) can be extremely effective in pinpointing the pain generators. In this setting, the authors have safely employed discography to establish a definitive diagnosis to tailor the course of a rehabilitation program to that specific diagnosis. Moreover, simply validating the patient's pain can, at times, be a potent boost for the healing process. Obviously, the potential for complications should be considered in the decision-making process before the patient undergoes any spinal injection procedure.

PREPROCEDURAL EVALUATION

Patient education is the most crucial element of the intake evaluation. It serves not only to fulfill requirements of informed consent, but most importantly to allay anxiety and allow the patient to become actively involved in the overall process. The patient is informed of what to expect before, during, and following the procedure. An anatomic model is used to explain the technical aspects of the procedure and to answer questions or concerns accordingly. Screening information obtained from the patient should include history of allergy, recent instrumentation, dental procedures or surgery, and untreated illness or infection. Vital signs are assessed, and the patient completes a pain diagram, a Dallas Pain Questionnaire,[61] and a baseline Visual Analogue Scale (VAS) for pain.

The Dallas Pain Questionnaire affords a basic understanding of how profoundly the patient's condition has impacted his or her physical and psychosocial function. This tool can provide a basis for understanding the patient's response to pain, a cardinal element of the study.

The postprocedural VAS is compared with the preprocedural one. The pain diagram, history (e.g., mechanism of injury), physical examination, and review of imaging studies aid the physician in selecting appropriate levels to study.

TECHNICAL PERFORMANCE OF LUMBAR DISCOGRAPHY

Three to five milligrams of intravenous midazolam (Versed) is administered preprocedurally over 3–5 minutes. The dose is titrated according to the patient's response. This allows an adequate level of sedation (because the patient is responsive and able to converse throughout) and prevents the recognized threat of profound respiratory depression associated with benzodiazepines.[47] Nonetheless, immediate ventilatory support must be available.

Most lumbar discs are readily and safely cannulated by a postero-oblique, extrapedicular approach. This technique, which has been described by Trosier[108] and modified by Aprill,[6] prevents the potential complications associated with thecal puncture from a transdural approach.[68]

Contraindications to an extrapedicular approach (in general) include bilateral severe lateral stenosis, bilateral conjoint nerve root sleeve anomalies, cystic nerve root dilatation, and obstruction of posterolateral fusion mass or instrumentation.[6]

Lateral approaches render the segmental nerves more vulnerable,[25,30,34] as evidenced by studying the nerve pathway[26,48,84] in relation to the proposed needle trajectories for these techniques. Bowel perforation is another complication associated with the lateral approach.[9]

High-resolution, thin-section computed tomography (CT) or high–field strength MRI should be studied prior to the procedure to allow the technical performance to accommodate the patient's anatomy.

The first task in performing a lumbar diagnostic disc injection is to select the level(s) and side of entry. If an anterior lumbar fusion is proposed for a patient with an L4–5 disc prolapse, the L3–4 and L5–S1 levels must also be studied to exclude the possibility of a symptomatic fissure at an adjacent level. Failure to appreciate this potential scenario may prevent a successful surgical outcome (if all affected levels are not included in the fusion mass).

The side of the patient from which to approach the disc(s) in question must be selected prior to the procedure. A left postero-oblique approach is used for a right posterolateral prolapse (and vice versa) to allow maximal visualization of the lesion following nucleography. The side contralateral to the patient's symptoms is also preferred to prevent needle-induced nociception from conflicting with the provocation response.

Once the patient is adequately sedated and sterilely prepped and draped, a segmentation count is undertaken in the prone position. Anomalous lumbosacral junctions or hemivertebrae must be identified and numbered accordingly, as these anomalies may lead to surgery at the wrong level.

C-arm fluoroscopy does not involve complex patient positioning maneuvers and allows adjustments for the lordotic curve. The patient usually lies prone with the face turned to either side. When the disc is accessed by a left postero-oblique approach, a foam wedge is placed under the left side of the patient to optimize visualization of the disc. This maneuver is necessary because the C-arm will not rotate past 45° to the left of the patient in the axial plane. Depending on the patient's lordotic curve, the clinician selects needle trajectory angles congruent with the lordosis at each level (Fig. 25-1A). The operator's attention is then directed to the subjacent superior articular process of the disc to be studied. Slowly, the C-arm fluoroscope is rotated in an axial plane, from a direct anteroposterior position into an

oblique position, until the superior articular process of the subjacent vertebra bisects the disc space under study. Tilting the C-arm fluoroscope in a cephalocaudad direction will superimpose the lateral margins of the end plates and open up the disc space for needle entry. Sometimes the patient may need to be gently rotated into a slight prone oblique position to discern the optimum angle for approach.

When using an overhead fluoroscopy unit, a "preview" of the patient's lordotic curve is initially obtained in the lateral decubitus position. Then, the patient is slowly rolled forward from a lateral decubitus position to a modified Sims' or prone oblique position (Fig. 25-1B). The patient's arm closest to

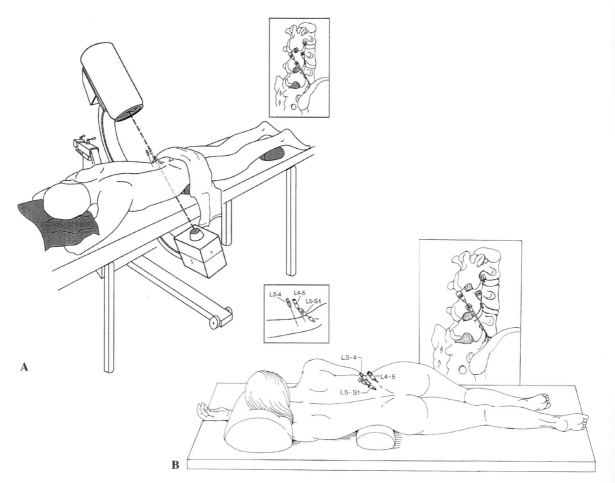

FIGURE 25-1. Technical performance of lumbar disc injection. *A,* Prone position for lumbar diagnostic disc injection using the C-arm fluoroscope. The patient lies prone with the head turned to one side; a small foam wedge is positioned under the abdomen to decrease the lumbar lordosis. The C-arm is rotated in an axial plane and is tilted cephalocaudad commensurate with the inclination of the spinal needle. Insets reveal the relationship of needles to bony landmarks and to each other (*top*) and the change in inclination of the needles to the skin surface from L3–4 to L5–S1 (*bottom*). Note the L5–S1 needle is inferior and medial to the L4–5 needle. *B,* Modified Sims' position for lumbar diagnostic disc injection. The arm adjacent the table is outstretched under a pillow. A figure-of-four position is assumed for the lower extremities. Note the progressive inclination of the needles to the skin surface from L3–4 to L5–S1. The inset discloses the relationship of needles to anatomic landmarks (e.g., superior articular processes and angle of respective interspaces) and to each other from an oblique projection. *C,* Preinjection oblique radiograph. Compare this plain film with *A* and *B.* The L4–5 interspace is marked with arrows to identify landmarks for optimal patient position (see text). A bent-needle technique was employed at L5–S1 (3, 4, 5, 1 = respective pedicles).

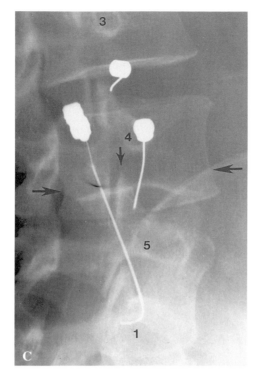

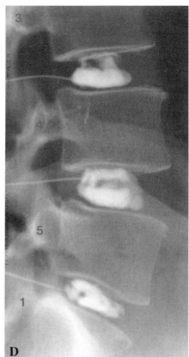

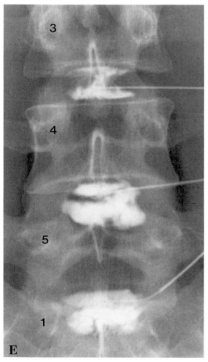

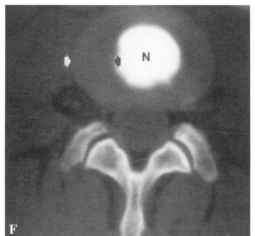

FIGURE 25-1 *(Cont.).*   *D,* Lateral nucleography. Smooth margins and spherical configurations attest to the integrity of these discs. The needles are in the mid to lower portions of the root canals. *E,* Posteroanterior nucleography. Again at each level contrast is well contained by the nuclear envelope. *F,* Normal L4–5 lumbar post-discography-CT. A classic circular configuration documents that contrast medium is within the central nuclear zone (*n*). The strength and integrity of the annular "ligament" is underscored by its thickness (*arrowheads*).

the table should be outstretched overhead and a pillow fashioned between the outstretched arm and the patient's head. The lower limbs are oriented in a near figure-of-four.

Under fluoroscopic visualization, a marker is placed laterally on the back at the site of proposed needle entry site in the skin. The needle will access the disc through a postero-oblique approach. With a 25-gauge, 3.5-inch spinal needle, local anesthetic (1% lidocaine) is dispersed down to the superior articular process along the proposed needle track. If 25-gauge needles are to be employed for the disc

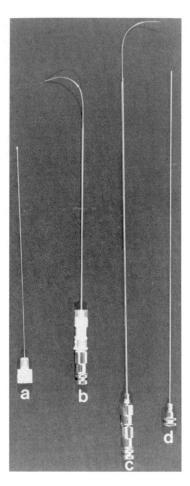

FIGURE 25-2.   Primary tools of the discography trade. A 25-gauge, 3.5-inch spinal needle (a). This is routinely used for anesthetic infiltration prior to passing a larger procedure needle and is also employed as a procedure needle for cervical and thoracic discography. A 20-gauge, 3.5-inch outer trocar-25-gauge, 5.5-inch inner bent procedure needle (b). The bend is greater than in c. This is the conventional set-up for L5–S1. An 18-gauge, 6-inch outer trocar, 25-gauge, 8-inch inner bent procedure needle (c). This combination is necessary for very large or obese patients. A 22-gauge, 6-inch spinal needle (d), the workhorse of lumbar discography.

injection, local anesthesia is not necessary because the dysesthetic "sting" associated with local anesthesia is often more painful than needle-induced nociception.

Lumbar discography can often be accomplished with 25-gauge needles; however, the needle should be selected according to the patient's body habitus (Fig. 25-2). For large, muscular, or tense patients, a 25-gauge needle may not provide enough tensile strength for "steering." A 22-gauge needle will allow ample maneuverability. Six-inch needles are adequate in length for most patients, although the authors have used 10-inch needles for a few obese patients. Lumbar discs in thin patients may be

accessible by the same 3.5-inch, 25-gauge needles used for cervical discography.

Guided by the fluoroscopic beam, the spinal needle penetrates the skin, subcutaneous adipose, lumbodorsal fascia, and muscle and passes along the lateral aspect of the tip of the superior articular process, through the annulus, and into the nuclear region. At the lumbosacral junction, the sensitive iliotransverse ligament must also be penetrated. Before the needle enters the "spongy" nucleus, it passes through the distinctive "springy" yet coarse annular ligament. On piercing the annulus, the patient will experience an abrupt, unsustained pang of back pain. If the needle deflects off the superior articular process laterally, directing the needle tip inward (toward the disc) and the bevel outward will reorient it toward the nucleus.

As noted above, the tip of the superior articular process is a general reference point, but the needle position is adjusted according to the height of the superior articular process in relationship to the segmental nerve root and end plates. The tip of a long, narrow superior articular process may lie dangerously close to the dorsal root ganglion or anterior ramus of the segmental nerve. Conversely, a needle directed along a stubby superior articular process may find its path interrupted by the lower end plate, unless adjusted upward. In general, the discography needle should be kept within the lower one-third of the root canal.[48] A careful preprocedural review of the CT and MRI will allow accurate identification of the pertinent anatomic relationships.

The ease and proficiency by which the L5–S1 disc injection is accomplished is the litmus test of any discographer's skill. The lumbosacral inclination and iliac crest provide a challenge unique to this level. Except in patients with a low intercrestal line, the anatomy of this level necessitates a bent-needle approach. The technique employed has been likened to Laredo's chemonucleolysis technique.[6,59]

Selecting a method and angle of approach for cannulating the L5–S1 disc should ultimately be a function of the "safe window" available for a given trajectory. A "window" is the potential three-dimensional pathway of tissue that would allow a needle to pass from the skin to its target point safely and uninterrupted. The body habitus, iliac crest, lordosis, L5 segmental nerve, and L5 transverse process all must be factored into the trajectory selection.

With the patient in a slight prone-oblique orientation (approximately 25°), a trocar is positioned to act as a guide for advancement of an inner, bent procedure needle (Fig. 25-3). A 3.5-inch, 20-gauge outer trocar with a 6-inch, 25-gauge inner needle is the usual combination, except for very large or rotund patients, who may require a 6-inch, 18-gauge outer trocar and an 8-inch, 22- or 25-gauge inner needle combination (see Figure 25-2).

The bony notch between the sacral ala and superior articular process of S1 is the target for the guide (Fig. 25-3A). In the sagittal plane, the percutaneous site must be congruent with the lumbosacral angle, and in the axial plane it must be lateral enough to ensure the trocar will direct the bent needle medially (avoiding the L5 segmental nerve). On occasion, bony obstacles such as the iliac crest or L5 transverse process will not allow the operator to select the optimal trajectory. Such predicaments can be assuaged by skill in maneuvering the two-needle system and selecting an appropriate bend for the inner needle.

Once the trocar has been advanced to the aforementioned notch, its position is observed in the lateral projection relative to the lumbosacral angle and L5 nerve root canal (Fig. 25-3B). The tip of the trocar

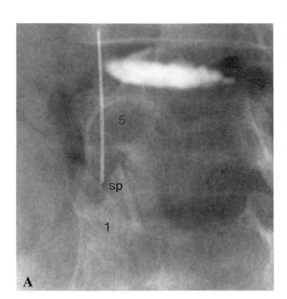

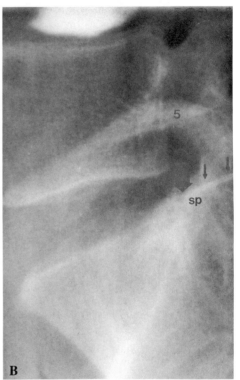

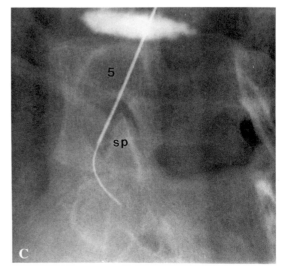

FIGURE 25-3. L5–S1 disc injection technique. *A*, A 20-gauge, 3.5-inch trocar is in position, abutting the S1 superior articular process. (5 = pedicle of L5; 1 = pedicle of S1.) *B*, Lateral view demonstrates position of trocar (*arrows*). Note the trocar is in the inferior aspect of the root canal and advanced to the anterior margin of the S1 superior articular process (*large arrow*). *C*, A 25-gauge, 6-inch bent spinal needle has been railroaded through the trocar. It was successfully directed around the superior articular process and under the L5 segmental nerve and is in the central nuclear zone.

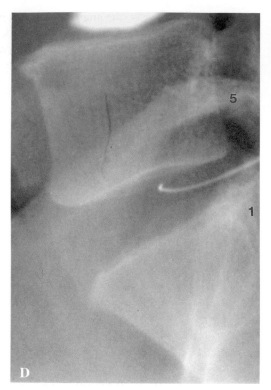

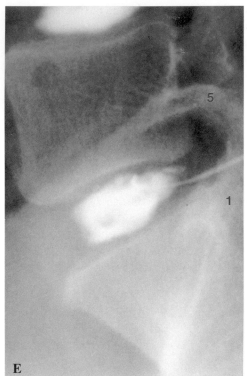

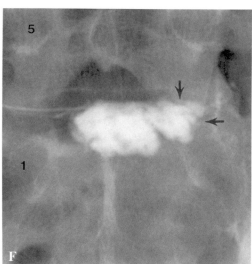

FIGURE 25-3 *(Cont.).*   *D,* The bent needle is in the center of the disc space. *E,* Normal L5–S1 nucleogram in the lateral projection. *F,* An L5–S1 nucleogram in AP projection. There is a slight lateral annular fissure (*arrows*) to the midannulus on the right. This was asymptomatic.

should rest at the posterior inferior border of the lateral canal. Again, the angle of the needle should be concordant with the lumbosacral inclination.

If the trocar bevel is opened medially toward the disc, it will allow the bent needle to pass accordingly. Two other factors inherent to the bent needle itself act synergistically with the trocar to impart a medial moment on the inner needle: (1) the bend that is oriented toward the disc and (2) the bevel that faces lateral to allow the tip to move medial on purchasing soft tissue such as the annulus.

Bending the inner needle affords the diagnostician an opportunity to customize the needle shape to the patient's body habitus and impart one's personalized flair to the procedure. Commercially bent needles are available. The first consideration is to bend the needle so the bevel faces away from the direction of the bend. Bending approximately 1.5 inches from the end of the needle around the thumbnail becomes rather easy after a limited amount of experience. Running the thumb tangentially along the needle shaft (with the index finger under the needle) and swiftly arcing the end of the needle back on its shaft can create a gentle, long bend. Once the initial bend is established, applying equal and simultaneous three-point pressure with thumb, index finger, and middle finger can be used to increase the degree of arc of the bend. The key to a good bend is to have a smooth turn and tip in the same plane as the needle shaft (see Figure 25-2). The degree of bend should be determined according to where the trocar tip lies in relation to the central nuclear zone.

With the trocar anchored firmly with one hand, the bent needle is carefully passed through it until resistance is met. The resistance indicates the bent needle has engaged the bevel of the guide. While the C-arm fluoroscope beam is directed postero-obliquely and tilted in a cephalocaudad orientation, the bent needle is advanced so it will "steer" around the S1 superior articular process, pass under the L5 nerve root, and purchase the annulus before turning into the midnuclear zone (Fig. 25-3C). Retracting the guide slightly while advancing the procedure needle may ensure that the target point is safely and accurately reached.

The needle position is then assessed in the antero-posterior (AP) and lateral projection before injecting contrast (Figs. 25-3D and 25-3F). If the injection is annular, the contrast dispersion pattern should be examined in several planes so the needle position can be adjusted accordingly (Fig. 25-4). Slight needle advancement or retracting and redirecting

usually suffice. Rarely, the angle or position of the trocar will need to be altered. Occasionally, the procedure needle loses its bend on initial pass, and it must be withdrawn and a new bent needle inserted.

INTERPRETING THE THREE FACETS OF DISCOGRAPHY

There are three cardinal components to a diagnostic disc injection: (1) provocation/analgesia, (2) discometry, and (3) nucleography. Each facet yields data that should be recorded separately yet viewed collectively. For example, an isolated, nonpainful, radial annular fissure may be only as significant as any other incidental imaging finding. Conversely, if this same fissure is associated with an unequivocal pain response, it will need to be treated aggressively to prevent further pain and disability. The provocation aspect is not always the pivotal factor, however. A nonpainful yet dynamically incompetent disc (i.e., discometry yields poor end-point resistance and the annulus is grossly marred by fissuring) adjacent to a proposed fusion level needs to be factored into the surgical decision algorithm if stability is the ultimate goal.

Provocation/Analgesia Assessment

The striking structural information garnered by high-resolution, multiplanar CT and high–field

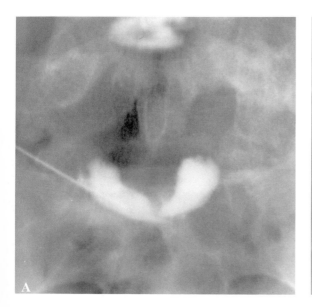 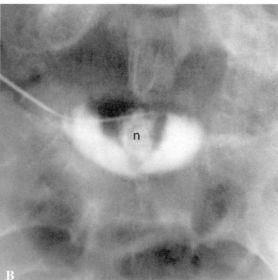

FIGURE 25-4.   *A,* An injection into the transitional or innermost annular substance provides hydrodynamic feedback at the syringe stopper, which is deceptively similar to a true nuclear injection. Even the annulogram (shown here), as it folds into the spongy nuclear region, can be mistaken for a nucleogram. *B,* Following a manipulation of the needle into the nucleus, the nuclear region is filled with contrast (*n*).

strength MRI has an allure likened to trompe l'oeil artistic works. Yet, this eye-catching anatomic information does not obviate the need for physiologic and functional correlation. Accordingly, the marked incidence of false-positive imaging data (whether it is myelography, CT, or MRI) warrants a provocation assessment to determine whether a structural finding is indeed a physiologic pain source.[10,53,113] Discography is the sole direct method to distinguish symptomatic from asymptomatic discs; hence, provocation/analgesia is the sine qua non of diagnostic disc injection.

Provocation (P) is recorded as follows:

P0   No pain response is noted upon injection or distention of the disc with contrast or saline.

P+/- An equivocal response; vague, uncharacteristic, or discordant pain both by nature and location.

P+   Definite, convincing pain provocation that is familiar to the patient yet only reproduces part of the symptom complex.

P++   Exact pain reproduction, concordant with the symptom complex.

Analgesic data is codified with symbology comparable to provocation (denoted R for "response"):

R0   No response to the instillation of anesthetic following a provocation elicitation.

R+/- A vague, uncertain response. An improvement of 2 or less on VAS of 0–10 (i.e., 0 = no pain; 10 = suicidal level of pain).

R+   Symptomatic relief greater than 2 on VAS of 0–10.

R++   Complete ablation of symptoms.

Analgesic responses should be interpreted relative to the duration of anesthesia employed. If 1% lidocaine is used for subcutaneous anesthetization, grading is withheld for 1.5–2.0 hours to allow any residual effect to be eliminated. The longer acting intradiscal agent should continue to act at least for its usual duration.

Accurately interpreting the provocation pain response is a vital component of discography. In general, injection into disrupted discs causes pain, whereas injection into nondisrupted discs does not. A significant relationship has been demonstrated between pain and disc deterioration. Similar or exact pain reproduction accompanies internal disc disruption, unlike disc degeneration, which elicits a dissimilar pain response.[73,109]

However, superimposed confounding factors such as psychological factors and delayed pain response pose a diagnostic dilemma. For instance, patients with elevated scores on hypochondriasis, hysteria, and depression scales of Minnesota Multiphasic Personality Inventory tend to overreport pain. Discordant pain response in such patients should be cautiously interpreted even with concordant CT or discographic images.[12] Occasionally, a patient will have a convincing provocation response, a definite provocation negative control level, and no or temporizing relief with anesthesia. This dilemma occurs most commonly in patients with a chronic condition and significant psychosocial overlay.

Delayed pain response experienced 2–12 hours after discography has been reported in some patients. In such cases, the disc usually has a normal morphology; because it is discrete or incomplete, the annular tear does not fill up at the time of injection. At follow-up, this delayed pain is likely to be missed unless the clinician specifically questions the patient; the patient will not report it, expecting discomfort after the procedure to be normal.[62]

A high-intensity zone (HIZ) in the posterior annulus is never seen on MRI in a morphologically normal disc.[85] Its presence often indicates painful annular fissures, as evidenced on provocative discography. Roughly 90% of the discs with HIZ have a concordantly painful response.[7,95]

Discometry

Discometry is an estimate of the hydrodynamic competence of a disc. This information is obtained by monitoring resistance at the syringe stopper during fluid distention of a disc and measuring the volume injected. Although exact measurements in pascals can be obtained by employing a pressure manometer,[32,74,75,80,82,83,111] the amount of annular resistance monitored in a static situation is by no means an accurate reflection of annular performance in daily activities. An intact annulus, however, has a firm, characteristically resilient end point; any experienced discographer is able to distinguish a competent from a grossly incompetent annulus. In fact, an exercise the senior author commonly prompts residents to undertake is to distend the disc with their eyes closed and the image intensifier off in order to gain an appreciation for this sensation. If the needle tip is inadvertently in the annulus and not in the central nuclear zone, the diagnostician will discern a rigid "end-feel" without the unmistakable "bounce back" resilience of a nuclear injection. Conversely, if the annulus is disrupted, diminished resistance at the needle hub will be recognized.

Discographers have long considered the mechanism of pain provocation in discs with poor resilience. How can such discs be provoked upon dynamic challenge? Is it likely that discs that are markedly disrupted and offer little to no resistance are incapable of providing a pain response upon "distention"? Paradoxically, Derby et al. found that most discs are provoked at low pressures.[32] They proposed chemical stimulation of attenuated outer annular fibers as the mechanism of pain generation. The pain experienced in the buttock, hip, groin, or lower limbs can arise from the posterior annulus of the intervertebral discs without direct nerve root involvement.[92]

Some suspect that end-plate deflections during discography are a possible source of pain.[49] Disc injections with contrast medium distend the disc and transiently increase the vertical and horizontal dimensions of the disc. In the vertical plane, the end plates are displaced by about 0.3 mm, while in the horizontal plane the disc bulges by 0.5 mm. It is speculated that the stretch induced by disc distention causes pain or is caused secondarily by provoking adjacent pain generators. There is, however, no evidence on immediate or delayed MRI of new end-plate changes after discography.[93] Similarly, there is no evidence to substantiate the concept of chemical irritation of bone or microfractures of subchondral trabeculae as a potential cause of postprocedure pain.[92] Vertebral end-plate changes, such as Modic changes seen on MRI in 20–50% of low back pain patients, are relatively specific but insensitive signs of a painful lumbar disc in discogenic back pain.[17]

Normal lumbar discs accept less than 3.0 ml of contrast medium.[1,36,83,110] Volumetric data should be compared level to level as well as against the norm, since occasionally one encounters an individual with "megadiscs," normal lumbar discs that accept 4.0 ml or greater of contrast medium.

Nucleography

As the physician instills contrast medium into the disc, a direct contrast view of the internal architecture of the disc is obtained (see Figures 25-1D and 25-1E). Frontal and lateral plain films are routine for both cervical and lumbar disc injections.

In a normal disc, contrast should be well contained within the nuclear region and have smooth round margins (see Figures 25-1D–F). Lumbar nucleograms are spherical (see Figure 25-1D). They may appear slightly oblong or binucleated following

appearance of nuclear clefts with age.[1] Contrast extravasating beyond the central nuclear zone indicates disruption of the annulus (Figs. 25-5 and 25-6; see also Figure 25-3F).

A profound correlation between radiographic and cadaveric nuclear contrast dye dispersal patterns was first demonstrated by Pierre Erlacher.[36] Sachs et al. then devised a grading system for nucleographic patterns using postdiscography-CT,[90] and Vanharanta et al. compared each pattern with provocation data.[109,110] Yu devised a grading system of annular fissures according to cadaveric injection study.[122] Other authors similarly have published their own nucleographic scoring methods. These systems all may foster communication between physicians but do not obviate the need for accurately detailing the exact relationship of contrast to the nuclear zone, annular region, and neural elements. The presence of nociceptors within the mid to outer annulus should also be considered when interpreting postdiscography-CT nucleograms (see Figure 25-1F).

Diagnostic disc injections must be followed by postdiscography-CT within 1–3 hours. Postdiscography-CT enhances diagnostic accuracy to 99.55%[69] and provides the diagnostician valuable information to complement findings on plain film nucleograms.[70,90,110] Moreover, postdiscography-CT is more sensitive than MRI for detecting annular fissures (Figs. 25-7 and 25-8).[10,58,102,105,121] The authors and others have disclosed painful radial, annular fissures on diagnostic disc injections in patients with normal MRI who have electrodiagnostically irrefutable radiculopathy (see Figure 25-7). Discography can also be applied to resolve conflicting findings among clinical presentation, MRI, and CT (Fig. 25-9; see also Figure 25-7).

Beyond acquiring postdiscography-CT data within the necessary time frame, exercising care and precision in determining CT examination parameters is essential to garner an optimal study. Axial sections of 5 mm from pedicle to pedicle with 3–4 mm table increments suffice for the lumbar spine. Additional selected gantry-angled slices through the L5–S1 interspace may improve spatial resolution of the posterior annulus to neural structures.

Bone and soft tissue window and level settings should be individually selected to optimally visualize contrast medium in relation to annular detail, neural elements, and vertebral body margins. Dosimetry (i.e., kilovolts [kV], milliamperes [mA], and time of exposure) are likewise customized to the body habitus.

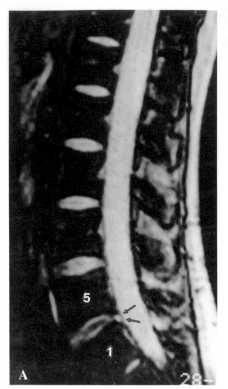

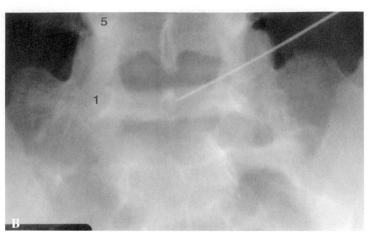

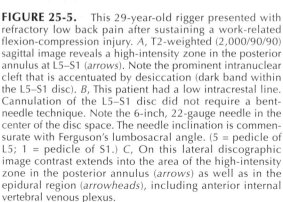

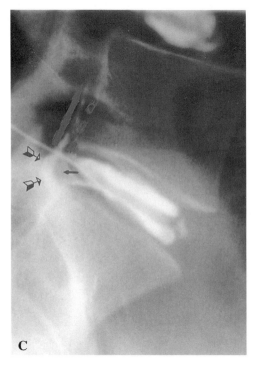

FIGURE 25-5. This 29-year-old rigger presented with refractory low back pain after sustaining a work-related flexion-compression injury. *A,* T2-weighted (2,000/90/90) sagittal image reveals a high-intensity zone in the posterior annulus at L5–S1 (*arrows*). Note the prominent intranuclear cleft that is accentuated by desiccation (dark band within the L5–S1 disc). *B,* This patient had a low intracrestal line. Cannulation of the L5–S1 disc did not require a bent-needle technique. Note the 6-inch, 22-gauge needle in the center of the disc space. The needle inclination is commensurate with Ferguson's lumbosacral angle. (5 = pedicle of L5; 1 = pedicle of S1.) *C,* On this lateral discographic image contrast extends into the area of the high-intensity zone in the posterior annulus (*arrows*) as well as in the epidural region (*arrowheads*), including anterior internal vertebral venous plexus.

BEYOND THE DURA MATER

Technically difficult situations can be fulfilling if the skill and ingenuity of the discographer rises to the challenge. However, new techniques or unfamiliar regions should not be explored until the clinician has the necessary skill level and a thorough understanding of the anatomy and potential for complications. Moreover, even the most basic spinal injection procedures should not be attempted without a keen grasp of orthogonal imaging (MRI and CT), pathophysiology of pain, and applied spinal biomechanics. Cadaveric dissection to investigate anatomy and the technical performance of fluoroscopically controlled procedures on cadavers forms a solid

foundation for accruing new skills. MRI and multiplanar CT provide a segue for mentally reconstructing the planar fluoroscopic image into a three-dimensional image.

Discography Following Posterolateral Fusion

Most patients who have had posterior lumbar fusion require a translumbar (interpedicular) approach to the lumbar disc, which punctures the theca twice and places the patient at risk for a postprocedure headache. A double-needle technique has been employed by the senior author to circumvent the dura in some patients with posterolateral

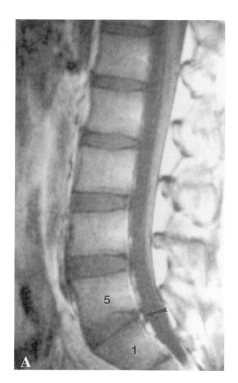

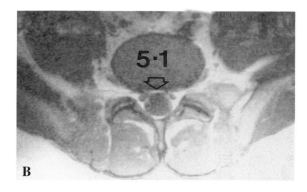

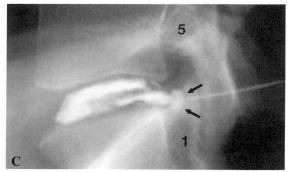

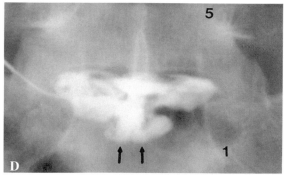

FIGURE 25-6. *A,* T1-weighted (600/20/90) sagittal image (postadministration of gadolinium) discloses a subtle area of enhancement in the posterior annulus of L5–S1 (*arrow*). *B,* T1-weighted (1150/40/90) axial MR at L5–S1 (postgadolinium) demonstrates a transverse "rim" of posterior annular enhancement. Could this be an inflammatory outer annular fissure? *C,* Lateral plain film nucleogram demonstrates a large concentric outer annular fissure (small prolapse). *D,* AP view of the same lesion on plain film nucleography; posteroinferior concentric fissure is demonstrated (*arrows*). *E,* Postdiscography-CT. Compare this image with the axial MRI section (postgadolinium). The lesion abuts the anterior theca and posteriorly displaces the right S1 nerve root in its entry zone (axillary take-off point). Parenthetically, contrast from a facet arthrogram is noted in the right posterior joint and adjacent the lamina.

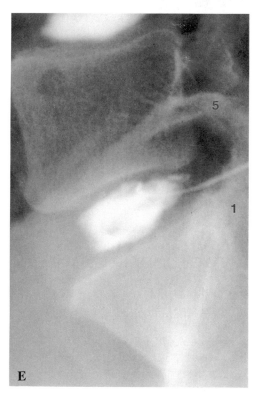

fusion and pedicle screw fixation (Fig. 25-10). The bent inner needle courses extradurally through the central canal; complications associated with thecal puncture, such as cephalgia, are thereby eliminated.

Thoracolumbar and Thoracic Discography

Information on dorsal diagnostic injections is scarce. Simmons and Segil detailed their technique

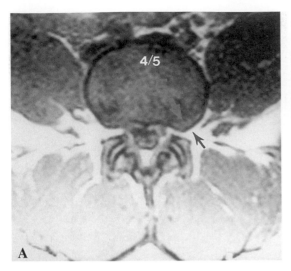

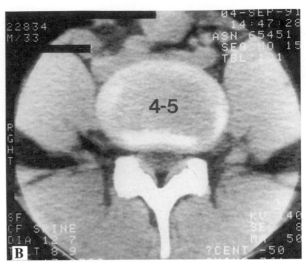

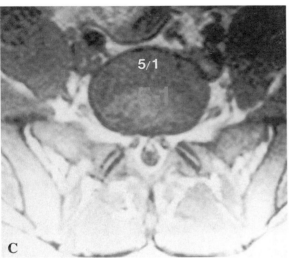

FIGURE 25-7. CT, MRI, and postdiscography-CT from a 33-year-old offshore worker who was thrown about the deck during high seas. He presented with a left L5 radiculopathy. His imaging studies were nondiagnostic and confounding. Discography, however, definitely diagnosed the physiologic pain generator and the structural pathology. *A*, Axial T1 (617/16/90) MRI section demonstrates a left posterolateral prolapse at L4–5 (*arrow*). This lesion may abut the L4 anterior ramus (extraforaminally) but does not appear to affect the L5 segmental nerve. *B*, L4–5 axial CT delineates no convincing findings. *C*, L5–S1 axial T1-weighted (617/16/90) MR section is within normal limits.

of thoracic discography for evaluating thoracic discogenic pain in 1975.[99] Symptoms of midthoracic band-like radicular pain and hypoesthesias in T5 distribution in a 42-year-old man were reproduced with T5–6 disc injection; the nucleography indicated a T5–6 posterior annular fissure.[99]

In chronic refractory thoracic pain, discography may reveal the source of pain and thus allow precise and effective treatment.[116] It is possible to cannulate thoracic and thoracolumbar discs with a single 3.5-inch spinal needle or a bent-needle approach; however strict adherence to guidelines and a meticulous technique are essential to avoid puncture of the pleura, theca, cord, or conus medullaris. Furthermore, beam hardening from overlying structures (e.g., ribs) and a narrow interspace make the procedure technically challenging. Despite possible pitfalls, Schellhas et al. performed 250 thoracic discograms without complication and concluded

that, in experienced hands, thoracic discography is safe and effective in evaluating dorsal pain and disc degeneration.[94]

The authors approach thoracic disc injections similar to lumbar discography with a few key anatomic accommodations. The C-arm is rotated or, when using the overhead fluoroscopy unit, the technician positions the patient so that the superior articular process falls just short of bisecting the interspace and passes the needle posterior to the head of the rib (Fig. 25-11A) to avoid entering the pleural space. An axial MRI or CT section of the thorax at the appropriate level(s) aids in defining specific anatomic relationships. Where the pleura may be jeopardized by a direct approach, a bent-needle technique is utilized. The senior author's bent-needle technique is similar to the L5–S1 technique, except for the guide that is adjusted to the kyphotic angulation of the disc space; a gentler bend on the

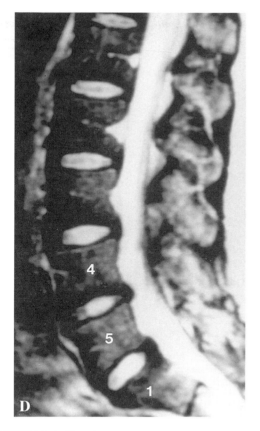

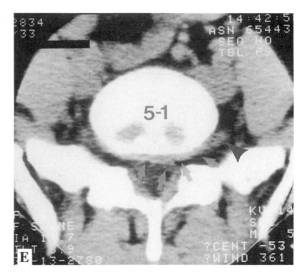

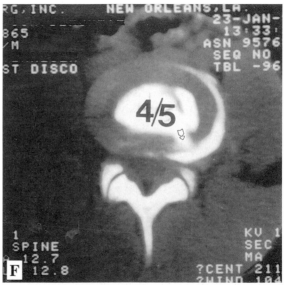

FIGURE 25-7 *(Cont.).* *D*, Long T2 sagittal MR (1800/80/80) section provided compelling evidence for intact annuli and normal state of disc hydration. *E*, Axial CT at L5–S1 (soft tissue window setting) demonstrates a broad-based left posterolateral prolapse (*arrows*) that abuts the L5 segmental nerve extraforaminally (*arrowhead*). *F*, L4–5 postdiscography discloses a radial fissure (*arrow*) from the central nuclear zone extending into a large circumferential outer annular fissure. *G*, An expansile fissure was revealed at this level that obliterates the left L5–S1 root canal (compare the right canal with the left). This lesion is also contiguous with the L5 epiradicular sheath. Contrast these startling findings with the L5–S1 axial MRI (above). On initial injection, the patient's left lower extremity radicular-type pain was reproduced and subsequently ablated upon direct intradiscal instillation of bupivacaine.

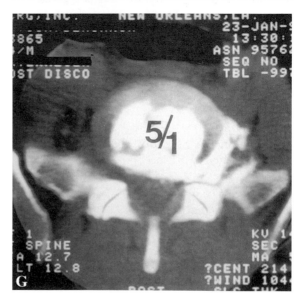

inner needle protects it from entering the central canal (Fig. 25-11B). Post dorsal discography-CT yields data similar to that in the lumbar region (Fig. 25-12); thinner transaxial sections may be necessary in the mid to upper thoracic regions.

COMPLICATIONS

Strict adherence to a preprocedural screening protocol and impeccable technique in the performance of discography will ensure a low morbidity rate.

Chemical irritation or injury to the disc or adjacent vertebral bodies has been speculated to be

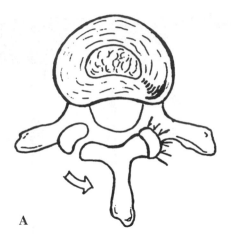
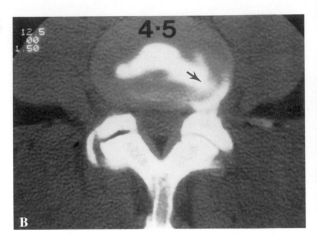

FIGURE 25-8. *A,* The components of a lumbar torsion injury.[37] Note the series of circumferential annular fissures extending to the outer annulus. There is a distraction-impaction injury to the posterior joints with strain of the capsular ligaments. (Adapted from Fortin JD: Enigmatic causes of spine pain in athletes. In Watkins RG (ed): The Spine in Sports. Chicago, Mosby, 1994.) *B,* Lumbar postdiscography-CT of a torsion injury. This patient, a 40-year-old registered nurse, sustained a work-related slip and fall on the left buttock with her right leg twisted under herself. She complained of aching and stabbing central lumbosacral pain with paresthesias in a left L4 distribution. The same facets of the torsion injury complex illustrated above are noted on this axial scan. A posterolateral radial fissure is indicated by the arrow. The right posterior joint is wider than the left, and there is right capsular calcification, owing to distraction-impaction (deformation of the neural arch), and severe capsular strain.

responsible for pain at discography or intractable low back pain thereafter. DeSéze alluded to a chemical discitis causing aseptic necrosis of the disc and secondary intervertebral arthrodesis.[33] According to DeHaene, this destructive evolution may have been from the concentrated iodine product DeSéze employed.[31] Crock also has presented the possibility of an aseptic or chemical form of discitis.[27] Currently available evidence does not support chemical discitis,

chemical irritation of bone, or microfracture of subchondral trabeculae to be the cause of pain at discography.[93] Vertebral end-plate changes following uncomplicated discography were evaluated in 20 consecutive patients. Pre- and postdiscography MRI scans revealed no new changes in end-plate signal intensity, suggesting that any changes in the vertebral end plates following discography were indicative of infectious discitis.[93]

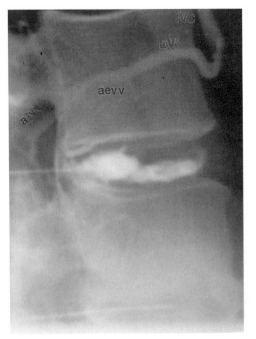

FIGURE 25-9. When Harry Crock first described internal disc disruption syndrome, he alluded to a systemic/immunologic response.[27] Patients with this syndrome often experienced generalized malaise, chronic fatigue, poor appetite, and depression. As revealed on this radiograph of injection of contrast medium into the disc space, inflammatory contents from a disrupted disc may have direct or immediate communication with the circulatory system. There is rapid clearance of contrast into the epidural and lumbar veins upon injection. Could this be one physiologic link between disc disruption and constitutional changes in some patients? (aaiv = anterior internal vertebral venous plexus [portions of]; aevv = anterior external vertebral venous plexus [portions of]; LV = lumbar vein; IVC = inferior vena cava.)

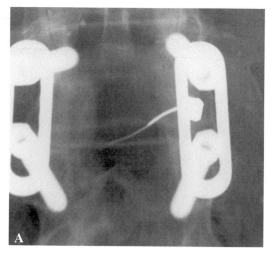
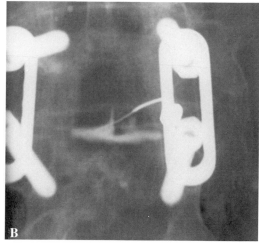
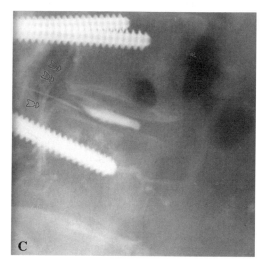

FIGURE 25-10. Circumventing the thecal sac while performing a disc injection at a level with pedicle screw instrumentation and a posterolateral fusion mass. *A*, Posteroanterior view. A bent needle has successfully been passed around the outer margin of the central canal (i.e., extradurally). Confirmation that the dura had not been violated was evidenced by absence of cerebrospinal fluid when the needle was withdrawn in slow increments with the fluoroscopy table at a 45° (upright) position. *B*, Postinjection posteroanterior nucleogram. *C*, Lateral nucleogram. Epidural venous continuity with the nucleus (*arrows*) indicated a complete annular rent. This level was symptomatic.

Fraser's experimental discitis sheep model provides compelling evidence for an infectious etiology.[41] Bacterial discitis is a widely recognized complication that follows discography; the incidence, however, is reportedly low (0.1–1.3%).[27,41,42,66,68,114] The avascularity of the disc provides an excellent culture medium for bacterial growth and infection. Bacterial inoculation occurs with skin or gut flora such as *Staphylococcus*, *Streptococcus*, and *Escherichia coli*. The latter can be seeded from the hypopharynx and esophagus (in cervical injections)[22] or the bowel (in lumbar injections)[2,42,45] following needle puncture in cases where technical guidelines are ignored.

Attempting to isolate organisms in patients with discitis has proven difficult. It appears that in many cases the offending organism has run its natural course and neovascularization from end-plate tributaries has provided rapid immunologic ablation before isolation is customarily attempted.[41,42] Moreover, some cases with a relatively benign and self-limited form of discitis from low-virulence, indolent organisms go undetected.[27,96] These factors do not obviate the need for an appropriate index of suspicion because sequelae such as epidural or retropharyngeal (cervical region) abscesses can occur.[57,66]

Preventive measures combine a meticulous, strict aseptic technique with prophylactic antibiotics (cefazolin). Experimental and clinical trials support the role of intravenous or intradiscal antibiotics in effectively preventing clinical, radiologic, and histopathologic signs of discitis.[78]

Patients with a dramatic increase in pain and stiffness or a change in the character of symptoms are initially screened with a sedimentation rate. An elevated sedimentation rate should prompt urgent confirmation by MRI.[39,65,107] Although radionuclide scans are significantly more sensitive than plain radiographs,[20,76] MRI is the gold standard in detection of discitis.[8,72,104] In a comparative experimental rabbit model, MRI was found to be superior to

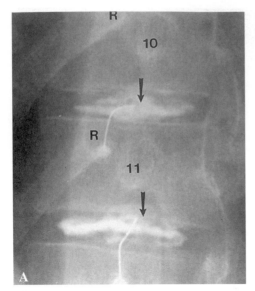

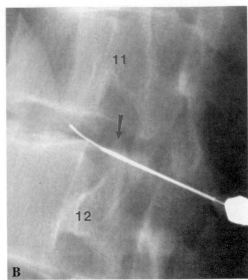

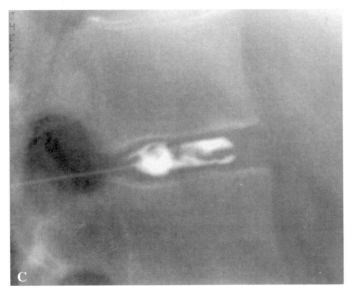

FIGURE 25-11. Thoracolumbar discography. *A,* Oblique view illustrates position of 25-gauge, 3.5-inch spinal needles in relation to rib heads (*r*) and tip of superior articular processes (*arrows*). (10 = pedicle of T10; 11 = pedicle of T11.) *B,* Compare this oblique view of a bent-needle technique at the thoracolumbar junction to the L5–S1 disc injection technique seen in Figure 25-3. The angulation of the guide corrects for the kyphotic dorsal curve, and the needle bend is gentler than at L5–S1. (11 = pedicle of T11; 12 = pedicle of T12; arrow = tip of T12 superior articular process.) *C,* Lateral view of a thoracolumbar disc injection provides a view of the typical oblong or elliptical nuclear configuration at this region.

bone scanning with a 92% sensitivity, 97% specificity, and 95% overall accuracy.[104]

In patients with nonspecific presenting symptoms, a premorbid psychiatric history, or a low pain threshold, the clinical diagnosis of discitis may be delayed or obscured. Furthermore, cost-containment measures that limit the use of screening modalities add to the challenge of rapidly establishing or excluding the diagnosis.

Other potential complications from discography include neural injury from direct needle trauma (either an impaled segmental nerve root from a misguided lumbar procedure or a cord injury from a cervical or thoracic discography needle), pneumothorax from a misguided C7–T1 or thoracic approach, and thecal puncture headache. Post–thecal puncture cephalgia or cord injury can occur when a cervical discography needle penetrates to a dangerous depth in the AP plane.[60] It is also possible to invade the subarachnoid space at L5–S1 if the inner needle is excessively bent or the trocar malpositioned. Again, these complications can be prevented with rigid technique.

A rare fatal case of pulmonary embolism following discography has been described.[97] The subject developed a systemic reaction accompanied by spasmodic extension of the back and legs following lumbar discography. Nucleus pulposus emboli into the lungs and acute herniations of disc material into vertebral marrow spaces were revealed on autopsy studies. It is uncertain whether this was primarily a complication of discography per se or was from the

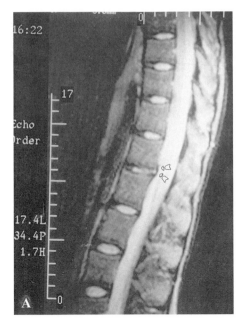

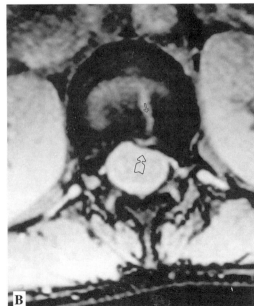

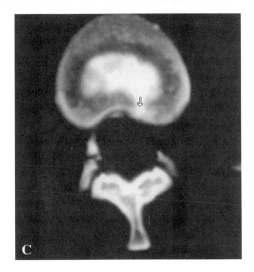

FIGURE 25-12.   *A*, This 24-year-old patient presented with thoracolumbar pain after having been involved in a rear-end motor vehicle accident. Note the slight diminution in signal intensity as well as the posterior annular protrusion or small prolapse (*arrows*) at T12–L1 on this T2-weighted (2,000/90/90) sagittal MRI image. *B*, Gradient echo axial image (650/18/26) through T12–L1 demonstrates a radial fissure (*small arrow*) extending from the central nuclear zone into a mild posterior left paracentral prolapse, which causes slight, angular effacement of the anterior theca (*large arrow*). *C*, Thoracolumbar post-discography-CT. Compare this image with the gradient echo MR axial image above. The same pathology is seen.

spasmodic arching of the back and legs that forced nuclear and disc contents into vertebral marrow spaces.[97]

POSTPROCEDURE CARE

Patients are attended to in an observation area following the procedure. Vital signs are obtained immediately. If stable, the patient is transported via gurney or wheelchair to CT (as indicated). Fluids are encouraged immediately, and the patient is provided a meal 1 hour after the procedure.

Postprocedural instructions include (1) education on the application of ice to the affected area; (2) information on the usual postprocedural symptoms such as increased local pain, stiffness, and dysphagia (for cervical procedures); and (3) instructions to avoid driving or operating machinery for the remainder of the day; patients should be accompanied by a responsible driver to and from the procedure site. An instruction sheet is also reviewed that includes the above information and an emergency telephone number to call for any sign of infection (detailed therein), sudden increased pain, sustained progressive increase in pain, or marked change in the character of symptoms.

Narcotic analgesics are dispensed judiciously, and a 2-day supply on an as required basis is sufficient. This is often a good opportunity to provide the uninformed patient with education concerning the physiology of addiction. Patients can be safely discharged 2 hours following the procedure.

HAS NEW TECHNOLOGY ECLIPSED DISCOGRAPHY?

Despite its edge in providing unsurpassed diagnostic information, discography and postdiscography-CT are invasive, operator dependent, and potentially hazardous. Conventional clinical examination methods unfortunately cannot reliably identify subjects with internal disc disruption[98] let alone discriminate between symptomatic and asymptomatic discs. There is a constant search for noninvasive means of screening subjects with disc pathology and distinguishing a pain-generating disc from other painless discs. To this end, ultrasound and bony vibration tests have been employed to complement the physical examination.[106,118–120] Initial reports suggest that these screening modalities may hold some promise in assessing intradiscal pain in selected cases, but they have yet to withstand the rigors of scientific scrutiny and validation before their induction.

Controversy surrounding the overall diagnostic efficacy of discography versus other imaging modalities such as MRI and CT is superfluous and belies the awareness necessary to properly apply any given one. Such unfortunate comparisons are perpetuated by reports that draw sweeping conclusions without understanding the fundamental application of the test in question.

For example, in a 1986 study comparing MRI to discography, Gibson et al. concluded that "MRI was shown to be more accurate than discography in the diagnosis of disc degeneration. It has several major advantages, which should make it the investigation of choice."[43] The authors did not employ postdiscography transverse CT imaging to enhance nucleographic findings on plain films, although postdiscography-CT scanning modality was routinely available in 1986.[70,90] If Gibson and coworkers had used a state-of-the-art protocol, they might have reached opposite conclusions. Furthermore, the technical expertise employed in the study may be suspect as evidenced by the statement: "the reproduction of symptoms by discography should be one of its main advantages in helping with localization. Unfortunately, this does not seem to be a particularly reliable sign and in a patient under sedation it can be difficult to interpret."[43] As noted above, such statements were discredited by Walsh et al.[111] When concluding that a particular modality is the "investigation of choice" one should clearly indicate what clinical scenario(s) should preempt that choice. Obviously, discography is not the study of choice as a screening tool for patients with low back pain. Conversely, discography is indicated for determining if an internally deranged disc is painful in a patient with refractory axial pain who has failed aggressive conservative care. The provocation data garnered from a poorly conducted study are meaningless (Fig. 25-13).

Each test should be viewed as an extension of the overall clinical context. The clinician who understands the strengths and weaknesses of each is collectively armed with a powerful diagnostic armamentarium. A well-recognized application of this axiom is the additive benefit of combining CT and myelography.[115]

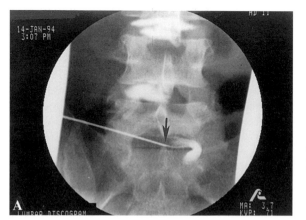 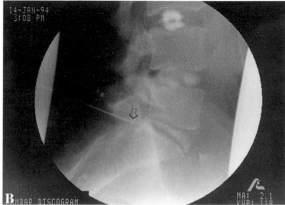

FIGURE 25-13. Lack of experience, poor training, and improper technique may all contribute to the duplicitous reputation of discography. The author was asked to reviews these films on a patient who reportedly was transported (via gurney) to the emergency room with intractable right leg pain following this procedure. *A*, Posteroanterior view of an attempted L5–S1 disc injection. The tip of the guide (*arrow*) has been advanced to midline, well beyond where it should be (see Figure 25-3). An annular contrast pattern suggests the bent needle has purchased the annulus. *B*, A lateral projection documents the guide position in the central canal (*arrows*). The bent inner needle has been manipulated superomedially to the L5–S1 annulus.

High-resolution, multiplanar CT, especially when combined with intrathecal enhancement, can provide an impressive view of the annular contour of the disc and its spatial relationship to canals (root and central), neural elements, and posterior joints.[115] Owing to superior osseous resolution, CT conveys the best view of end plates. However, CT comparatively provides little information regarding the internal integrity, biochemical constituency, and state of hydration of the disc. CT subjects the patient to ionizing radiation, and CT-myelography is an invasive procedure with certain morbidity.

High–field strength MRI is the Stradivarius imaging modality; it is superlative in its depiction of soft tissue anatomy, noninvasive, and without the risk of radiation. Some discs that appear normal on CT may clearly demonstrate various internal derangements such as desiccation, fissuring, or inflammation on MRI (see Figures 25-5 and 25-6). Painful, inflammatory annular fissures may be enhanced with gadolinium[87] or yield a focal high signal on T2-weighted images[7] (Fig. 25-14). The ever-expanding applications of MRI and a trend toward greater cost containment have encouraged some centers to forego conventional T2 spin echo sequences. These slow acquisition images are being replaced by speedier gradient echo and fast T2 pulses. Equating information on the nuclear matrix and annulus from the newer pulse sequences with true spin echo images must be done with caution.[51] For instance, annular signal intensity changes on T2 images that seem to correlate with pain on provocation may not be as conspicuous on the modern sequences. Moreover, studies that compared diagnostic disc injections to MRI employed conventional spin echo sequences. Therefore, the observations from these investigations may not extrapolate to the fast acquisition images.[7,55]

The limitations of MRI must be understood as well. MRI cannot consistently identify painful discs; the findings on MRI do not always correlate with discography. There is only a 55% correlation between MRI and discography. Simmons reported that 7% of discs that appeared normal on MRI were abnormal on discography and 13% of abnormal-looking discs on MRI were normal on discography.[101] Another study reported on 7 patients with surgically proven lumbar disc disruption, normal MRI, and abnormal discograms.[18] Roughly a third of the discographically abnormal discs can be normal on MRI, and a third of abnormal discs on MRI are asymptomatic.[79]

As an imaging modality, discography, when combined with axial CT, surpasses MRI in detecting

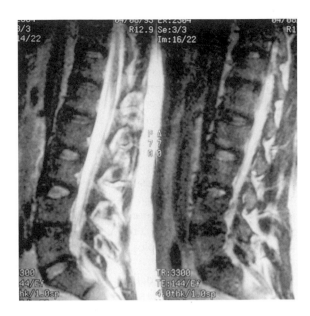

FIGURE 25-14. The right parasagittal portion of the L4–5 disc appears suspicious on these fast T2-weighted sagittal images (TR 3000, TE 144 EF), but without the signal intensity characteristics of true T2 weighting, it is difficult to discern the state of hydration of discs. Further confounding this issue is the chemical shift misregistration artifact appearing as dark horizontal bands adjacent to the end plates.

annular fissures.[122] Discography, however, is an invasive procedure and should be reserved for those patients who have unrelenting axial pain, no definite neurocompressive lesion, and failed aggressive functional restoration.[3,35,88]

CONCLUSION

Despite the recent exponential growth of noninvasive spinal technology, diagnostic disc injection remains the sole direct method for definitively determining if a disc is a physiologic pain generator. When indicated and impeccably performed, discography is a safe and sometimes powerful complement to the overall clinical context. This diagnostic tool may also enhance information obtained from other imaging modalities or reveal new and otherwise enigmatic findings.

REFERENCES

1. Adams MA, Dolan P, Hutton WC: The stages of disc degeneration as revealed by discograms. J Bone Joint Surg 68B:36–41, 1986.
2. Agre K, Wilson RR, Brim M, et al: Chymodiactin postmarketing surveillance: Demographic and adverse experience data in 29,075 patients. Spine 9:479–485, 1984.
3. Alexander AH: Nonoperative management of herniated nucleus pulposus: Patient selection by the extension sign long-term follow-up. Orthop Rev 21:181–188, 1992.

4. Amundsen P: The evolution of contrast media. In Sackett J, Strother C (eds): New Techniques in Myelography. Hagerstown, MD, Harper & Row, 1979, pp 2–5.

5. Antti-Poika I, Soini J, Tallroth K, et al: Clinical relevance of discography combined with CT scanning. A study of 100 patients. J Bone Joint Surg 72B:480–485, 1990.

6. Aprill CN III: Diagnostic disc injection. In Frymoyer JW (ed): The Adult Spine: Principles and Practice, 2nd ed. Philadelphia, Lippincott-Raven, 1996, pp 539–562.

7. Aprill C, Bogduk N: High intensity zones in the disc annulus: A sign of painful disc on magnetic resonance imaging. Br J Radiol 65:361–369, 1992.

8. Arrington JA, Murtagh FR, Silbiger ML, et al: Magnetic resonance imaging of post-discogram discitis and osteomyelitis in the lumbar spine: Case report. J Fla Med Assoc 73:192–194, 1986.

9. Benoist M: Positioning alternatives for chemonucleolysis: Current concepts in chemonucleolysis. J R Soc Med 72:47–53, 1984.

10. Bernard TN Jr: Lumbar discography followed by computed tomography: Refining the diagnosis of low-back pain. Spine 15:690–707, 1990.

11. Bernard TN Jr: Repeat lumbar spine surgery. Factors influencing outcome. Spine 18:2196–2200, 1993.

12. Block AR, Vanharanta H, Ohnmeiss DD, et al: Discographic pain report: Influence of psychological factors. Spine 21:334–338, 1996.

13. Blumenthal S, Baker J, Dosett A, Selby DK: The role of anterior lumbar fusion for internal disc disruption. Spine 13:566–569, 1988.

14. Boden SD, Davis DO, Dina TS, et al: Abnormal magnetic resonance scans of the lumbar spine in asymptomatic subjects. J Bone Joint Surg 72A:403–408, 1990.

15. Bogduk N, Tynan W, Wilson AS: The nerve supply to the human lumbar intervertebral discs. J Anat 132:39–56, 1981.

16. Bogduk N, Modic MT: Lumbar discography. Spine 21:402–404, 1996.

17. Braithwaite I, White J, Saifuddin A, et al: Vertebral endplate (Modic) changes on lumbar spine MRI: Correlation with pain reproduction at lumbar discography. Eur Spine J 7:363–368, 1998.

18. Brightbill TC, Pile N, Eichelberger RP, et al: Normal magnetic resonance imaging and abnormal discography in lumbar disc disruption. Spine 19:1075–1077, 1994.

19. Brodsky AE, Binder WF: Lumbar discography: Its value in diagnosis and treatment of lumbar disc lesions. Spine 4:110–120, 1979.

20. Bruschwein DA, Brown ML, McLeod RA: Gallium scintigraphy in the evaluation of disc-space infections: Concise communications. J Nucl Med 21:925–927, 1980.

21. Buirski G, Silberstein M: The symptomatic lumbar disc in patients with low-back pain: Magnetic resonance imaging appearances in both a symptomatic and control population. Spine 18:1808–1811, 1993.

22. Cloward RB: Cervical discography defended [letter]. JAMA 233:862, 1975.

23. Colhoun E, McCall IW, Williams L, et al: Provocation discography as a guide to planning operations on the spine. J Bone Joint Surg 70B:267–271, 1988.

24. Collis JS Jr, Gardner WJ: Lumbar discography: An analysis of 1,000 cases. J Neurosurg 19:452–461, 1962.

25. Crawshaw C: Needle insertion techniques for chemonucleolysis: Current concepts in chemonucleolysis. J R Soc Med 72:55–59, 1984.

26. Crock HV: Normal and pathological anatomy of the lumbar spinal nerve root canals. J Bone Joint Surg 63B:470–490, 1981.

27. Crock HV: Practice of Spinal Surgery. New York, Springer-Verlag, 1983, pp 1–319.

28. Curry TS, Dowdey JE, Murry RC: Christensen's Physics of Diagnostic Radiology, 4th ed. Philadelphia, Lea & Febiger, 1990, pp 165–166.

29. Dabezies EJ, Murphy CP: Dural puncture using the lateral approach for chemonucleolysis. Spine 10:93–96, 1985.

30. Day PL: Lateral approach for lumbar diskogram and chemonucleolysis. Clin Orthop 67:90–93, 1969.

31. DeHaene R: La discographie. J Belg Radiol 36:131, 1953.

32. Derby R, Kine G, Schwarzer A, et al: Relationship between intradiscal pressure and pain provocation during discography. Presented at the 8th Annual Assembly of the North American Spine Society, San Diego, 1993.

33. DeSéze S, Levernieux J: Les accidents de la discographie. Rev Rheum 19:1027–1033, 1952.

34. Edholm P, Fernstrom I, Lindblom K: Extradural lumbar disc puncture. Acta Radiol Scand 6:322–328, 1967.

35. Ellenberg MR, Ross ML, Honet JC, et al: Prospective evaluation of the cause of disc herniations in patients with proven radiculopathy. Arch Phys Med Rehabil 74:3–8, 1993.

36. Erlacher PR: Nucleography. J Bone Joint Surg 34B:204–210, 1952.

37. Farfan HF, Cossette JW, Robertson GH, et al: The effects of torsion of the lumbar intervertebral joints: The role of torsion in the production of disc degeneration. J Bone Joint Surg 52A:468–497, 1970.

38. Feinberg SB: The place of discography in radiology as based on 2320 cases. Am J Radiol 92:1275–1281, 1964.

39. Fernand R, Lee CK: Postlaminectomy disc space infection: A review of the literature and a report of three cases. Clin Orthop 209:215–218, 1986.

40. Flanagan MN, Chung B: Roentgenographic changes in 188 patients 10–20 years after discography and chemonucleolysis. Spine 11:444–448, 1986.

41. Fraser RD, Osti OL, Vernon-Roberts B: Discitis following chemonucleolysis: An experimental study. Spine 11:679–687, 1986.

42. Fraser RD, Osti OL, Vernon-Roberts B: Discitis after discography. J Bone Joint Surg 69B:26–35, 1987.

43. Gibson MJ, Buckley J, Mawhinney R, et al: Magnetic resonance imaging and discography in the diagnosis of disc degeneration. J Bone Joint Surg 68B:369–373, 1986.

44. Groen G, Baljet B, Drukker J: The nerves and nerve plexuses of the human vertebral column. Am J Anat 188:282–296, 1990.

45. Guyer RD, Collier R, Stith W, et al: Discitis after discography. Spine 13:1352–1354, 1988.

46. Guyer RD, Ohnmeiss DD: Lumbar discography: Position statement from the North American Spine Society Diagnostic and Therapeutic Committee. Spine 20:2048–2059, 1995.

47. Hall SC, Ovassapian A: Apnea after intravenous diazepam therapy. JAMA 238:1052, 1977.

48. Hasue M, Kunogi J, Konno S, Kikuchi S: Classification by position of dorsal root ganglia in the lumbosacral region. Spine 14:1261–1264, 1989.

49. Heggeness MH, Doherty BJ: Discography causes endplate deflection. Spine 18:1050–1053, 1993.

50. Heggeness MH, Waters WC, Gray PM: Discography of lumbar discs after surgical treatment for disc herniation. Spine 22:1606–1609, 1997.

51. Hendrick RE, Russ PD, Simon JH: MRI: Principles and Artifacts. New York, Raven Press, 1993, pp 83–89.

52. Hirsch C: An attempt to diagnose level of disc lesion clinically by disc puncture. Acta Orthop Scand 18:131–140, 1948.

53. Hitselberger WE, Whitten R: Abnormal myelograms in asymptomatic patients. J Neurosurg 28:204–206, 1968.

54. Holt EP Jr: The question of lumbar discography. J Bone Joint Surg 50A:720–726, 1968.

55. Horton W, Daftar T: Which disc as visualized by MRI is actually a source of pain? Spine 17:S164–S171, 1992.

56. Ito M, Incorvaia KM, Yu SF, et al: Predictive signs of discogenic lumbar pain on magnetic resonance imaging with discography correlation. Spine 23:1252–1258, 1998.

57. Junila J, Ninimaki T, Tervonen O: Epidural abscess after lumbar discography: A case report. Spine 22:2191–2193, 1997.

58. Kornberg M: Discography and magnetic resonance imaging in the diagnosis of lumbar disc disruption. Spine 14:1368–1372, 1989.

59. Laredo J, Busson J, Wybier M, Bard M: Technique of lumbar chemonucleolysis. In Bard M, Laredo J (eds): Interventional Radiology in Bone and Joint. New York, Springer-Verlag, 1988, pp 101–122.

60. Laun A, Lorenz R, Angnoli AL: Complications of cervical discography. J Neurosurg Sci 25:17–22, 1981.

61. Lawlis GF, Cuencas R, Selby D, et al: The development of the Dallas Pain Questionnaire: An assessment of the impact of spinal pain on behavior. Spine 14:511–515, 1989.

62. Lehmer SM, Dawson MH, O'Brien JP: Delayed pain response after lumbar discography. Eur Spine J 3:28–31, 1994.

63. Lindblom K: Protrusions of the discs and nerve compression in the lumbar region. Acta Radiol Scand 25:195–212, 1944.

64. Lindblom K: Diagnostic puncture of the intervertebral discs in sciatica. Acta Orthop Scand 17:231–239, 1948.

65. Lindholm TS, Pylkkanen P: Discitis following removal of intervertebral disc. Spine 7:618–622, 1982.

66. Lownie SP, Ferguson GG: Spinal subdural empyema complicating cervical discography. Spine 14:1415–1417, 1989.

67. Malinsky J: The ontogenetic development of nerve terminations in the intervertebral discs of man. Acta Anat 38:96–113, 1959.

68. Milette PC, Melanson D: A reappraisal of lumbar discography. J Assoc Can Radiol 11:176–182, 1982.

69. Min K, Leu HJ, Perrenoud A: Discography with manometry and discographic CT: Their value in patient selection for percutaneous lumbar nucleotomy. Bull Hosp Joint Dis 54:153–157, 1996.

70. Mital MA, Thompson WC III: Role of discography enhanced by CT scanning in investigation of low back pain with sciatica. Presented at the Meeting of the Federation of Spine Associations, New Orleans, February 19–30, 1986.

71. Mixter WJ, Barr JS: Ruptures of the intervertebral disc with involvement of the spinal canal. N Engl J Med 211:210–215, 1934.

72. Modic MT, Feiglin D, Pirano D, et al: Vertebral osteomyelitis: Assessment using MR. Radiology 157:157–166, 1985.

73. Moneta GB, Videman T, Kaivanto K, et al: Reported pain during lumbar discography as a function of anular ruptures and disc degeneration: A re-analysis of 833 discograms. Spine 19:1968–1974, 1994.

74. Nachemson A: Lumbar intradiscal pressure. Acta Orthop Scand Suppl 43:1–104, 1960.

75. Nachemson A, Elfstrom G: Intravital dynamic pressure measurement in lumbar discs. Scand J Rehab Med Suppl 1:1–40, 1970.

76. Norris S, Ehrlich MG, Keim DE, et al: Early diagnosis of disc space infection using gallium-67. J Nucl Med 19:384–386, 1978.

77. North American Spine Society: Position statement on discography. The Executive Committee of the North American Spine Society. Spine 13:1343, 1988.

78. Osti OL, Fraser RD, Vernon-Roberts B: Discitis after discography: The role of prophylactic antibiotics. J Bone Joint Surg 72B:271–274, 1990.

79. Osti OL, Fraser RD: MRI and discography of annular tears and intervertebral disc degeneration: A prospective clinical comparison. J Bone Joint Surg 74B:431–435, 1992.

80. Panjabi MM, Brown M, Lindahl S, et al: Intrinsic disc pressure as a measure of integrity of the lumbar spine. Spine 13:913–917, 1988.

81. Pease CN: Injuries to the vertebrae and intervertebral discs following lumbar puncture. Am J Dis Child 49:849–860, 1935.

82. Quinnell RC, Stockdale H: Pressure standardized lumbar discography. Br J Radiol 53:1031–1036, 1980.

83. Quinnell RC, Stockdale HR, Willis DS: Observations of pressures within normal discs in the lumbar spine. Spine 8:166–169, 1983.

84. Rauschning W: Normal and pathologic anatomy of the lumbar root canals. Spine 12:1008–1019, 1987.

85. Ricketson R, Simmons JW, Hauser BO: The prolapsed intervertebral disc: The high intensity zone with discography correlation. Spine 21:2758–2762, 1996.

86. Roofe PG: Innervation of the annulus fibrosus and posterior longitudinal ligament. Arch Neurol Psychiatry 44:100–103, 1940.

87. Ross JS, Modic MT, Masaryk TJ: Tears of the annulus fibrosus: Assessment with Gd-DTPA-enhanced MR imaging. AJNR Am J Neuroradiol 10:1251–1254, 1989.

88. Saal JA, Saal JS: The nonoperative treatment of herniated nucleus pulposus with radiculopathy: An outcome study. Spine 14:431–437, 1989.

89. Saal JS, Franson RC, Dobrow R, et al: High levels of inflammatory phospholipase A_2 activity in lumbar disc herniations. Spine 15:674–678, 1990.

90. Sachs BL, Vanhararnta H, Spivey MA, et al: Dallas discogram description: A new classification of CT/discography in low-back disorders. Spine 12:287–294, 1987.

91. Sachs BL, Spivey MA, Vanharanta H, et al: Techniques for lumbar discography and computed tomography/discography in clinical practice. Orthop Rev 19:775–778, 1990.

92. Saifuddin A, Emanuel R, White J, et al: An analysis of radiating pain at lumbar discography. Eur Spine J 7:358–362, 1998.

93. Saifuddin A, Renton P, Taylor BA: Effects on the vertebral end-plate of uncomplicated lumbar discography: An MRI study. Eur Spine J 7:36–39, 1998.

94. Schellhas KP, Pollei SR: Thoracic disc degeneration: Correlation of MR imaging and discography. Presented at the 8th Annual North American Spine Society Assembly, San Diego, 1993.

95. Schellhas KP, Pollei SR, Gundry CR, et al: Lumbar disc high-intensity zone: Correlation of magnetic resonance imaging and discography. Spine 21:79–86, 1996.

96. Schofferman L, Schofferman J, Zucherman J, et al: Occult infections causing persistent low-back pain. Spine 14:417–419, 1989.

97. Schreck RI, Manion WL, Kambin P, et al: Nucleus pulposus pulmonary embolism: A case report. Spine 20:2463–2466, 1995.

98. Schwarzer AC, Aprill CN, Derby R, et al: The prevalence and clinical features of internal disc disruption in patients with chronic low back pain. Spine 20:1878–1883, 1995.

99. Simmons EH, Segil CM: An evaluation of discography in the localization of symptomatic levels in discogenic disease of the spine. Clin Orthop 108:57–69, 1975.

100. Simmons JW, Aprill CN, Dwyer AP, et al: A reassessment of Holt's data on "The question of lumbar discography." Clin Orthop 237:120–124, 1988.

101. Simmons JW, Emery SF, McMillin, et al: Awake discography: A comparison study with magnetic resonance imaging. Spine 16:S216–S221, 1991.

102. Smith BM, Hurwitz EL, Solsberg D, et al: Interobserver reliability of detecting lumbar intervertebral disc high-intensity zone on magnetic resonance imaging and association of high-intensity zone with pain and anular disruption. Spine 23:2074–2080, 1998.

103. Steindler A, Luck J: Differential diagnosis of pain low in the back: Allocation of the source of pain by procaine hydrochloride method. JAMA 110:106–113, 1938.

104. Szypryt E, Hardy J, Hinton C, et al: A comparison between magnetic resonance imaging and scintigraphic bone imaging in the diagnosis of disc space infection in an animal model. Spine 13:1042–1048, 1988.

105. Tervonen O, Lahde S, Rydberg J: Lumbar disc degeneration. Correlation between CT and CT/discography. Acta Radiol 31:551–554, 1990.

106. Tervonen O, Lahde S, Vanharanta H: Ultrasound diagnosis of lumbar disc degeneration: Comparison with computed tomography/discography. Spine 16:951–954, 1991.

107. Thibodeau AA: Closed space infection following removal of lumbar intervertebral disc. J Bone Joint Surg 50A:400–410, 1968.

108. Troiser O: Technique de la discographie extra-durale. J Radiol 63:571–578, 1982.

109. Vanharanta H, Sachs BL, Spivey MA, et al: The relationship of pain provocation to lumbar disc deterioration as seen by CT/discography. Spine 12:295–298, 1987.

110. Vanharanta H, Sach BL, Ohnmeiss DD, et al: Pain provocation and disc deterioration by age: A CT/discographic study in a low back pain population. Spine 14:420–423, 1989.

111. Walsh TR, Weinstein JN, Spratt KF, et al: Lumbar discography in normal subjects: A controlled prospective study. J Bone Joint Surg 72A:1081–1088, 1990.

112. White AA, Panjabi MM: Clinical Biomechanics of the Spine, 2nd ed. Philadelphia, Lippincott-Raven, 1990, p 390.

113. Wiesel SW, Tsourmas N, Feffer HL, et al: A study of computer assisted tomography. I. The incidence of positive CAT scans in an asymptomatic group of patients. Spine 9:549–556, 1984.

114. Wiley J, McNab I, Wortzman G: Lumbar discography and its clinical applications. Can J Surg 11:280–289, 1968.

115. Wilmink JT: CT morphology of intrathecal lumbosacral nerve root compression. Am J Neuroradiol 10:233–248, 1989.

116. Winter RB, Schellhas KP: Painful adult thoracic Scheuermann's disease: Diagnosis by discography and treatment by combined arthrodesis. Am J Orthop 25:783–786, 1996.

117. Yoshizawa H, O'Brien JP, Thomas-Smith W, et al: The neuropathology of intervertebral discs removed for low back pain. J Pathol 132:95–104, 1980.

118. Yrjama M, Vanharanta H: Bony vibration stimulation: A new, non-invasive method for examining intradiscal pain. Eur Spine J 3:233–235, 1994.

119. Yrjama M, Tervonen O, Vanharanta H: Ultrasonic imaging of lumbar discs combined with vibration pain provocation compared with discography in the diagnosis of internal anular fissures of the lumbar spine. Spine 21:571–575, 1996.

120. Yrjama M, Tervonen O, Kurunlahti M, et al: Bony vibration stimulation test combined with magnetic resonance imaging: Can discography be replaced? Spine 22:808–813, 1997.

121. Yu SW, Haughton VM, Sether LA, et al: Comparison of MR and discography in detecting radial tears of the annulus: A post-mortem study. Am J Neuroradiol 10:1077–1081, 1989.

122. Yu SW, Sether LA, Ho PS, et al: Tears of the annulus fibrosus: A correlation between MR and pathologic findings in cadavers. Am J Neuroradiol 9:367–370, 1988.

123. Zucherman J, Derby R, Hsu K, et al: Normal magnetic resonance imaging with abnormal discography. Spine 13:1355–1359, 1988.

26

Sacroiliac Joint Injection and Arthrography with Imaging Correlation

Joseph D. Fortin, D.O., and Nalini Sehgal, M.D.

Life is uncharted territory. It reveals its story one moment at a time.

— Leo Busgaglia

Sacroiliac joint (SIJ) dysfunction as a primary source of low back pain is a resurgent topic. Metabolic, inflammatory, infectious, traumatic, degenerative, and structural etiologies of sacroiliac joint pain have all been described.[1,2,8,11–13,16,22,36,47,53,59,60] Still, the concept of mechanical SIJ pain has yet to gain widespread recognition in the differential diagnosis of low back pain.

A host of factors has impeded modern scientific interest in validating the sacroiliac joint as a generator of mechanical low back pain. Paradoxically, at the turn of the century the SIJ was considered the most common cause of sciatica.[6,29] This theory fell from favor in 1934 when Mixter and Barr described herniated nucleus pulposus in subjects with sciatica.[45] Other reasons for overlooking the SIJ as a potential pain generator include meager information on SIJ-mediated pain, deep inaccessible location of the joint, nonspecific physical examination tests, and technically demanding SIJ injections.

Major medical texts fail to discuss the widespread neural innervation,[55] anatomic variability,[5,35,59] and unique biomechanical properties[3,13,30–32,45,57,60] of the SIJ. The limited number of reports that provide basic science and clinical information pertinent to the SIJ are scattered among osteopathic, chiropractic, physiotherapy, biomechanic, radiology, and spine journals. Hence, even the scant information that is available has not been widely disseminated.

Until recently, there were no studies to demonstrate that reproducible pain could be elicited by stimulating a normal SIJ. True intra-articular injections were considered difficult, if not impossible,[4,35] and arthrography had not been described[34,43] except in cadavers.[35] The existence of pain patterns that could be ascribed to the SIJ was also questioned.

Clinical tests believed to evaluate SIJ dysfunction are in fact pelvic motion tests. These tests indicate pelvic girdle dysfunction and do not distinguish the various causes of pelvic girdle pain including SIJ pain. By themselves, these tests cannot reliably predict symptomatic sacroiliac dysfunction.[14,15] It is no surprise that the clinical presentation of sacroiliac joint dysfunction has been nebulous.

There is now compelling evidence for the sacroiliac joint to be a putative source of mechanical low back pain. Radionuclide scans attest to the high metabolic activity at the sacroiliac joint.[18] Like other synovial joints,[5,59] the sacroiliac joint moves,[7,10,17,27,38,48,52,54,56,63,64] although the amplitude of motion is small. Strategic placement of the sacroiliac joint between the spine and the hip joints subjects it to enormous mechanical stressors.[33,42,54,57,58,60,61] In addition, its rich innervation provides an anatomic substrate for pain.[55] A recent study on human cadavers suggests that the sacroiliac joint is predominantly innervated by the dorsal sacral rami of S1–S2 roots.[23] Ongoing research on surgically removed specimens of human SIJ capsule indicates the existence of mechanoreceptors and nociceptors in the periarticular tissues of the sacroiliac joint.[23] Proximity of the SIJ to the lumbosacral plexus ventrally, sacral nerve roots dorsally, and the L5 nerve root superiorly provides a potential nociceptive pathway.[26]

The author and coworkers have applied provocative injections and arthrography to (1) describe SIJ pain referral patterns in asymptomatic volunteers,[19] (2) predict symptomatic sacroiliac joints in patients with suspected lumbar discogenic or zygapophyseal joint pain,[20] (3) describe morphologic features of the SIJ capsule,[24,25] and (4) define contrast extravasation patterns on SIJ arthrography and postarthrography–computed tomography (CT) in subjects with low back or groin pain. Tracking of contrast medium from capsular rents along adjacent nerve roots and nerve plexuses may provide an explanation for groin and lower limb referred pain frequently seen with SIJ dysfunction.[26]

PATIENT SELECTION AND DIAGNOSTIC CONSIDERATIONS

While interest in sacroiliac joint pain has been rekindled, the steps toward its diagnosis remain enigmatic. The challenge for the clinician is to distinguish patients with sacroiliac joint dysfunction from those with other causes of low back pain.[14,15,33,36]

Sacroiliac joint dysfunction is suspected when a patient presents with a suggestive mechanism of injury. Common mechanisms include a direct fall on the buttocks, a rear-end motor vehicle accident (with the ipsilateral foot on the brake at the moment of impact), a broadside-type motor vehicle accident (with a blow to the lateral aspect of the pelvic ring), and a fall in a hole (with one leg in the hole and the other extended outside).[18] The diagnosis is further supported if the patient points with one finger to an area of pain just inferomedial to the posterior superior iliac spine (PSIS); this exercise (the Fortin finger test) has a high correlation with provocation positive injections when other causes of low back pain have been excluded.[18,24] This area of the back and the SIJ are innervated by the dorsal rami of the sacral nerve roots. Cadaveric dissections of adult and fetal sacroiliac joints by Kissling reveal an almost exclusive innervation of the SIJ by nerve twigs derived from S1–S4 dorsal rami. It is suggested that stimulation of these nerve fibers during SIJ arthrography refers sensory symptoms in the distribution of dorsal sacral rami.[23] Pain diagrams, which document a predominant pain zone extending from the PSIS to the caudal portion of the joint, can accurately predict which patients with suspected discogenic or posterior element pain have symptomatic sacroiliac joints upon provocative injection.[19,20] Tangentially, all patients with suspect presentations should have the necessary laboratory and radiologic work-up to exclude spondyloarthropathic, metabolic, or infectious etiology of sacroiliac joint pain.

Physical examination findings include a positive seated flexion–standing flexion test or Gillet test for aberrant sacroiliac motion, pain provocation with Patrick's maneuver, positive Gaenslen's test, positive distraction and compression tests, and tenderness over the ipsilateral sacroiliac joint, sacrotuberous ligament, piriformis muscle, and pubic symphysis.[4,18,21,24,37]

Screening imaging modalities such as bone scan and CT scan may prove helpful[28,39,42,51,62]; however, a cost-effective clinical algorithm for their use has not been identified. A radionuclide scan may reflect misleading or indiscernible metabolic changes,[28] but asymmetric radioisotope uptake sometimes can be a credible clinical indicator.[18,41] One study suggests that bone scintigraphy has a viable role as a noninvasive method of diagnosing mechanical sacroiliac joint pain.[41] Mild degenerative changes of the sacroiliac joint on CT scan are common after the age of 30 years.[51] Degenerative changes may be found earlier in athletes and workers who repetitively stress the joint; characteristic morphologic changes in response to stress develop.[22,62] Subtle CT changes, such as asymmetric joint width or sacral torsion, in the overall clinical context may manifest a greater clinical significance.[18]

Reproduction of symptoms upon distention of the joint capsule by provocative injection and subsequent mitigation with an analgesic block confirm the diagnosis.[19,20] The ligamentous integrity of the joint is established arthrographically.[25]

Because diagnostic injections are invasive, patient selection should be reserved for patients who have the above profile for a potentially painful sacroiliac joint and have failed to respond to aggressive functional restoration or who have reached a plateau in physical therapy. In these cases, sacroiliac joint injection can be applied for diagnostic affirmation and for the therapeutic benefit of the intra-articular injection of anesthetic and long-acting corticosteroid.

In experienced hands, SIJ injections can be performed safely without complications. A low morbidity rate does not, however, obviate the need for preprocedural patient education and the same precautions and preparation necessary for any spinal invasive technique. For details, see chapter 25.

RADIOLOGIC EQUIPMENT AND MATERIALS

Sacroiliac joint injections at or above the level of the PSIS are commonly performed as routine office procedures without the advantage of image intensifier control.[4] Because of the thickness of the dorsal sacroiliac and interosseous ligaments as well as the tortuous opposing surfaces of the medial iliac wing and dorsal sacrum, these injections most likely result in ligamentous or subligamentous deposit of solutions.[35] Even at the relatively accessible inferior portion of the joint, a "blind" injection is unlikely to find its way to the joint space, because the needle is deflected by the irregular and convoluted joint surface or slips off the posterolateral margin of the iliac bone (deep to the gluteus muscle).

Fluoroscopic control is essential to ensure an intra-articular injection. Suitable equipment options include (1) a routine fluoroscopy suite with an overhead tower or C-arm, (2) a special procedures suite with a C-arm or angio unit, or (3) an operating room with a C-arm.

Most patients can be studied with standard 25-gauge, 3.5-inch spinal needles without local infiltration. Skin and subcutaneous tissues are infiltrated with 1% lidocaine (Xylocaine) for larger diameter needles. The tensile strength of a 22-gauge needle can be useful, on occasion, to gain entry into narrow and tortuous joints. Rarely, a 6-inch needle is required.

Luer-Lok 3-ml syringes allow the greatest sensitivity to change in resistance at the needle hub. Larger syringes require substantially greater pressure to inject, even without obstruction.

Contrast medium is used for needle position verification, provocation, and arthrography. Nonionic contrast agents such as iohexol and iopamidol are more expensive but less allergenic and irritating than their ionic counterparts (e.g., methylgucamine-isothalamate), so they are preferred over the ionic contrast agents routinely used. A concentration of 240–300 mg per ml is recommended.

THE PROCEDURE

The patient is sterilely prepped and draped in the prone position (Fig. 26-1). Under image intensifier control, a 25- or 22-gauge, 3.5-inch spinal needle is directed into the inferior aspect of the sacroiliac joint using a posterior approach. The usual portal of entry is the inferior one-third of the joint. There is often a lucency in the inferior aspect of the joint, which allows the least resistance upon needle passage (Fig. 26-2). There may be two or more "limbs" of the joint, because the joint is laterally divergent from its posterior to anterior borders and has interdigitations. In this instance, the medial or posterior division is the most amenable to cannulation. Where the inferior aspect of the joint cannot be entered, the joint is accessed through the deeper more rostral aspect of the joint. Rolling the patient obliquely 5–10° from side to side when using an overhead fluoroscopy unit or rotating the C-arm side to side in an axial plane will permit a better three-dimensional perspective of the joint and enable selection of the "window" for optimal needle trajectory. With few exceptions, a direct posterior approach is used. Once the dorsal sacroiliac and interosseous ligaments are engaged, the needle often takes a characteristic bend because it conforms with the interdigitating contours of the diarthrodial joint (see Figure 26-2). This phenomenon is often preceded by a subtle tactile sensation of a "giving way"

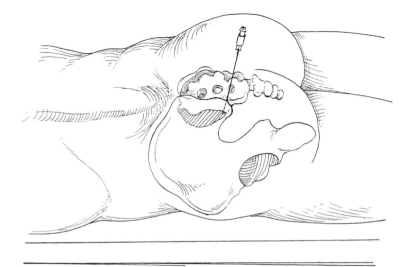

FIGURE 26-1. Sacroiliac joint injection. The patient is in a prone position, and the needle has been guided into the inferior aspect of the joint employing a direct posterior approach.

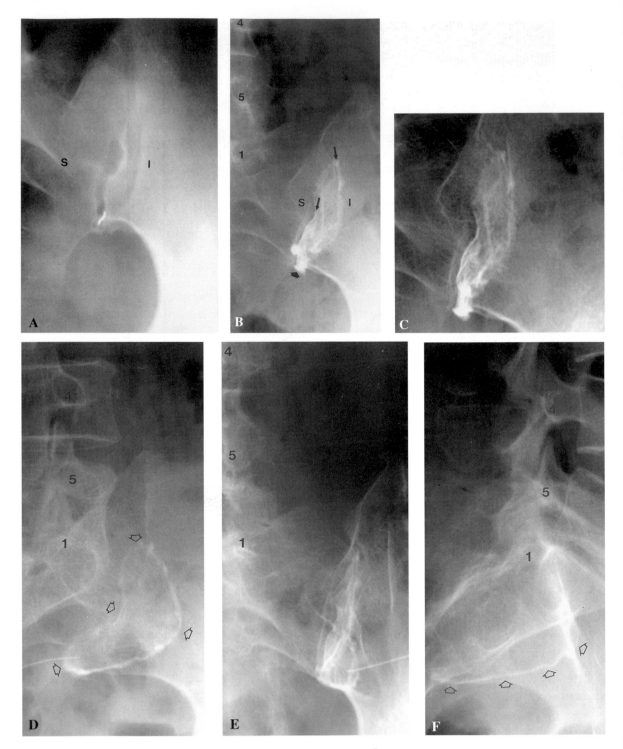

FIGURE 26-2. Sacroiliac joint arthrography. *A,* Preinjection spot film documents the needle, with a characteristic bend, within the inferior aspect of the joint. Note the lucent area around the needle. *B,* Posteroanterior arthrogram of the right sacroiliac joint. Divergent joint surfaces appear as distinct beads of contrast (*arrows*) or "separate" joint cavities. A 25-gauge, 3.5-inch spinal needle is in the inferior aspect of the joint. (Arrowhead = coin-shaped inferior recess; S = sacrum; I = ilium.) *C,* Magnified posteroanterior projection spot film. *D,* Oblique view of the right sacroiliac joint. This en-face view delineates the auricular shape of the synovial joint (*arrowheads*). (4 = pedicle of L4; 5 = pedicle of L5; 1 = pedicle of S1.) *E,* Opposite oblique arthrogram contiguously demarcates the vertical extent of the joint space. Compare with Figure 26-2B. *F,* Lateral view of the right sacroiliac joint capsular margin. The ventral capsular border is demarcated by contrast medium (*arrowhead*). (5 = pedicle of L5; 1 = pedicle of S1.)

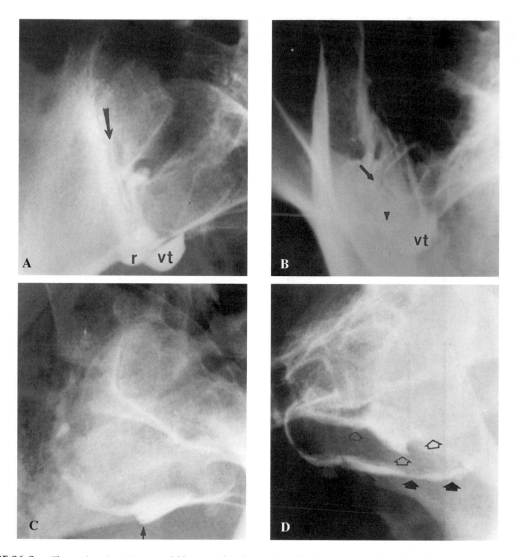

FIGURE 26-3. The patient is a 37-year-old housewife who was involved in a rear-end motor vehicle accident with her left foot planted firmly on the brake at the moment of impact. She presented with left hip, thigh, and groin pain. Because the lumbosacral plexus is immediately anterior to the SIJ, these findings may help to explain the lower extremity symptoms in some patients with SIJ pain. *A,* A posteroanterior arthrogram. (r = inferior recess; vy = collection of contrast escaping through a ventral tear arrow-bead of contrast within joint margins.) *B,* Opposite oblique view. This confirms that the needle tip (*arrowhead*) is remote to ventral tear (vt). Arrow-bead of contrast is within joint space. *C,* Oblique view. The smooth line of contrast medium outlining the capsular margins (*arrow*) is interrupted by an anterior capsular and anterior sacroiliac ligamentous rent.

(*Figure continued on next page.*)

at the needle hub as the needle purchases and then penetrates through the ligaments to enter the joint. If bony resistance is met after the ligaments are engaged, and the needle is not yet within the joint margin, the needle should be withdrawn slightly without becoming disengaged. Subsequent needle advancement, while simultaneously rotating it around its own longitudinal axis, will allow it to deflect and conform to the joint margins. The initial instillation of a small amount of contrast medium should outline the coin-shaped inferior recess of the joint. This landmark on the anteroposterior (AP) projection, together with the auricular shape of the diarthrodial joint in the oblique view, should allow definitive evaluation of proper needle position.

Following verification of initial needle position, further contrast is instilled to a volume commensurate with firm end-point resilience or fluoroscopically visualized extravasation. Provocation responses are recorded at this time and anesthesia administered accordingly (see Codifying Provocation/Analgesia Responses, below). If arthrographic resolution is diluted by anesthesia, 0.2–0.4 ml of additional contrast will serve to bolster the image.

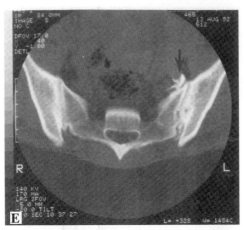

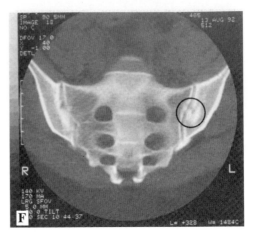

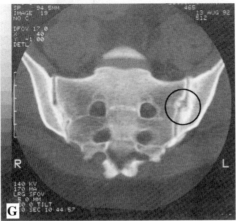

FIGURE 26-3 (Cont). *D*, Offset lateral of bilateral arthrograms discloses an intact right ventral capsule (*closed arrowheads*) in contrast to disrupted left capsule (*open arrowheads*). *E*, Postarthrography axial CT at the proximal S2 level (bone window/level settings). Contrast medium is present within both sacroiliac joints. A presacral collection of contrast medium is clearly noted, evidencing a ventral tear (arrow). Contrast solution contacts the lumbosacral plexus elements. *F* and *G*, Two coronal views through the sacroiliac joint in the same patient. Note the area of joint margin cortical irregularity on the left. These changes are similar to osteochondritis dissecans commonly seen in appendicular joints. The opposing areas of bony prominence on the iliac (most remarkable) and sacral surfaces suggest a partially detached subchondral fragment with a surrounding lucent area and adjacent iliac sclerosis (*areas encircled*). This combination of eburnation, macroporosity, and sclerosis may be the osseous footprints of stress hardening secondary to trauma. Similar changes may be occurring on the right to a lesser extent.

PLAIN FILM EVALUATION

The AP view demonstrates the inferior recess of the joint, contrast within the joint margins, and any subligamentous or inferior recess extension (see Figure 26-2). The oblique (en-face) view is essential to delineate precisely where the contrast is in relation to the joint borders (see Figure 26-2). This view will reveal diverticula and ventral capsular tears to vantage (Fig. 26-3; see also Figure 26-2). The lateral view also demonstrates posterior ligamentous extravasation, diverticula, or ventral tears (see Figure 26-3). If bilateral arthrograms are obtained, an "offset" lateral (10–20° from a true lateral projection) will allow one to compare both capsular borders on one film (see Figure 26-3). As a result of beam attenuation in the lateral projection, the ventral tears or diverticula are not as sharply resolved as on the en-face view. At times, the opposite oblique view can add additional information including a clear view of the contrast within the superior joint space, superior recess extravasation, an outline of some diverticula, and confirmation of any extravasation from the inferior recess or

anteroinferior capsule (noted on other projections) (see Figure 26-3).

CODIFYING PROVOCATION/ ANALGESIA RESPONSES

Provocation

For the grading system, see chapter 25.

Fortin et al. arthrographically studied the sacroiliac joints of 10 asymptomatic volunteers. Upon direct intra-articular injection and under fluoroscopic visualization, these volunteers experienced unsustained, pressure-type buttock discomfort—in contrast to intense buttock pain evoked upon stimulating a symptomatic SIJ.[19] This suggests that the disparity between an asymptomatic and symptomatic joint should be easily distinguished by an experienced operator.

Analgesia

Following a provocation positive injection, 0.6–1.0 ml of a long-acting anesthetic (e.g., 0.75% bupivacaine) is instilled. A long-acting corticosteroid

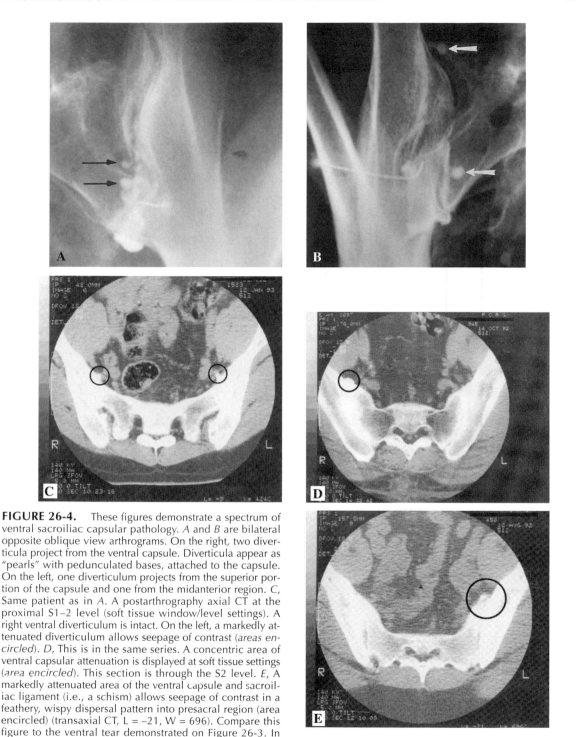

FIGURE 26-4.   These figures demonstrate a spectrum of ventral sacroiliac capsular pathology. *A* and *B* are bilateral opposite oblique view arthrograms. On the right, two diverticula project from the ventral capsule. Diverticula appear as "pearls" with pedunculated bases, attached to the capsule. On the left, one diverticulum projects from the superior portion of the capsule and one from the midanterior region. *C,* Same patient as in *A.* A postarthrography axial CT at the proximal S1–2 level (soft tissue window/level settings). A right ventral diverticulum is intact. On the left, a markedly attenuated diverticulum allows seepage of contrast (*areas encircled*). *D,* This is in the same series. A concentric area of ventral capsular attenuation is displayed at soft tissue settings (*area encircled*). This section is through the S2 level. *E,* A markedly attenuated area of the ventral capsule and sacroiliac ligament (i.e., a schism) allows seepage of contrast in a feathery, wispy dispersal pattern into presacral region (area encircled) (transaxial CT, L = –21, W = 696). Compare this figure to the ventral tear demonstrated on Figure 26-3. In contrast to a contained, attenuated area, schisms generally extend greater than a single 5-mm axial CT section. However, both contained attenuations and schisms are inconspicuous on plain film.

such as betamethasone (Celestone) can be combined with the local anesthetic in 2:1 proportion. Volumes are small (less than 2.0 ml of contrast and anesthetic), commensurate with the joint's capacity. This ensures a focal anesthetic effect (i.e., limited dispersal to adjacent structures). In a study of 74 SIJ injections, the mean volume of contrast injected was determined to be 1.08 ml (standard deviation 0.29 ml).[25]

Some patients with a convincing mechanism of injury, pain diagram, physical examination, and

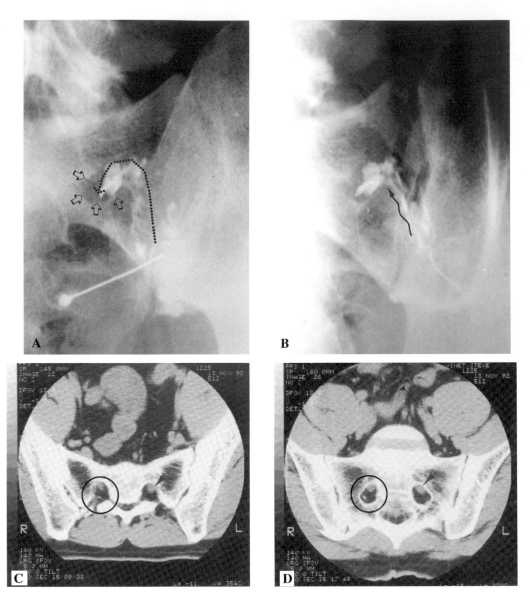

FIGURE 26-5.   This case, involving a 33-year-old offshore worker with a prolonged right H-reflex (on electrodiagnostics), illustrates a third arthrographic link between the SIJ and neural elements. Posterior subligamentous extension of contrast into the S1 dorsal foramina (*arrowheads*) is shown on the right. *A*, Posteroanterior arthrogram. Contrast is seen extending into the S1 dorsal foramina (*curved arrow*). *B*, Opposite oblique view in same patient demonstrates pathway of contrast from the joint margins into the S1 dorsal foramina (*wavy arrow*). *C* and *D*, Axial and direct coronal postarthrography CT through the S1 dorsal foramina (soft tissue window settings). Contrast is visualized in the S1 dorsal foramina on both scans (*areas encircled*). (Arrowheads = contralateral S1 anterior ramus).

provocative injection fail to respond favorably to anesthetization of SIJ.[20] The reason for this is unclear but may involve supervening factors such as central neurogenic facilitation or psychosocial modifiers.

PLAIN FILM AND CT ARTHROGRAPHIC FINDINGS

Before describing morphologic capsular findings in the SIJ as "pathologic," the developmental and maturational changes of the normal sacroiliac joint must first be elucidated. The morphologic characteristics of 74 sacroiliac joint arthrograms were described by Fortin and Tolchin[25]; the findings on plain film arthrograms were classified and compared to their postarthrography-CT counterparts. After carefully scoring anterior, posterior, superior, and inferior aspects of the capsule, they found a significant direct correlation between data recorded from both modalities. This study demonstrated that a detailed analysis of the SIJ capsule is possible by plain film arthrography or postarthrography CT, with excellent agreement between the two techniques. Moreover, each test has specific regional benefits: the plain film displayed diverticula to optimal advantage, and postarthrography-CT was superior in resolving anterior capsular "pathology."

Sacroiliac joint arthrography has disclosed abnormalities in capsular morphology that encompasses discrete attenuated areas, schisms, frank tears (Figs. 26-3 and 26-4), and diverticula varying in size, shape, and number (see Figure 26-3).[25] Arthrographic findings indicate three potential pathways of communication between the SIJ and the neural elements.[25,26] These are (1) posterior subligamentous extension into the dorsal sacral foramina (Fig. 26-5), (2) superior recess extravasation at the alar level into the L5 epiradicular sheath (Fig. 26-6), and (3) leakage from a ventral tear to the lumbosacral plexus

(see Figure 26-3). Extravasation of inflammatory mediators from a dysfunctional sacroiliac joint to adjacent neural tissues may explain the radicular pain in some patients. Electrodiagnostic correlation is needed; however, compelling anecdotal cases of impaired nerve function in patients with sacroiliac joint pain have been observed.[25,26]

The current combined information on sacroiliac joint injection and arthrography represents a mere first approximation. Most likely because of the limited number of data points in any given category, no single arthrographic finding has been definitively correlated with pain provocation on injection.[25] Accordingly, the relevance of all the arthrographic findings as they pertain to patient care is in question.

Currently, we are resigned to extrapolate findings on SIJ arthrography to what is "normal" and "abnormal" in other joints. For instance, a full-thickness ligamentous tear often renders a joint unstable.

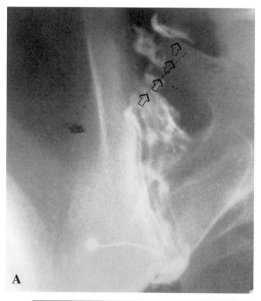

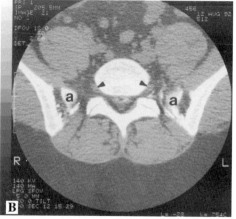

FIGURE 26-6. Another putative pathway between the SIJ and neural elements is visualized in this case of a 19-year-old clerk with a pain diagram suggestive of a left L5 radiculopathy. *A,* Posteroanterior arthrogram demonstrates contrast extravasating from the superior recess (*arrows*). *B,* Postarthrography axial CT at the level of L5–S1. Contrast has extended from the superior recess to the L5 epiradicular sheath at the alar level. (a = sacral ala; arrowheads = anterior rami of L5.)

In a weight-bearing joint, this instability is manifest as (1) intermittent and often painful sounds such as clicking, popping, grinding, or clunking, (2) a sudden "giving way," (3) a sense of apprehension or being "off-balance," (4) an inability to fully bear weight on the affected side, or (5) the inability to load the joint in a manner that stresses the involved structure. Hence, like some patients with knee meniscal tears, these symptoms in a patient with a sacroiliac ventral capsular rent may be the result of instability. Conversely, some asymptomatic patients, or those whose knee pain is attributable to other causes, may have incidental meniscal tears,[46] and some patients with or without back pain may have incidental SIJ ventral capsular tears.[25] Extrapolations must be made circumspectly because, when compared to other joints, the sacroiliac joint is unique in its configuration, mechanics, and histology. Arthrographic patterns aside, sacroiliac joint provocative injection remains the sole direct method to distinguish between a symptomatic and an asymptomatic joint. Such tests are needed to predicate treatment on the correct diagnosis.

POSTPROCEDURE CARE

Patients are observed in a holding area following the procedure. Vital signs are obtained, and the patient is provided fluids. If an arthrography-CT is indicated, the patient is transported to the CT scan within 1–2 hours.

Postprocedural instructions include education on the application of ice to the affected area and information on the usual postprocedural symptoms such as increased local pain and stiffness. In a study of asymptomatic volunteers, no pain was reported 48 hours after sacroiliac joint injections.[19] On occasion, a 2-day supply of narcotic analgesics are judiciously dispensed. Driving, manual labor, and sports activities are discouraged the day of the procedure. Most patients resume their usual activities within 24 hours. An instruction sheet provides emergency phone numbers and details the warning signs of infection. Patients can be safely discharged 1–2 hours following the procedure.

SUMMARY

Basic science research has enhanced our awareness on SIJ morphology and neurophysiology. Further study to identify the type of nerve endings within the SIJ capsule and inflammatory mediators within a dysfunctional sacroiliac joint may lend credence to the basis of provocative injections and help to explain referred pain.

Although MRI is invaluable in assessing other joints (e.g., shoulder or knee), where it provides exquisite details of soft tissue anatomy and articular surfaces, its role in evaluating SIJ pathology is yet to be established. CT remains superior to MRI in depicting sacroiliac joint abnormalities. Both CT and MRI are, however, limited by their failure to identify convincingly the pain generator. Currently, provocative-analgesic injections combined with postarthrographic CT imaging are the only means to confirm whether the SIJ is a valid pain generator. The statistical temperament of all SIJ diagnostic tests must be carefully investigated and compared with a more substantial basic science database. This information in turn should be coalesced into a paradigm that is practical for clinical application.

REFERENCES

1. Ahlstrom H, Feltelius N, Nyman R, et al: Magnetic resonance imaging of sacroiliac joint inflammation. Arthritis Rheum 33:1763–1769, 1990.
2. Bakalim G: Results of radical evacuation and arthrodesis in sacroiliac tuberculosis. Acta Orthop Scand 37:375–386, 1966.
3. Beal MC: The sacroiliac problem: Review of anatomy, mechanics, and diagnosis. J Am Osteopath Assoc 81:667–679, 1982.
4. Bernard TN, Cassidy JD: Sacroiliac joint syndrome: Pathophysiology, diagnosis and management. In Frymoyer JW (ed): The Adult Spine: Principles and Practice, 2nd ed. Philadelphia, Lippincott-Raven, 1997, pp 2343–2366.
5. Bowen V, Cassidy JD: Macroscopic and microscopic anatomy of the sacroiliac joint from embryonic life until the eighth decade. Spine 6:620–628, 1981.
6. Brooke R: The sacroiliac joint. J Anat 58:299–305, 1924.
7. Brunner CH, Kissling RO, Jacob HAC: The effects of morphology and histopathology on the mobility of the sacroiliac joint. Spine 16:1111–1117, 1991.
8. Carrera GF, Foley WD, Kozin F, et al: CT of sacroiliitis. Am J Radiol 136:41–46, 1981.
9. Chafetz N, Genant HK, Gillespy T, et al: Magnetic resonance imaging. In Kricun ME (ed): Imaging Modalities in Spinal Disorders. Philadelphia, W.B. Saunders, 1988, p 499.
10. Colachis SC, Worden RE, Bechtol CD, et al: Movement of the sacroiliac joint in the adult male: A preliminary report. Arch Phys Med Rehabil 44:491–498, 1985.
11. Cossermelli-Messina W, Festa Neto C, Cossermelli W: Articular inflammatory manifestations in patients with different forms of leprosy. J Rheumatol 25:111–119, 1998.
12. Coy JT, Wolf CR, Brower JD: Pyogenic arthritis of the sacroiliac joints. J Bone Joint Surg 5A:845–849, 1976.
13. DonTigny R: Function and pathomechanics of the sacroiliac joint. Phys Ther 65:35–44, 1985.
14. Dreyfuss P, Dreyer S, Griffin J, et al: Positive sacroiliac screening tests in asymptomatic adults. Spine 19:1138–1143, 1994.
15. Dreyfuss P, Michaelsen M, Pauza K, et al: The value of history and physical examination in diagnosing sacroiliac joint pain. Spine 21:2594–2602, 1996.
16. Dunn EJ, Byron DM, Nugent JT: Pyogenic infections of the sacroiliac joint. Clin Orthop 118:113–117, 1976.

17. Egund N, Olsson TH, Schmid H, Selvik G: Movements in the sacroiliac joint demonstrated with roentgenstereophotogrammetry. Acta Radiol Diagn 19:833–846, 1978.

18. Fortin JD: The sacroiliac joint: A new perspective. J Back Musculoskel Rehabil 3:31–43, 1993.

19. Fortin JD, Dwyer A, West S, et al: Sacroiliac joint pain referral patterns upon application of a new injection/arthrography technique. Part I: Asymptomatic volunteers. Spine 19:1475–1482, 1994.

20. Fortin JD, Dwyer A, Aprill C, et al: Sacroiliac joint pain referral patterns. Part II: Clinical evaluation. Spine 19:1483–1489, 1994.

21. Fortin JD, Falco F: The Fortin finger test: An indicator of sacroiliac joint pain. Am J Orthop 7:477–480, 1997.

22. Fortin JD, Falco F: Enigmatic causes of spine pain in athletes. Phys Med Rehabil State Art Rev 11:445–464, 1997.

23. Fortin JD, Kissling RO, O'Connor BL, et al: Sacroiliac joint innervation and pain. Am J Orthop 28(12), 1999.

24. Fortin JD, Pier J, Falco F: Sacroiliac joint injection: Pain referral mapping and arthrographic findings. In Vleeming A, Mooney V, Dorman T, et al (eds): Movement, Stability, and Low Back Pain: The Essential Role of the Pelvis. New York, Churchill-Livingstone, 1997, pp 271–285.

25. Fortin JD, Tolchin R: Sacroiliac arthrograms and post-arthrography CT. Arch Phys Med Rehabil 74:1259, 1993.

26. Fortin JD, Washington WJ, Falco F: Three pathways between the sacroiliac joint and neural structures exist. Am J Neuroradiol 20:1429–1434, 1999.

27. Frigerio NA, Stowe RR, Howe JW: Movement of the sacroiliac joint. Clin Orthop 100:370–377, 1974.

28. Goldberg RP, Genant HK, Shimshak R, Shames D: Applications and limitation of quantitative sacroiliac joint scintigraphy. Radiology 128:683–686, 1978.

29. Goldthwaite GE, Osgood RB: A consideration of the pelvic articulations from an anatomical, pathological, and clinical standpoint. Boston Med Surg J 152:593–601, 1905.

30. Greenman PE: Clinical aspects of sacroiliac function in walking. J Manual Med 5:125–129, 1990.

31. Grieve E: Lumbopelvic rhythm and mechanical dysfunction of the sacroiliac joint. Physiotherapy 67:171–173, 1981.

32. Grieve E: Mechanical dysfunction of the sacroiliac joint. Int Rehabil Med 5:46–52, 1982.

33. Gunterbert B, Romanus B, Stener B: Pelvic strength after major amputation of the sacrum: An experimental approach. Acta Orthop Scand 47:635–642, 1976.

34. Hendrix RW, Lin PP, Kane WJ: Simplified aspiration of injection technique for the sacroiliac joint. J Bone Joint Surg 64A:1249–1252, 1982.

35. Kissling RO: Zur arthrographie des iliosacralgelenks. Z Rheumat 51:183–187, 1992.

36. Kuslich SD, Ulstrom CL, Michael CJ: The tissue origin of low back pain and sciatica. Orthop Clin North Am 22:181–187, 1991.

37. Laslett M, Williams M: The reliability of selected pain provocation tests for sacroiliac joint pathology. Spine 19:1243–1249, 1994.

38. Lavignolle B, Vital JM, Senega S, et al: An approach to the functional anatomy of the sacroiliac joints in vivo. Anat Clin 5:169–176, 1982.

39. Lawson TL: The sacroiliac joint: Anatomic plain roentgenographic and computed tomographic analysis. J Comput Assist Tomogr 6:307–314, 1982.

40. Maigne JY, Aivaliklis A, Pfefer F: Results of sacroiliac joint double block and value of sacroiliac pain provocation tests in 54 patients with low back pain. Spine 21:1889–1892, 1996.

41. Mierau D: Scintigraphic analysis of sacroiliac pain. In Program of the 7th Annual Meeting of the North American Spine Society. Rosemont, IL, North American Spine Society, 1992.

42. Miller JAA, Schultz AM, Anderson GBJ: Load-displacement behavior of sacroiliac joints. J Orthop Res 5:92–101, 1987.

43. Miskew DB, Block RA, Witt PF: Aspiration of infected sacroiliac joints. J Bone Joint Surg 32A:1591–1597, 1979.

44. Mitchell SL, Moran PS, Pruzzo NA: An Evaluation and Treatment Manual of Osteopathic Muscle Energy Procedures. Manchester, MO, Mitchell, Moran and Pruzzo Assoc., 1979.

45. Mixter WJ, Barr JS: Rupture of the intervertebral disc with involvement of the spinal canal. N Engl J Med 211:210–215, 1934.

46. Negendank WG, Fernandez-Madrid FR, Heilbrom LK, et al: Magnetic resonance imaging of meniscal degeneration in asymptomatic knees. J Orthop Res 8:311–320, 1990.

47. Norman GF, May A: Sacroiliac conditions simulating intervertebral disc syndrome. West J Surg 64:461–462, 1956.

48. Pitkin HC, Pheasant HC: Sacrarthrogenic telalgi II: A study of sacral mobility. J Bone Joint Surg 18:365–374, 1936.

49. Porterfield JA, Oerosu C: The sacroiliac joint. In Gould JA (ed): Orthopaedic and Sports Physical Therapy, 2nd ed. St. Louis, Mosby, 1990, pp 553–559.

50. Remy M, Bouillet P, Bertin P, et al: Evaluation of magnetic resonance imaging for the detection of sacroiliitis in patients with early seronegative spondyloarthropathy. Rev Rhum Engl Ed 63:577–583, 1996.

51. Resnick E, Niwayama G, Georgen TG: Degenerative disease of the sacroiliac joint. Invest Radiol 10:608–621, 1975.

52. Reynolds HM: Three-dimensional kinematics in the pelvic girdle. J Am Osteopath Assoc 80:277–280, 1980.

53. Roland MR, Morris RM: A study of the natural history of low back pain. Spine 8:145–150, 1983.

54. Scholten PJM, Schultz AB, Luchies CW, et al: Motions and loads within the human pelvis: A biomechanical model study. J Orthop Res 6:840–850, 1988.

55. Solonen KA: The sacroiliac joint in the light of anatomical, roentgenological and clinical studies. Acta Orthop Scand Suppl 27:1–127, 1957.

56. Sturesson B, Selvik G, Uden A: Movements of the sacroiliac joints: A roentgenstereophotogrammetric analysis. Spine 14:162–165, 1989.

57. Vleeming A, et al: Load application to the sacrotuberous ligament: Influences on sacroiliac joint mechanics. Clin Biomech 4:204–209, 1989.

58. Vleeming A, Stoeckart TR, Snijders CJ: The sacrotuberous ligament: A conceptual approach to its dynamic role in stabilizing the sacroiliac joint. Clin Biomech 4:201–203, 1989.

59. Vleeming A, Stoeckart R, Volkers ACW, et al: Relation between form and function in the sacroiliac joint. Part I: Clinical anatomical aspects. Spine 15:130–132, 1990.

60. Vleeming A, Volkers ACW, Snijders CJ, et al: Relation between form and function in the sacroiliac joint. Part II: Biomechanical aspects. Spine 15:133–135, 1990.

61. Vleeming A, Pool-Goudzwaard AL, Hammudoghlu D, et al: The function of the long dorsal sacroiliac ligament. Spine 21:556–562, 1996.

62. Vogler JB, Brown WH, Helms CA, Genant HK: The normal sacroiliac joint: A CT study of asymptomatic patients. Radiology 151:433–437, 1984.

63. Weisl H: The movements of the sacroiliac joint. Acta Anat 23:80–90, 1955.

64. Wilder DG, Pope MH, Frymoyer JW: The functional topography of the sacroiliac joint. Spine 5:575–579, 1980.

27

Zygapophyseal Joint Injection Techniques in the Spinal Axis

Paul Dreyfuss, M.D., Michael Kaplan, M.D.
and Susan J. Dreyer, M.D.

Injections to diagnose and control pain originating from the zygapophyseal joints (z-joints) should be used as an adjunct to active and conservative spine care. These injections have become an important aspect of nonsurgical spine care. Although their value has been disputed,[27,57,74,75,88] when appropriately used they can provide both diagnostic information and potentially therapeutic benefit. Fluoroscopically guided, contrast-enhanced z-joint injection procedures help to specifically evaluate the z-joint as a source of spinal and referred extremity pain.[6,7,10,14–16,23,28,29,32,33,37–39,41, 42,53,54,58,76,79,83,84,89,90,98–100,109,111,132] These injection procedures also may provide short- and long-term pain relief through the effects of the anesthetic and corticosteroid, respectively.[18,47,48] Pain relief may allow patients to advance through their rehabilitation program more rapidly, resulting in improved function.

The lumbar z-joints were first identified as a source of pain in 1911.[64] In 1933, the term facet syndrome was coined to refer to the low back and leg symptom complex associated with pain emanating from these joints.[64] Subsequently, various types of localized, pseudoradicular, and somatic referred pain states have been described from these joints in the lumbar and later in the cervical and thoracic spine.[2,23,52,56,61,62–64,72,94,98,133]

Although this chapter reviews the general considerations and indications for z-joint injection techniques (intra-articular or medial branch blocks), it focuses on pertinent z-joint anatomy and block techniques in the cervical, thoracic, and lumbar spine. This chapter will not critique the literature related to the potential therapeutic efficacy of these procedures from the use of intra-articular corticosteroids; this topic is available for review elsewhere.[42,47,48,84]

GENERAL CONSIDERATIONS AND INDICATIONS

Before any z-joint injection, a patient should have a thorough regional musculoskeletal and neural examination that focuses on the painful spinal segments and any associated secondary sites of pathology within the kinetic chain. The authors support the use of plain films before z-joint injections to rule out fractures, infection, or neoplasm. Because there are no pathognomonic findings specific for z-joint-mediated pain, additional spinal imaging studies (e.g., computed tomography [CT], CT-myelography, magnetic resonance imaging [MRI], bone scans) and ancillary testing (laboratory and electrodiagnostic testing) help determine whether other sites of pathology exist (e.g., intrinsic disc disease, nerve root compression). Such pathology can mimic z-joint pain. Although no universally accepted treatment algorithm exists for cervical, thoracic, or lumbar z-joint pain, active conservative care should precede any injection procedure. Conservative care may include oral medications, modalities, traction, instruction in body mechanics, strengthening, flexibility training, specialized manual physical therapy (e.g., direct and indirect articular mobilization techniques, facilitated soft tissue stretching and positional release), aerobic conditioning, and restoration of optimal movement patterns. The specific details of any therapeutic intervention should be sought before one assumes that therapy was administered as prescribed. Patient compliance also should be assessed.

Because the vast majority of low back pain appears to be self-limited, the authors advocate z-joint injection procedures only after a minimum of 4 weeks of appropriate and directed conservative care. If pain is inhibiting progress in physical or manual therapy, the clinician may elect for earlier use of z-joint injection procedures.

Currently, z-joint injection procedures are the gold standard in the diagnosis of z-joint–mediated pain. Radiographs, history, physical examination, or a combination of these findings are not specific for cervical, thoracic, or lumbar z-joint-mediated pain. Diagnostically, z-joint injection procedures (intra-articular or medial branch blocks) are useful in confirming a suspected z-joint as either the sole source of or a contributor to a patient's pain complex. Either intra-articular or medial branch blocks can be used; this depends on the preference of the operator because they are believed to be equally diagnostic.[6,15,16,37,44,77,92] If joint entry is not possible, appropriate medial branch blocks should be performed to block the nerve supply to the suspected painful joint. To obtain both diagnostic and potentially therapeutic value, the z-joint may be injected with both anesthetic and corticosteroid. If medial branch blocks are used, corticosteroid should not be added routinely, because these injections are predominantly diagnostic. Confirming the z-joint(s) as a significant pain source focuses the patient's rehabilitation program and allows for z-joint neurotomy if the pain does not respond to other treatment measures.

Imaging studies provide only anatomic information and cannot independently determine whether particular structures are painful. Thus, abnormal CT or MRI scans demonstrating disc pathology are not a contraindication to z-joint injection procedures if the clinical evaluation provides sufficient evidence to investigate the z-joints.[47,100,109,131] Furthermore, absence of degenerative z-joint changes on plain radiographs, CT, or MRI do not contraindicate injection of these joints.[29,37,89,100,109,117] Bone and single photon emission computed tomography (SPECT) scans do not need to be abnormal to consider the z-joints as putatively painful.[108,122] However, with regard to response to intra-articular corticosteroids, a study of 58 patients with low back pain found that those with facetal uptake on SPECT scans had a 95% response rate at 1 month and a 79% response rate at 3 months to z-joint injections with steroid and anesthetic. In contrast, subjects with negative SPECT scans were unchanged after corticosteroid injections of their facet joints.[40]

Pain-inhibited weakness, subjective nondermatomal sensory loss, and extremity complaints should not be a contraindication to z-joint injections because these findings can occur with z-joint–mediated pain.[58,98]

Prior to z-joint injection procedures, bleeding disorders, infections, drug allergies, and current medications should be noted. There is no consensus as to the importance of discontinuing nonsteroidal anti-inflammatory drugs (NSAIDs) and aspirin before z-joint injection procedures. NSAIDs may be stopped 2–3 days before and aspirin 7–10 days before these injection procedures. Warfarin (Coumadin) should be discontinued 4–6 days before the scheduled injection. Patients on newer low-molecular-weight heparins (e.g., enoxaparin [Lovenox], ardeparin [Normiflo], or other antithrombotics such as danaparoid [Orgaran]) are at increased risk of bleeding and generally should not receive injections while on these agents. Antiplatelet agents such as ticlopidine (Ticlid) and clopidogrel (Plavix) are also contraindicated. Preinjection coagulation parameters can be used for patients on Coumadin.[43]

Patients with diabetes mellitus should monitor their blood glucose after corticosteroid injection and have a plan to treat a significant increase in their blood glucose. Patients with artificial heart valves may require the use of antibiotics before and after the procedure as determined by their surgeon or cardiologist. Because these are sterile procedures, preprocedural antibiotics are rarely needed for patients with mitral valve prolapse or artificial limbs. Patients being treated with antibiotics for any active infection should generally not undergo z-joint injection procedures. Febrile patients and those who are hemodynamically unstable with a significantly high or low blood pressure should not be injected. Many injectionists prefer that the patient neither eats nor drinks 3 hours before the procedure.

Intra-articular z-joint injections should not be used in treatment isolation. Analgesia from z-joint injections may facilitate treatment to advance recovery.[47,48,50] Duration of pain relief from intra-articular z-joint corticosteroids has been quite variable in open, noncontrolled clinical trials.[23,28,29,38,39,41,54,73,79,87,89,90,98,100,111,132,133] This likely represents variability in selection criteria, heterogeneity of the patient populations studied and the lack of uniformity in controlling any postinjection rehabilitation programs prescribed. Additionally, controlled trials have concluded that minimal to no benefit is gained from isolated z-joint injection[9,27,88]; these trials were randomized, controlled studies but did not meet all of the criteria for reporting of such trials.[1] A critique of the randomized, controlled trials in the lumbar spine exists.[42,48] When administered with other cointerventions in a noncontrolled fashion, substantial, lasting beneficial effects have been observed with z-joint corticosteroid injections versus placebo.[27] Further research is necessary to validate such combined therapies. Additionally, good to excellent long-term results have been reported following intra-articular corticosteroid injections in patients with synovial cysts and radicular pain.[104]

No agreement or available studies exist regarding the appropriate dose or type of corticosteroid used in z-joint injections; these decisions are left to the physician. The most common agents used are methylprednisolone acetate, triamcinolone diacetate, and betamethasone. Most clinicians use a mixture of 25–50% corticosteroid to 50–75% anesthetic for injection into the z-joints. The authors prefer to use stronger anesthetics (e.g., 0.75% bupivacaine or 4% lidocaine) in the hope that the false-negative rate decreases with these diagnostic injections. The agent used is dictated by the number of medial branch nerves or z-joints injected so that the total volume used remains safe if erroneous uptake were to occur in the venous system.

For purely diagnostic medial branch blocks, there is no rationale to simultaneously inject corticosteroids.[92,101] There are no reports of extended pain relief following anesthetic and corticosteroid medial branch blocks. If entrapment of the medial branch of the dorsal ramus under the mamilloaccessory ligament with symptomatic nerve irritation indeed exists, then corticosteroid medial branch blocks are theoretically attractive in this instance.

After informed consent is obtained, a precautionary heplock or open intravenous line is recommended for cervical and thoracic injections. Intravenous access is not routinely performed for lumbar spine z-joint blocks but is the authors' preference. Judicious premedication with sedatives or anxiolytics instead of analgesics may be required, especially for cervical and thoracic injections in order to minimize the risk of patient movement. However, the physician must consider the results of a recent study supporting the notion that conscious sedation prior to diagnostic spinal injections may have a clinically significant effect on the patients' pain reports. That is, patients will report less pain on a Visual Analogue Scale (VAS) tool even before the procedure.[5]

Blood pressure measurements are recommended for all z-joint procedures. Pulse oximetry is generally recommended for cervical and thoracic procedures, because it may warn of those patients who become vasovagal. Resuscitation equipment should be available, and personnel must be knowledgeable of its location and use.

Prior to a diagnostic injection, the patient should be examined to find maneuvers or provocative tests that reproduce typical pain and record the pain level. Provocative testing may include manual mobilization, range of motion testing, activities of daily living, and postures believed to stress regional z-joint(s). If the patient is pain-free before the scheduled injection, it generally should not be performed because it will be impossible to make any diagnostic conclusions. Postinjection pain level and response to provocative tests also should be noted.

All z-joint block procedures should be performed under sterile conditions with the skin appropriately prepped. Fluoroscopic imaging and contrast medium is absolutely necessary to achieve proper needle placement and injectant flow. Venous uptake occurs at a rate of 6.1% with intra-articular lumbar zygapophyseal joint blocks.[127] Contrast is necessary to avoid this, which potentially may yield a false-negative diagnostic result. One study on non–fluoroscopically guided ("blind") paravertebral injections concluded that such injections should not be performed without fluoroscopy due to potential complications and the lack of any diagnostic accuracy.[105] After joint entry is perceived with any spinal axis z-joint injection, the minimal amount of contrast necessary to document intra-articular spread and exclude extra-articular spread or venous uptake is instilled (Figs. 27-1 and 27-2). This may be a little as 0.2 ml in the cervical and thoracic spine. Continued contrast injection will outline the superior and inferior capsular recesses that exist in all spinal z-joints. Although a radiographically appealing arthrogram may be obtained, it usually provides little to no additional diagnostic information and serves only to limit the amount of subsequent anesthetic/corticosteroid that can be injected before reaching joint capacity. Exceptions include synovial cysts, which can be visualized by a detailed arthrogram.[113] With a communicating lumbar pars defect, > 1 ml of contrast may need to be injected before spread from one z-joint across the pars defect to an adjoining z-joint can be appreciated (Fig. 27-3).[91,103]

A minimal amount of contrast medium should be injected at the target location for medial branch blocks to exclude venous uptake (even with a negative aspiration) and ensure appropriate injectant flow (Fig. 27-4). This guards against false-negative responses that can occur with venous uptake even after needle redirectioning and subsequent lack of venous uptake.[51,77]

Because epidural spread potentially can occur following z-joint injections, it is prudent to use the least neurotoxic, nonionic contrast agents, such as Omnipaque. Contrast allergic reactions are less common with nonionic agents. Premedication for contrast allergies has been shown to decrease minor contrast reactions but may not reduce anaphylactoid reactions.

When a firm capsular endpoint is perceived with routine z-joint injections, the injection should cease. If excessive volume is injected or a ventral capsular defect exists, epidural spread can occur, thereby limiting the diagnostic specificity of the block. Throughout the injection and when capsular distension is perceived by the physician, the patient may be asked whether concordant pain is reproduced for all or a specific part of his or her pain pattern. Pain generally occurs with capsular distention.[52,56,61–63] The diagnostic value of this subjective response has not been established.[120]

Because of the increased risks in the cervical and thoracic spine, it is recommended that the injectionist demonstrate meticulous fluoroscopically guided needle techniques in the lumbar spine before any cervical or thoracic injection. Needle control can be improved by using the cutting edge or bevel. If the injectionist positions the needle's bevel opening opposite the desired direction of travel and concurrently bends the exposed shaft with the convexity toward the bevel opening, one can obtain improved needle guidance away from the bevel opening and toward the target. This prevents the need to withdraw the needle and redirect it through additional soft tissues, which may cause a temporary increase in patient discomfort. The nuances of bevel control have been documented elsewhere.[46] In addition, applying a distal 15° curve near the tip of the needle with the convexity of the curve to the bevel opening further enhances needle guidance.[59]

The investigation of suspected painful z-joints usually begins based on clinical evaluation, which may include: (1) determining the sites of maximal segmental or direct articular tenderness; (2) mechanical, segmental, provocative testing causing concordant pain; (3) determination of "articular restriction" in company with localized soft tissue findings such as facilitated muscle tone[69]; (4) recognizing the most commonly involved joints (e.g., C2–C3, C5–C6 and L4–L5, L5–S1)[23,29,79,82,84,100,121]; and (5) evaluating for recognized z-joint referral zones[52,56,61-63,94,98] Each clinician relies on a combination of these and other findings to determine at which levels to begin z-joint injections. A recent study explored potential indicators of z-joint pain on physical examination and found that pain

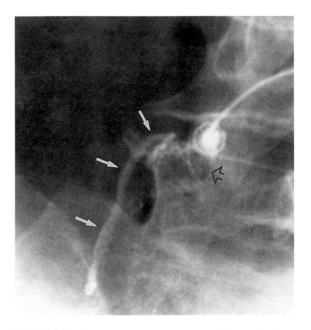

FIGURE 27-1. Anteroposterior (AP) radiograph of an L4–L5 z-joint injection with venous uptake despite perceived joint entry. The black arrow denotes the inferior aspect of the L4–5 z-joint, and the three white arrows denote venous filling with contrast.

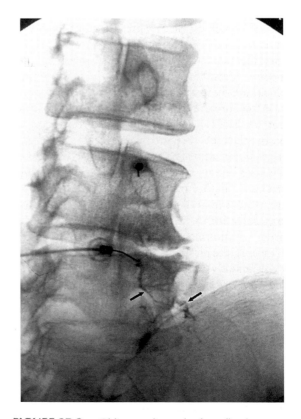

FIGURE 27-2. Oblique radiograph of needle placements for L3 and L4 medial branch blocks. Contrast is seen to flow into a regional vein as denoted by the black arrows with the L4 medial branch injection.

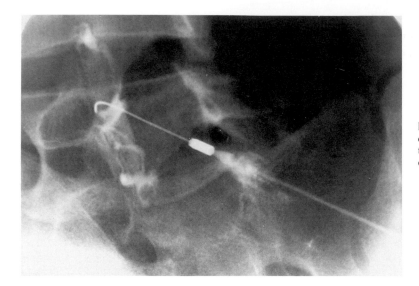

FIGURE 27-3. Oblique radiograph of an L4–L5 z-joint injection with contrast demonstrating filling across a pars defect to the ipsilateral L5–S1 z-joint.

provocation produced by passive rotation combined with extension (quadrant loading) had a high sensitivity and could thus appropriately be used as a "screening" test.[121]

After the expected onset of anesthesia from a z-joint block, the patient is questioned regarding pain relief. After diagnostic blocks the patient is reexamined with the provocative tests or maneuvers that previously caused concordant pain before the block. Any change in the patient's pain and quality of spinal motion is noted. Depending on the findings after the block(s), further levels above or below the original segment may need to be blocked. Most clinicians will follow the patient with some form of an objective, self-reported "pain diary," which typically asks for numerical ratings on pain reduction or VAS pain ratings over a period of several hours and then over a 7–10-day period after the block.

The patient is observed in a well-equipped recovery area for 15–60 minutes, depending on the location of the block (cervical blocks require the longest observation), total anesthetic dosage, any procedural complications, and if sedatives or anxiolytics were administered. The patient should be given discharge instructions and asked to keep a pain diary.

During the ensuing 24–72 hours, an occasional patient may experience an increase in pain that usually abates with acetaminophen and local ice application. If fevers, positional headaches, or neurologic symptoms develop or if unusual pain persists, patients should be promptly evaluated. Typically, physical and manual therapy programs do not need to be interrupted following the injection.[50,47] The patient should be reevaluated 10–14 days after the

procedure by phone, and if residual pain exists, the patient should be reexamined in the office.

Controversy exists regarding the number and frequency limitations of z-joint injections. As in peripheral joint injections, most clinicians use no more than three intra-articular corticosteroid injections

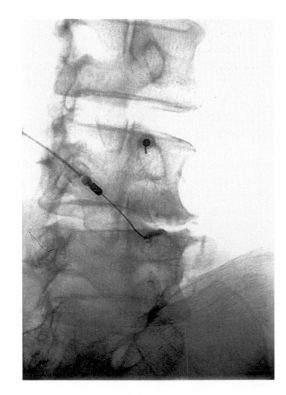

FIGURE 27-4. Oblique radiograph of the patient in Figure 27-2. The L4 medial branch needle has been redirected so there is appropriate contrast flow along the target nerve in the groove between the superior articular and transverse processes.

per year, although no study has determined a safe or maximum frequency or number of injections. The efficacy of individual blocks should be evaluated; if no prolonged corticosteroid response occurs (e.g., 3 months of relief) to the initial injection, additional use of corticosteroids should be withheld. Routine serial blocks should not be performed.

Repeat diagnostic z-joint blocks to confirm a particular joint as the pain generator are often performed on a different day with a different strength anesthetic.[7,37] Dual blocks of the joints or their nerve supply are recommended to obtain a secure diagnosis of z-joint pain due to a false-positive rate of single z-joint injection procedures in the lumbar and cervical spine of 38% and 27%, respectively.[7,8,118] In one double-blind, controlled study, subjects with chronic neck pain underwent dual medial branch blocks (lidocaine and bupivacaine [Marcaine]) and a placebo block with saline.[80] The false-negative rate of time-contingent relief (longer relief with Marcaine than lidocaine) with dual medial branch blocks was high (46%) against placebo, but the false-negative rate of non–time contingent relief (not necessarily having longer relief with Marcaine than lidocaine) with dual medial branch blocks was 0% (100% sensitivity). Eighty-eight percent (12% false-positive rate) of those with and 65% (35% false-positive rate) of those without time contingent relief after dual medial branch blocks withstood (no pain relief) a placebo challenge. Dual medial branch blocks (lidocaine vs. bupivacaine) substantially reduce the likelihood of a false-positive response; however, only a placebo injection can absolutely exclude a true placebo response. The authors contend that non–time contingent relief following dual medial branch blocks is a reasonable diagnostic compromise between single medial branch blocks with their unacceptably high false-positive rate and triple blocks (comparative blocks and a placebo block) that incur additional time and expense. With this approach, sensitivity remains high (near 100%), and specificity is greatly improved compared to single intra-articular or medial branch blocks.

Different possibilities exist for the confirmatory second set of blocks. If a therapeutic steroid response to the first set of intra-articular injections occurred, two options exist: (1) the second set of injections can be performed with intra-articular corticosteroid alone and concomitant medial branch blocks (immediate pain relief would be due to the medial branch blocks); or (2) another set of intra-articular z-joint injections may be repeated with anesthetic and corticosteroid. If only an immediate, temporary response occurred from the anesthetic (no corticosteroid response) with the first set of z-joint injections, two options exist for the confirmatory second set of blocks: (1) medial branch blocks or (2) intra-articular injections with only anesthetic. Repeat corticosteroid injections in the absence of a sustained response (> 4 weeks) to the first injection are not recommended. The authors do not perform more than two z-joint corticosteroid injections in a 12-month period. If pain persists, the patient is evaluated for medial branch radiofrequency neurotomy with medial branch blocks.

Many clinicians prefer to make a more definitive diagnosis of z-joint–mediated pain through successful completion of two sets of z-joint block procedures, including at least one set of medial branch blocks, before considering medial branch nerve denervation.[37,45,49] In this methodology, the nerves targeted for subsequent neurotomy are tested, and the diagnosis is more secure (fewer false-positives) with the use of two z-joint block procedures and adequate temporary pain relief. Medial branch denervation has been reported with phenol, cryoanalgesia, and radiofrequency techniques.[49,60,78,110,112,115,123]

CERVICAL ZYGAPOPHYSEAL JOINT INJECTION TECHNIQUES

The cervical z-joints have been shown to be a potential source of pain.[23,41,54,56,62,111,132] Pain can be referred anywhere from the cranium to the midthoracic spine.[23,56,62] It was not until 1981 that a z-joint injection technique was first described.[102] Recently, interest has increased in the role of the cervical z-joints in the production of clinical pain syndromes and in the ability to diagnose this entity through selective blocking procedures.[23,41,54,56,73,82,111,132]

An initial report of 128 patients undergoing single z-joint blocks suggested that at least 26% of neck pain was z-joint mediated.[2] Subsequent prevalence reports were on a homogenous population of patients following whiplash injury. A cohort of 50 patients underwent comparative blocks under double-blind conditions. Time contingent relief was required. Even using these relatively insensitive criteria[82] the lowest possible prevalence of cervical z-joint pain was 54%.[10] A separate group of 68 whiplash-injured patients were studied under randomized, double-blind, placebo-controlled triple blocks. The worst case prevalence of z-joint pain below C2–C3 was 46% (95% CI:34–57%).[84] In a similar study in whiplash-injured patients in whom headache was the main complaint, the headache was related to the C2–C3 joint in 53% of cases (95% CI:37–68%).[83] One study reported a 41% incidence of combined z-joint and disc pain as elucidated through discography and noncontrolled medial branch blocks in a population of 56 patients with chronic neck pain.[17]

Anatomy

The cervical z-joints are paired, diarthrodial, synovial joints located between the superior and inferior articular pillars in the posterior cervical column.[12] Cervical z-joints extend from C2–C3 to C7–T1. The atlanto-occipital and lateral atlantoaxial synovial joints are by definition not zygapophyseal joints because of their anterior location. Each z-joint is lined with hyaline cartilage and contains a meniscus.[137] The joints may contain a variety of intra-articular inclusions, with fibroadipose meniscoids being the most common. They are located at the dorsal and ventral poles of the joint where they cover the portion of the articular surface that becomes exposed during normal gliding of the joint.[97] A fibrous joint capsule exists that is richly innervated with both mechanoreceptors and nociceptors.[95,134,135]

The superior aspect of the joint is the inferior articular process of the more superior vertebral segment and faces forward and downward at 45°. The inferior aspect of the joint is the superior articular process of the more inferior vertebral segment and faces backward and upward at 45° (Fig. 27-5). The inclination of the lower joints is steeper.[55] C2–C3 is more oblique in its orientation and, at times, steeper than its subjacent counterpart due to its transitional nature both anatomically and biomechanically.[24] The z-joint's articular surfaces are generally flat with only minimal concavity and convexity.[70]

The joint volume is usually ≤ 1 ml.[15,16,56,82] Both superior and inferior capsular recesses exist with the superior recess adjacent to the neuroforamina and the dorsal root ganglia.

Each cervical z-joint from C3–C4 to C7–T1 is innervated from the medial branches of the dorsal rami with each joint supplied from the branch above and below that joint. C2–C3 is largely innervated from the third occipital nerve (TON), which is the superficial medial branch of the C3 dorsal ramus. The deep medial branch of the C3 dorsal ramus is referred to as the C3 medial branch proper. Articular branches also may arise from a communicating loop that crosses the back of the joint between the TON and the C2 dorsal ramus.[13,24] Each C3–C7 dorsal ramus crosses the same segment's transverse process and divides into lateral and medial branches. The medial branch curves around the "waist" of the articular pillar of the same numbered vertebra. The medial branch nerves are bound by fascia, held against the articular pillar and covered by the tendinous slips of the origin of the semispinalis capitis.[82] Articular branches arise as the nerve approaches the posterior aspect of the articular pillar. An ascending branch innervates the joint above and a descending branch innervates the joint below. At C7 the base of the transverse process occupies most of the lateral aspect of the articular pillar and pushes the medial branch higher than typical cervical medial branch nerves.[14,81]

The TON continues around the lower lateral and dorsal surface of the C2–3 joint embedded in connective tissue that invests the joint capsule.[13,24] The TON provides muscular branches to the semispinalis capitis and becomes cutaneous over the suboccipital region. C4–C7 medial branch nerves typically lack any cutaneous branches.[13,81]

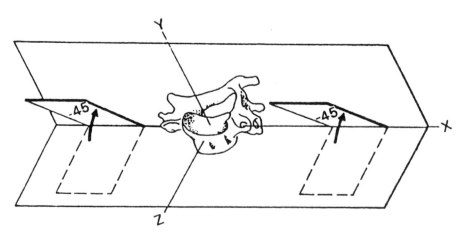

FIGURE 27-5. The plane of the articular facets in a typical cervical z-joint. (From White AW 3d, Panjabi MM: The basic kinematics of the human spine. Spine 3:12–20, 1978, with permission.)

The radiographic anatomy has been evaluated on lateral and anteroposterior imaging of the TON and the C3-C7 medial branch nerves of 10 dissected cadavers.[85] The courses of the C4 and C5 medial branch nerves was relatively constant following the waist of their respective articular pillars. C3, C6, and C7 showed more variation. Although in each cadaver the TON was rostral to the C3 medial branch, with the variation of the C3 medial branch nerve (more superior location at the upper third of the C3 articular pillar), it often overlapped the TON. The C6 medial branch nerves coursed around the waist of the articular pillar or above it, between the waist and the superior articular process. Most of the C7 medial branches (7 of 10) were located high on the C7 articular pillar and crossed the lateral image of the C6–C7 z-joint. A few were lower on the C7 transverse process. The distance between the osseous articular pillar and the medial branches was greater than expected. Although some nerves were adjacent to the bone, others were separated by 2–3 mm.[85]

The anteriorly located vertebral artery ascends through the foramina transversaria of C1–C6. It passes directly superior in the neck until the transverse process of the axis where it then courses upward and laterally to the foramina transversaria of the atlas.[114] The vertebral artery at C2–C7 is located anterior to the z-joints from both a posterior and lateral injection approach.

Third Occipital Nerve Block Techniques

To block the nerve supply to the C2–C3 z-joint, the TON should be blocked. The C2 communicating loop can additionally be blocked, but this is not standard practice.[14] Although both techniques (posterior and lateral) are presented, the authors prefer a lateral approach because it is faster and more patient friendly.

Posterior Approach Third Occipital Nerve

The target site for blockade of the TON is at the posterolateral margin of the C2–C3 joint. Because the TON is large (approximately 1.5–2.0 mm) compared to typical medial branch nerves (approximately 1.0 mm),[81,85] it is believed necessary to block it at three separate sites. Under anteroposterior (AP) imaging, it may be necessary to move the mandible and teeth so that the joint image is not obscured. A 25-gauge spinal needle is inserted into the skin slightly below the joint line and angled cephalad. Care must be taken to avoid medial stray toward the spinal canal. After the posterolateral aspect of the C2–C3 z-joint is reached, the needle is then directed to each of three sites along the posterolateral margin of the joint (Figs. 27-6 and 27-7). The first site is opposite the equator of the joint, the second is at its lower margin, and the third is midway between the first and second sites. Adequate blockade of the nerve is achieved using a total of 1.5 ml of anesthetic: 0.5 ml of anesthetic is delivered per site.[24] More recent recommendations use of a total volume of approximately 1.0 ml.[14]

Lateral Approach Third Occipital Nerve

With the patient in the lateral position a 25- or 26-gauge spinal needle is inserted toward the target

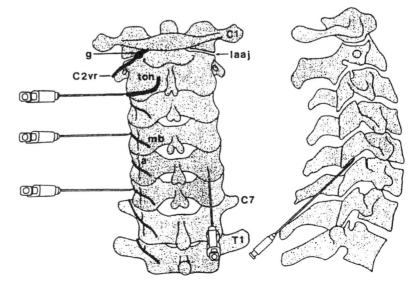

FIGURE 27-6. Proper needle placements for a posterior approach to a third occipital nerve (TON) block, C5–C6 intra-articular z-joint injection, and C4 and C6 medial branch blocks. The second cervical ganglia *(g)*, C2 ventral ramus *(C2vr)*, and the lateral atlantoaxial joint *(laaj)* are noted. (From Bogduk N: Back pain: Zygapophyseal blocks and epidural steroids. In Cousins MJ, Bridenbaugh PO (eds): Neural Blockade in Clinical Anesthesia and Management of Pain, 2nd ed. Philadelphia, J.B. Lippincott, 1988, pp 935–954, with permission.)

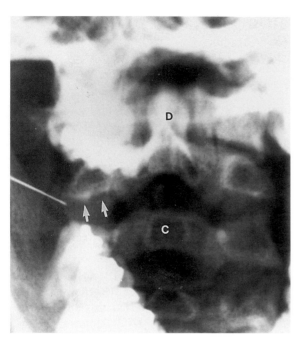

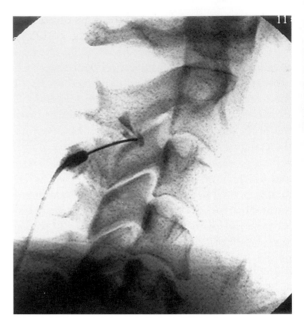

FIGURE 27-7.   Open mouth AP radiograph showing a posterior approach to a third occipital nerve block. The needle tip rests on the posterolateral aspect of the C2–C3 z-joint at its equator. The white arrows denote the C2–C3 joint line. The dens *(D)* and the C3 spinous process *(C)* are noted.

FIGURE 27-9.   Lateral radiograph of a lateral approach to a third occipital nerve block. The needle is placed at the middle of three injection sites used for a third occipital nerve block with adequate contrast flow to incorporate the target nerve.

locations for a TON block. These target sites are located along a vertical line bisecting the articular pillar of C3. Injections are made (1) directly above the subchondral plate of the C2 inferior articular process at the level of the apex of the C3 superior articular pillar, (2) immediately below the subchon-

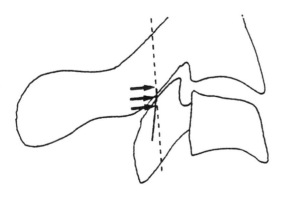

FIGURE 27-8.   The target points for a third occipital nerve block using a lateral approach. Three injections are placed along a vertical, midline through the C3 articular pillar *(dotted line)*. The injections are placed over the joint line *(middle arrow)*, immediately above the subchondral plate of the inferior articular facet of C2 *(upper arrow)* and immediately below the subchondral plate of the superior articular facet of C3 *(lower arrow)*. (From Barnsley L, Bogduk N: Medial branch blocks are specific for the diagnosis of cervical zygapophyseal joint pain. Reg Anesth 18:343–350, 1993, with permission.)

dral plate of the C3 superior articular process at the level of the bottom of the C2–3 intervertebral foramen, and (3) at a point midway between these two sites, usually on the subchondral plate of the superior articular process of C3 (Fig. 27-8).[6,7,14,24,83] At each of these three locations 0.5 ml of anesthetic is injected.[6] More recent recommendations specify the use of 0.3 ml at each of the three target locations.[14]

At times, the authors use a slight variation to the reported technique. One can evaluate the spread of contrast at the first target, being the middle needle position (Fig. 27-9). If flow covers all three target locations, the total injectant volume (1.0 ml) may be delivered at this one site if contrast dispersal also is seen over all three target locations upon injection of the anesthetic. If this modified technique is successful, it limits procedural soreness from repeated needle redirections. With a successful TON block, a small patch of numbness will occur over the suboccipital area.[7,24]

Lateral Approach C2 Communicating Loop

No formal description exists nor is there a validated needle placement for this nerve block. Using published descriptions and drawings of this nerve,[13,24,82] it seems appropriate to block this nerve on a vertical line that bisects the junction of the middle of the C3 articular pillar. The nerve will be blocked on the lateral edge of the mass of C2 at its concavity as viewed on AP imaging (Fig. 27-10).

Cervical Medial Branch Block Techniques

To block the nerve supply to the C3–C4 to C7–T1 z-joints the medial branches above and below the joint should be blocked. For example, to block the C4–C5 z-joint's nerve supply the C4 and C5 medial branches should be blocked. Although both techniques (posterior and lateral) are described, the authors prefer a lateral approach because fewer soft tissues are penetrated; it is therefore faster and more comfortable for the patient.

Posterior Approach C3–C8 Medial Branches

The patient is positioned prone on the x-ray table with the head and chest supported by pillows. The mouth is left free to move. An AP image of the cervical spine will show a scalloped lateral margin. The convexities of this margin represent the z-joints, and the concavities represent the waists of the articular pillars. Moving the intensifier slightly caudad provides better visualization of the waist of the articular pillar. The C3–C7 medial branches lie at the deepest point in this concavity.

After the target location is established, the skin is punctured up to 1 cm lateral to this radiographic point. A 25-gauge spinal needle is then directed ventrally and medially onto the back of the articular pillar just medial to its lateral concavity. Initially, directing the needle medially to bone ensures that the needle is not placed too deeply. The needle is then directed laterally until the tip reaches the lateral margin of the waist of the articular pillar. The needle should be felt to barely slip off the bone laterally in a ventral direction at the deepest point of articular pillar's concavity (Fig. 27-11).[15,16] Lateral imaging should be obtained to ensure the needle tip rests at the centroid of the articular pillar (Fig. 27-12). The centroid is found at the intersection of the two diagonals of the diamond-shaped pillar.[6]

For a C8 medial branch block the needle is first placed onto the transverse process of T1 and then directed until it lies at the superolateral border of the transverse process analogous to thoracic medial branch blocks.

Lateral Approach C3–C6 Medial Branches

The patient lies on his or her side, and a 25- or 26-gauge spinal needle is inserted toward the centroid of the articular pillar as seen on a true lateral

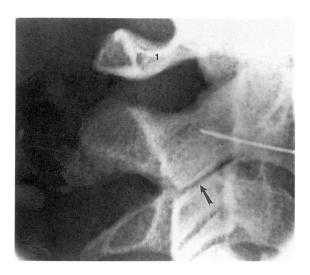

FIGURE 27-10. Lateral radiograph of a C2 communicating branch nerve injection. The black arrow denotes the C2–C3 z-joint, and the number 1 indicates the C1 segment.

radiograph (Fig. 27-13).[6–8] If necessary, the uppermost articular pillar can be distinguished from the opposite side either by moving the C-arm or by

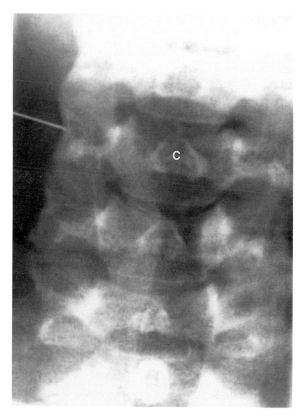

FIGURE 27-11. AP radiograph of a posterior approach to a C4 medial branch block. The needle tip rests at the deepest point of the articular pillar's concavity. The letter C denotes the spinous process of C4.

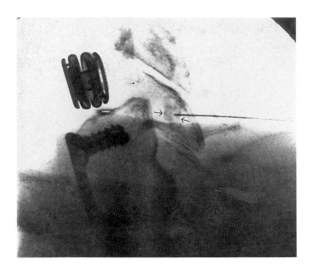

FIGURE 27-12. Lateral radiograph of a cervical medial branch block using a posterior approach. The needle is at the centroid of the articular pillar. The black arrows denote appropriate anterior and posterior extension of contrast on the articular pillar.

rolling the patient. The needle will be seen to travel with the uppermost articular pillar as the two articular pillars separate on the fluoroscopic image.

Lateral Approach C7 Medial Branch

The needle is advanced so that it stays within the confines of the C7 superior articular process, which prevents excessive advancement into the C8 foramen and toward the vertebral artery. After the superior articular process is contacted, AP imaging should verify that the needle lies against the lateral aspect of the superior articular process. If not, the needle tip usually will lie lateral to the target against the upper aspect of the large C7 transverse process. If this occurs, the needle should be repositioned under lateral imaging to a more superior location on the superior articular process. After contrast is

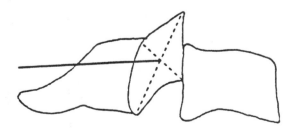

FIGURE 27-13. The target point for C3–C7 medial branch blocks using a lateral approach. The target point for injection is the centroid of the articular pillar as seen in a true lateral view of the cervical spine. The dotted lines intersect at the centroid. (From Barnsley L, Bogduk N: Medial branch blocks are specific for the diagnosis of cervical zygapophyseal joint pain. Reg Anesth 18:343–350, 1993, with permission.)

injected (0.1–0.2 ml), 0.3 ml of anesthetic should be injected over the target nerve to ensure adequate flow. The needle should then be withdrawn about 4 mm and another 0.3 ml of anesthetic should be injected after contrast reveals nonvascular flow. This additional injection allows for variation in the location of the C7 medial branch nerve, which may at times be displaced away from bone by a bundle of the semispinalis capitis muscle.[14]

With both the posterior and lateral medial branch block approaches, 0.1–0.2 ml of contrast is injected after proper needle location is visualized to ensure injectant spread over the target tissues without inadvertent venous uptake or flow away from the articular pillar. AP imaging may help ensure the contrast is placed against the articular pillar and not in a more lateral soft tissue plane (Fig. 27-14). If less than optimal flow occurs, the needle should be repositioned for reinjection of contrast medium and interpretation. After appropriate flow is achieved, 0.5 ml of anesthetic (e.g., 2–4% lidocaine) is injected around the nerve.[6,7,14] With proper technique, the injectant

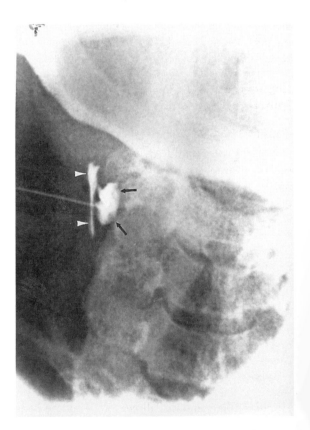

FIGURE 27-14. AP radiograph of a cervical medial branch injection using a lateral approach. The white arrows denote initial contrast spread in a fascial plane lateral to the medial branch nerve. The black arrows denote appropriate contrast spread at the waist of the articular pillar.

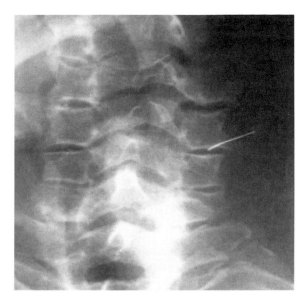

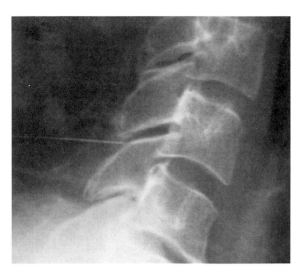

FIGURE 27-15.   Pillar view of needle position for a C5–C6 z-joint injection using a posterior approach. (Courtesy of Garrett Kine, M.D.)

FIGURE 27-16.   Lateral radiograph demonstrating needle position for a C5–C6 z-joint injection using a posterior approach. (Courtesy of Garrett Kine, M.D.)

reaches the target nerve and does not affect any other diagnostically important structures such as the ventral ramus.[6] With accurate needle placement, 0.5 ml adequately diffuses to achieve a successful block.[6]

Intra-articular Cervical Z-joint Injection Techniques

Posterior Approach

With the posterior approach the patient is placed prone on the x-ray table and a cushion is placed under the chest to allow for neck flexion. Positioning the head with slight rotation to the opposite side may allow for easier joint penetration. This is recommended by some clinicians,[111] but not all.[16] The skin entry point lies approximately two segments below the target joint. It is determined either by directing an imaginary line to the skin along the plane of the joint (as determined by a lateral view) or, preferably, by direct visualization of the joint via a tangential view (pillar view) and making a skin mark along the plane of the x-ray beam into the center of the joint lucency.[16] While advancing at approximately a 45° angle, one must proceed cautiously to ensure that the needle is directed over the articular pillars and not allowed to stray medially toward the interlaminar space or excessively lateral. The needle is advanced until it strikes the articular pillar, preferably below the target site. Switching to lateral imaging can confirm proper location and that the needle is not advanced too deeply. The needle is

then directed into the joint space, which may require a combination of posterior, pillar, and lateral imaging. The needle should be seen in the joint space laterally and in the mid portion of the joint on posterior or pillar imaging (Figs. 27-15 and 27-16). Infiltration with contrast medium should confirm intra-articular spread (Figs. 27-17 and 27-18). The joint is injected with a mixture of anesthetic and steroid in a volume not to exceed 1 ml. The posterior approach is often required for the C7–T1 z-joint where the lateral approach may involve risk of contacting the lung apex or inferior neurovascular structures.

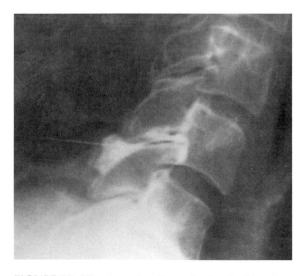

FIGURE 27-17.   Lateral radiograph of a C5–C6 arthrogram. Needle placement is via a posterior approach. (Courtesy of Garrett Kine, M.D.)

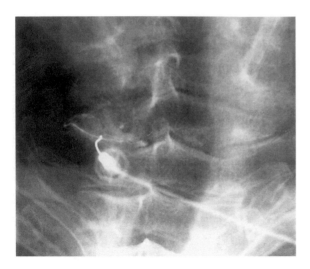

FIGURE 27-18. AP radiograph of a C7–T1 arthrogram with needle placement via a posterior approach. Contrast outlines a very thin joint space.

C3–C4 to C6–C7 (C7–T1) Joint Injection Lateral Approach

The lateral approach to the cervical z-joint was first described by Okada[102] and later by Dwyer.[56] Proponents of the lateral versus the posterior approach argue that it is technically less demanding, it may be performed with a smaller 25- or 26-gauge, and it is more comfortable for the patient because less soft tissue is traversed. The authors prefer this approach.

The patient is positioned on the side with the affected target joint uppermost or closest to the fluoroscopic intensifier. It is helpful to pull the shoulders down (to avoid obscuring the joints under fluoroscopy) and slightly rotate the plane of the upper torso and shoulders posteriorly about 25° and have the patient's contralateral ear lie flat against a pillow in a neutral position. Occasionally, the head may need to be slightly rotated toward the table, particularly for C2–C3 joint injections. Infrequently, slight lateral flexion toward the side being injected is necessary, varying the pillow height to maximally visualize the joint's silhouette under fluoroscopy, which is occasionally true for C2–C3 (Fig. 27-19).

Straight lateral fluoroscopic imaging visualizes both the ipsi- and contralateral joints at the target level. In order to differentiate the uppermost from the contralateral joints, certain maneuvers are used. A 25- or 26-gauge needle can be inserted toward the z-joints at the target level to the superior articular process. The patient is then slightly rolled with the neck and upper torso as one unit. The image of the

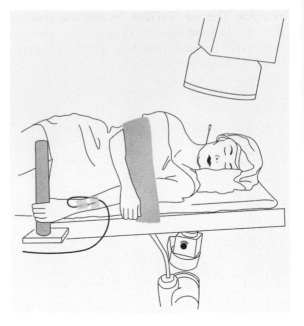

FIGURE 27-19. Patient, needle, and C-arm positioning during a C3–C4 z-joint injection using a lateral approach.

target joint and needle will then move in the same direction on the fluoroscopic screen as the overlying joint images separate.

Alternatively and preferably, the patient may remain stationary and the intensifier is rotated so that the ipsi- and contralateral joints separate on the screen (Figs. 27-20 and 27-21). Depending on the fluoroscopic unit, anterior rotation of the image intensifier usually causes the uppermost target joint to move posteriorly on the screen. The movement of the needle in relation to the target joints helps to distinguish the two sides. The relative motion of the uppermost target joint will be greater than the contralateral z-joint because it is closer to the intensifier and the x-ray beams undergo greater dispersion. With a C-arm, better definition of the joint space (increased joint line lucency) can be obtained with a variable amount of cephalad-to-caudad tilt of the C-arm, depending on the segmental level (see Figure 27-21). The two sides should be separated no further after the neuroforamen begins to become visible. Ideally, the C-arm is rotated no further than the point at which both articular pillars may be seen separately (see Figure 27-21).

Correct identification of the two sides is absolutely critical to avoid directing the needle toward the contralateral joint and potentially through the intervertebral foramina. After the correct joint is clearly identified, the needle is advanced until the superior articular process is contacted just above the joint line. The needle is then directed and advanced through the joint capsule. Typically, the z-joint is more easily entered if one begins slightly superior to the joint and angles the needle inferiorly along the plane of the articular surfaces until the joint is entered. The resistance of the joint capsule can be minimal to negligible. Therefore, switching between lateral and posteroanterior (PA) imaging is occasionally required to prevent excessive medial needle placement. Using the lateral approach, the needle remains posterior to the ventral ramus and the vertebral artery.

Depending on the size of the patient's neck and shoulders, C7–T1 may not be reached from a lateral approach and requires the posterior pillar view approach. If C7–T1 is attempted from a lateral approach in patients with long necks and smaller shoulders, it is better to start with a much steeper superior-to-inferior approach than is typical for midcervical levels to minimize the possibility of contacting more inferior neurovascular and pleural structures.

Lateral Approach C2–C3 Joint Injection

The C2–C3 joint is technically more difficult to both visualize and enter because of its unique anatomy. It is not as flat as the more caudal joints and tends to be more vertically and medially angulated. Having the patient rotate his chin downward to the opposite side may facilitate needle entry. The joint is best entered posterolaterally. Using a lateral approach after the uppermost and opposite C2–C3 articular pillars have been "separated" by the above methods, the C-arm is angled until the joint line is appreciated. This may require more medial and downward tube angulation.[14] Because of the more vertical orientation of this joint, at times the joint line cannot be seen unless the tube is excessively angled so that skin entry path along the x-ray beam would begin in the skull. Obviously, this is not feasible. If the joint line cannot be easily visualized laterally or only with excessive tube angulation, a postero-oblique visualization is necessary. The needle is advanced down to the articular pillar where the injectionist believes that the joint space exists based on visualization either of the C3–C4 joint or of the C2–C3 joint space via the previous "excessive" tube angulation. The C-arm is returned to a lateral position, and then the intensifier is slowly rotated posteriorly until an oblique joint line is clearly seen (Fig. 27-22). The needle is then guided into the superior aspect of the joint using this view (Figs. 27-23 and 27-24). Usually the needle

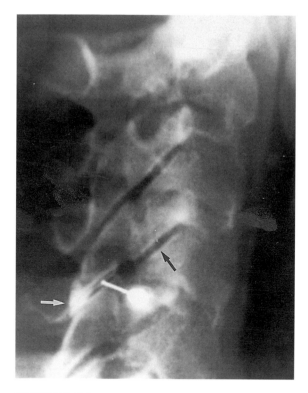

FIGURE 27-20.   Lateral radiograph demonstrating needle placement in a midcervical z-joint. A small amount of contrast has been injected *(white arrow)* to ensure intra-articular placement. The C-arm has been rotated anteriorly so that the uppermost and contralateral *(black arrow)* joints appear separated. Slight angulation of the C-arm has provided improved definition of the joint line.

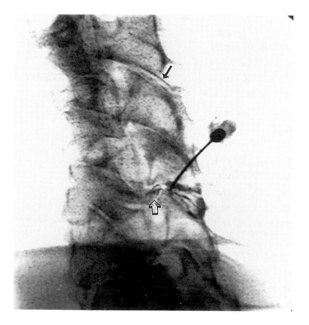

FIGURE 27-21.   Slightly oblique radiograph of a cervical z-joint injection using a lateral approach. The solid black arrow denotes a z-joint two segments cephalad, and the open black arrow denotes the superior articular recess.

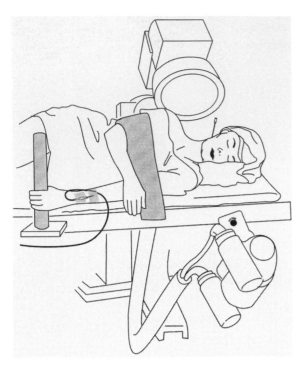

FIGURE 27-22. Patient, needle, and C-arm positioning during a C2–C3 z-joint injection using a lateral approach and oblique visualization of the joint.

is advanced superiorly into the superior capsule of the joint margin under this postero-oblique view.

After joint entry is perceived, infiltration with a small amount of contrast medium (e.g., 0.2 ml)

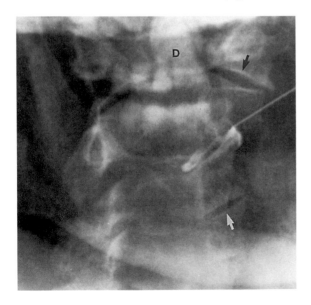

FIGURE 27-23. Oblique radiograph of a C2–C3 z-joint arthrogram with needle placement in the superior aspect of the joint. A lateral needle approach was used. The dens *(D)*, lateral atlantoaxial joint *(black arrow)* and C3–C4 z-joint *(white arrow)* can be seen.

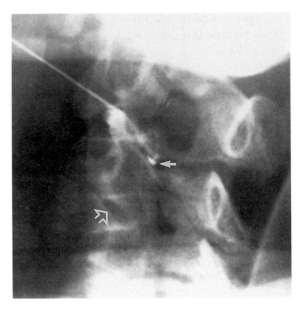

FIGURE 27-24. Oblique radiograph of a C2–C3 z-joint arthrogram with needle placement in the superior aspect of the joint. A lateral approach was used. The inferior extent of the joint *(solid white arrow)* and the C3–C4 z-joint *(open white arrow)* can be seen.

should confirm intra-articular spread (Fig. 27-25). The joint is injected with a mixture of anesthetic and corticosteroid in a volume not to exceed 1 ml.

The posterior approach typically requires more time than the lateral approach for two reasons: (1) it is necessary to switch between an AP and lateral view, and (2) the needle must be advanced through additional soft tissues, which may divert the path of the needle and require redirection. For an experienced operator using a lateral approach, the use of an additional AP view to judge depth generally is unnecessary because he or she (1) accesses needle depth by contacting the articular pillar, (2) determines minimal joint entry by learning the particular, delicate "feel" of entering the cervical z-joint capsule, and (3) avoids excessive medial needle placement after gaining precision control of the needle.

If volumes > 1 ml or forceful rapid injections are used in cervical z-joint injections, the joint capsule may rupture and result in spread of the injectant.[56] A series of 142 arthrograms documented a communicating pathway in 80% of subjects between the z-joint and the interlaminar space, interspinous space, contralateral z-joint, paraextradural space, or cervical extradural space when volumes in excess of 1 ml were used.[102] Most recommend ≤ 1 ml.[14,42,73] Even when smaller volumes are used, extra-articular leakage has been observed in up to 17% of cases.[41,73,132]

Attempts should be made to avoid extra-articular spread because this decreases the specificity of the z-joint block.

Potential Complications from Cervical Zygapophyseal Joint Injection Techniques

Medial branch and TON blocks have fewer risks than intra-articular z-joint blocks. Serious complications from cervical z-joint block techniques are uncommon when meticulous technique is followed by an experienced physician and regional anatomy is respected. Minor transient problems such as local postinjection pain and light-headedness occasionally may occur. At times, ataxia and dizziness due to interruption of the postural tonic-neck reflexes and proprioceptive input to the cervical muscles may occur, which is more common if superfluous anesthetic is used at more proximal segments. This side effect should not outlast the effect of the anesthetic.[15] Excessive volumes or misplaced anesthetics could result in sympathetic blockade. The vertebral artery and ventral ramus are susceptible to injury during a lateral approach if the needle strays anterior to the z-joints. If the vertebral artery is entered and anesthetic is injected, seizures may occur with as little as 0.5–1.0 ml.[36] If air is injected into the vertebral artery, an air embolus may cause severe neurologic sequelae.[106] If overdistension of the z-joints occurs with large volumes, anesthetic leakage into the epidural space may occur with its subsequent effects. Overzealous insertion into the z-joints from a lateral or posterior approach may result in penetration of the epidural or even the subdural or subarachnoid spaces.

THORACIC ZYGAPOPHYSEAL JOINT INJECTION TECHNIQUES

Attention to the thoracic z-joints as a source of pain has greatly lagged behind investigation of the cervical and lumbar counterparts. It was not until 1987 that injection of the thoracic z-joints was reported[133] and only recently that a detailed description of the technique was outlined in several case reports.[53] Although cervical and lumbar z-joint–mediated pain appears to be more common, these joints are capable of mediating both local and referred pain. Patterns of pain induced by distending the thoracic zygapophyseal joint's capsule during injection under fluoroscopy has been reported at all thoracic facet segmental levels in normal volun-

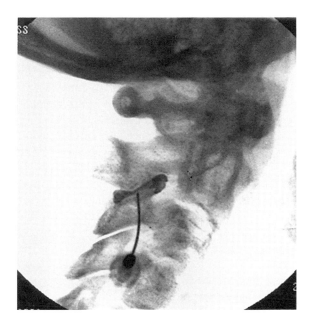

FIGURE 27-25. Lateral radiograph of a C2–C3 z-joint arthrogram using a lateral approach.

teers.[52,61] The prevalence of thoracic z-joint–mediated pain remains unknown.

Anatomy

The thoracic z-joints are paired diarthrodial joints that extend from C7–T1 to T12–L1. The joint's articular surfaces are inclined 60° from the horizontal to the frontal plane and rotated 20° from the frontal to the sagittal plane in a medial direction (Fig. 27-26). The lateral aspect of the joint is located anterior while the medial aspect is posterior.[55] The superior articular facet is almost flat and faces posterior, superior, and slightly lateral, whereas the inferior articular facet is oriented in a reciprocal manner. Some variation in the inclination of the joints exists with the midthoracic joints approximately 60° off the horizontal

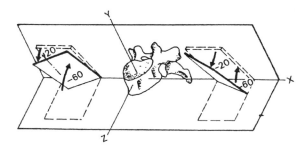

FIGURE 27-26. The plane of the articular facets in a typical thoracic z-joint. (From White AW 3d, Panjabi MM: The basic kinematics of the human spine. Spine 3:12–20, 1978, with permission.)

plane, whereas the upper segments are more vertically oriented. The lower thoracic segments show a joint angle that approaches the sagittal plane.[130]

The capsules of the z-joints are attached to the margins of the articular processes. The anterior capsule is formed by the capsular fibers of the ligamentum flavum and the posterior ligamentous complex blends with the posterior capsule.[130] Intra-articular meniscoid structures have been reported.[69] The joints generally hold only a volume of 0.5–0.6 ml.[52]

A detailed microdissection and histologic study of the human thoracic z-joint and capsule has not been performed. In the primate, the fibrous capsule of the thoracic z-joint has been shown to contain variously sized axons.[124] It seems logical that the human thoracic z-joint capsule is likewise innervated. It has been shown that the human thoracic z-joints have encapsulated nerve ending believed to be primarily mechanoreceptive.[96]

The thoracic z-joints are likely innervated from branches of the posterior rami. Limited early human dissections reveal that the thoracic dorsal rami pass posteriorly through an osseoligamentous tunnel bound by the transverse process, the neck of the rib below, the medial border of the superior costotransverse ligament, and the lateral border of the zygapophyseal joint.[26] The nerve then runs laterally through the space formed between the anterior lamella of the superior costotransverse ligament anteriorly, the costolamellar ligament, and the posterior lamella of the superior costotransverse ligament posteriorly. At the end of this space the nerve divides into medial and lateral branches. The medial branch crosses the transverse process obliquely and runs caudomedially between the multifidus and semispinalis muscles. The thoracic medial branch nerve is reported to be consistently related to the subjacent costotransverse joint at its posteromedial border.[26] The medial branch divides into three branches, two of which enter the latter two muscles. Articular branches are proposed to arise from the medial branch of the dorsal ramus running above and below each joint.[26]

Dissections of 84 thoracic medial branch nerves from seven sides of four adult cadavers has been performed.[31,32] The nerves were traced upon leaving the intertransverse space crossing the superolateral corner of transverse process and then passing medially and inferiorly across the transverse process before ramifying into the multifidus muscle at the T1–T4 and T9–T10 levels. Exceptions to this occurred at midthoracic levels (T5–T8) where the nerve did not always assume contact with the trans-

verse process. Although the nerve curved in a similar fashion, sometimes the inflection occurred at a point superior to the superolateral corner of the transverse process so that the nerve did not run upon the transverse process but was suspended in the intertransverse space separated from the transverse process by the fascicles of the multifidus. The T11 and T12 medial branches were unique because of their different osseous anatomy. The T12 transverse process is much shorter; the T11 medial branch ran across the lateral surface of the root of the superior articular process of T12. The T12 medial branch assumed a course analogous to lumbar medial branch nerves (Figs. 27-27 and 27-28). Each medial branch nerve gave off a short, ascending branch that entered the inferior aspect of the z-joint as it passed caudal to the joint. A slender descending branch arose from the medial branch at the superolateral aspect of transverse process. It has a sinuous course through the multifidus to enter the superior aspect of z-joint below. The T1–T7 medial branches are musculocutaneous, whereas the lower thoracic medial branches have a muscular distribution only.[26]

Thoracic Medial Branch Block Technique

Currently, no validated thoracic medial branch block technique exists for use in the cervical and lumbar spine.[6,51,77] Based on anatomic dissections, Chua recommends for diagnostic blocks of the medial branch nerves that the superolateral aspect of the transverse process serve as the target for archetypical levels (T1–T4 and T9–T10). Recommendations for all levels have been issued by the International Spinal Injection Society (ISIS).[14] Apparently previous recommendations to block the nerve in analogous fashion to the lumbar spine were erroneous.[125,126]

Medial Branch Blocks at T1–T4 and T9–T10

The skin entry point is directly over the target nerve at the superolateral aspect of the transverse process. The transverse process should be differentiated from the rib, lung, and lamina. The transverse process may, at times, be very difficult to image, and the superolateral aspect usually can be more easily appreciated with a slight degree (approximately 10°) of contralateral rotation of the image intensifier. The needle is advanced to bone resting on the superolateral corner of the transverse process. After contrast (0.1–0.2 ml) reveals flow over the location of the target nerve, 0.5 ml of anesthetic should be injected

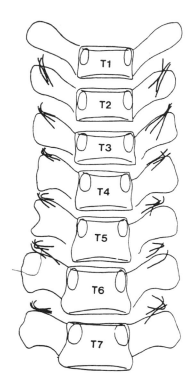

FIGURE 27-27. Diagram of the T1–T6 medial branch nerves in relation to the transverse processes. (From Chua WH: Clinical Anatomy of the Thoracic Dorsal Rami [thesis]. Newcastle, Australia, University of Newcastle, 1994, with permission.)

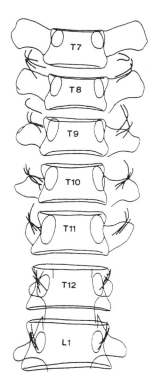

FIGURE 27-28. Diagram of the T7–T12 medial branch nerves in relation to the transverse processes. (From Chua WH: Clinical Anatomy of the Thoracic Dorsal Rami [thesis]. Newcastle, Australia, University of Newcastle, 1994, with permission.)

(Fig. 27-29).[14] In theory, the bevel should open medially to maximize medial flow over the course of the nerve. Both medial branch nerves that innervate the target joint should be anesthetized. The numerical relationship of the nerves, transverse processes, and joints are analogous to those in the lumbar spine.

Medial Branch Blocks at T5–T8

At these levels the local anesthetic needs to reach not only the superolateral corner of the transverse process for those nerves that have a similar position to T1–T4 and T9–T10 nerves, but also just above and medial to the superolateral corner of the transverse process.

The anesthetic should be placed at the same depth of the transverse process and the height of the injection should be opposite the upper border of the rib at the target level.[14]

After osseous contact is made at the superolateral aspect of the transverse process, the bevel should open superiorly and medially and contrast should then be injected to ensure flow over the superolateral aspect of the transverse process as well as

superior and medial for those nerves assuming an analogous superiorly displaced course. If the contrast does not flow in this fashion, the needle tip can be repositioned and bevel direction altered with reinjection of contrast to ensure adequate flow. These steps almost always suffice. However, if flow occurs only over the transverse process, 0.3 ml may be injected at this location with the needle advanced carefully superiorly to the target location to rest in the intertransverse space at the same depth. The depth may be determined by marking the original depth to reach the transverse process on the shaft of the needle. Not advancing past this mark of the needle shaft prevents overzealous anterior placement toward the pleura. Contrast should be reinjected at this position to ensure that inadvertent venous uptake does not occur.

Medial Branch Blocks at T11–T12

Injection technique is essentially the same as in the lumbar spine. The T11 medial branch is blocked at the T12 transverse process. The T12 transverse process is short and may not easily be seen on AP imaging. On the oblique view (as used for lumbar

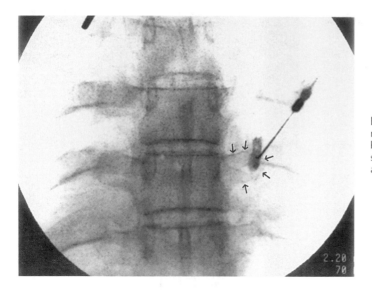

FIGURE 27-29. AP radiograph of a thoracic medial branch block. The arrows denote the border of the target transverse process. Contrast is seen to appropriately spread over the superolateral aspect of the transverse process.

medial branch blocks) a "Scottie dog" with a stub nose is seen. The target is high on the "eye" that appears between 2 and 4 o'clock on the right and between 8 and 10 o'clock on the left. For T12, the nerve is targeted at L1 just as with L1–L4 medial branch blocks.[14]

Intra-articular Thoracic Z-Joint Injection Technique

The patient is positioned prone in the fluoroscopy suite. Initially, AP imaging is used. No rotation should be seen at the levels to be injected. Cephalad and caudad tilt is used to bring the image of the intervertebral discs at the target levels parallel to the end plates to maximally open the disc space. Under intermittent AP imaging, the first joint to be injected is identified, and the skin overlying the inferior margin of the vertebrae is marked. For example, if the T6–T7 z-joint is to be blocked the inferior aspect of that z-joint will be located at the superior aspect of the T7 pedicle. For a T6–T7 z-joint injection, a skin mark is placed over the inferior portion of the T7 vertebral body while under AP imaging (Fig. 27-30). A 3.5-inch, 25-gauge spinal needle is inserted angling up approximately 45-60° off the plane of the skin toward the target joint. More proximal segments may require an angle more perpendicular to the skin. Under intermittent AP imaging, the needle is advanced cephalad toward the superior articular process of T7. The needle should remain on an imaginary vertical line connecting the midportion of the T7 and T8 pedicles. If the needle does not stray medial or lateral to this line, it should be safely over bone. At times, the needle may need

to be placed at the medial aspect of the joint where it is more posterior and accessible. The needle should not be placed medial to the most medial aspect of the pedicle on AP imaging or risk entry into the epidural or subarachnoid spaces. After approximately 4-5 cm of needle is inserted or the needle tip is seen to lie at the mid to inferior aspect of the T7 pedicle, the intensifier is rotated away from the side being injected until the outline of the joint is first clearly visible. This may require near-lateral imaging. Minor rotational changes to align the x-ray

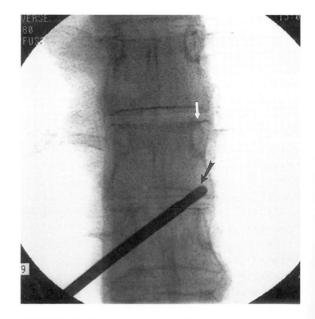

FIGURE 27-30. AP radiograph of the typical approach to a thoracic z-joint injection. The tip of the thick metal marker *(black arrow)* pertains to the skin starting position for injection of the z-joint one segment superior. The inferior aspect of the target z-joint is denoted by the white arrow.

beam with the plane of the joint may be required. On oblique, near-lateral imaging the needle tip should be at or near the inferior aspect of the target joint. The needle is then advanced through the capsule into the inferior aspect of the joint (Fig. 27-31). If upon oblique, near-lateral imaging the needle appears but does not contact osseous structures, it should be slightly withdrawn and the intensifier returned to a AP view. The needle should be viewed to ensure it has not wrongly strayed too far medial or lateral. Again, in this example of a T6–T7 z-joint injection, an AP image of the needle tip should be at the mid to slightly medial aspect of the T7 pedicle and not outside the border of the T7 pedicle (Fig. 27-32). Complications may occur if the needle is quickly advanced and strays from the target location. After the needle is inserted into the inferior aspect of the joint, a minimal amount of contrast should be injected (Fig. 27-33). The contrast should be seen to fill the joint space and/or the inferior or superior capsular recesses (Fig. 27-34). The total volume injected into the joint generally should not exceed 0.6 ml to prevent rupturing the joint capsule (Fig. 27-35).

At more superior levels (T1–T2 to T5–T6) generally a more perpendicular approach to the z-joints is needed. At these more superior levels on AP imaging, skin entry is usually at the midportion of the vertebral body rather than its inferior aspect.

Entry into the joint may be impeded by a large laminar ridge, particularly in older patients. When this ridge is present, the needle tends to sky off the ridge dorsally and cannot be advanced anteriorly back into the joint. When this occurs, a more perpendicular approach is required to avoid needle placement inferior to the inferior aspect of the joint where this laminar ridge resides. Therefore, some clinicians prefer to mark the level of the target joints and begin with oblique imaging that allows direct visualization of the joint and the needle angle required. The optimal skin entry angle to the joint(s) are marked based on the inferior angulation of the joint (which can have an acute angle prohibiting an inferior traditional approach) and the presence of a large laminar ridge (Fig. 27-36). The horizontal level required that allows for a direct approach to each joint is marked and the C-arm in returned to AP imaging. The needle is then advanced along the midpedicular line starting at the marked horizontal line. After adequate depth is obtained, the C-arm is returned to the oblique view to image the joint and guide the needle into the inferior aspect of the joint to ensure that medial-to-lateral

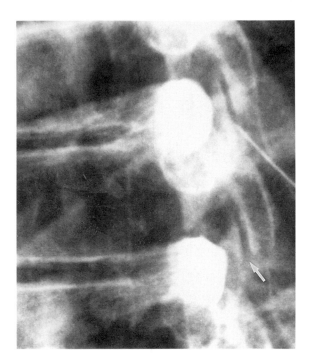

FIGURE 27-31. Near lateral radiograph of needle placement in the inferior aspect of the T6–T7 z-joint. The white arrow denotes the target needle location (inferior aspect of the z-joint) for a T7–T8 z-joint injection.

stay does not occur or that bone is contacted. A distal curved tip on the needle is useful to steer into

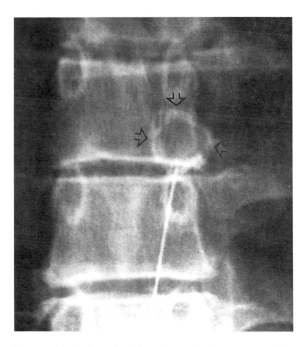

FIGURE 27-32. An AP radiograph of a T6–T7 z-joint arthrogram. The black arrows denote the margins of the joint capsule. The needle tip is in the optimal position in line with the midposition of the T7 pedicle.

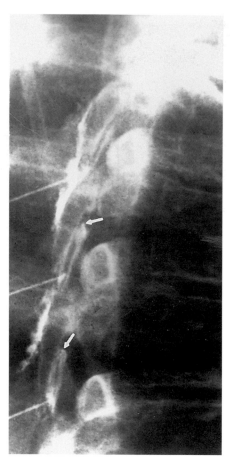

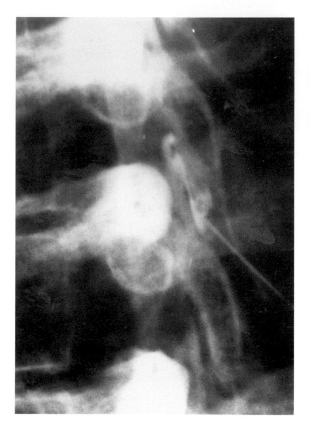

FIGURE 27-34. Near lateral radiograph of a T6–T7 z-joint arthrogram. Small superior and inferior capsular recesses are seen.

FIGURE 27-33. Near lateral (far oblique) radiograph of injection of three sequential thoracic z-joints. Despite similar and adequate-appearing needle placement in each z-joint, differences in contrast flow is appreciated. Contrast does not fill the most superior z-joint but spreads posteriorly. Contrast is seen in the middle z-joint in addition to posterior extravasation. Contrast is contained within the most inferior z-joint injection with no extravasation

tighter and more tortuous joints, especially in those with inferior spurring.[59]

Potential Complications from Thoracic Zygapophyseal Joint Injection Techniques

Although certain clinicians believe that intra-articular thoracic z-joint injections cannot be performed without pleural puncture,[125] complications from thoracic z-joint injections are uncommon when appropriately performed by skilled injectionists. Most problems are minor and self-limited, such as local postinjection pain or regional muscle spasm. If regional anatomy is not respected or appreciated, misplaced needles can theoretically result in epidural, subarachnoid, or pleural puncture.

LUMBAR ZYGAPOPHYSEAL JOINT INJECTION TECHNIQUES

The lumbar z-joints are well accepted pain generators that are evidenced by clinical studies, experimental observations on asymptomatic subjects, and a mass of anatomic and histologic literature supporting the nociceptive ability of these joints.[3,4,11,25,30,63,65,94,98,128] Clinically, lumbar z-joint pathology can cause both local and referred extremity pain. The prevalence of lumbar z-joint pain based on single diagnostic blocks has been reported to range broadly from 7.7% to 75%.[27–29,38,58,71,79,87, 89,98–100,107,109] Recent inquiry using a double-block diagnostic paradigm places the prevalence at approximately 15% in younger, injured workers.[119,121] In older patients with chronic low back pain the prevalence of lumbar z-joint pain was 40% using placebo-controlled blocks.[116] One study in 92 consecutive patients undergoing both discography and blocks of the z-joints has shown that the combination of pain from both structures was only 3%.[119]

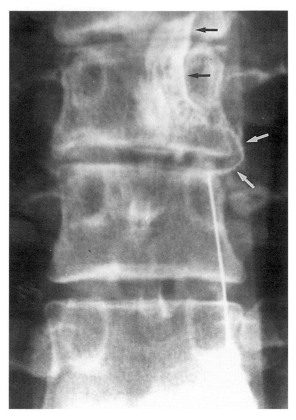

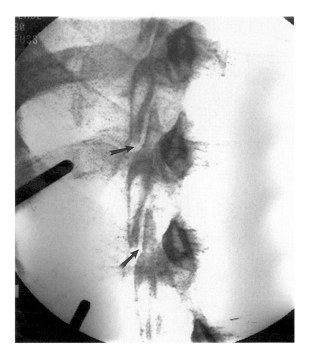

FIGURE 27-36. Near lateral (far oblique) radiograph of the thoracic z-joints. Thick metal pointers are placed on the skin such that the needle trajectory from this skin entry site would allow for cannulation of the inferior aspect of the target z-joints. The black arrows denote the unique trajectory needed for each of the two targeted thoracic z-joints based on the presence or absence of a ridge from the base of the superior articular process.

FIGURE 27-35. AP radiograph of a T8–T9 z-joint injection demonstrating epidural spread when an excessive amount of contrast was injected. The lateral capsular margin *(white arrows)* and subsequent epidural spread *(black arrows)* are both demonstrated.

Anatomy

The lumbar z-joints are paired synovial joints that vary in both shape and orientation.[25] The joints may be flat or curved in a **C** or **J** shape. The average orientation of the L4–L5 and L5–S1 z-joints with respect to the sagittal plane is 45° (Fig. 27-37). The more superior joints tend to be oriented in the sagittal plane. The more inferior joints may be oriented in the frontal plane.

The articular surface is covered with hyaline cartilage, and meniscus structures exist in these joints.[20] The dorsal, superior, and inferior margins of the joint are enclosed by a strong, 1-mm–thick fibrous capsule.[34,35,136] At the superior and inferior poles of the joint this capsule creates two subcapsular recesses containing adipose tissue. Anteriorly, the capsule is replaced by the ligamentum flavum. Fascicles of the multifidus muscle attach to the joint capsule, potentially preventing the capsule from being compressed by moving articular surfaces.[25,86] The capsule of the lumbar z-joints is richly innervated with

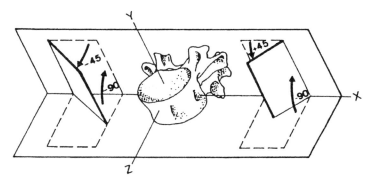

FIGURE 27-37. The plane of the articular facets in a typical lumbar z-joint. (From White AW 3d, Panjabi MM: The basic kinematics of the human spine. Spine 3:12–20, 1978, with permission.)

encapsulated, unencapsulated, and free-nerve endings.[3,4,65,96] Nociceptive nerves have been reported in the joint capsule[65] and nerves containing substance P have been isolated in the subchondral bone of degenerative lumbar z-joints.[11] Mechanoreceptors also have been isolated in the capsule of lumbar z-joints.[96] The capacity of the lumbar z-joint is approximately 1–2 ml.[66,107]

The lumbar z-joints are innervated by the medial branches of the dorsal rami of L1–L5.[21,22,25,128] Each z-joint is supplied by the two medial branches located at the transverse processes of the same levels comprising that z-joint. The L1–L4 dorsal rami divide off the spinal nerves and then divide into lateral, intermediate, and medial branches. The fifth dorsal ramus divides into medial and intermediate branches only. The intermediate and lateral branches of the L1–L5 dorsal rami enter the erector spinae muscles of the back. Each L1–L4 medial branch nerve crosses the base of the superior articular process at its junction with the transverse process (Fig. 27-38). Within 1 cm, the medial branch enters the mamilloaccessory notch under the

mamilloaccessory ligament.[37] After exciting this notch, the medial branch supplies articular branches to the z-joint above. It then courses inferiorly across the lamina to supply the interspinous ligament and muscles, the multifidus muscle, and the superior aspect of the z-joint below. The L5 dorsal ramus crosses the ala of the sacrum rather than the transverse process. It then runs in a groove formed by the junction of the sacral ala and the root of the superior articular process of S1. The L5 dorsal ramus divides into medial and intermediate branches at the base of the L5–S1 z-joint. The medial branch wraps around the base of this joint before supplying it and then enters the multifidus. Each L1–L4 lumbar medial branch nerve lies across the transverse process of the vertebra below. For example, the L3 medial branch is located at the junction of the superior articular process and transverse process of L4.[21,22,25]

Lumbar Medial Branch Block Techniques

To block the nerve supply to each lumbar z-joint, two medial branch blocks are necessary because of its dual innervation.[14–16,37] For example, L4–L5 is blocked by anesthetizing the L3 medial branch at the transverse process of L4 and L4 at the transverse process of L5. To anesthetize the nerve supply to the L5–S1 z-joint, the L4 medial branch should be blocked at the transverse process of L5 and the L5 dorsal ramus at the ala of the sacrum. It has been suggested that a communicating branch from the dorsal ramus of S1 may provide additional supply to the L5–S1 joint and can be blocked just above its exit from the S1 posterior foramina.[37] A recent study suggests that blockade of the L4 medial branch and the L5 dorsal rami alone adequately protects the L5–S1 z-joint from an experimental stimulus without the need for blockade of a potential ascending branch from S1.[77]

L1–L4 Medial Branch Blocks

The nerve should be blocked proximal to the mamilloaccessory ligament and notch for L1–L4 medial branch blocks.[51] The target location for L1–L4 medial branches is at the junction of the superior articular process and the transverse process that the nerve crosses, midway between the superior border of the transverse process and the location of the mamilloaccessory notch (see Figures 27-4 and 27-38). This point is not associated with an

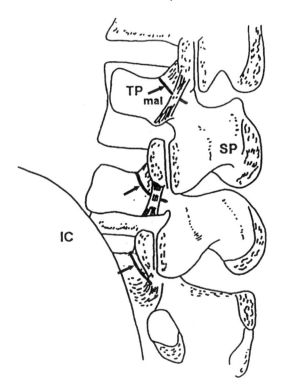

FIGURE 27-38. Oblique diagram of the L3 and L4 medial branch nerves and the L5 dorsal ramus. *SP* denotes the spinous process, *TP* the transverse process, *IC* the iliac crest, and *mal* the mamilloaccessory ligament. The black arrows, from cephalad to caudad, denote appropriate needle placement over the L3 medial branch, L4 medial branch, and L5 dorsal ramus, respectively.

inadvertent spread of injectant into the intervertebral foramen or epidural space for L1–L4 medial branch blocks.[51] On oblique views, the target point lies high on the "eye" of the "Scottie dog" (see Figure 27-4).[14] Placement more superior at the most superior junction of the superior articular process and transverse process as previously recommended[15] leads to an unacceptable incidence of spread into the foramen.[51]

A 22- or 25-gauge spinal needle may be used. A slight superior-to-inferior and lateral-to-medial needle approach to medial branch blocks has been validated.[51] If an inferior-to-superior needle approach is used, the injected anesthetic theoretically may spread toward the spinal nerve root or the sinuvertebral nerve, thereby substantially decreasing the block's specificity.[51]

From the skin entry point using AP imaging (usually just above the tip of the target transverse process), the needle is advanced toward the back of the root of the transverse process to ensure safe needle depth away from the ventral ramus. Alternatively, a direct oblique view may be used and the needle advanced "down the beam" toward the target using a slightly superior starting position to the final target. In general, for L1–L4 medial branch blocks approximately a 25–35° angle is necessary (depending on the level) to maximally visualize the osseous landmarks of the "Scottie dog." Thus, the needle will be directed anterior, medial, and caudad to reach the target location. The needle is then directed to the target location. Switching to an AP view is necessary to ensure that the needle is placed medial enough despite osseous contact on the oblique view, and an oblique view is necessary to ensure needle placement on the target if the needle was initially advanced on AP imaging (Figs. 27-39 and 27-40).

On AP imaging, the tip of the needle should be at least in line with the lateral margin of the silhouette of the superior articular process and, if possible, medial to this margin. The superior articular process frequently bulges laterally, overlapping the target point dorsally. If the needle tip is lateral to this point, it has contacted a thick transverse process instead of the superior articular process. In this case, the needle usually needs to be adjusted dorsally until correct position is obtained on both AP and oblique views.[14] Before injection the bevel opening should be medial and slightly inferior to reduce lateral and superior flow to the intervertebral foramen, especially if the needle is placed inadvertently higher than the target position.[51]

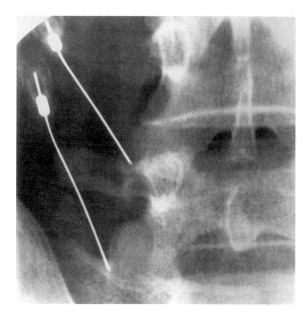

FIGURE 27-39. AP radiograph demonstrating needle placement for an L4 medial branch block and an L5 dorsal ramus block.

L5 Dorsal Ramus Blocks

The target point for the L5 dorsal ramus is at the junction of the ala of the sacrum with the superior articular process of the sacrum. This target point is recognized as a notch between these two bones with a minor amount of ipsilateral obliquity. The target

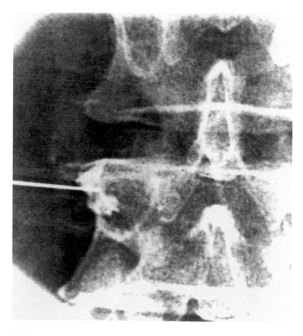

FIGURE 27-40. AP radiograph of an L3 medial branch block showing adequate medial placement of the needle and appropriate contrast flow along the path of the target nerve.

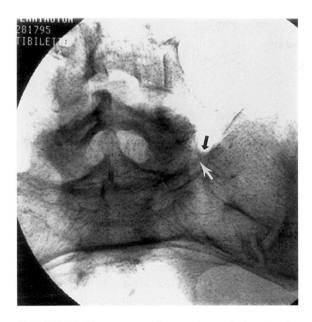

FIGURE 27-41. A 15° oblique radiograph showing the osseous groove between the S1 superior articular process and the sacral ala where the L5 dorsal ramus resides. The black arrow denotes the most superior aspect of this groove, and the white arrow denotes the appropriate location for needle placement for an L5 dorsal ramus block.

point lies opposite the middle of the base of the superior articular process and thus slightly below the silhouette of the top of the sacral ala (Fig. 27-41; see also Figure 27-39). Higher placement is associated with spread into the L5–S1 epidural space and lower placement with spread to the S1 posterior sacral foramen.[51]

A 22- or 25-gauge spinal needle may be used. For an L5 dorsal ramus block, an approximately 10–15° oblique view can be helpful to optimally view the junction of the sacral ala and the superior articular process of S1 (Fig. 27-42; see also Figure 27-41). Further obliquity usually places the medial iliac crest in front of the trajectory to the target position. The needle is advanced directly "down the beam" to the target position on slight oblique imaging. A superior-to-inferior approach is not used. AP imaging is then obtained to verify that the needle is placed at or preferably medial to the lateral silhouette of the S1 superior articular process (Figs. 27-43 and 27-44). After the needle is in the proper location, the bevel opening should be medial. This has been shown to reduce inadvertent

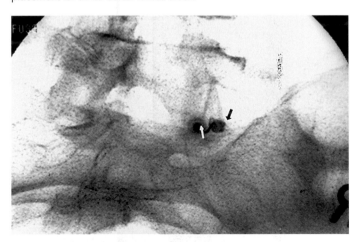

FIGURE 27-42. A 15° oblique radiograph depicting an L5 dorsal ramus block with appropriate contrast flow. The white arrow depicts the base of the L5–S1 z-joint, and the black arrow denotes the superior aspect of the junction between the S1 superior articular process and the sacral ala.

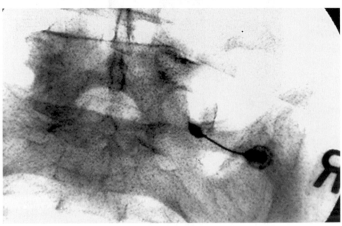

FIGURE 27-43. AP radiograph of an L5 dorsal ramus block with appropriate contrast flow.

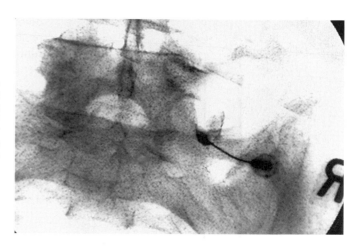

FIGURE 27-44. AP radiograph of needle placement for an L5 dorsal ramus block. The needle was advanced under a 20° oblique view such that it could be directed anteriorly and appropriately under the large overhanging wall of the S1 superior articular process where the target nerve resides. The arrows denote the lateral border of the superior articular process.

spread to the S1 posterior foramen or the L5 intervertebral foramen.[51]

For L1–L4 medial branch blocks and L5 dorsal rami blocks, 0.5 ml of anesthetic should be injected over the target nerve.[19,51,77] The authors use more potent anesthetics (e.g., 4% lidocaine and 0.75% bupivacaine) to minimize the risk of false-negative medial branch blocks, which can occur at a 10% rate with 2% lidocaine.[77] Failure to obtain relief with lumbar medial branch blocks in a case in which venous uptake of contrast dye is observed (despite needle redirection with avoidance of subsequent venous uptake) carries a 50% risk for false-negative results.[77] Contrast dye (usually 0.1–0.3 ml) is necessary for medial branch dorsal ramus blocks to confirm selective osseous flow along the location of the nerves and that no inadvertent venous uptake has occurred, which is observed 8% of the time with medial branch blocks.[51]

Intra-articular Lumbar Z-joint Injection Techniques

With the patient prone on the fluoroscopy table, pillows may be placed under the abdomen to attempt to "open" the z-joints and make needle entry easier. The cephalad lumbar z-joints are more sagittally oriented and often can be visualized on direct AP views. The more inferior z-joints generally require oblique imaging to visualize the joint space. If necessary, either the patient or the C-arm may be rotated with ipsilateral obliquity until the posterior joint space is first visualized. This can be achieved easily by rotating the image intensifier to the ipsilateral side or bending the ipsilateral knee to roll the patient onto his or her contralateral side. In more C-curved joints, rotating the C-arm to the point where the joint space is best seen likely images the

anterior rather than the posterior aspect of the joint where needle entry occurs (Figs. 27-45 and 27-46).[37,44] After the joint is visualized a skin mark is made, and in the line of the x-ray beam a needle is directed toward the z-joint. If the superior or

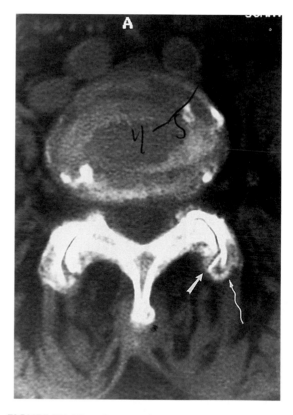

FIGURE 27-45. CT scan of an L4–L5 z-joint showing an acute medial angulation and opening *(straight white arrow)* at the most posterior aspect of the joint. The curved arrow depicts the typical needle trajectory used for a lumbar z-joint injection. Obviously, this trajectory would not be effective. Contralateral rotation in line with the straight white arrow would be necessary to image the posterior opening of this z-joint. The trajectory would be almost perpendicular to the usual trajectory used at this level.

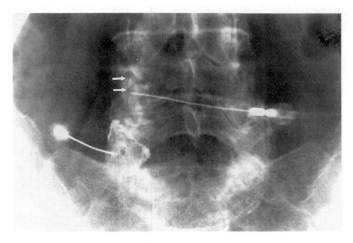

FIGURE 27-46. AP radiograph of an L5–S1 z-joint arthrogram after using the typical needle trajectory (lateral to medial) and an L4–L5 z-joint arthrogram after using a medial-to-lateral trajectory owing to a pronounced medial opening of the L4–L5 z-joint as seen in Figure 27-45. The white arrows depict the L4–L5 z-joint silhouette, but this faint silhouette does not represent the most posterior aspect of the joint.

inferior articular processes are encountered, safe needle depth can be determined. The needle is then gently repositioned until it is felt to enter the joint space. The posterior joint capsule is relatively firm and there is a characteristic "feel" when the needle penetrates this capsule. The needle need not be advanced completely into the joint but just a few millimeters past the joint capsule. If the needle is advanced too firmly it is possible to wedge the needle in the articular cartilage, which may potentially damage the articular cartilage and/or impede the flow of the injectant.

At times it is anatomically impossible to advance the needle into the posterior joint space. When this occurs, options still remain to obtain intracapsular placement of the injectant. While remaining near the posterior joint margin the needle can be advanced slightly medially or laterally so that the needle tip penetrates the joint capsule medial to its attachment on the articular processes (Fig. 27-47). This may require slight rotations of

the bevel to obtain an arthrogram with contrast injection. The needle also can be directed into either the superior or inferior capsular pockets. The needle should be carefully "walked off" either the superior or inferior aspect of the articular processes into the capsular pockets, but not excessively, or overpenetration through these recesses is possible. Upon contrast injection with the above techniques, filling of the entire joint cavity should occur (Figs. 27-48 and 27-49).

Occasionally the L4–L5 or, more frequently, the L5–S1 z-joint is in or near the frontal plane so that highly oblique or lateral imaging is needed to visualize the joint space. The skin entry point that correlates with the direction of the x-ray beam is then located over the iliac crest that obstructs use of this approach (Fig. 27-50). If this occurs, a direct posterior approach can be used.[113] A lateral skin mark is placed pertaining to the inferior aspect of the joint on highly oblique or lateral imaging, and the C-arm is then brought back to AP imaging. A

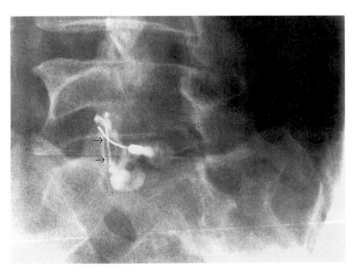

FIGURE 27-47. Oblique radiograph of an L5–S1 z-joint arthrogram. The needle is just under the lateral extension of the joint's capsule rather than in the osseous joint space depicted by the black arrows.

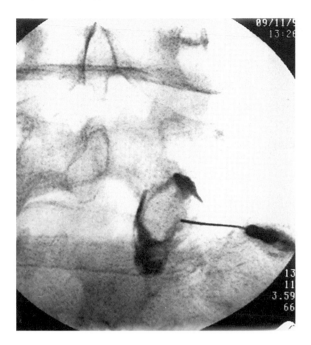

FIGURE 27-48. AP radiograph of a needle placed into the middle of the L5–S1 z-joint with an appropriate confirmatory arthrogram.

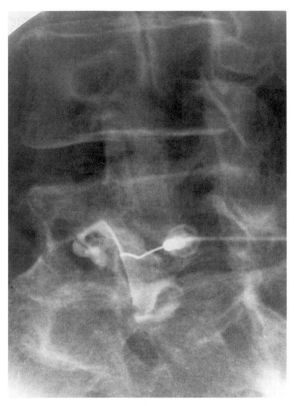

FIGURE 27-49. Oblique radiograph of an L5–S1 z-joint arthrogram. Superior and inferior capsular recesses are demonstrated.

horizontal line is drawn perpendicular to the long axis of the spine that intersects this lateral skin mark. On AP imaging, a medial skin mark is placed along this horizontal line or just inferior to it and also should be located lateral to the interlaminar space where the midportion of the inferior aspect of the z-joint should exist. Under AP imaging, the needle is then inserted directly down or down with a slight superior tilt (if the medial skin mark was placed just inferior to the horizontal line) to the inferior aspect of the joint (Fig. 27-51). The needle should not be allowed to stray too far medial into the interlaminar space, too far lateral away from the z-joint, or too far inferior toward the posterior S1 foramen. When bone is contacted, the C-arm is rotated until the joint space is seen; the needle is then directed into either the inferior aspect of the joint or the inferior capsular recess (Fig. 27-52). When appropriately placed, injection of contrast will reveal spread throughout the joint space (Figs. 27-53 and 27-54). If appropriate contrast spread does not occur, switching between AP and highly oblique or lateral imaging helps to guide the needle into the target location.

Alternatively, when the iliac crest occludes the L5–S1 z-joint (see Figure 27-50), sometimes it is possible to provide a caudad tilt to "throw" the iliac crest away so that a clear, direct trajectory is appreciated to the more superior aspect of the L5–S1 z-joint

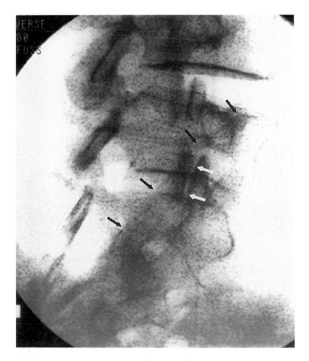

FIGURE 27-50. Oblique radiograph of the L5–S1 z-joint showing the iliac crest occluding the potential path of the needle to the joint opening. The white arrows denote the joint space, and the black arrows denote the iliac crest.

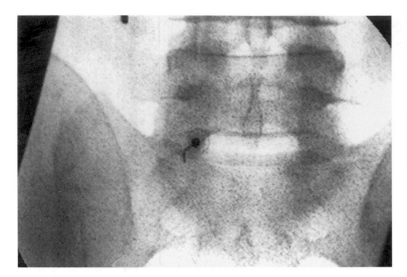

FIGURE 27-51. AP radiograph of a needle placed into the most inferior aspect of the L5–S1 z-joint using a direct posterior approach.

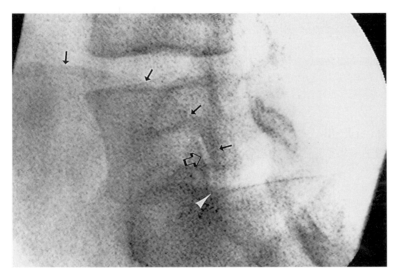

FIGURE 27-52. Far oblique radiograph showing the L5–S1 z-joint occluded by the iliac crest when imaging in line with the joint plane is visualized. This is the same patient as in Figure 27-51. A needle is placed in the most inferior aspect of the joint *(white arrow)*. The open black arrow denotes the joint line, and the closed black arrows denote the iliac crest.

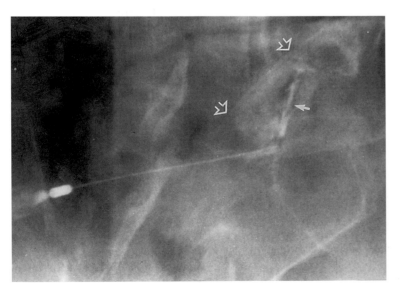

FIGURE 27-53. Near lateral radiograph of an L5–S1 z-joint arthrogram using a direct posterior approach. The needle is placed in the inferior aspect of the joint. Contrast is seen in the joint *(closed white arrow)*, and the margin of the iliac crest is appreciated *(open white arrows)*.

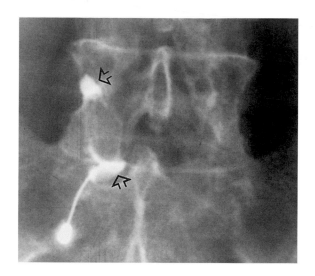

FIGURE 27-54. AP radiograph of an L5–S1 z-joint arthrogram using a direct posterior approach. The needle is placed in the inferior capsular recess. Superior and inferior capsular recesses *(open black arrows)* are demonstrated.

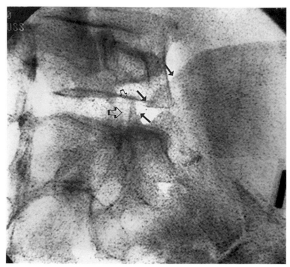

FIGURE 27-55. Oblique radiograph of the same patient as in Figure 27-50. Cephalad angulation has now been introduced, "throwing" the iliac crest out of the way so that a needle could enter the L5–S1 z-joint without hitting the iliac crest. The open black arrows denote the joint opening, and the solid black arrows denote the iliac crest.

(Fig. 27-55). The needle is directed "down the beam." Then the needle is directed in a superior-to-inferior approach with slightly more medial angulation than is typical.

After joint entry is perceived, 0.2–0.3 ml of contrast is instilled to ensure proper intra-articular placement. A complete arthrogram need not be produced at the expense of reducing the volume of the subsequent active injectant. The lumbar z-joints generally should not be injected with > 1.5 ml of volume to avoid spread of the injectant posterior to the joint or into the epidural space.[14,37] If pressure is generated before this volume, the injection should cease to avoid rupturing the joint capsule and causing extravasation of the injectant.

Potential Complications from Lumbar Zygapophyseal Joint Injection Techniques

Complications from lumbar z-joint block procedures are rare. The majority of problems are self-limited and usually are restricted to increased z-joint pain and local needle site pain. Chemical meningism from penetration of the dural cuff leading to subarachnoid entry with two level z-joint injections and a one-level medial branch block has been reported. In such cases large volumes of injectant were used and the descriptions of needle placement and contrast flow under fluoroscopic imaging prior to injection were not discussed.[129] With the use of fluoroscopy and contrast in experienced

hands, damage to a spinal nerve root or needle placement into the epidural or subarachnoid spaces should not occur. Cases of spinal anesthesia following lumbar facet injections, however, have been reported.[67,93] Only one case report exists regarding an infection associated with z-joint injections.[33]

CONCLUSION

The z-joints may be a source of local and referred pain in patients with spinal axis and extremity pain. The definitive diagnosis of z-joint–mediated pain relies on properly performed controlled z-joint block techniques. These techniques maintain an important diagnostic and potentially therapeutic role in the management of spinal pain and should not be performed in isolation but rather in the context of other diagnostic and therapeutic methods. Many questions remain regarding the clinical role of z-joint techniques in the daily practice of spinal medicine. Answers to these questions will be obtained only through future research.

REFERENCES

1. The Standards of Reporting Trials Group: A proposal for structured reporting of randomized controlled trials. JAMA 272:1926–1931, 1994.
2. Aprill C, Bogduk N: The prevalence of cervical zygapophyseal joint pain: A first approximation. Spine 17:744–747, 1992.

3. Ashton IK, Ashton BA, Gibson SJ, et al: Morphological basis for back pain: The demonstration of nerve fibers and neuropeptides in the lumbar facet joint capsule but not in the ligamentum flavum. J Orthop Res 10:72–78, 1992.

4. Avramov AI, Cavanaugh JM, Ozaktay CA, et al: The effect of controlled mechanical loading on group II, III, and IV afferent units from the lumbar facet joint and surrounding tissue. An in vitro study. J Bone Joint Surg 74A:1464–1471, 1992.

5. Bainbridge JS, Wright RE: The effect of conscious sedation on subjective pain ratings in patients undergoing diagnostic/therapeutic spinal injection. Presented at the 5th annual meeting of the International Spinal Injection Society, Denver, October, 1997.

6. Barnsley L, Bogduk N: Medial branch blocks are specific for the diagnosis of cervical zygapophyseal joint pain. Reg Anesth 18:343–350, 1993.

7. Barnsley L, Lord S, Bogduk N: Comparative local anaesthetic blocks in the diagnosis of cervical zygapophyseal joint pain. Pain 55:99–106, 1993.

8. Barnsley L, Lord S, Wallis B, Bogduk N: False-positive rates of cervical zygapophyseal joint blocks. Clin J Pain 9:124–130, 1993.

9. Barnsley L, Lord SM, Wallis BJ, Bogduk N: Lack of effect of intraarticular corticosteroids for chronic pain in the cervical zygapophyseal joints. N Engl J Med 330:1047–1050, 1994.

10. Barnsley L, Lord SM, Wallis BJ, et al: The prevalence of chronic cervical zygapophyseal joint pain after whiplash. Spine 20:20–26, 1995.

11. Beaman DN, Graziano GP, Glover RA, et al: Substance P innervation of lumbar spine facet joints. Spine 18:1044–1049, 1993.

12. Bland JH: Anatomy and biomechanics. In Disorders of the Cervical Spine. Philadelphia, W.B. Saunders, 1987, pp 9–63.

13. Bogduk N: The clinical anatomy of the cervical dorsal rami. Spine 7:319–330, 1982.

14. Bogduk N: International Spinal Injection Society guidelines for the performance of spinal injection procedures. Part 1. Zygapophyseal joint blocks. Clin J Pain 13:285–302, 1997.

15. Bogduk N: Back pain: Zygapophyseal joint blocks and epidurals. In Cousins MJ, Bridenbaugh PO (eds): Neural Blockade in Clinical Anesthesia and Pain Management, 2nd ed. Philadelphia, J.B. Lippincott, 1990, pp 935–954.

16. Bogduk N: Back pain: Zygapophyseal joint block and epidural steroids. In Cousins MJ, Bridenbaugh PO (eds): Neural Blockade in Clinical Anesthesia and Pain Management. Philadelphia: J.B. Lippincott, 1996, pp 935–954.

17. Bogduk N, Aprill C: On the nature of neck pain, discography and cervical zygapophyseal joint blocks. Pain 54:213–217, 1993.

18. Bogduk N, Aprill C, Derby R: Diagnostic blocks of spinal synovial joints. In White AH (ed): Spine Care Diagnosis and Conservative Treatment, Vol. 1. St. Louis, Mosby, 1995, pp 298–321.

19. Bogduk N, Aprill C, Derby R: Lumbar zygapophyseal joint pain: Diagnostic blocks and therapy. In Wilson DJ (ed): Interventional Radiology of the Musculoskeletal System. London, Edward Arnold, 1995, pp 3–86.

20. Bogduk N, Engel R: The menisci of the lumbar zygapophyseal joints: A review of their anatomy and clinical significance. Spine 9:454–460, 1984.

21. Bogduk N, Long DM: The anatomy of the so-called articular nerves and their relationship to facet denervation in the treatment of low back pain. J Neurosurg 51:172–177, 1979.

22. Bogduk N, Long DM: Percutaneous lumbar medial branch neurotomy. A modification of facet denervation. Spine 5:193–200, 1980.

23. Bogduk N, Marsland A: The cervical zygapophyseal joints as a source of neck pain. Spine 13:610–617, 1988.

24. Bogduk N, Marsland A: On the concept of third occipital headache. J Neurol Neurosurg Psychiatry 49:775–780, 1986.

25. Bogduk N, Twomey LT: Clinical Anatomy of the Lumbar Spine, 2nd ed. London, Churchill Livingstone, 1991.

26. Bogduk N, Valencia F: Innervation and pain patterns of the thoracic spine. In Grant R (ed): Physical Therapy of the Cervical and Thoracic Spine. Edinburgh, Churchill Livingstone, 1988, pp 27–37.

27. Carette S, Marcoux S, Truchon R, et al: A controlled trial of corticosteroid injections into the facet joints for chronic low back pain. N Engl J Med 325:1002–1007, 1991.

28. Carrera GF: Lumbar facet joint injection in low back pain and sciatica: Preliminary results. Radiology 137:665–667, 1980.

29. Carrera GF, Williams AL: Current concepts in evaluation of the lumbar facet joints. CRC Crit Rev Diagn Imag 21:85–104, 1984.

30. Cavanaugh JM, Ozaktay AC, Yamashita T, et al: Mechanisms of low back pain: A neurophysiological and neuroanatomic study. Clin Orthop 335:166–180, 1997.

31. Chua WH, Bogduk N: The surgical anatomy of thoracic facet denervation. Acta Neurochir 136:140–144, 1995.

32. Chua WH: Clinical Anatomy of the Thoracic Dorsal Rami [thesis]. Newcastle, Australia, University of Newcastle, 1994.

33. Cook NJ, Hanrahan P, Song S: Paraspinal abscess following facet joint injection. Clin Rheumatol 18:52–53, 1999.

34. Cyron BM, Hutton WC: The tensile strength of the capsular ligaments of the apophyseal joints. J Anat 132:145–150, 1981.

35. Cyron BM, Hutton WC: The tensile strength of the capsular ligaments of the apophyseal joints. J Anat 132:145–150, 1981.

36. Derby R: [Personal communication]. 1998.

37. Derby R, Bogduk N, Schwarzer A: Precision percutaneous blocking procedures for localizing spinal pain. Part 1: The posterior lumbar compartment. Pain Digest 3:89–100, 1993.

38. Destouet JM, Gilula LA, Murphy WA, Monsees B: Lumbar facet joint injection: Indication, technique, clinical correlation and preliminary results. Radiology 145:321–325, 1982.

39. Destouet JM, Murphy WA: Lumbar facet block: Indications and technique. Orthop Rev 14:57–65, 1985.

40. Dolan AL, Ryan PJ, Arden NK, et al: The value of SPECT scans in identifying back pain likely to benefit from facet joint injection. Br J Rheumatol 35:1269–1273, 1996.

41. Dory MA: Arthrography of the cervical facet joints. Radiology 148:379–382, 1983.

42. Dreyer SJ, Dreyfuss P: Low back pain and the zygapophyseal (facet) joints. Arch Phys Med Rehabil 77:290–300, 1996.

43. Dreyer S, Dreyfuss P: Injection therapy. In Cole A (ed): Low Back Pain: Diagnosis and Treatment: A Symptom Based Approach [in press].

44. Dreyer SJ, Dreyfuss P, Cole A: Zygapophyseal (facet) joint injections: Intra-articular and medial branch block techniques. Phys Med Rehabil Clin North Am 6:715–742, 1995.

45. Dreyer S, Dreyfuss P, Cole A: Posterior elements (facet and sacroiliac joints) and low back pain. Phys Med Rehabil State Art Rev 13:443–471, 1999.

46. Dreyfuss P: The power of bevel control. ISIS Sci Newsl 13(1):16, 1998.

47. Dreyfuss PH, Dreyer SJ, Herring SA: Contemporary concepts in spine care: Lumbar zygapophyseal (facet) joint injections. Spine 20:2040–2047, 1995.

48. Dreyfuss P, Dreyer S: Lumbar facet injections. In Gonzalez EG, Materson RS (eds): The Nonsurgical Management of Acute Low Back Pain. New York, Demos Vermande, 1997, pp 123–126.

49. Dreyfuss P, Halbrook B, Pauza K, et al: Lumbar radiofrequency neurotomy for chronic zygapophyseal joint pain: A pilot study using dual medial branch blocks. ISIS Sci Newsl 3(2):13–33, 1999.
50. Dreyfuss P, Michaelsen M, Horne M: MUJA: Manipulation under joint anesthesia/analgesia: A treatment approach for recalcitrant low back pain of synovial joint origin. J Manipulative Physiol Ther 18:537–546, 1995.
51. Dreyfuss P, Schwarzer AC, Lau P, Bogduk N: The target specificity of lumbar medial branch and L5 dorsal ramus blocks: A computed tomography study. Spine 22:895–902, 1997.
52. Dreyfuss P, Tibiletti C, Dreyer S: Thoracic zygapophyseal joint pain patterns: A study in normal volunteers. Spine 19:807–811, 1994.
53. Dreyfuss P, Tibiletti C, Dreyer S, Sobel J: Thoracic zygapophyseal joint pain: A review and description of an intra-articular block technique. Pain Digest 4:44–52, 1994.
54. Dussault RG, Nicolet VM: Cervical facet arthrography. J Can Assoc Radiol 36:79–80, 1985.
55. Dvorak J, Dvorak V: Biomechanics and functional examination of the spine. In Manual Medicine-Diagnostics, 2nd ed. New York, Thieme, 1990, pp 1–34.
56. Dwyer A, Aprill C, Bogduk N: Cervical zygapophyseal joint pain patterns 1: A study in normal volunteers. Spine 15:453–457, 1990.
57. Esses SI, Moro JK: The value of facet blocks in patient selection for lumbar fusion. Spine 18:185–190, 1993.
58. Fairbank J CT, Park WM, McCall IW, O'Brien JP: Apophyseal injection of local anesthetic as a diagnostic aid in primary low-back pain syndromes. Spine 6:598–605, 1981.
59. Finch PM, Racz GB, McDaniel K: A curved approach to nerve blocks and radiofrequency lesioning. Pain Digest 7:251–257, 1997.
60. Fox JL, Rizzoli HV: Identification of radiologic co-ordinates for posterior articular nerve of Luschka in the lumbar spine. Surg Neurol 1:343–346, 1973.
61. Fukui S, Ohseto K, Shiotani M: Patterns of pain induced by distending the thoracic zygapophyseal joints. Reg Anesth 22:332–336, 1997.
62. Fukui S, Ohseto K, Shiotani M, et al: Referred pain distribution of the cervical zygapophyseal joints and cervical dorsal rami. Pain 68:79–83, 1996.
63. Fukui S, Ohseto K, Shiotani M, et al: Distribution of referred pain from the lumbar zygapophyseal joints and dorsal rami. Clin J Pain 13:303–307, 1997.
64. Ghormley RK: Low back pain with special reference to the articular facets, with presentation of an operative procedure. JAMA 101:1773–1777, 1933.
65. Giles LG, Harvey AR: Immunohistochemical demonstration of nociceptors in the capsule and synovial folds of human zygapophyseal joints. Br J Rheumatol 26:362 364, 1987.
66. Glover JR: Arthrography of the joints of the lumbar vertebral arches. Orthop Clin North Am 8:37–42, 1977.
67. Goldstone JC, Pennant JH: Spinal anaesthesia after facet joint injection. Anaesthesia 42:754–756, 1987.
68. Goldthwaith JE: The lumbosacral articulation: An explanation of many cases of lumbago, sciatica and paraplegia. Boston Med Surg J 164:365–372, 1911.
69. Grieve GP: Common Vertebral Joint Problems, 2nd ed. Edinburgh, Churchill Livingstone, 1988.
70. Grieve GP: Applied anatomy--regional. In Common Vertebral Joint Problems, 2nd ed. London, Churchill Livingstone, 1988, p 7.
71. Helbig T, Lee CK: The lumbar facet syndrome. Spine 13:61–64, 1988.
72. Hirsch D, Ingelmark B, Miller M: The anatomical basis for low back pain. Acta Orthop Scand 33:1–17, 1963.
73. Hove B, Gyldensted C: Cervical analgesic facet joint arthrography. Neuroradiology 32:456–459, 1990.
74. Jackson RP: The facet syndrome: Myth or reality? Clin Orthop 279:110–121, 1992.
75. Jackson RP, Jacobs RR, Montesano PX: Facet joint injection in low back pain: A prospective statistical study. Spine 13:966–971, 1988.
76. Jeffries B: Facet steroid injections. Spine State Art Rev 2:409–417, 1988.
77. Kaplan M, Dreyfuss P, Halbrook B, Bogduk N: The ability of lumbar medial branch blocks to anesthetize the zygapophyseal joint: A physiologic challenge. Spine 23:1847–1852, 1998.
78. Kline MT: Radiofrequency techniques in clinical practice. In Waldman S, Winnie A (eds): Interventional Pain Management. Philadelphia, W.B. Saunders, 1996, pp 185–217.
79. Lau LSW, Littlejohn GO, Miller MH: Clinical evaluation of intra-articular injections for lumbar facet joint pain. Med J Aust 143:563–565, 1985.
80. Lord SM, Barnsley L, Bogduk N: The utility of comparative local anesthetic blocks versus placebo-controlled blocks for the diagnosis of cervical zygapophyseal joint pain. Clin J Pain 11:208–213, 1995.
81. Lord S, Barnsley L, Bogduk N: Percutaneous radiofrequency neurotomy in the treatment of cervical zygapophyseal joint pain: A caution. Neurosurgery 36:732–739, 1995.
82. Lord SM, Barnsley L, Bogduk N: Cervical zygapophyseal joint pain in whiplash injuries. Spine State Art Rev 12:301–322, 1998.
83. Lord S, Barnsley L, Wallis B, et al: Third occipital nerve headache: A prevalence study. J Neurol Neurosurg Psychiatry 57:1187–1190, 1994.
84. Lord S, Barnsley L, Wallis BJ, et al: Chronic cervical zygapophyseal joint pain after whiplash: A placebo-controlled prevalence study. Spine 22:1737–1744, 1996.
85. Lord SM: Cervical Zygapophyseal Joint Pain after Whiplash Injury, Precision Diagnosis, Prevalence, and Evaluation of Treatment by Percutaneous Radiofrequency Neurotomy [doctoral thesis]. Newcastle, Australia, University of Newcastle, 1996.
86. Lewin T, Moffet B, Viidik A: The morphology of the lumbar synovial intervertebral joints. Acta Morphol Nederlando-Scand 4:299–319, 1962.
87. Lewinnek GE, Warfield CA: Facet joint degeneration as a cause of low back pain. Clin Orthop 213:216–222, 1986.
88. Lilius G, Laasonen EM, Myllynen P, et al: Lumbar facet joint syndrome: A randomised clinical trial. J Bone Joint Surg 71B:681–684, 1989.
89. Lippit AB: The facet joint and its role in spine pain: Management with facet joint injections. Spine 9:746–750, 1984.
90. Lynch MC, Taylor JF: Facet joint injection for low back pain. J Bone Joint Surg 68B:138–141, 1986.
91. Maldague B, Mathurin P, Malghem J: Facet joint arthrography in lumbar spondylolysis. Radiology 140:29–36, 1981.
92. Marks RC, Houston T: Facet joint injection and facet nerve block: A randomized comparison in 86 patients. Pain 49:325–328, 1992.
93. Marks R, Semple AJ: Spinal anesthesia after facet joint injection. Anaesthesia 43:65–66, 1988.
94. McCall IW, Park WM, O'Brien JP: Induced pain referral from posterior lumbar elements in normal subjects. Spine 4:441–446, 1979.
95. McClain RF: Mechanoreceptor endings in human cervical facet joints. Spine 19:495–501, 1994.
96. McClain RF, Pickar JG: Mechanoreceptor endings in human thoracic and lumbar facet joints. Spine 23:168–173, 1998.

97. Mercer S, Bogduk N: Intra-articular inclusion of the cervical synovial joints. Br J Rheumatol 32:705–710, 1993.

98. Mooney V, Robertson J: Facet joint syndrome. Clin Orthop 115:149–156, 1976.

99. Moran R, O'Connell D, Walsh MG: The diagnostic value of facet joint injections. Spine 12:1407–1410, 1986.

100. Murtagh FR: Computed tomography and fluoroscopy guided anesthesia and steroid injection in facet syndrome. Spine 13:686–689, 1988.

101. Nash TP: Facet joints—intra-articular steroids or nerve block? Pain Clinic 3:563–564, 1990.

102. Okada K: Studies on the cervical facet joints using arthrography of the cervical facet joint. J Jpn Orthop Assoc 55:563–580, 1981.

103. Park WM, McCall IW, Benson D, et al: Spondylarthrography: The demonstration of spondylosis by apophyseal joint arthrography. Clin Radiol 36:427–430, 1985.

104. Parlier-Cuau C, Wybier M, Nizard R, et al: Symptomatic lumbar facet joint synovial cysts: Clinical assessment of facet joint steroid injection after 1 and 6 months using long-term follow-up in 30 patients. Radiology 210:509–513, 1999.

105. Purcell-Jones G: Paravertebral somatic nerve block: A clinical, radiographic and computed tomographic study in chronic pain patients. Anesth Analg 68:32–39, 1989.

106. Racz G: [Personal communication]. 1994.

107. Raymond J, Dumas JM: Intra-articular facet block: Diagnostic tests or therapeutic procedure? Radiology 151:333–336, 1984.

108. Raymond J, Dumas JM, Lisbona R: Nuclear imaging as a screening test for patients referred for intra-articular facet block. J Can Assoc Radiol 35:291–292, 1984.

109. Revel ME, Listrat VM, Chevalier XJ, et al: Facet joint block for low back pain: Identifying predictors of a good response. Arch Phys Med Rehabil 73:824–828, 1992.

110. Rossi V, Pernak J: Low back pain: The facet syndrome. Adv Pain Res Ther 13:231–244, 1990.

111. Roy DF, Fleury J, Fontaine SB, Dussault RG: Clinical evaluation of cervical facet joint infiltration. J Can Assoc Radiol 36:118–120, 1988.

112. Saberski LR: Cryoneurolysis in clinical practice. In Waldman S, Winnie A (eds): Interventional Pain Management. Philadelphia, W.B. Saunders, 1996, pp 172–184.

113. Sarazin L, Chevrot A, Pessis E, et al: Lumbar facet joint arthrography with the posterior approach. Radiographics 19:93–104, 1999.

114. Schaeffer JP (ed): Morris' Human Anatomy: A Complete Systematic Treatise. New York, Blankiston, 1953, pp 657, 664–665.

115. Schuster GD: The use of cryoanalgesia in the painful facet syndrome. J Neurol Orthop Surg 3:271–274, 1982.

116. Schwarzer AC, Wang SC, Bogduk N, et al: Prevalence and clinical features of lumbar zygapophyseal joint pain: A study in an Australian population with chronic low back pain. Ann Rheum Dis 54:100–106, 1995.

117. Schwarzer AC, Wang SC, O'Driscoll D, et al: The ability of computed tomography to identify a painful zygapophyseal joint in patients with chronic low back pain. Spine 20:907–912, 1995.

118. Schwarzer AC, Aprill CN, Derby R, et al: The false positive rate of uncontrolled diagnostic blocks of the lumbar zygapophyseal joints. Pain 58:195–200, 1994.

119. Schwarzer AC, Aprill CN, Fortin J, et al: The relative contributions of the disc and zygapophyseal joint in chronic low back pain. Spine 19:801–806, 1994.

120. Schwarzer AC, Derby R, Aprill C, et al: The value of the provocation response in lumbar zygapophyseal joint injections. Clin J Pain 10:309–313, 1994.

121. Schwarzer AC, Aprill CN, Derby R, et al: Clinical features of patients with pain stemming from the lumbar zygapophyseal joints. Is the lumbar facet syndrome a clinical entity? Spine 19:1132–1137, 1994.

122. Schwarzer AC, Scott AM, Wang S, et al: The role of bone scintigraphy in chronic low back pain: Comparison of SPECT and planar images and zygapophyseal joint injection. Aust N Z J Med 22:185, 1992.

123. Silvers HR: Lumbar percutaneous facet rhizotomy. Spine 15:36–40, 1990.

124. Stillwell DL: The nerve supply of the vertebral column and its associated structures in the monkey. Anat Record 125:139–162, 1956.

125. Stolker RJ, Vervest AC, Groen GJ: Percutaneous facet denervation in chronic thoracic spinal pain. Acta Neurochir (Wein) 122:82–90, 1993.

126. Stolker RJ, Vervest AC, Groen GJ: Parameters in electrode positioning in thoracic percutaneous facet denervation: An anatomical study. Acta Neurochir (Wein) 128:32–39, 1994.

127. Sullivan WJ, Willick SE, Chira-Adisai W, et al: Incidence of vascular uptake in lumbar spinal injection procedures. Spine [in press].

128. Suseki K, Takahashi Y, Takahashi K, et al: Innervation of the lumbar facet joints. Origins and functions. Spine 22:477–485, 1997.

129. Thompson SJ, Lomax DM, Collett BJ: Chemical meningism after lumbar facet joint block with local anesthetic and steroids. Anaesthesia 46:563–564, 1991.

130. Valencia F: Biomechanics of the thoracic spine. In Grant R (ed): Physical Therapy of the Cervical and Thoracic Spine. Edinburgh, Churchill Livingstone, 1988, pp 39–50.

131. Weishaupt D, Zanetti M, Hodler J, Boos N: MR imaging of the lumbar spine: Prevalence of intervertebral disk extrusion and sequestration, nerve root compression, end plate abnormalities, and osteoarthritis of the facet joints in asymptomatic volunteers. Radiology 209:661–666, 1998.

132. Wedel DJ, Wilson PR: Cervical facet arthrography. Reg Anesth 10:7–11, 1985.

133. Wilson PR: Thoracic facet joint syndrome: A clinical entity? Pain Suppl 4:S87, 1987.

134. Wyke B: Neurology of the cervical spinal joints. Physiotherapy 65:72–75, 1979.

135. Wyke B: Articular neurology: A review. Physiotherapy 58:563–580, 1981.

136. Yahia LH, Garzon S: Structure on the capsular ligaments of the facet joints. Anat Anz 175:185–188, 1993.

137. Yu S, Sether L, Haughton VM: Facet joint menisci of the cervical spine: Correlative MR imaging and cryomicrotomy study. Radiology 164:79–82, 1987.

28

Atlanto-occipital and Atlantoaxial Joint Injections

Kevin Pauza, M.D., and Paul Dreyfuss, M.D.

Upper cervical pain and headache may be caused by muscles,[20,63] ligaments,[31,49] discs,[12,58] dura and nerve roots,[8] vertebral arteries,[52] joints,[6] or other structures within the upper cervical spine.[9] Cervical joints potentially responsible for these symptoms include the atlanto-occipital (AO), atlantoaxial (AA), and the C2–C3 zygapophyseal joints.[1,2,6–11,30,49] Previous studies describe symptom referral patterns of the AO[25,26,33,35] and AA joints.[25,33] Because no known radiographic, laboratory, or clinical examination method exists to confirm or eliminate these joints as pain generators, an intra-articular injection of local anesthetic serves as the only means available to establish the diagnosis. In addition, the instillation of corticosteroid may serve to decrease intra-articular inflammation and provide sustained relief.[15,26,48,51] However, no controlled trials validate the efficacy of intra-articular corticosteroids for AO or AA joint-mediated pain. This chapter addresses the pertinent anatomy, pathophysiology, clinical presentation, evaluation, and treatment of the atlanto-occipital and atlantoaxial joints.

ANATOMY

The AO and AA joints are not zygapophyseal (facet) joints. Hence, they differ from these synovial joints in the vertebral column in many respects.[14,16] AO and AA joints are in series with the small uncovertebral joints on the sides of the bodies of the other cervical vertebrae, not with the zygapophyseal joints on the vertebral arches. They are therefore positioned anterolateral to the spinal canal and cord (not posterolateral).[51]

Anatomy of the Atlanto-occipital Articulation (C0–C1)

The AO joints are paired synovial articulations that form the connection between the occipital condyles, the superior articular facets of the atlas.

Their sensory innervation comes from the ventral rami of C1.[6] The joint's shape is bean-like with its two long axes converging anteriorly and medially and its lateral edges sloping superiorly. The joint's orientation, on average, lies 28° from the sagittal plane and 62° from the frontal plane.[29] A loose synovial membrane surrounds the joint with pronounced laxity at its anterior, posterior, and lateral joint margins.[22] Occasional capsular extensions to the odontoid and transverse ligaments have been described.[54] The AO joint is relatively large compared to the lower cervical facet joints. The surface area of the superior facet of C1 ranges from 103.2 to 277.4 mm², and the area of the occipital condyle ranges from 109.76 to 329.0 mm².[53] Computed tomography (CT) evaluation reveals an average joint space of 1 mm.[21] This articulation predominately allows not only extension (approximately 20°), but also flexion, lateral bending, and axial rotation to a much lesser extent (3–8°).[29]

Anatomy of the Atlantoaxial Articulation (C1–C2)

The AA joints are paired synovial articulations formed by the superior articular facet of the axis and the inferior articular facet of the lateral mass of the atlas. The articular surface of the axis is convex and faces superolaterally, whereas the articular surface of the atlas is slightly concave or flat and faces inferomedially.[28,57] The long axis of the joint is oriented obliquely, with its medial aspect more ventral and its lateral aspect more dorsal. The superior facet of C2 (axis) and the inferior facet of C1 (atlas) slope slightly so that the lateral aspect is more caudal than the medial aspect.[21] There may be an anterior to posterior joint gap of approximately 3.5 mm,[29] but the main articulation is 1 mm wide.[21] The joint capsule is lax, allowing significant rotation. Synovial folds exist that project beyond the medial aspect of the joint approximately 1–5 mm and tapering laterally.[17] The axis has the characteristic odontoid process around which the atlas can rotate. This allows axial rotation of approximately 40° to either side of the midline. It also allows some flexion, extension, and lateral bending.[4]

Vascular Anatomy

Vertebral Artery Anatomy

The vertebral artery initially ascends through the foramina transversaria of the upper six cervical vertebrae, accompanied by a large branch derived from the inferior cervical sympathetic ganglion and a plexus of veins that unite to form the vertebral vein at the lower part of the neck. It lies in front of the anterior primary rami of the C2–C6 spinal nerves and pursues an almost vertical course as far as the transverse process of the axis, through which it runs upward and lateral to the foramen transversarium of the atlas. It exits the foramina transversarium, curving posteriorly behind the lateral mass of the atlas, traveling immediately lateral to the anterior primary ramus of the first cervical nerve. It lies within a groove on the upper surface of the posterior arch of the atlas and enters the vertebral canal by passing below the lower, arched border of the posterior AO membrane.[41] The posterior primary ramus of the first cervical nerve lies between the artery and the posterior arch of the atlas.[56] With true lateral imaging of the AA joint, the vertebral artery lies at the middle-to-posterior aspect of the joint. A study of 558 vertebral angiograms demonstrated that the vertebral artery traversed posterior to the mid-portion of the joint on all occasions when viewed laterally.[19] However, with rotation, the anteroposterior (AP) relationship of the vertebral artery to the AA joint changes. For example, with cervical rotation to the right, the left vertebral artery is displaced anteriorly over the AA joint. With rotation to the left, the left vertebral artery may be displaced posteriorly.[34]

Internal Carotid Artery, External Carotid Artery, Internal Jugular Vein, and Occipital Artery Anatomy

The internal carotid artery (ICA) passes superiorly in front of the transverse processes of the upper cervical vertebrae, lying along the surface of the rectus capitis anticus major muscle from the C1 to the C3 segmental level until it enters the carotid foramen in the temporal bone. At C1–C2, the internal jugular vein lies slightly posterior to the ICA. The ICA is separated anteriorly from the external carotid artery (ECA) by the stylopharyngeus muscle, glossopharyngeal nerve, and pharyngeal branch of the vagus nerve.[56] Transverse sectional anatomy reveals that the ICA rests at or anterior to the atlantodental space when viewed laterally.[3,46] No angiographic reference exist that reviews the anterior-posterior relation of the ICA to the C1–C2 interval in normal or anomalous situations. To evaluate this relationship, the authors reviewed 50 lateral ICA angiograms performed for evaluation of atherosclerotic disease at a regional medical facility. A substantial degree of variation existed in the anteroposterior position of the ICA. In most instances, the artery was visualized at or anterior to the atlantodental interval, but on occasion arterial loops or curves in the ICA brought it to rest at the anterior portion of the AA joint, thus posterior to the atlantodental interval. In no instance was the ICA at the mid or posterior portion of the AA joint. The occipital artery was seen on multiple occasions to cross the anterior to mid-lateral silhouette of the AA joint after it branched posteriorly from the ECA. Rarely, loops in the ECA were seen to cross the anterior aspect of the AA just posterior to the atlantodental interval.

Neuroanatomy

On the posterior aspect of the AA and AO joints the dura extends laterally to the joint's mid-portion, and the spinal cord extends to the joint's most medial aspect.[3,46] Both the C1 ventral rami and posterior rami are situated between the posterior arch of C1 and the vertebral artery. The ventral rami curves anteriorly, around the lateral aspect of the atlas to innervate the AO joint.[4] Directly inferior to the mid-portion of the posterior aspect of the AO joint are the C1 ventral and dorsal rami and the vertebral artery. The C1 rami and vertebral artery lie closer to the posterior aspect of the AO joint at its medial aspect relative to their location at the joint's lateral aspect. Posteriorly, the vertebral artery is farthest from the AO joint at the most superior and lateral margin of the joint.[56]

The C2 nerve roots are intimately related to the posterior aspect of the AA joint. They leave the dural sac medial to the AA joint and travel inferiorly and obliquely across the posterior aspect of the joint. The C2 spinal nerve is short and quickly divides into its ventral and dorsal rami. The ventral ramus passes laterally across both the joint and vertebral artery to merge with the cervical plexus. The AA joint's sensory innervation comes from the ventral rami of C2.[6] The dorsal rami passes inferiorly and posteriorly. The C2 spinal nerve and rami are bound to the AA joint capsule by investing fascia and are surrounded by a venous plexus and a variable amount of fat.[5,38] Anatomically the C2 ganglion lies opposite the medial half of the AA joint, but from a posteroanterior (PA) radiographic view the ganglion lies opposite the midpoint of the joint's silhouette.[5] Also, from a PA radiographic view the dural sac covers the medial half of the AA joint.[5]

PATHOPHYSIOLOGY

As previously mentioned, earlier studies describe symptom referral patterns of the AO[25,26,33,35] and AA joints[25,33] into other regions of the head and neck. This referral mechanism has been demonstrated in many clinical experiments. In one study, pain was produced in the orbit, frontal region, and vertex with electrical stimulation of the C1 dorsal root.[42] In another study, injecting 4% saline into posterior cervical muscles close to their insertions near the occiput produced pain in the forehead. Stimulating the same muscles 1–2 inches caudally produced pain in the vertex. Stimulation of the sternocleidomastoid referred pain to the temporal region.[20]

Insight to these referral patterns may be gained by understanding the innervation of the structures within this region. Referred pain transmission is characterized by the synapse of afferents from one region of the body onto neurons in the central nervous system that also receive afferents from another region of the body. As previously mentioned, the ventral rami of C1 innervates the AO joint[4] and the ventral rami of C2[6] innervates the AA joint. Recognizing the interrelationship of these sensory fibers with other regionally innervated structures helps to explain symptom referral patterns. More specifically, terminals of the upper three cervical nerves and the trigeminal nerve ramify in a continuous column of gray matter formed by the pars caudalis of the spinal nucleus of the trigeminal nerve and the dorsal horns of the upper three cervical segments. Within this column, the pars caudalis of the trigeminal nucleus cannot be differentiated from the gray matter on the basis of intrinsic cytoarchitecture or on the basis of the afferents received. Therefore this region of gray matter should be considered as a single or combined nucleus and appropriately can be labeled the trigeminocervical nucleus.[6] The

trigeminal nucleus consistently extends caudally to the C2 level, but portions may extend as far as the C4 level.[40,43,61,62] The trigeminocervical nucleus functions as the nociceptive nucleus for the entire upper cervical spine and head because it possesses the essential central nervous structures responsible for the transmission of pain and receives afferents from the upper cervical and trigeminal nerves.[10]

CLINICAL PRESENTATION

Cervical stiffness, "tired neck," restricted movement, and a constant or intermittent headache are common complaints of patients with AO or AA joint dysfunction. Episodic pain may occur and is greatly influenced by external mechanical factors. Unusual complaints, such as visual disturbances, dizziness, nausea, tongue numbness, ear pain, and a variety of autonomic complaints, also have been attributed to AO and AA joint dysfunction.[6,9,47,48]

Atlanto-occipital Pain

Patients with AO pain complain primarily of unilateral suboccipital pain. Pain may spread toward the frontal area slightly anterior to the vertex. Laterally, pain approaches, but does not reach, the ear. Rarely, the whole hemicranium or supraorbital regions are involved.[35] Recently, a referral map was produced for the AO joint (Fig. 28-1).[25] This study involved pressurization of the AO joint with iothalamate meglumine (Conray) under fluoroscopy in 5 asymptomatic subjects. With capsular distention, the predominant referral pattern was suboccipital pain and occasionally occipital and temporal pain that approached, but did not include,

OA LEFT

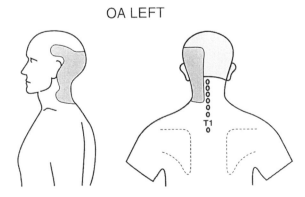

FIGURE 28-1. Composite referred pain map for the atlanto-occipital joint. (From Dreyfuss P, Michaelsen M, Fletcher D: Atlanto-occipital and lateral atlanto-axial joint pain patterns. Spine 19:1125-1131, 1994, with permission.)

the vertex. In 1 subject, pain extended caudal to the C5 segmental level, and in another subject isolated temporal pain occurred. All AO joint referral patterns were ipsilateral.[25] The referral map of 10 AO joint injections was obtained in a study of symptomatic patients undergoing cervical joint of dorsal rami injections. Pain was seen in the upper posterolateral cervical spine with all injections, and in 30% pain extended into the posterior occipital region.[33] These referral maps correlate with clinical observations.[15,26]

Atlantoaxial Pain

Patients with symptomatic AA joints complain primarily of pain localized to the retromastoid, suboccipital, postauricular or the C1–C2 segmental level.[32,33,59] A referral map generated for this joint (Fig. 28-2) corresponds well with these observations and primarily demonstrates pain localized to the C1–C2 segmental level laterally and posterolaterally. All AA joint referral patterns were ipsilateral.[25,33] These referral maps also correlate with clinical observations.[32,36,37,51,59]

TREATMENT

No universally accepted treatment algorithm exists for suspected AO or AA joint pain, although an algorithm for the treatment of cervical zygapophyseal joint pain exists.[24] This algorithm for treating the cervical zygapophyseal joint parallels the AO and AA joint pain treatment plan.

A comprehensive approach addressing both mechanical and inflammatory abnormalities within the articulations and adjacent soft tissues should be used. Most clinicians attempt at least 3–6 weeks of

C1-2 RIGHT

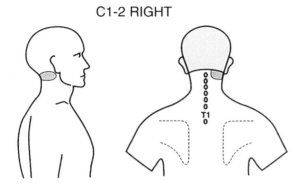

FIGURE 28-2. Composite referred pain map for the lateral atlanto-axial joint. (From Dreyfuss P, Michaelsen M, Fletcher D: Atlanto-occipital and lateral atlanto-axial joint pain patterns. Spine 19:1125-1131, 1994, with permission.)

conservative care before performing diagnostic and therapeutic AO or AA joint intra-articular injections. Less invasive treatment options include physical, manual, or occupational therapy. Pharmacologic, psychological, or ergonomic intervention also should be considered. Deviation from the algorithm may be necessary when severe pain precludes normal function or the ability of the patient to participate in a conservative program. This may indicate that the procedure should be performed earlier than normal.

If conservative care fails, the clinical history and physical examination may dictate which joints to treat. The aforementioned pain referral patterns[13] may assist with this determination as may a segmental examination of the upper cervical spine.[57] After intra-articular injection with local anesthetic, pain relief concordant to or longer than the expected duration of the anesthetic used confirms the joint's role as a pain generator. Therapeutic injection of these joints uses both local anesthetic and corticosteroid. After injection, a period of significant pain relief may facilitate other treatment options, such as manual or physical therapy. There is no role for a series of AA joint injections given without regard to corticosteroid response of the initial injection, and an AA joint injection should never be repeated in a patient who experienced no significant relief during the anesthetic phase of a prior AA joint injection.

AO AND AA JOINT INJECTION TECHNIQUE

AO and AA joint injections possess significant potential risks and require both excellent hand–eye coordination and substantial experience with fluoroscopically guided spinal injections. A thorough understanding of the regional anatomy and ability to diagnose and treat potential injection complications is imperative.

Preparation

Absolute contraindications to the procedure include bacterial infection (systemic or localized) and bleeding diathesis due to anticoagulants or hematologic disease. Relative contraindications include allergy to injectants, steroid psychosis, pregnancy, nonsteroidal anti-inflammatory drugs (NSAIDs), aspirin and other antiplatelet agents (e.g., Ticlid, Plavix), hyperglycemia, adrenal suppression, immune compromise, and congestive heart failure.

The person performing the injection must obtain written informed consent before administering sedation or performing the procedure. Intravenous access should be established, and if sedation is used, it should be short acting to prevent an analgesic effect while still minimizing inadvertent patient movement. The patient should remain responsive. Blood pressure, pulse, and O_2 saturation should be continuously monitored; full resuscitation equipment and appropriate pharmacologic agents should be available. The skin overlying the target joint should be prepared sterilely and draped. Occasionally, it may be necessary to shave the inferior aspect of the occiput. See Table 28-1 for materials.

Atlanto-occipital Joint Injection Technique

This modified approach replaces previously described injection techniques[23,26,55] because of its relative technical ease, patient comfort, and safety issues. This approach differs from others[15,55] because it involves a more lateral starting position in line with the long axis of the target joint. Cross-sectional and cadaveric dissections studies of the greater occipital nerve[13,46] demonstrate that the more lateral starting position of this modified approach substantially decreases the chance of greater occipital nerve injury.

The patient is placed prone on the procedure table with the head slightly flexed and supported in an adjustable head-holder. A head-holder stabilizes the patient while providing him or her with comfort and unobstructed breathing and communication. The C-arm is rotated approximately 25–30° ipsilateral oblique. This angle of rotation minimizes the likelihood of needle penetration of vital neural or vascular structures, as determined by anatomic cross-sectional analysis.[46] Additionally, this places the needle trajectory in line with the long axis of the joint (28° oblique). This minimizes the risk encountered with inadvertent advancement of the needle past the posterior margin of the joint because the needle will remain contained within the joint. It may be necessary to rotate the C-arm in a rostral to caudal direction until the AO joint is unobscured by the occipital brim. The joint will appear medial to the mastoid process and immediately beneath the occipital brim (Fig. 28-3).

The tip of a metal marker is placed gently on the skin (without traction) 1–2 mm superior to the most superior of the AO joint line just inside its most lateral margin in what is known as the target location. The target is slightly above the visualized joint line

TABLE 28-1. Materials for AO and AA Joint Injection

Equipment and Supplies
1. Fluoroscopy (mandatory)
2. 24–26-gauge spinal needle (recommended). Avoid using curved tip.
3. Medication and contrast syringes
4. Connection tubing so that contrast can be injected during fluoroscopic visualization to confirm proper anatomic and extravascular needle placement.
5. Physiologic monitor
6. Skin marker (optional)

Medications
1. Sedation and antibiotics (optional)

Agents (total volume up to 1.0 ml/joint)
1. **Contrast medium:** Radiographic contrast medium is essential to confirm extravascular and intra-articular needle placement and is used to obtain an arthrogram prior to any subsequent injection. A nominal amount (0.1–0.3 ml) is sufficient. Examples include Omnipaque 240 and Isovue 300/370.
2. **Local anesthetics** (combined with the corticosteroid in a 2:1 or 1:1 ratio): Agents commonly used include lidocaine 1–2% and bupivacaine 0.25–0.50%.
3. **Corticosteroids:** Employed to decrease intra-articular inflammation and may facilitate more active conservative care.

because the visualized joint line actually represents the anterior aspect of the AO joint, which is more inferior than the posterior aspect of the joint, which is the target. The posterior aspect of the joint is the target because the joint is approached posteriorly. Because the anterior aspect of the AO joint is broader with a greater PA-AP dimension, it will be more easily apparent on a PA-AP radiograph than the posterior aspect of the joint space.

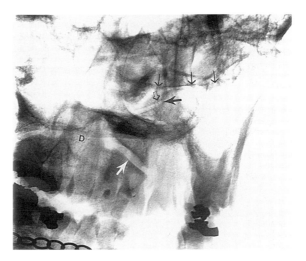

FIGURE 28-3. A 25-30° ipsilateral oblique with the appropriate amount of tilt such that the AO joint is seen under the occipital brim. The target for needle entry is at the tip of the small, open black arrow. The most lateral edge of the AO joint is at the tip of the solid, thick black arrow. The white arrow denotes the AA joint, the letter *D* denotes the dens, and the occipital brim is identified by the three small, thin black arrows.

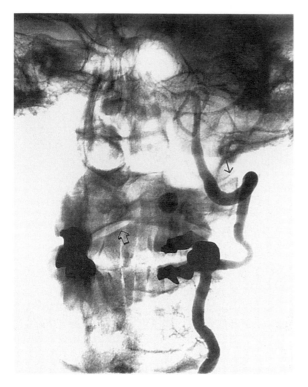

FIGURE 28-4. A 20° ipsilateral oblique radiograph of a vertebral arteriogram. The vertebral artery is well visualized in relation to the AO joint. The target for needle entry into the AO joint is denoted by the thin black arrow. The open black arrow denotes the AA joint on the contralateral side.

The skin entry point is directly over the target using the ipsilateral oblique imaging with the necessary degree of C-arm tilt, as described above. Occasionally, it may be necessary for the skin entry sight to be slightly inferior to the target point to avoid contact with the occipital brim. A lidocaine skin wheal is raised, and a 3.5-inch, 25- or 26-gauge

spinal needle punctures the skin directly over the target. The shaft of the needle is directed along the axis of the x-ray beam under intermittent fluoroscopy toward and into the target location in the AO joint. The needle must not deviate medially or inferiorly. The only relatively safe direction of deviation is toward the occiput superiorly. An ascending loop of the vertebral artery may course laterally to the AO joint, and the space medial to the juncture of the medial two-thirds and lateral one-third of the joint contains the spinal canal and vertebral artery again as it crosses over the AO joint toward the foramen magnum (Fig. 28-4). As the needle approaches the target, osseous contact is perceived. If the radiograph reveals that the needle should have made osseous contact but did not, the needle may have strayed too far laterally. When osseous contact is perceived (Fig. 28-5), the C-arm is rotated to an approximately 25° contralateral oblique view. This view is approximately perpendicular to the posterior joint plane and will best reveal the superior and inferior orientation of the needle tip with respect to the most posterior (target) aspect of the joint space (Figs. 28-6 and 28-7). Alternating between this contralateral and ipsilateral oblique views allows needle placement into the joint without complication.

Usually the oblique and contralateral oblique views are the only views necessary to obtain safe joint entry and subsequent injection of contrast (Figs. 28-8, 28-9, 28-10, and 28-11). However, lateral and AP views can provide additional information if

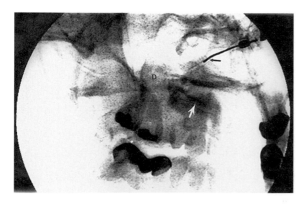

FIGURE 28-5. A 25° ipsilateral oblique showing a needle appropriately placed into the AO joint approximately 3 mm inside its most lateral edge (tip of the black arrow). The white arrow denotes the AA joint, and the letter *D* denotes the dens.

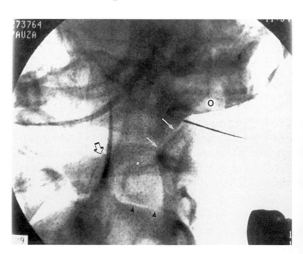

FIGURE 28-6. A 25° contralateral oblique depicting a needle placed into the AO joint at its most posterior, superior, and lateral aspect. The white arrows denote the target AO joint, the open black arrow shows the dens, the small triangular black arrows point to the AA joint, and the letter *O* identifies the occiput.

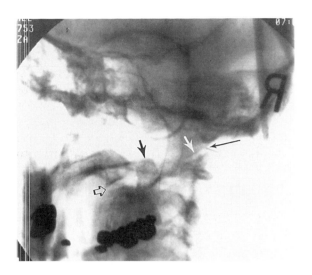

FIGURE 28-7. A 25° contralateral oblique radiograph of needle placement into the AO joint prior to contrast injection. The tip of the needle is shown as the long, thin black arrow; the AO joint is denoted by the white arrow; the top of the dens is denoted by the thicker, short black arrow; and the contralateral AA joint is marked by the open black arrow.

joint entry was not easily obtained with oblique imaging. A lateral radiograph serves to demonstrate that the needle has not deviated too far anteriorly but provides little value in the actual directing of the needle (Figs. 28-12 and 28-13). One reason for a more anterior location than desired is that the needle strayed laterally past the target posterior aspect of the joint space. On a lateral view the

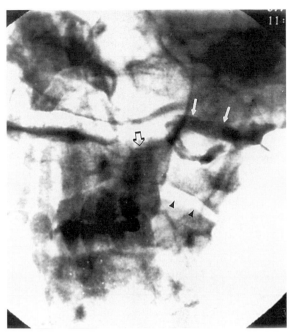

FIGURE 28-9. A 25° contralateral oblique radiograph of an AO joint arthrogram. The top of the dens is noted by the open black arrow, the AA joint by the small triangular black arrows, and the superior aspect of the AO joint arthrogram by the white arrows.

needle tip is located at the posterior juncture of the occiput and atlas (see Figure 28-12). AP imaging can

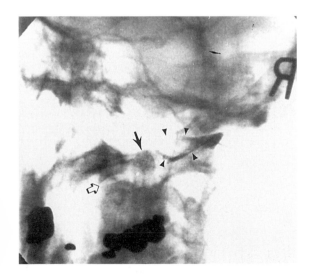

FIGURE 28-8. A 25° contralateral oblique radiograph of needle placement into the AO joint after contrast injection. This is the same patient as in Figure 28-7. The margins of the arthrogram are noted by four small triangular black arrows, the top of the dens is identified by the thicker solid black arrow, and the lateral margin of the contralateral AA joint is identified by the open black arrow.

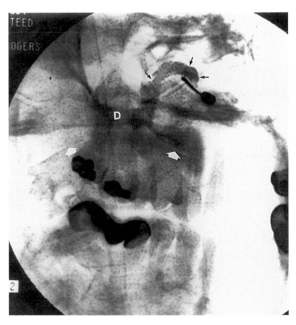

FIGURE 28-10. A 25° ipsilateral oblique of an AO joint arthrogram. The needle is appropriately placed approximately 3 mm inside the lateral margin of the joint. The lateral margins of the arthrogram are noted by three black arrows. The white arrows denote the AA joints, and the letter *D* denotes the dens.

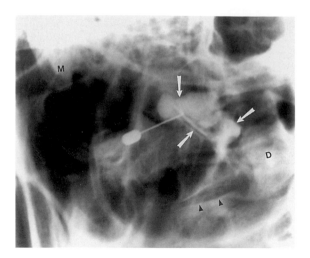

FIGURE 28-11. A 25° ipsilateral oblique demonstrating appropriate needle placement for obtaining an AO joint arthrogram. The arthrogram is outlined by three white arrows. The letter *M* denotes the mastoid process, *D* the dens, and the small, triangular black arrows the AA joint.

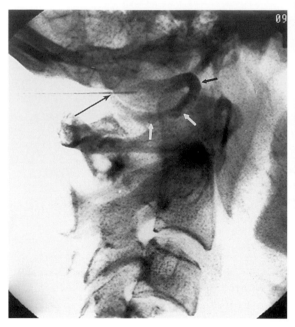

FIGURE 28-13. Lateral radiograph of an AO joint arthrogram. The needle has been advanced farther into the joint than is typically necessary to obtain an arthrogram. A needle should not be advanced more anterior than where this needle rests. The lateral margin of the arthrogram is denoted by the three short arrows. The most posterior aspect of the joint is marked by a long, thin black arrow.

help to image the lateral and superior aspect of the joint and the proximity of the needle tip to those osseous margins (Figs. 28-14 and 28-15).

After capsular penetration is perceived by a subtle loss of resistance, a trace amount of nonionic, water-soluble contrast media is injected through a small connection tubing during fluoroscopic visualization to confirm intra-articular placement. If vascular or soft tissue contrast flow occurs, the needle is rotated or redirected. Occasionally, minimal contrast in-

jection elicits pain; however this pain provocation possesses no known diagnostic value. Next, medication is introduced until resistance is met or 1.0 ml is injected, whichever occurs first. Anesthetic and corticosteroid in a 2:1 or 1:1 volume is recommended. Possible injectants include 0.5% bupivacaine, 1.5% lidocaine, betamethasone (40 mg/ml), and triamcinolone (6 mg/ml). Connection tubing

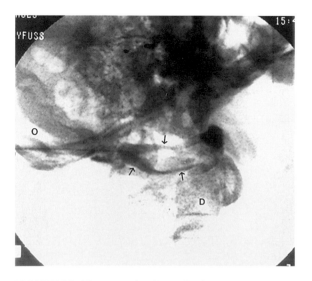

FIGURE 28-12. Lateral radiograph of an AO joint arthrogram. The needle is placed just inside the most posterior aspect of the joint. The letter *D* indicates the dens, the black arrows show the margins of the AO joint arthrogram, and *O* marks the occiput.

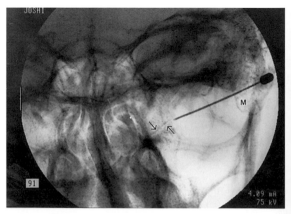

FIGURE 28-14. AP radiograph of a needle placed into the superior, lateral, and posterior aspect of the AO joint. The AO joint is noted by the small black arrows, and the mastoid process is identified by the letter *M*.

between the syringe and needle hub facilitates injection without needle movement. The needle is removed and the patient's pain relief is assessed in the recovery room during the next 30 minutes. Blood pressure, pulse, and O_2 saturation should be intermittently monitored during the recovery phase. In addition, the patient should rate his or her pain while his or her usual symptoms are provoked. The patient should be instructed to record pain relief hourly for the remainder of that day and daily during the next week.

Atlantoaxial Joint Injection Technique

The AA joint may be injected by either a posterior[23,51] or lateral[18] approach. The posterior approach is preferable because fewer vital vascular and neural structures reside between the skin and joint capsule with this trajectory. Sectional anatomy reveals the vertebral artery and other structures located directly lateral to the AA joint, including the external and internal carotid veins, parotid gland, superior cervical ganglion, hypoglossal nerve, and cranial nerves IX–XI.[3,46] Sectional anatomy reveals that from a posterior approach the only structures encountered upon anterior advancement toward the AA joint are regional muscles and the C2 ganglia and nerves. Therefore, discussion will be limited to this safer posterior approach.

The patient is positioned prone on the procedure table with his or her head in an adjustable head-holder in a neutral or slightly flexed posture. Image absolute AP and maximally visualize the AA joint silhouette. This may require slight tilt of the image intensifier in either a caudad or cephalad direction. Slight repositioning of the head or the C-arm in various degrees of flexion may be necessary to prevent the occiput, sinuses, mandible, teeth, or metallic dental work from obscuring the joint. Occasionally, opening the patient's mouth will remove the obscuring dental artifact. The target is the juncture of the medial two-thirds and the lateral one-third of the joint silhouette on the symptomatic side (Fig. 28-16). This target site is lateral to the spinal cord, thecal space, and C2 ganglion, and medial to the ascending vertebral artery. Others have recommended targeting the mid-aspect of the joint,[51] but this is not advisable because the C2 ganglion on the inferior aspect of the AA joint is located here.[5,38,50]

The tip of a metal marker is placed gently, without traction, on the skin over this target and a skin wheal is raised with lidocaine. The needle punctures

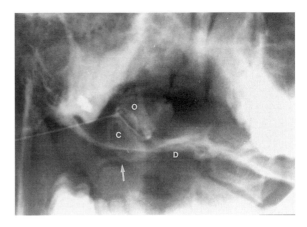

FIGURE 28-15. AP radiograph of an AO joint arthrogram. The letter *O* denotes the occiput, *C* the C1 segment, and *D* the dens. (From Dreyfuss P, Michaelsen M, Fletcher D: Atlanto-occipital and lateral atlanto-axial joint pain patterns. Spine 19:1125-1131, 1994, with permission.)

the skin directly over the target and the shaft of the needle is directed along the axis of the x-ray beam. The image intensifier may be rotated to lateral projection to determine needle depth. The needle should not stray toward the mid-portion of the joint or the C2 ganglion may be irritated. Additionally, the needle should not stray toward the medial aspect of the joint or risk entering the spinal canal. If the needle strays lateral to the joint margin, the vertebral artery may be injured. Initially penetrating the skin slightly superior to the joint line may help avoid irritating the C2 ganglion in case the needle inadvertently strays toward the middle of the

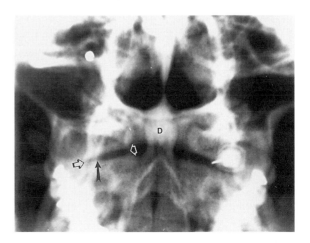

FIGURE 28-16. PA radiograph of a needle placed into the AA joint just lateral to the location of the C2 ganglia. It would be more appropriate to place the needle as depicted on the contralateral side at the tip of the solid black arrow. The open black arrow denotes the lateral margin of the AA joint, and the open white arrow denotes the medial edge of the joint. The letter *D* denotes the dens.

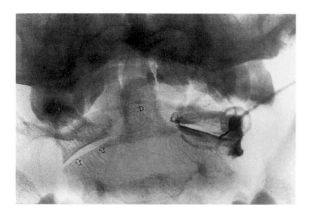

FIGURE 28-17. AP radiograph of an AA joint arthrogram. The needle is appropriately placed at the junction of the lateral one-third and medial two-thirds of the joint's osseous margin. *D* represents the dens, and the open black arrows denote the contralateral AA joint.

joint, because this ganglion often lies on the inferior aspect of this joint's midpoint.

After the osseous borders of the joint are contacted or adequate depth is perceived, a lateral view should be obtained to confirm needle depth. This prevents anterior placement because one can inappropriately advance the needle entirely through the AA joint capsule. Once the clinician believes that the needle should be or is at the joint capsule a lateral image should be obtained. If the needle is greater than approximately 1.0 cm posterior from the target point, AP imaging should be re-obtained and the needle advanced further toward the target. Capsule penetration is perceived with a subtle change of resistance. Injecting a trace amount of contrast during fluoroscopic visualization confirms intra-articular needle placement (Figs. 28-17, 28-18, and 28-19). It is not necessary to obtain a complete arthrogram. After confirmation, injectant is introduced until

resistance is perceived or up to 1.0 ml of injectant is introduced, whichever comes first. The needle is removed and the patient's pain relief is assessed in the recovery room during the next 30 minutes. Blood pressure, pulse, and oxygen saturation should be intermittently monitored during the recovery phase. The patient should rate his or her pain and should record pain relief hourly for the remainder of the day and daily over the next week.

Potential Risks

Risks associated with (but not limited to) these injections include exacerbation of usual pain, bleeding, allergic reaction, infection, venous or arterial penetration with hemorrhage, and C1 or C2 nerve root irritation. If the vascular system is erroneously injected, seizures or other central neurologic events could occur. Epidural or intrathecal spread may result in partial blockade of the upper cervical cord function with respiratory compromise. Spinal cord penetration could cause paralysis or death. At the time of this writing, no serious complication caused by AO or AA joint injections has been reported.

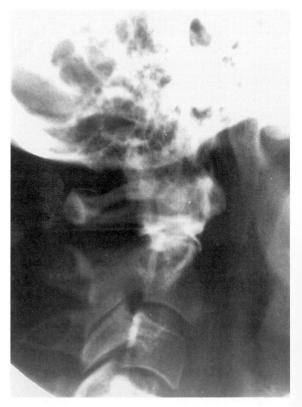

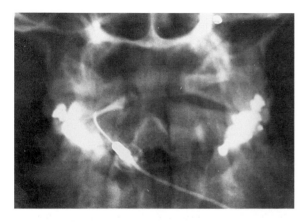

FIGURE 28-18. PA radiograph of an AA arthrogram using a posterior approach with the needle at the target location.

FIGURE 28-19. Lateral radiograph of a posterior approach to the AA joint with an arthrogram.

Postinjection Recovery

On the day of the injection the patient should be excused from work and not allowed to drive or operate machinery. Occasionally, a temporary increase of pain may occur during the first few days following the injection. If this occurs, ice (not heat) should be placed over the injection site. Pain should abate. The corticosteroids typically exert their effect within approximately 3 days. The patient should avoid any increase in his or her usual activities during the first week. Thereafter, activity may be increased slowly. Currently, no literature exists regarding the long-term clinical response to injection of these joints. Anecdotally, the authors have observed relief ranging from brief pain relief lasting for the duration of the anesthetic to 100% relief remaining at 4-year follow-up.

OTHER THERAPEUTIC OPTIONS

Other options for recalcitrant AA pain include partial radiofrequency denervation of the C2 ganglia,[44] C2 ganglionotomy,[60] partial posterior rootlet rhizotomy,[27,39] greater occipital nerve stimulation,[64] regional prolotherapy, or surgical fusion. Options for recalcitrant AO joint pain are posterior surgical fusion, greater occipital nerve stimulation,[64] upper cervical partial rootlet rhizotomy,[27,39] chemical or radiofrequency C1 root neurotomy,[45] and regional prolotherapy, which pose a greater risk to the patient compared to intra-articular injections. The success of these interventions is poorly studied.

CONCLUSION

The atlanto-occipital and atlantoaxial joints can cause pain and other symptoms. The physician's ability to identify these structures as pain generators is a valuable part of the patient's diagnostic algorithm. Because of their proximity to vital structures, the risk-to-benefit ratio must be considered closely. It is of utmost importance that these procedures are performed only by clinicians who possess significant experience, skill, and understanding of the relevant anatomy.

REFERENCES

1. Aprill C, Bogduk N: The prevalence of cervical zygapophyseal joint pain: A first approximation. Spine 17:744–747, 1992.
2. Aprill C, Dwyer A, Bogduk N: Cervical zygapophyseal joint patterns: A clinical evaluation. Spine 15:458–461, 1990.
3. Bergman RA, Afifi AK, Jew JY, Reimann PC: Atlas of Human Anatomy in Cross Section. Munich, Urban & Schwarzenberg, 1991.
4. Bogduk N: The clinical anatomy of the cervical dorsal rami. Spine 7:319–330, 1982.
5. Bogduk N: Local anesthetic blocks of the second cervical ganglia: A technique with application in occipital headache. Cephalalgia 1:41-50, 1981.
6. Bogduk N: Cervical causes of headache and dizziness. In Grieve GP (ed): Modern Manual Therapy of the Vertebral Column. London, Churchill Livingstone, 1987, pp 289–302.
7. Bogduk N: Back pain: Zygapophyseal blocks and epidural steroids. In Cousins MJ, Bridenbaugh PO (eds): Neural Blockade in Clinical Anesthesia and Management of Pain. Philadelphia, J.B. Lippincott, 1988, pp 935–954.
8. Bogduk N: Neck pain: An update. Aust Fam Physician 17:75–80, 1988.
9. Bogduk N, Corrigan B, Kelly P, et al: Cervical headache. Med J Aust 143:202–207, 1985.
10. Bogduk N, Marsland A: On the concept of the third occipital headache. J Neurol Neurosurg Psychiatry 49:775–780, 1986.
11. Bogduk N, Marsland A: The cervical zygapophyseal joints as a source of neck pain. Spine 13:610–617, 1988.
12. Bogduk N, Windsor M, Inglis A: The innervation of the cervical intervertebral discs. Spine 13:1–8, 1988.
13. Bovim G, Bonamico L, Fredriksen TA, et al: Topographic variations in the peripheral course of the greater occipital nerve: Autopsy study with clinical correlations. Spine 16:475–478, 1991.
14. Breathnach AS (ed): Frazer's Anatomy of the Human Skeleton, 5th ed. London, J&A Churchill, 1958, pp 19–20.
15. Busch E, Wilson PR: Atlanto-occipital and atlanto-axial injections in the treatment of headache and neck pain. Reg Anesth Pain Med 14(S2):45, 1989.
16. Cave AJ: Anatomical notes on the occipito-atlanto-axial articulations. J Anat 68:416–423, 1934.
17. Chang H, Found EM, Clark CR, et al: Meniscus-like synovial fold in the atlantoaxial (C1–C2) joint. J Spinal Disord 5:227–231, 1992.
18. Chevrot A, Cermakova E, Vallee C, et al: C1–2 arthrography. Skeletal Radiol 24:425–429, 1995.
19. Cox TCS, Stevens JM, Kendall BE: Vascular anatomy in the suboccipital region and lateral cervical puncture. Br J Radiol 54:572–575, 1981.
20. Cyriax J: Rheumatic headache. Br Med J 2:1367–1368, 1938.
21. Daniels DL, Williams AL, Haughton VM: Computed tomography of the articulation and ligaments at the occipito-atlantoaxial region. Radiology 146:709–716, 1983.
22. Dirheimer Y, Ramsheyi A, Reolon M: Positive arthrography of the craniocervical joints. Neuroradiology 12:257–260, 1977.
23. Dreyfuss P: Atlanto-occipital and lateral atlanto-axial joint injections. In Lennard T (ed): Physiatric Procedures in Clinical Practice. Philadelphia, Hanley & Belfus, 1995, pp 227–237.
24. Dreyfuss P: Cervical facet pain. In Ramamurthy S, Rogers JN (eds): Decision Making in Pain Management. St. Louis, Mosby, 1993, pp 96–99.
25. Dreyfuss P, Michaelsen M, Fletcher D: Atlanto-occipital and lateral atlanto-axial joint pain patterns: A study of five normal subjects. Spine 19:1125–1131, 1994.
26. Dreyfuss P, Rogers J, Dreyer S, Fletcher D: Atlanto-occipital joint pain: A report of three cases and description of intraarticular block technique. Reg Anesth Pain Med 19:344–351, 1994.
27. Dubuisson D: Treatment of occipital neuralgia by partial posterior rhizotomy at C1–3. J Neurosurg 82:581–586, 1995.
28. Duckworth J: Anatomy of the suboccipital region. In Vernon H (ed): Upper Cervical Syndrome: Chiropractic Diagnosis and Treatment. Baltimore, Williams & Wilkins, 1988, p 7.

29. Dvorak J, Dvorak V: Biomechanics and functional examination of the spine. In Dvorak J, Dvorak V: Manual Medicine-Diagnostics, 2nd ed. New York, Thieme, 1990, pp 8–19.

30. Dwyer A, Aprill C, Bogduk N: Cervical zygapophyseal joint pain patterns I: A study of normal volunteers. Spine 15:453–457, 1990.

31. Edmeads J: The cervical spine and headache. Neurology 38:1874–1878, 1988.

32. Ehni G, Benner B: Occipital neuralgia and the C1-2 arthrosis syndrome. J Neurosurg 61:961–965, 1984.

33. Fukui S, Ohseto K, Shiotani M, et al: Referred pain distribution of the cervical zygapophyseal joints and cervical dorsal rami. Pain 68:79–83, 1996.

34. Fielding JW: Cineroentgenography of the normal cervical spine. J Bone Joint Surg 39A:1280–1288, 1957.

35. Grieve GP: Common patterns of clinical presentation. In Grieve GP: Common Vertebral Joint Problems. London, Churchill Livingstone, 1981, pp 206–208.

36. Halla JT, Hardin JG: Atlantoaxial (C1–2) facet joint osteoarthritis: A distinctive clinical syndrome. Arthritis Rheum 30:577–582, 1987.

37. Harata S, Kawagishi T: Osteoarthritis of the atlanto-axial joint. Int Orthop 5:277–282, 1981.

38. Ho PS, Yu S, Sether L, et al: MR and cryomicrotomy of C1 and C2 roots. AJNR Am J Neuroradiol 9:829–831, 1988.

39. Horowitz MB, Yonas H: Occipital neuralgia treated by intradural dorsal nerve root sectioning. Cephalalgia 13:354–360, 1993.

40. Humphrey T: The spinal tract of the trigeminal nerve in human embryos between 7 and 8 weeks of menstrual age and its relation to early fetal behavior. J Comp Neurol 97:143–209, 1952.

41. Johnston TB, Whillis J (eds): Gray's Anatomy Descriptive and Applied, 30th ed. Philadelphia, Longmans, Green, 1949.

42. Kerr FW: A mechanism to account for frontal headache in cases of posterior fossa tumors. J Neurosurg 18:605–609, 1961.

43. Kerr FW: Structural relation of the trigeminal spinal tract to upper cervical roots and the solitary nucleus in the cat. Exp Neurol 4:134–148, 1961.

44. Kline MT: Radiofrequency techniques in clinical practice. In Waldman SD, Winnie AP (eds): Interventional Pain Management. Philadelphia, W.B. Saunders, 1996, pp 185–217.

45. Koch D, Wakhloo AK: CT-guided chemical rhizotomy of the C1 root for occipital neuralgia. Neuroradiology 34:451–452, 1992.

46. Koritke JG, Sick H: Atlas of Sectional Human Anatomy, 2nd ed. Munich, Urban & Schwarzenberg, 1988.

47. Lance JW, Anthony MS: Neck-tongue syndrome on sudden turning of the head. J Neurol Neurosurg Psychiatry 43:97–101, 1980.

48. Lamer TJ: Ear pain due to cervical spine arthritis: Treatment with cervical facet injection. Headache 31:682–683, 1991.

49. Lord S, Barnsley L, Wallis B, et al: Third occipital nerve headache: A prevalence study. J Neurol Neurosurg Psychiatry 57:1187–1190, 1994.

50. Lu J, Ebraheim NA: Anatomic considerations of C2 nerve root ganglia. Spine 23:649–652, 1998.

51. McCormick CC: Arthrography of the atlanto-axial (C1-C2) joints: Techniques and results. J Interventional Radiol 2:9–13, 1987.

52. Mokri B, Houser OW, Sandok BK, Piepgras DG: Spontaneous dissections of the vertebral arteries. Neurology 38:880–885, 1988.

53. Mysorekar VR, Nandedkar AN: Surface area of the atlanto-occipital articulations. Acta Anat 126:223–225, 1986.

54. Poirier P, Charpy A, Nicolas A: Traite d'anatomie humanine. Tome 1: Arthrologie. Paris, Masson, 1926.

55. Racz GB, Sanel H, Diede JH: Atlanto-occipital and atlantoaxial injections in the treatment of headache and neck pain. In Waldman SD, Winnie AP (eds): Interventional Pain Management. Philadelphia, W.B. Saunders, 1996, pp 219–222.

56. Schaeffer JP (Ed.): Morris' Human Anatomy: A Complete Systematic Treatise. New York, Blankiston, 1953, pp 657, 664–665.

57. Schafer RC, Faye LJ: The cervical spine. In Schafer RC, Faye LJ: Motion Palpation and Chiropractic Technique: Principles of Dynamic Chiropractic. Huntington Beach, CA, Motion Palpation Institute, 1990, p 93.

58. Schellhas KP, Smith MD, Gundry CR, Pollei SR: Cervical discogenic pain: Prospective correlation of magnetic resonance imaging and discography in asymptomatic subjects and pain sufferers. Spine 21:300–312, 1996.

59. Star MJ, Curd JG, Thorne RP: Atlantoaxial lateral mass osteoarthritis: A frequently overlooked cause of severe occipitocervical pain. Spine 17S:S71–S76, 1992.

60. Stechison MT, Mullin BB: Surgical treatment of greater occipital neuralgia: An appraisal of strategies. Acta Neurochir (Wien) 131:236–240, 1994.

61. Taren JA, Kahn EA: Anatomic pathways related to pain in face and neck. J Neurosurg 19:116–121, 1962.

62. Torvik A: Afferent connections to the sensory trigeminal nuclei, the nucleus of the solitary tract and adjacent structures. J Comp Neurol 106:51–141, 1956.

63. Travell JG, Simons DG: Myofascial Pain and Dysfunction: The Trigger Point Manual, Vol. 2. Baltimore, Williams & Wilkins, 1992, pp 8–11.

64. Weiner RL, Reed KL: Peripheral neurostimulation for control of intractable occipital neuralgia. Int Neuromodulation [in press].

29

Interventional Sympathetic Blockade

Robert E. Windsor, M.D., Herman Gore, M.D., and
Marcie A. Merson, M.D.

The sympathetic nervous system is implicated in numerous pain syndromes. Interruption of sympathetic pathways has proven efficacy in relieving pain. An aggressive multimodal approach is essential for successful diagnosis and treatment. The pain physician is encouraged to become familiar with the indications, techniques, and potential complications of interventional sympathetic blockade procedures.

Pain associated with sympathetic dysfunction has been given various names, from causalgia to shoulder-hand syndrome. The nomenclature has alternated between clinical and pathophysiologic. In 1994, the International Association for the Study of Pain (IASP) reviewed the literature and agreed that a consensus of opinion as to the causality of the condition did not exist and that a pathophysiologic description was not warranted. It also agreed that a clinical entity does exist and that it may be characterized by several distinct clinical conditions. As a result, they recommended usage of the term *complex regional pain syndrome* (CRPS) type 1 and type 2 (Table 29-1).[38]

The sympathetic nervous system is thought to be involved in sympathetically maintained pain (SMP), despite the fact that not all of the criteria are present to label SMP a CRPS. Sympathetically independent pain (SIP) is a pain syndrome believed to exist in the absence of involvement by the sympathetic nervous system and is unaffected by sympathetic blockade. In this chapter, pain syndromes treatable by sympathetic blockade are referred to as sympathetically mediated pain (SMedP).

Sympathetically mediated pain may occur in response to or play a role in a wide spectrum of clinical disorders, including peripheral nerve injury, limb trauma or surgery, repetitive stress injury, central nervous system (CNS) insult (stroke or traumatic brain injury), myocardial infarction, phantom limb pain, herpes zoster, occlusive vascular disease, or Raynaud's syndrome.[11,12,26,29]

Although the pathophysiology of SMedP is not fully understood, several theories have been advanced to explain the mechanisms of SMP.[26,29,48] It is believed that either peripheral or central factors cause distorted information processing in the sympathetic neuronal pools of the dorsolateral spinal cord, which leads to inappropriate response to afferent sensory input and overexcitation of efferent sympathetic outflow.[48] Classically it is described as a severe burning discomfort that may occur spontaneously or secondary to painful (hyperesthesia) or nonpainful (allodynia) stimuli. Often it is associated with other signs or altered sympathetic tone, including erythema, edema, altered skin temperature, discoloration, and dystrophic changes of the skin, nails, and underlying bone and joints.[12,26,29,48,49]

Recent investigations suggest that the current constructs used to describe the autonomic nervous system may be inaccurate. There also is evidence that patients with generalized autonomic dysfunction have an increased incidence of SMedP.

Sympathetically maintained pain may be difficult to treat and requires early intervention. The condition may be suspected when common limb disorders have been excluded and patients complain of pain in association with signs or symptoms suggestive of altered sympathetic tone. The condition may be present without signs of autonomic disturbance and also should be suspected in any patient who reports subjective pain out of proportion to objective pathology. SMP is a clinical diagnosis that may be supported by the presence of characteristic findings on physical examination, plain radiographs, triple-phase bone scan, thermogram, or significant pain relief with sympathetic blockade.[12,23,26,45,48,49,59] At the time of this writing (1999), no agreement on a

TABLE 29-1. Diagnostic Features of CRPS Type 1 and Type 2

Type 1	Type 2
1. An initiating noxious event 2. Continued pain, allodynia, or hyperalgesia* 3. Evidence of edema, vasomotor changes, or temperature changes* 4. Exclusion of other conditions that may explain symptoms*	1. The presence of continuing pain, allodynia, or hyperalgesia after a nerve injury that is not necessarily confined to the distribution of the injured nerve 2. Evidence of edema, vasomotor changes, or temperature changes

* Diagnosis of CRPS type 2 is excluded by the existence of conditions that otherwise account for the degree of pain and dysfunction.

From Racz GB, Heavener JE, Noe CE: Definitions, classifications and taxonomy: An overview. Phys Med Rehabil State Art Rev 10:195–206, 1996.

gold standard laboratory examination has yet been reached.

Aggressive treatment protocols are required to obtain successful lasting pain relief and prevent chronic dystrophic changes. Local or regional sympathetic blockade is the cornerstone of treatment for SMedP and is thought to help by interrupting and disorganizing the inappropriate sympathetic activity.[29,48] However, treatment protocols should be multidimensional.[41] Medications may decrease central and peripheral sympathetic tone. Physical therapy may be beneficial for analgesic modalities, for reduction of edema, and to promote active mobilization and reconditioning of involved extremities. Additionally, psychological support may help to assess and treat comorbid conditions such as anxiety, depression, and personality disorders. Recalcitrant cases unresponsive to traditional techniques may respond to stimulation of the dorsal column.[39] Surgical sympathectomy is reserved for confirmed SMedP that has failed all other forms of treatment.[31]

In spite of the controversy surrounding the concept of SMP, these blocks remain clinically useful. Neurolytic sympathetic block is often well tolerated, because numbness and motor weakness are uncommon and neuritis rarely develops. The classic targets for sympatholysis are the stellate or cervicothoracic ganglion for facial and upper extremity pain, celiac plexus for abdominal pain, the superior hypogastric plexus for pelvic pain, the lumbar sympathetic chain for lower extremity pain, and the ganglion of Impar for perineal pain. In addition, the thoracic ganglion occasionally is blocked for the treatment of hyperhidrosis and of pain emanating from the pleura or esophagus.

Patient preparation before the procedure includes appropriate laboratory studies and execution of an informed consent document. Intravenous access is recommended prior to the procedure to allow rapid management of potential complications and permit administration of preoperative intravenous sedation. Patients should be monitored for heart rate, blood pressure, and oxygen saturation. A full complement of resuscitative equipment and medications should be available, and the attending physician should be familiar with current advanced cardiac life support protocols.[3,19]

The patient is positioned on the procedure table and is then prepped and sterilely draped. Light sedation (1–4 mg intravenous midazolam) may be given to increase patient comfort and promote patient compliance. Patients are not allowed to drive themselves home after sedating procedures; following an uncomplicated postprocedure recovery, the patient is discharged to the care of a responsible friend or family member for transportation home.

SPHENOPALATINE GANGLION BLOCK

Current indications for blockade of the sphenopalatine ganglion include the management of acute migraine, acute and chronic cluster headache, and a variety of facial neuralgias. Permanent destruction of the sphenopalatine ganglion may be accomplished by creating a radiofrequency lesion in the ganglion.[22]

Anatomy

The sphenopalatine (pterygopalatine) ganglion is found in the pterygopalatine fossa, which is located posterior to the middle nasal concha and anterior to the pterygoid canal. It is adjacent to and inferior to the maxillary nerve, a branch of the trigeminal nerve, and connects with it via the pterygopalatine nerves. Only the parasympathetics are believed to synapse in the ganglion. Parasympathetic nerves arise from the facial nerve synapse in the ganglion via fibers of the nerve of the pterygoid canal and the greater petrosal nerve. Postganglionic fibers then continue to the lacrimal, palatine, and nasal gland via orbital branches of the maxillary, lacrimal, and zygomatic nerves. Postganglionic sympathetic fibers originating in the internal carotid plexus pass through the ganglion (without synapsing) via the nerve of the pterygoid canal and the deep petrosal nerve. Sensory fibers connect the maxillary nerve to the ganglion by way of branches of the ganglion (primarily maxillary nerve fibers) that extend from the nasopharynx, nasal cavity, palate, and orbit. There are five branches. The pharyngeal branch supplies the sphenoidal sinus and the mucosa of the roof of the pharynx; via the palatine canal, the greater palatine nerves extend posterior inferior nasal branches that supply the palate via the greater palatine foramen (with components of the maxillary and facial nerves). The tonsil and soft palate are supplied via the lesser palatine nerve as it arises from the lesser palatine foramen. The nasopalatine nerve emerges through the sphenopalatine foramen, passes along the nasal septum, and emerges through the median incisive foramen to reach the hard palate. The posterior ethmoidal and sphenoidal sinuses below the periosteum of the orbit are supplied via the orbital branches. The nasal cavity is supplied via the posterior superior nasal branches.

In addition to sensory fibers, the nasopalatine, palatine, and nasal nerves contain vasomotor fibers and secretory fibers to the palatine and nasal glands. Also, fibers related to taste can be found in the palatine nerves that pass via the greater petrosal nerve to reach the facial nerve.[16]

Technique

A cotton-tipped applicator soaked with cocaine or viscous lidocaine is advanced through the nares, along the middle turbinate posteriorly until it comes in contact with the posterior wall of the nasopharynx. The zygomatic arch may be used as a landmark because it corresponds to the level of the middle turbinate (Fig. 29-1A). A second applicator is then generally placed somewhat posterior and superior to the initial one. A response is seen in 5–10 minutes, although it may be left in position for 30–45 minutes for an adequate evaluation of the block's effectiveness. Common side effects are tearing or lacrimation, bleeding, light-headedness, generalized discomfort, and complaints of numbness of the posterior oropharynx.[13,42]

Pterygopalatine fossa anesthetic block typically is done under fluoroscopy with the patient in the supine position. Beginning with a lateral view, the head is rotated so that the right and left rami of the mandible zygoma and lateral pterygoid plates are superimposed, confirming a perfect lateral view.

The pterygopalatine fossa is most clearly visualized in this view. A 22-gauge B-bevel needle is inserted anterior to the mandible and under the zygoma and directed in a medial and slightly posterior direction with continuous visualization under fluoroscopy as it is advanced into the pterygopalatine fossa until it comes in contact with the pterygoid plate. Paresthesias may be elicited if the needle impinges on the nasopalatine, greater or lesser palatine, or maxillary nerves. The C-arm is rotated in the anteroposterior view so that the tip of the needle is seen just under the lateral nasal mucosa. Approximately 1 ml of contrast agent may then be injected to check for venous runoff, because this is a highly vascular area. Needle position may be additionally confirmed by passing a small amount of electrical current through the needle using a frequency of 50 Hz (sensory) and 2 Hz (motor) and low voltage (< 1 volt). Stimulation may provoke some palatal or facial paresthesia but should not cause muscular twitching or paresthesia in other areas. Following successful stimulation 1 ml of 1% or 2% lidocaine with epinephrine is injected. Elimination of pain confirms the diagnosis.

Radiofrequency Thermoregulation (RFTC) Lesioning

An 88-mm, 22-gauge SMK probe with a 2-mm active electrode tip is placed in the same way as described for pterygopalatine fossa anesthetic block (Figs. 29-1B and 29-1C). After needle contact with the pterygoid plate in the pterygopalatine fossa, electrical stimulation is conducted for sensory stimulation at 1 volt at 50 Hz. Correct stimulation is obtained when the patient reports the sensation to be within or just posterior to the nose. If stimulation is achieved in the soft palate, the needle should be advanced slightly medially. To confirm that the probe is placed in an extravascular position, a 1-ml volume of contrast is injected. After confirmation of the extravascular position a 1-ml volume of 1% lidocaine is injected. Following successful relief of symptoms, radiofrequency lesioning may be carried out for 60 seconds while maintaining the probe temperature above 65°C. The probe is then advanced 1 mm medially and the process is repeated.

Generally the patient should be kept for observation after the procedure for approximately 2 hours, because 10–20% of patients experience epistaxis. Discomfort for 10 days to 2 weeks is expected. Loss of sensation on the soft palate also may occur. Additional complications are rare.[22]

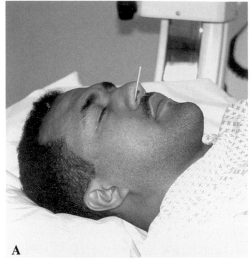

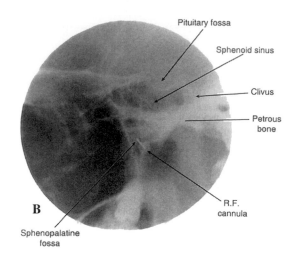

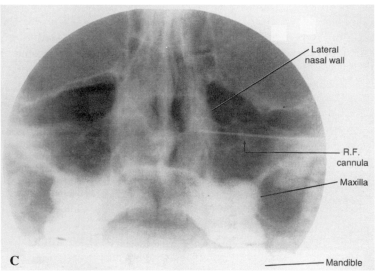

FIGURE 29-1. Sphenopalatine ganglion. *A,* Blockade of the sphenopalatine ganglion via the transnasal approach. *B* and *C,* Note the relative positions of the identified structures. The RF cannula is in the lateral wall of the nasal cavity (middle turbinate) where the sphenopalatine ganglion resides.

GASSERIAN GANGLION BLOCKADE

Indications for gasserian ganglion block using local anesthetic and/or radiofrequency nerve lesioning include management of trigeminal neuralgia, cluster headache, intractable ocular pain due to persistent glaucoma, and palliation of cancer pain.[6,24,54,56] Contraindications to the procedure include local infection, sepsis, coagulopathy, and significantly increased intracranial pressure.[15]

Anatomy

The trigeminal nerve is the largest of the cranial nerves and is a mixed somatic nerve with primarily sensory function.[9] It arises from the base of the pons and sends sensory fibers to the crescent-shaped gasserian ganglion. The gasserian ganglion is formed from two roots that exit the ventral surface of the brain stem at the midpontine level.[21] These roots pass in a forward and lateral direction in the posterior cranial fossa across the border of the petrous temporal bone. They then enter a recess called Meckel's cave, which is formed by an invagination of the surrounding dura mater into the middle cranial fossa. The dural pouch that lies just behind the ganglion is called the trigeminal cistern and contains cerebrospinal fluid. The gasserian ganglion's three sensory divisions, the ophthalmic (V1), maxillary (V2), and mandibular (V3) exit the anterior convex aspect of the ganglion. A smaller motor root joins the mandibular division as it exits the cranial cavity via the foramen ovale.

Ophthalmic Division

The ophthalmic branch is the smallest division of the trigeminal nerve and is purely sensory in function.[30] It enters the orbit via the superior orbital fissure. The branch is divided into the frontal, nasociliary, and lacrimal nerves.

Maxillary Division

The maxillary division is a pure sensory nerve. It exits the middle cranial fossa via the foramen rotundum and crosses the pterygopalatine fossa.[30] Passing through the inferior orbital fissure, it enters the orbit, emerging on the face via the infraorbital foramen. The nerve provides sensory innervation of the dura mater of the medial cranial fossa, temporal and lateral zygomatic region, much of the upper mouth, conjunctiva of the upper eyelid, and the skin inferior to the eye, lateral nose, and upper lip.

Mandibular Division

The large sensory root and smaller motor root of the mandibular division leave the middle cranial fossa together via the foramen ovale.[30] They then join to form the mandibular nerve. This combined trunk gives off two branches—the nervus spinosus, which runs superiorly with the middle meningeal artery through the foramen spinosum to supply the dura mater and the mucosal lining of the mastoid sinus, and the internal pterygoid, which supplies the internal pterygoid and gives off branches to the otic ganglion.

Technique of Neural Blockade

The patient is placed in the supine position with the cervical spine extended over a rolled towel. The skin and subcutaneous tissues are then anesthetized with 1% lidocaine with epinephrine approximately 3 cm lateral to the corner of the mouth.[9] A 3½-inch, 25-gauge spinal needle is advanced through the anesthetized area toward the auditory meatus in the plane that contains the ipsilateral pupil and the entrance site of the needle.[15] The needle is advanced until contact is made with the infratemporal surface of the wing of the sphenoid bone immediately anterior to the foramen ovale. The needle tip is withdrawn slightly and "walked" posteriorly into the foramen ovale (Fig. 29-2). Paresthesia of the mandibular nerve may be encountered as the needle enters the foramen ovale.[60]

After entry into the foramen ovale the stylet of the Hinck needle is removed. A careful aspiration for blood should then be carried out. A free flow of cerebrospinal fluid (CSF) is usually encountered. Failure to observe a free flow of CSF does not necessarily mean that the needle tip is not properly located within the central nervous system in proximity to the gasserian ganglion; it simply may indicate that the needle lies within Meckel's cave anterior to the trigeminal cistern.[15] Fluoroscopic guidance with process occasionally may be helpful. A small amount of nonionic contrast agent (1–2 ml) should be injected under fluoroscopic visualization and a spot film should be obtained for documentation purposes before the injection of any local anesthetic or neurolytic substance. After needle position is confirmed, 0.1-ml aliquots of a preservative-free local anesthetic, such as 1% lidocaine for diagnostic blocks and 0.5% bupivacaine for therapeutic blocks with an average volume of 0.4 ml is carefully injected.[6] This approach to the gasserian ganglion may be used to place a radiofrequency probe. Standard radiofrequency precautions and lesion parameters should be followed.

Because of the highly vascular nature of the pterygopalatine space as well as its proximity to the middle meningeal artery, significant hematoma of the face and subscleral hematoma of the eye are possible sequelae. As mentioned previously, because the ganglion lies within cerebrospinal fluid, small amounts of local anesthetic injected through the needle may lead to total spinal anesthesia.[15] As a result, it is imperative that small, incremental doses of local anesthetic are injected with time allowed after each dose to observe the effect of prior doses.[6] Chemical neurolysis and neurodestructive procedures on the gasserian ganglion should be carried out under fluoroscopic guidance and only by persons familiar with the anatomy and the technique of gasserian ganglion block.

The potential complications and unwanted side effects of blockade of the gasserian ganglion include stroke, spinal blockade, respiratory arrest, cardiac arrest, corneal anesthesia, activation of herpes labialis and herpes zoster, and postprocedure dysesthesias including anesthesia dolorosa, abnormal motor function including weakness, facial asymmetry, Horner's syndrome, facial ecchymosis and hematoma, ocular subscleral hematoma, local anesthetic toxicity, trauma to nerve, infection, and sloughing of skin and subcutaneous tissue.

The presence and extent of corneal anesthesia must be carefully evaluated in all patients undergoing gasserian ganglion block.[55] If corneal anesthesia is present, the patient must be instructed in the use of ocular lubricating ointment and drops as well as eye-patching techniques to avoid corneal injury. Eye care must be continued for the duration of the corneal anesthesia. Approximately 10% of patients who undergo procedures involving the gasserian

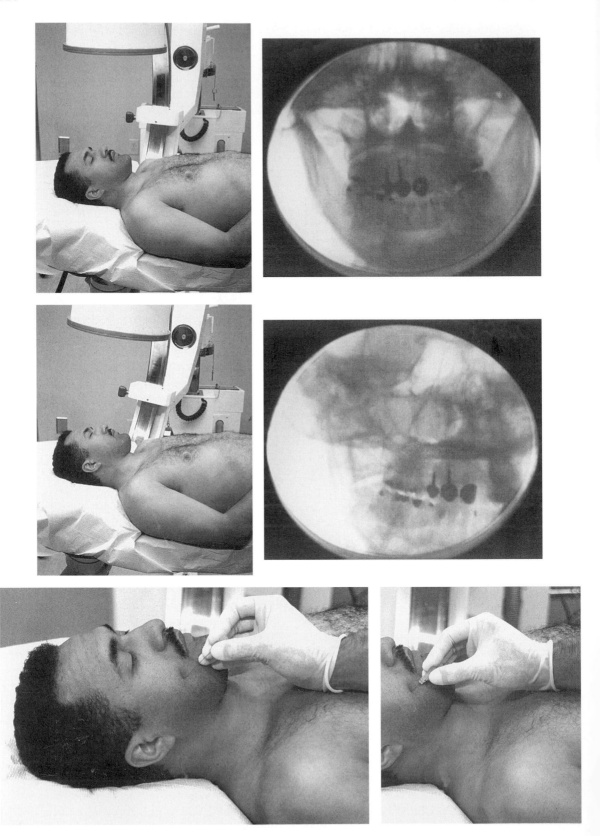

FIGURE 29-2. Gasserian sympathetic nerve blockade. A clinical and radiologic demonstration of a gasserian sympathetic nerve block.
(Continued on next page.)

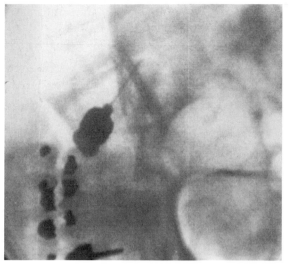
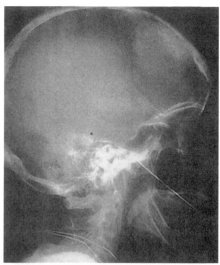
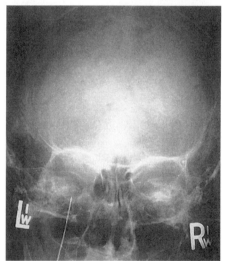

FIGURE 29-2 *(Continued)*.

ganglion experience an activation of herpes labialis and, occasionally, of herpes zoster in the distribution of the trigeminal nerve.

Approximately 6% of patients who undergo chemical neurolysis or neurodestructive procedures of the gasserian ganglion experience postprocedure dysesthesias in the area of anesthesia. Symptoms range from mild, uncomfortable burning or pulling sensations to severe pain. Severe postprocedure pain (anesthesia dolorosa) may be worse than the patient's original pain complaint and often is harder to treat. Sloughing of skin and subcutaneous tissue has been associated with anesthesia dolorosa.[24]

CERVICOTHORACIC (STELLATE GANGLION) BLOCKADE

Stellate ganglion block (SGB) is indicated for the diagnosis or treatment of SMedP involving the face or upper extremity. A thorough understanding of the regional anatomy, injection techniques, and potential complications is required due to the high density of vital structures in the cervical region. Stellate ganglion blockade is contraindicated in patients taking heparin or warfarin (Coumadin) and in patients with clinical blood dyscrasias associated with abnormal or prolonged bleeding.[26] Bilateral stellate ganglion block should not be performed because of the increased risk of complications, including aspiration secondary to bilateral recurrent laryngeal nerve block or hypoventilation secondary to bilateral phrenic nerve block.

The sympathetic innervation of the head and upper extremity receives preganglionic fibers from the upper 5–7 thoracic spinal segments.[17,19] These small, myelinated fibers have their cell bodies in the gray matter of the dorsolateral spinal cord and exit the spinal canal with the anterior primary rami as white rami communicans. The fibers ascend along the anterolateral surface of the spinal column to synapse in one of the three cervical sympathetic chain ganglia (superior, middle, and inferior). The superior and middle ganglia lie just anterior to the prevertebral fascia covering the longus colli and longus capitis muscles, posterior to the carotid sheath, and medial to the vertebral artery at the levels of the C2 and C6 vertebrae respectively.[11,17,19] The inferior cervical sympathetic ganglion lies just superior to the dome of the pleura and anterior to the neck of the first rib, where it often is fused with the first thoracic ganglia to form the stellate ganglion. Small, unmyelinated postganglionic fibers exit the superior cervical ganglion as gray rami communicans and supply the first four cervical spinal nerve roots and the cardiac plexus before ascending to the head along the internal and external carotid arteries. Postganglionic fibers from the middle cervical ganglion supply the fifth and sixth cervical nerve roots with additional contributions to the cardiac plexus and thyroid gland. Postganglionic fibers from the stellate ganglion supply the C7, C8, and T1 nerve roots and the vertebral plexus. In some cases, preganglionic fiber will pass through the cervical ganglia to synapse with the postganglionic neurons at distant sites. However, local anesthetic blockade of the cervical sympathetic chain at the C6 or C7 level will disrupt the efferent and afferent sympathetic innervation to the head and upper extremity.[11,26]

Stellate ganglion blockade may be safely performed by a trained physician in an outpatient setting with or without fluoroscopy; however, its use does increase the margin of safety. A variety of SGB techniques have been described. A fluoroscopic approach is described here.

The patient is positioned supine with the neck slightly extended and the jaw relaxed. The anterior cervical region is sterilely draped. Under fluoroscopic visualization, the C6 and C7 vertebral bodies are visualized. The carotid sheath is gently retracted laterally and the larynx is retracted medially to allow the index fingertip to palpate for the bony protuberance at the base of the C6 transverse process (Chassaignac's tubercle) or the anterior body of C7.[11,26] The skin and subcutaneous tissues are anesthetized with 13 ml of 1% lidocaine. Under fluoroscopic visualization, a short beveled 1½- or 3½-inch, 22- or 25-gauge needle is inserted until contact is made with the anterior vertebral body of C6 or C7 and then withdrawn 25 mm. Under fluoroscopic visualization, 3–5 ml of a nonionic contrast

agent is injected, and the contrast column should be seen to extend in both a cephalad and caudal direction on the ipsilateral side of the spine (Fig. 29-3). The column should extend down to the upper or mid-thoracic region; should not enter the canal through a foramen or any other route or demonstrate a fascial injection pattern other than that described; and should not be carried off by vascular uptake or outline an anterior ramus or other specific neural structure. If any such suboptimal injection patterns exist, the needle position is inadequate and must be moved. Following negative aspiration for CSF or blood in four quadrants, a small test dose of 0.2–0.5 ml of anesthetic solution is injected, and the patient is monitored closely for any signs of intravascular or intradural injection. If no signs of CNS toxicity, hypotension, or spinal block are observed, the remainder of local anesthetic is slowly injected. A total of 6–10 ml of 0.25% or 0.5% bupivacaine should be injected.[10,11,26,28,57] A smaller volume and lower concentration provide for a lower risk of complication and more specific sympathetic blockade; however, there also is a higher risk for incomplete sympathetic blockade.[28] Larger volumes and higher concentrations of local anesthetic may be considered in patients who have undergone previously failed SGB; conversely, smaller volumes should be used in patients who have undergone previous anterior cervical surgery, because the anatomy may be critically distorted. The contrast column described above will migrate in both a cephalad and caudal direction with the injection of the local anesthetic. After the contrast column has reached the mid-thoracic level, further injection of local anesthetic should be stopped. This method will permit the lowest dose of local anesthetic to be injected that will bathe the required region of the sympathetic trunk. The injection of local anesthetic should occur slowly in a stepwise manner, injecting only 2–3 ml of local anesthetic at one time and waiting 30–60 seconds while monitoring vital signs.

After the injections, patients should be observed for one hour to monitor their vital signs, observe for potential complications, and assess block outcome. Successful sympathetic blockade is indicated by the development of an ipsilateral Horner's syndrome (ptosis, miosis, and enophthalmos), conjunctival injection, and a temperature increase of the ipsilateral upper extremity of 2°C or an absolute temperature in excess of 34°C.[11,26,28]

Acute, potentially life-threatening complications may occur, including seizures, spinal block,

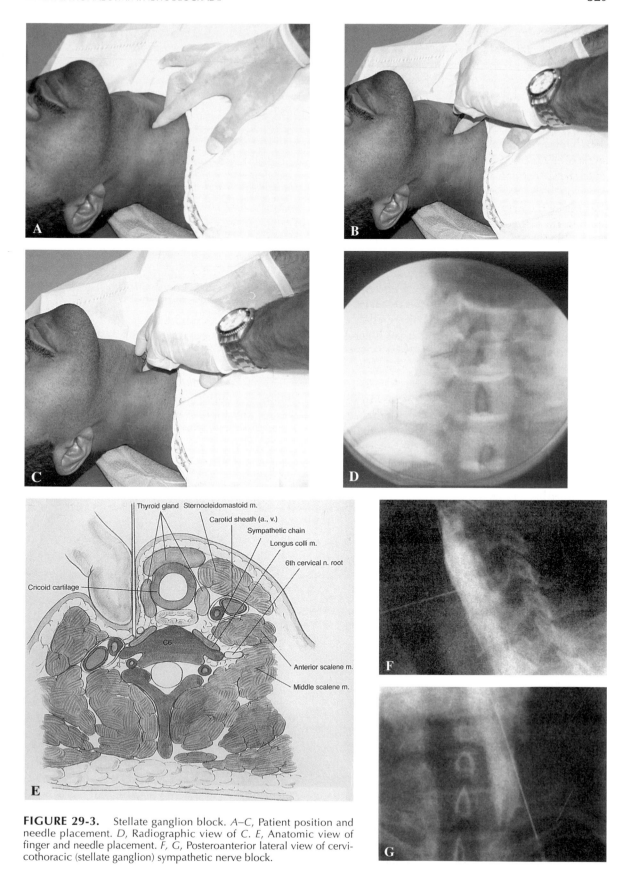

FIGURE 29-3. Stellate ganglion block. *A–C,* Patient position and needle placement. *D,* Radiographic view of *C. E,* Anatomic view of finger and needle placement. *F, G,* Posteroanterior lateral view of cervicothoracic (stellate ganglion) sympathetic nerve block.

hypotension, or pneumothorax.[11,26,28,44,57] Additional complications such as recurrent laryngeal nerve block, brachial plexus block, phrenic nerve block, or local hematoma also may occur. In addition to standard postprocedure protocol, patients are counseled not to eat or drink for the expected duration of anesthetic blockade due to the increased risk of aspiration from clinical or occult blockade of the recurrent laryngeal nerve.

PLEXUS AND SPLANCHNIC NERVE BLOCK

Indications

Indications for celiac plexus block include use as a diagnostic tool to determine whether flank, retroperitoneal, or upper abdominal pain is sympathetically mediated via the celiac plexus, to palliate pain secondary to acute pancreatitis and intraabdominal malignancies, and to reduce the pain of abdominal "angina" associated with visceral arterial insufficiency.[14,27,37,40,56]

Neurolysis of the celiac plexus with alcohol or phenol is indicated to treat pain secondary to malignancies of the retroperitoneum and upper abdomen and in some chronic benign abdominal pain syndromes, such as chronic pancreatitis, in carefully selected patients.[4,18,33,51]

Contraindications include anticoagulant therapy, coagulopathy, antiblastic cancer therapies, liver abnormalities, local or intra-abdominal infection and sepsis, and bowel obstruction.[3,40,53] The use of alcohol as a neurolytic agent should be avoided in patients on disulfiram therapy for alcohol abuse.

Clinically Relevant Anatomy

It is necessary to understand the anatomy of the autonomic nervous system as well as the relationship of the anatomic structures surrounding the celiac plexus in order to perform celiac plexus and splanchnic nerve block safely and effectively.

The sympathetic innervation of the abdominal viscera originates in the anterolateral horn of the spinal cord.[5] Preganglionic fibers from T5–T12 exit the spinal cord in conjunction with the ventral roots to joint the white communicating rami on their way to the sympathetic chain. Rather than synapsing with the sympathetic chain, these preganglionic fibers pass through it to ultimately synapse on the celiac ganglia.[25]

THE SPLANCHNIC NERVES

The greater, lesser, and least splanchnic nerves provide the major preganglion contribution to the celiac plexus.[8] The greater splanchnic nerve has its origin from the T5–T10 spinal roots. The nerve travels along the thoracic paravertebral border, through the crus of the diaphragm and into the abdominal cavity, ending on the celiac ganglion of its respective side. The lesser splanchnic nerve arises from the T10–T11 roots and passes with the greater nerve to end at the celiac ganglion. The least splanchnic nerve arises from the T11–T12 spinal roots and passes through the diaphragm to the celiac ganglion. Note that the greater, lesser, and least splanchnic nerves are preganglionic structures that synapse at the celiac ganglia.[40] Blockade limited solely to these nerves is properly termed *splanchnic nerve block*.

THE CELIAC GANGLIA

The three splanchnic nerves synapse at the celiac ganglia. The number of ganglia range from 1–5 and from 0.5–4.5 cm in diameter.[58] The ganglia lie anterior and anterolateral to the aorta. The ganglia located on the left are uniformly more inferior than their right-sided counterparts by as much as a vertebral level, but both groups of ganglia lie below the level of the celiac artery. In most instances, the ganglia lie approximately at the level of the first lumbar vertebra. Postganglionic fibers radiate from the celiac ganglia along the course of the blood vessels that innervate the abdominal viscera, which was derived from the embryonic foregut.[33] These organs are much of the distal esophagus, stomach, duodenum, small intestine, ascending and proximal transverse colon, the adrenal glands, pancreas, spleen, liver, and biliary system.

THE CELIAC PLEXUS

The celiac plexus arises from the preganglionic splanchnic nerves, vagal preganglionic parasympathetic fibers, sensory fibers from the phrenic nerve, and postganglionic sympathetic fibers.[5] The celiac plexus is anterior to the diaphragmatic crura.[61] It extends in front of and around the aorta, with the greatest concentration of fibers anterior to the aorta. Blockade of these neural structures, which include the afferent fibers carrying nociceptive information, is properly termed *celiac plexus block*. Note that the phrenic nerve also transmits nociceptive information from the upper abdominal viscera that may be perceived as poorly localized pain referred to the supraclavicular region.[5]

The normal configuration of these structures may be dramatically distorted owing to organomegaly or tumor. The aorta lies anterior and slightly to the left of the anterior margin of the vertebral body. The inferior vena cava lies to the right of the midline, and the kidneys are posterolateral to the great vessels. The pancreas lies anterior to the celiac plexus. All of these structures lie within the retroperitoneal space.

CELIAC PLEXUS BLOCKADE

The patient is placed in the prone position with a pillow beneath the abdomen to reverse the thoracolumbar lordosis, which increases the distance between the costal margins and the iliac crests as well as between the transverse processes of adjacent vertebral bodies. The patient's spine is surveyed under fluoroscopic visualization. The lumbar spine, lumbopelvic junction, thoracolumbar junction, and T12 ribs are located. Any anatomic anomaly is noted so that appropriate procedural adjustments may be made. The C-arm is rotated to a posterolateral projection. The ipsilateral L1 transverse process is watched as the C-arm is rotated. The angle of rotation is stopped after the tip of the transverse process has "disappeared" within the substance of the L1 vertebral body. This angle will be between 30° and 45° off the sagittal plane. At this point, the image of the ipsilateral T12 rib most likely will be superimposed on the L1 vertebral body. As a result, the C-arm should be rotated in a caudal to cephalad manner while maintaining the posterolateral angle described above. The C-arm should be rotated under active fluoroscopic visualization and should be stopped once the image of the T12 rib is no longer superimposed on the L1 vertebral body. A metallic pointer is used to mark the skin in the center of the fluoroscopic field. This point will represent the entrance point of the needle. The soft tissue should then be anesthetized beginning at the entrance point and extending in an *en pointe* fashion toward the anterior L1 vertebral body through the subcutaneous tissues and paraspinal muscles. At this point, a 3½- or 6-inch, 22- or 25-gauge spinal needle, with or without a 30° bend 1–2 cm from its distal tip with the convexity of the bend on the same side of the needle as the bevel, is advanced in an *en pointe* fashion down to the anterolateral border of the L1 vertebral body (Fig. 29-4). After the needle tip

contacts bone, the C-arm is rotated back to a sagittal projection. The needle tip should be seen to rest in the ipsilateral longitudinal interpedicular line. The C-arm is then rotated to a cross table lateral projection, and the needle tip should be seen to rest at the anterior vertebral body. At this point, the needle is aspirated in a quadrant fashion (the needle is rotated and aspirated in all four quadrants) and 4–6 ml of nonionic contrast agent is injected. The contrast should be seen to remain immediately anterior to the anterior vertebral line on cross table lateral view, superimposed upon the ipsilateral interpedicular line on sagittal view, and without vascular uptake. If the contrast column extends in an inferolateral projection on sagittal view, the needle tip remains too lateral and should be cautiously advanced 1–2 cm medially taking care not to penetrate a major vessel. A bend on the end of the needle as described above will aid appropriate placement of the needle in this situation. If the contrast column is whisked away in a longitudinal fashion, the needle tip is in a major vessel and should be backed up slightly and reinjected with contrast. If this does not correct the migration of the contrast column, the needle placement should be re-examined and probably repeated. If the contrast column runs off in a serpentine fashion, the needle tip lies within Batson's plexus and should be repositioned. If the needle tip cannot be repositioned to allow for appropriate contrast column as described above, the procedure should be repeated.

After the needle is appropriately placed as demonstrated by both contrast injection and radiographic evaluation, 12–15 ml of 1.0% lidocaine or 3.0% 2-chloroprocaine is administered through each needle. For therapeutic local anesthetic block, 10–12 ml of 0.5% bupivacaine is administered through each needle. Because of the potential for local anesthetic toxicity, all local anesthetics should be administered in incremental doses.[51] For treatment of the pain of acute pancreatitis, an 80-mg dose of depot methylprednisolone or 6 mg of betamethasone is recommended for the initial celiac plexus block and 40 mg given for subsequent blocks.[52]

SPLANCHNIC NERVE BLOCK

Splanchnic nerve block may provide relief of pain in a subset of patients who fail to obtain relief from celiac plexus block.[1,33] The splanchnic nerves transmit the majority of nociceptive information from the viscera[5] and are contained in a narrow compartment made up of the vertebral body and the pleura laterally, the posterior mediastinum ventrally, and the pleural attachment to the vertebra dorsally. This compartment is bounded caudally by the crura of the diaphragm. The volume of this compartment is approximately 10 ml on each side.[1]

The technique for splanchnic nerve block differs little from the approach to the celiac plexus, except that the needle is placed more cephalad to ultimately rest at the anterolateral margin of the T12 vertebral body. It is imperative that the needle is placed medially against the vertebral body to reduce the incidence of pneumothorax.

An alternate approach to splanchnic nerve block uses 3½- or 6-inch, 22-gauge spinal needles.[32] The needles are placed 3–4 cm lateral to the midline just below the 12th ribs. Their trajectory is slightly mesiad so that their tips come to rest at the anterolateral margin of the T12 body.

Complications of these techniques include hypotension, altered gastrointestinal motility, paresthesias or deficits of the lumbar somatic nerve, intravascular injection (venous or arterial), subarachnoid or epidural injection, diarrhea, renal and other visceral injury, paraplegia, pneumothorax, chylothorax, pleural effusion, vascular thrombosis or embolism, vascular trauma, perforation of cysts or tumors, injection of the psoas muscle, intradiscal injection, abscess, peritonitis, retroperitoneal hematoma, urinary abnormalities, ejaculatory failure, postprocedure pain, and failure to relieve pain.

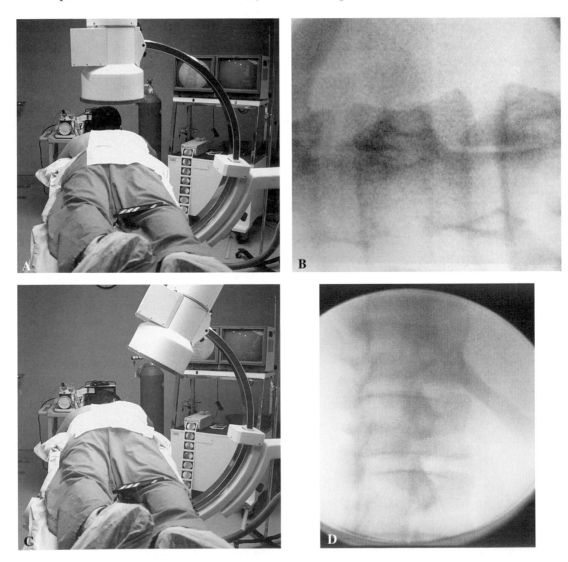

FIGURE 29-4. Celiac plexus nerve block. *A–D,* Correct position of patient and C-arm position, as well as fluoroscopic view.

(Continued on next page.)

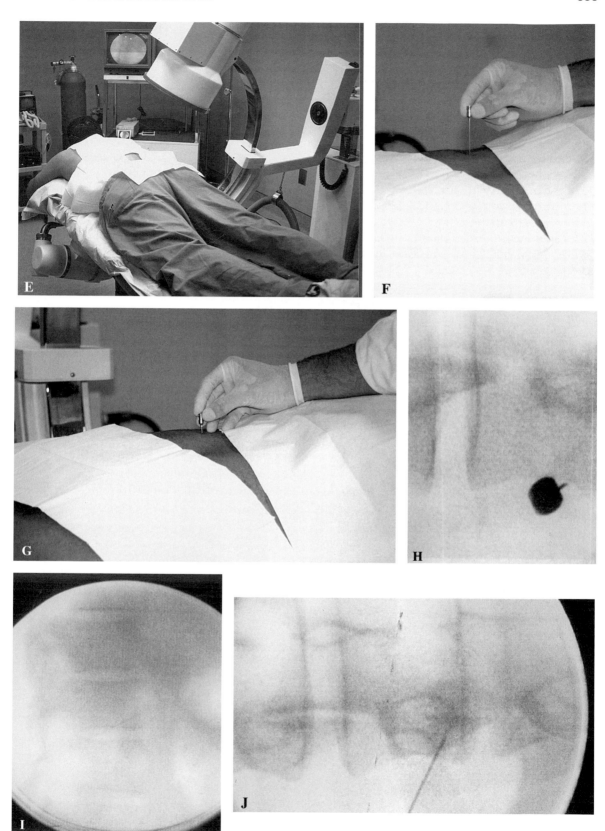

FIGURE 29-4 *(Continued).* *E–J*, Patient and C-arm position, needle placement, and fluoroscopic views.

LUMBAR SYMPATHETIC BLOCK

The preganglionic sympathetic outflow to the lower extremity originates in the neurons of the dorsolateral spinal cord corresponding to the lower thoracic and first two lumbar segments. From there, small myelinated fibers pass out of the spinal cord along with the anterior ventral rami as white rami communicans. These preganglionic fibers synapse with small unmyelinated fibers in the lumbar sympathetic chain ganglia. The lumbar sympathetic ganglia lie along the anterolateral surface of the lumbar vertebrae just anterior to the prevertebral fascia of the psoas muscle.[17,19,47] The number of lumbar sympathetic chain ganglia present varies considerably from one individual to another.[17,19] Postganglionic fibers exit the ganglia as gray rami communicans and supply one or more lumbar nerve roots. Deposition of local anesthetic along the sympathetic chain of the L2 or L3 levels will provide sympathetic denervation of the lower extremity.[50]

Lumbar sympathetic blockade (LSB) is contraindicated in anticoagulated patients or in patients with blood dyscrasias. Bilateral blockade is not recommended due to the potential for significant hypotension.

The patient's lower thoracic and upper lumbar region is prepped in a sterile fashion. The patient is positioned in either the prone or lateral decubitus position (block side up). The upper lumbar region is surveyed using fluoroscopy. The fluoroscopic beam is rotated until the tip of the ipsilateral L2 transverse process is completely superimposed on the substance of the L2 vertebral body. A metallic marker is used to place on the surface of the skin where the tip of the L2 transverse process meets the edge of the vertebral body. A 3½- or 6-inch, 22- or 25-gauge spinal needle is directed immediately caudal to the tip of the L2 transverse process using an *en pointe* approach under active fluoroscopic guidance. The needle is advanced until the needle tip gently contacts the inferior anterolateral L2 vertebral body[26,47,50] (Fig. 29-5). A cross table lateral view is taken, and the needle tip should be at the anterior vertebral line at the inferior L2 or superior L3 vertebrae. A sagittal view is obtained and the needle tip should be within the ipsilateral longitudinal interpedicular line. At this point 4–6 ml of nonionic contrast is injected, and the contrast column should extend up and down the ipsilateral thoracolumbar spine. On lateral view, the column remains immediately anterior to the anterior longitudinal line. A contrast column that extends in a caudal and lateral direction is outlining the psoas muscle, which generally will provide a suboptimal sympathetic block and often will also block the anterior rami of the upper lumbar region. As a result, when a psoas shadow is seen the needle should be advanced slightly and contrast should be reinjected. A vascular pattern should not be seen. If a suboptimal

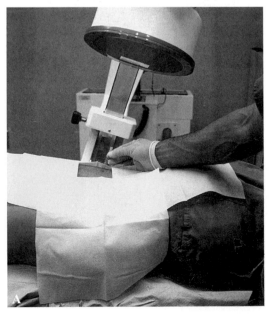
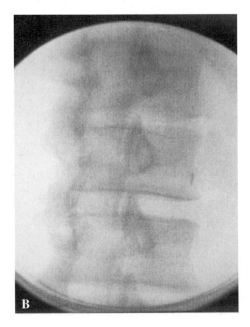

FIGURE 29-5. Lumbar sympathetic block. *A–F,* A clinical and radiologic demonstration of a lumbar sympathetic nerve block. *(Continued on next page.)*

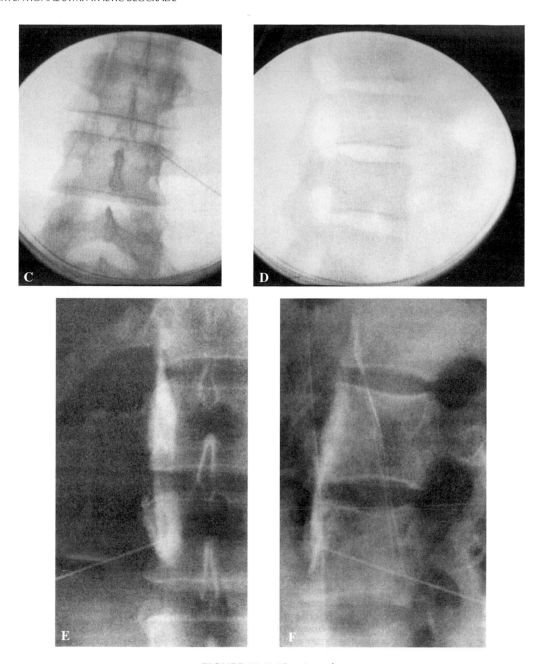

FIGURE 29-5 *(Continued).*

contrast column or a vascular pattern occurs then and the needle cannot be manipulated to obtain a correct needle placement, the procedure should be aborted.[43]

After both radiographic and contrast injection have confirmed correct needle placement, 10–15 ml of 0.25% or 0.5% bupivacaine is slowly injected.[12,26] Successful sympathetic blockade is indicated by a rise in lower extremity temperature of 3°C.[47]

Potential complications of LSB include intravascular injection, intradural injection with spinal anesthesia or postural headache, hypotension, lumbar plexus block, renal puncture, or genitofemoral neuralgia.[26,44,47]

After successful SGB or LSB has been performed, it is important to carefully examine the involved extremity for resolution of pain or pain-producing stimuli. Significant reduction of pain (> 50–75%) or painful stimuli in the absence of somatic blockade suggests the presence of SMedP. Serial diagnostic blocks may be required to rule out a placebo response.

Patients whose pain returns following a pain-free interval with SGB or LSB may be candidates for treatment with serial blocks. Additionally, arranging for the patient to participate in physical therapy for limb mobilization immediately following a successful block may greatly enhance the long-term treatment benefits of sympathetic blockade. Unfortunately, little controlled data exist to indicate the optimal frequency or ultimate number of serial blocks that are indicated in the management of SMedP.

SUPERIOR HYPOGASTRIC PLEXUS BLOCK

Indications for this procedure include the diagnosis and treatment of pelvic pain originating from malignancy, endometriosis, pelvic inflammatory disease, adhesions, and other pathologic processes. The block was introduced in 1990, and several studies show good relief of intractable pelvic pain.[36] Contraindications are similar to those listed for the aforementioned procedures and include infection, sepsis, and coagulopathy.

Anatomy

The superior hypogastric plexus is a retroperitoneal structure located bilaterally at the level of the lower third of the fifth lumbar vertebral body and upper third of the first sacral vertebral body at the sacral promontory and in proximity to the bifurcation of the common iliac vessels.[7,34,46,61] This plexus (sometimes referred to as the presacral nerve) is formed by the confluence of the lumbar sympathetic chains and branches of the aortic plexus that contains fibers that have traversed the celiac and inferior mesenteric plexuses. In addition, it usually contains parasympathetic fibers that originate in the ventral roots of S2–S4 and travel as slender nervi erigentes (pelvic splanchnic nerves) through the inferior hypogastric plexus to the superior hypogastric plexus.

The superior hypogastric plexus divides into the right and left hypogastric nerves that descend lateral to the sigmoid colon and rectosigmoid junction to reach the two inferior hypogastric plexuses. The superior plexus gives off branches to the ureteric and testicular (or ovarian) plexuses, the sigmoid colon, and the plexus that surrounds the common and internal iliac arteries. The inferior hypogastric plexus is a bilateral structure situated on either side of the rectum, lower part of the bladder,

and (in the male) prostate and seminal vesicles or (in the female) uterine cervix and vaginal fornices. In contrast to the superior hypogastric plexus, which is situated in a predominantly longitudinal plane, the configuration of the inferior hypogastric plexus is oriented more transversely, extending posteroanteriorly and parallel to the pelvic floor. Because of its location and configuration, the inferior hypogastric plexus does not lend itself to surgical or chemical extirpation.

Injection Technique

The patient assumes the prone position with padding placed beneath the pelvis to flatten the lumbar lordosis. The lumbosacral region is cleansed aseptically. The lumbar region is surveyed under fluoroscopy. The fluoroscopy tube is rotated approximately 45° for a posterolateral view of the L5 vertebral body. At this point, an image of the iliac crest will most likely be superimposed on the L5 vertebral body. The fluoroscopy tube is then rotated in a cephalad-caudad direction (the appropriate view is posterolateral and cephalad to caudad) so that the image of the iliac crest is no longer superimposed upon the L5 vertebral body (Fig. 29-6). At this point a 3½- or 6-inch, 22- or 25-gauge spinal needle is inserted using an *en pointe* method down to the anterolateral L5 vertebral body. The fluoroscopic image is rotated in a sagittal plane and cross table manner. In the sagittal plane, the needle tip should lie in the ipsilateral longitudinal interpedicular line, and in the cross table lateral view the needle tip should rest at the anterior longitudinal line. If the needle repeatedly encounters the L4 or L5 transverse processes, a slightly more axial trajectory requiring repetitive biplanar fluoroscopic views in order to properly place the needle may be necessary. If this method fails, a 30° bend should be placed in the needle 1–2 cm from the end of the needle with the convexity on the bevel side of the needle. By alternately rotating the needle while the needle is advanced, the needle tip may be skived around anatomic impediments. After fluoroscopic visualization confirms needle placement, 2–4 ml of nonionic contrast agent should be injected. The contrast column should remain along the midline or paramedian region in the sagittal view and the prevertebral space in the cross table lateral view. For diagnostic blocks, 8 ml of 0.25% or 0.5% bupivacaine or 1% lidocaine is injected.

Additional precautions include careful aspiration prior to injection and the use of "test" doses of local

FIGURE 29-6. Superior hypogastric plexus block. *A*, Patient is in a prone position, and the C-arm is positioned caudally to inject the superior hypogastric plexus. *B–E*, Radiographic views with proper needle placement confirmed by injected contrast material for blockade of the superior hypogastric plexus.

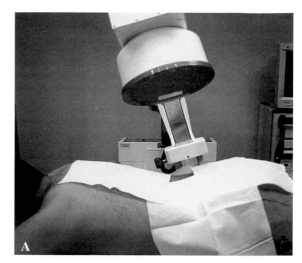

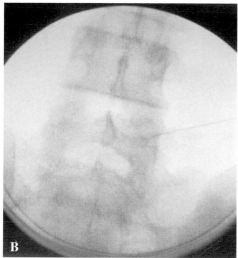

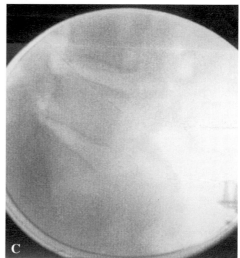

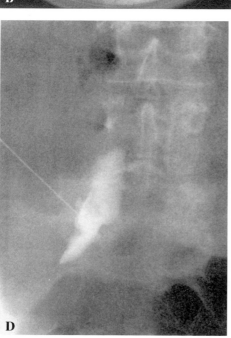

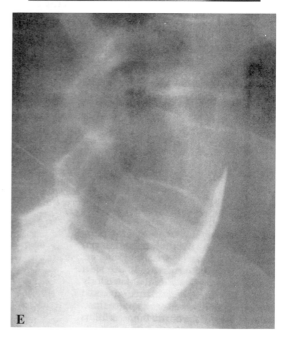

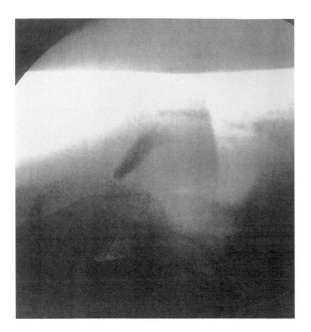

FIGURE 29-7. Ganglion impar blockade. Lateral radiograph demonstrating proper needle placement confirmed by the apostrophe-shaped contrast collection. The authors' preferred technique is to place the needle through the sacrococcygeal ligament.

anesthetic. Vascular puncture with a risk of subsequent hemorrhage and hematoma formation is possible because of the close proximity of the bifurcation of the common iliac vessels. Intramuscular or intraperitoneal injection may result from an improper estimate of needle depth. These and less likely complications (e.g., subarachnoid and epidural injection, somatic nerve injury, renal or ureteral puncture) can be avoided by careful observation of technique.

GANGLION IMPAR (GANGLION OF WALTHER) BLOCK

Blockade of the ganglion impar (ganglion of Walther) has been introduced as an alternative means of managing intractable neoplastic perineal pain of sympathetic origin.[35] The first report of interruption of the ganglion impar for relief of perineal pain appeared in 1990.[20] Characteristically, sympathetically maintained pain in the perineal region has distinct qualities: it tends to be vague and poorly localized and is commonly accompanied by sensations of burning and urgency. Although the anatomic interconnections of the ganglion impar rarely are described in any detail in the anatomic literature, the sympathetic component of these pain syndromes probably is derived, at least in part, from

this structure. The ganglion impar is a solitary retroperitoneal structure located at the level of the sacrococcygeal junction that marks the termination of the paired paravertebral sympathetic chains.

Technique

The patient is positioned in the prone position and the intergluteal cleft is prepared with Betadine while making sure to swab the skin toward the anus. The point of entrance is at the superior intergluteal cleft and the sacrococcygeal junction. A 1½-inch, 25-gauge needle is placed down to the posterior sacrum immediately above the sacrococcygeal ligament in the midline. The needle is then walked caudally until it touches the sacrococcygeal ligament. It then is advanced through the ligament taking care not to advance it more than 2 cm through the ligament (Fig. 29-7). Both sagittal and lateral fluoroscopic views are obtained to confirm needle placement. The needle tip should be in the midline on sagittal view and immediately anterior to the anterior longitudinal line. Between 2 and 4 ml of nonionic contrast is injected. The contrast column should remain in the midline and anterior to the anterior longitudinal line. The contrast column should resemble an apostrophe on lateral projection.

A 4-ml volume of 0.25% or 0.5% bupivacaine is injected for diagnostic and prognostic purposes. Alternatively, the procedure may be performed with a 3½-inch, 22-gauge radiofrequency probe with a 5-mm exposed tip.

Under most circumstances, needle placement is relatively straightforward. Local tumor invasion, particularly from rectal cancer, may prohibit the spread of injected solutions. Observation that the spread of contrast material is restricted to the retroperitoneum is essential. Potential complications include epidural spread within the caudal canal, perforation of the rectum, or periosteal injection. In addition, exaggerated anterior curvature of the sacrococcygeal vertebral column may inhibit access, in which case the needle may be further modified with an additional bend.

Acknowledgment is made to Jonathan P. Lester, M.D., for his contribution to this chapter in the first edition.

REFERENCES

1. Abram SE, Boas RA: Sympathetic and visceral nerve blocks. In Benumof JL (ed): Clinical Procedures in Anesthesia and Intensive Care. Philadelphia, J.B. Lippincott, 1992, p 787.

2. American Heart Association: Guidelines for Cardiopulmonary Resuscitation and Emergency Cardiac Care. JAMA 268:2171–2302, 1992.

3. American Heart Association: Textbook of Advanced Cardiac Life Support, 3rd ed, Dallas, AHA, 1993.

4. Bell SN, Cole R, Roberts-Thomson IC: Coeliac plexus block for control of pain in chronic pancreatitis. Br Med J 282:1604, 1980.

5. Bonica JJ: Autonomic innervation of the viscera in relation to nerve block. Anesthesiology 29:793–813, 1968.

6. Bonica JJ: Neurolytic blockade and hypophysectomy. In Bonica JJ (ed): The Management of Pain. Philadelphia, Lea & Febiger, 1990.

7. Brass A: Anatomy and physiology: Autonomic nerves and ganglia in pelvis. In Netter FH (ed): The Ciba Collection of Medical Illustrations. Vol. 1: Nervous System. Summit, NJ, Ciba Pharmaceutical, 1983, p 85.

8. Brown DL: Celiac plexus nerve block. In Brown DL (ed): Atlas of Regional Anesthesia. Philadelphia, W.B. Saunders, 1992, pp 245–247.

9. Brown DL: Trigeminal (gasserian) ganglion block. In Brown DL (ed): Atlas of Regional Anesthesia. Philadelphia, W. B. Saunders, 1992, p 140.

10. Bruyns T, Devulder J, Vermeulen H, et al: Possible inadvertent subdural block following attempted stellate ganglion blockade. Anaesthesia 46:747–749, 1991.

11. Carron H, Weller R: Treatment of post-traumatic sympathetic dystrophy. Adv Neurol 4:485, 1974.

12. Charlton J: Management of sympathetic pain. Br Med Bull 47:601–618, 1991.

13. Cousins M: Neural Blockade. Philadelphia, J.B. Lippincott, 1988, p 543.

14. Dale AW: Splanchnic block in the treatment of acute pancreatitis. Surgery 32:605, 1952.

15. Feldstein G: Percutaneous retrogasserian glycerol rhizotomy. In Racz G (ed): Techniques of Neurolysis. Boston, Kluwer, 1989, pp 126–128.

16. Gardner G, Gray AJ, O'Rahilly SF: Anatomy: A Regional Study of Human Structure, 5th ed. Philadelphia, W.B. Saunders, 1906, pp 676–677.

17. Gray H: The peripheral nervous system. In Clement C (ed): Anatomy of the Human Body. Philadelphia, Lea & Febiger, 1985, p 1149.

18. Hegedus V: Relief of pancreatic pain by radiography-guided block. AJR 133:1101–1103, 1979.

19. Hollinshead H: The nervous system. In Textbook of Anatomy. Hagerstown, MD, Harper & Row, 1984, p 37.

20. Kames LD, Rapkin AJ, Naliboff BD, et al: Effectiveness of an interdisciplinary pain management program for the treatment of chronic pelvic pain. Pain 41:41–46, 1990.

21. Katz J: Gasserian ganglion. In Katz J (ed): Atlas of Regional Anesthesia. Norwalk, CT, Appleton & Lange, 1994, pp 4–5.

22. Kline M: Stereotactic Radiofrequency Lesions as Part of the Management of Pain. Orlando, FL, Paul M Deutsch Press, 1992, p 54.

23. Kozin F, Soin J, Ryan L, et al: Bone scintigraphy in the reflex sympathetic dystrophy syndrome. Radiology 138:437–443, 1981.

24. Lipton S: Neurolysis: Pharmacology and drug selection. In Patt RB (ed): Cancer Pain. Philadelphia, J.B. Lippincott, 1993, pp 354–355.

25. Lofstrom JB, Cousins MJ: Sympathetic neural blockade. In Cousins MJ, Bridenbaugh PO (eds): Neural Blockade in Clinical Anesthesia and Management of Pain, 2nd ed. Philadelphia, J.B. Lippincott, 1988, pp 479–491.

26. Lofstrom J, Cousins MJ: Sympathetic neural blockade of upper and lower extremity. In Cousins MJ, Bridenbaugh PO (eds): Neural Blockade in Clinical Anesthesia and Management of Pain, 2nd ed. Philadelphia, J.B. Lippincott, 1988, p 461.

27. Loper KA, Coldwell DM, Leck J, et al: Celiac plexus block for hepatic arterial embolization: A comparison with intravenous morphine. Anesth Analg 69:398–399, 1989.

28. Malmqvist E, Bengtsson M, Sorenson J: Efficacy of stellate ganglion block: A clinical study with bupivacaine. Reg Anesth 17:340–347, 1992.

29. Mandel S, Rothrock R: Sympathetic dystrophies: Recognizing and managing a puzzling group of syndromes. Postgrad Med 87:213–214, 217–218, 1990.

30. Neill RS: Head, neck and airway. In Wildsmith JAW, Armitage EN (eds): Principles and Practice of Regional Anesthesia. New York, Churchill Livingstone, 1987.

31. Olcott C, Eltherington L, Wilcosky B, et al: Reflex sympathetic dystrophy—the surgeon's role in management. J Vasc Surg 14:488–492, 1991.

32. Parkinson SK, Mueller JB, Little WL: A new and simple technique for splanchnic nerve block using a paramedian approach and 3½-inch needles. Reg Anesth 14(suppl):41, 1989.

33. Patt RB: Neurolytic blocks of the sympathetic axis. In Patt RB (ed): Cancer Pain. Philadelphia, J.B. Lippincott, 1993, pp 393–411.

34. Pitkin G, Southworth JL, Hingson RA, Pitkin WM: Anatomy of the sympathetic trunk. In Conduction Anesthesia, 2nd ed. Philadelphia, J.B. Lippincott, 1953.

35. Plancarte R, Amescua C, Patt R, et al: Presacral blockade of the ganglion of Walther (ganglion impar). Anesthesiology 73:A751, 1990.

36. Plancarte R, Amescua C, Patt R, et al: Superior hypogastric plexus block for pelvic cancer pain. Anesthesiology 73:236–239, 1990.

37. Portenoy RK, Waldman SD: Recent advances in the management of cancer pain. Part I. Pain Management 4:23–29, 1991.

38. Racz GB, Heavener JE, Noe CE: Definitions, classifications and taxonomy: An overview. Phys Med Rehabil State Art Rev 10:195–206, 1996.

39. Raj B, Lewis R, Laros G, et al: Electrical stimulation analgesia. In Raj P (ed): Practical Management of Pain, 2nd ed. St. Louis, Mosby, 1991, p 922.

40. Raj PP: Chronic pain. In Raj PP (ed): Handbook of Regional Anesthesia. New York, Churchill Livingstone, 1985, pp 113–115.

41. Raja S, Davis K, Campbell J: The adrenergic pharmacology of sympathetically-maintained pain. J Reconstr Microsurg 8:63–69, 1992.

42. Ramamurthy R, Rogers JN: Decision Making in Pain Management. St. Louis, Mosby, 1993, pp 258–259.

43. Rocco AG: Radiofrequency lumbar sympatholysis. Reg Anesth 20:3–12, 1995.

44. Schmidt S, Gibbons J: Postdural puncture headache after fluoroscopically guided lumbar paravertebral sympathetic block. Anesthesiology 78:198–200, 1993.

45. Smith F, Powe J: Effect of sympathetic blockade on bone imaging. Clin Nucl Med 1:665–669, 1992.

46. Snell RS, Katz J: Clinical Anatomy for Anesthesiologists. Norwalk, CT, Appleton & Lange, 1988, p 271.

47. Sprague R, Ramamurthy S: Identification of the anterior psoas sheath as a landmark for lumbar sympathetic block. Reg Anesth 15:253–255, 1990.

48. Stanton-Hicks M: Upper and lower extremity pain. In Raj P (ed): Practical Management of Pain, 2nd ed. St. Louis, Mosby, 1991, p 312.

49. Tollison C, Satterthwaite J: Reflex sympathetic dystrophy: Diagnosis and treatment. Phys Assist July:51, 1992.

50. Umeda S, Arai T, Hatano Y, et al: Cadaver anatomic analysis of the best site for chemical lumbar sympathectomy. Anesth Analg 66:643–646, 1987.

51. Waldman SD, Portenoy RK: Recent advances in the management of cancer pain. Part II. Pain Management 4:19, 1991.

52. Waldman SD: Acute and postoperative pain management. In Weiner RS (ed): Innovations in Pain Management. Orlando, FL, PMD Press, 1993, pp 28–29.
53. Waldman SD: Celiac plexus block. In Weiner RS (ed): Innovations in Pain Management. Orlando, FL, PMD Press, 1990, pp 10–15.
54. Waldman SD: Cluster headache. Intern Med 13:31–32, 1992.
55. Waldman SD: Evaluation and treatment of common headache and facial pain syndromes. In Raj PP (ed): Practical Management of Pain. St. Louis, Mosby, 1992, p 217.
56. Waldman SD: Management of acute pain. Postgrad Med 18:15–17, 1992.
57. Wallace M, Milholland A: Contralateral spread of local anesthetic with stellate ganglion block. Reg Anesth 18:55–59, 1993.
58. Ward EM, Rorie DK, Nauss LA, et al: The celiac ganglion in man: Normal and anatomic variations. Anesth Analg 58:461–465, 1979.
59. Werner R, Davidoff G, Jackson MD, et al: Factors affecting the sensitivity and specificity of the three-phase technetium bone scan in the diagnosis of reflex sympathetic dystrophy syndrome in the upper extremity. J Hand Surg 14A:520–523, 1989.
60. Winnie AP: The early history of regional anesthesia in the United States. In Scott DB, McClure J (eds): Regional Anesthesia, 1884–1984. Sodertalje, Sweden, ICM Press, 1984, p 35.
61. Woodburne RT, Burkel WE: Essentials of Human Anatomy. New York, Oxford University Press, 1988, p 552.

30

Epidural Procedures in Spine Pain Management

Jeffrey L. Woodward, M.D., Stanley A. Herring, M.D.,
and Robert E. Windsor, M.D.

The use of epidural injections in the cervical, thoracic, and lumbosacral spine for both diagnostic and therapeutic purposes has developed as an important part of a comprehensive interdisciplinary approach to spinal pain. Diagnostic information garnered from epidural injections can be helpful in confirming hypotheses regarding the pain generators responsible for a patient's spine or extremity discomfort. It is well known that structural abnormalities seen on CT or MRI scans do not always cause pain, and diagnostic injections often can help correlate abnormalities on imaging studies with associated pain complaints. Therapeutically, epidural injections can provide significant pain relief, during which time recovery of disc and nerve root injuries can occur and patients also can progress their level of physical activity. Frequently, since the severe pain due to an acute disc injury with or without radiculopathy is often time-limited, therapeutic injections can help manage the patient's pain without reliance on oral analgesics. Epidural corticosteroid injections always are recommended in conjunction with a formal physical therapy program such as dynamic spine stabilization programs, which include spine mobility and strengthening exercises and postural and dynamic body mechanics training. A physician knowledgeable in the appropriate spine exercise programs and also trained in diagnostic and therapeutic spine injections can often best manage the medical care of patients with spine pain.

Historically, the first published reports of epidural injections for low back pain and sciatica occurred in 1901 and involved the injection of cocaine.[43,135,144,160,170] Viner[189] injected mixtures of procaine, Ringer's solution, saline, and liquid petrolatum using a caudal approach. In 1930, Evans[76] published good results in 22 of 40 patients with unilateral sciatica treated by caudal epidural injection of procaine and saline.

In 1955, Boudin et al.[27] became probably the first to inject corticosteroid into the subarachnoid space; this was followed in 1957 by Lievre[178] with the first published report of epidural corticosteroid injection with hydrocortisone for the treatment of low back pain. The literature contains many more reports on lumbar epidural injections than on cervical epidural injections for pain management. Papers by Shulman et al.[169] and Catchlove and Braha[42] published in 1984 are the earliest references for cervical epidural injections. A review of the literature has revealed no historical information on thoracic epidural corticosteroid injections.

ANATOMY

The spine is often divided anatomically into the anterior (the vertebral body and intervertebral disc), neuroaxial (structures within the epidural space and neural pathways), and posterior (zygapophyseal joints and associated bony vertebral arch structures) compartments.[24] Epidural injections are used to diagnose and treat abnormalities in both the anterior and the neuroaxial compartments. The spinal anatomy that is pertinent to epidural injections is discussed below.

Posterior Compartment

A knowledge of spine surface and bony anatomy is helpful in performing epidural injections. Important surface bony landmarks include the vertebra prominens at C7, base of scapular spine at T3, inferior angle of scapula at T7, inferoposterior T12 rib margins 10 cm from midline at L1, line between iliac crests at about L5 (Tuffier's line), and the posterior superior iliac spine at S1. The C7 spinous process, the vertebra prominens, can be felt to move with flexion and extension of the cervical spine, but the T1 spinous process remains fixed during cervical motion.

The orientation of the vertebral spinous processes is important for midline epidural approaches (Fig. 30-1). In the middle and lower cervical spine, the spinous processes are often bifid and are angled inferiorly at about 45° to the spine axis except at C7, which is less acutely angled.[46] With the cervical spine in a flexed position, the tip of each spinous process roughly overlies its lamina.[148] The thoracic spinous processes angulate sharply downward, often covering the entire interlaminar space below, thereby making the paramedian approach easiest. Lumbar spinous processes have only a slight downward angulation with the inferior border of the spinous process directly above the widest part of the interlaminar space, making both the midline and paramedian approach relatively easy. The widest interlaminar space is typically at the L4–5 interspace just below the inferior border of the L4 spinous process.

The bony anatomy of the sacrum and its sacral hiatus have a direct effect on the performance and success of caudal epidural injections. The sacral hiatus is an inverted V–shaped bony defect in the posterior and inferior surface of the sacrum covered by the sacrococcygeal ligament. The edges of the hiatus are bony prominences called the sacral cornu, which are remnants of the S5 articular processes. Needle placement through the sacral hiatus allows percutaneous access to the sacral canal, which forms the distal extent of the epidural space. Numerous anatomic variations in the bony structure of the sacrum have been documented. Black and Holyoke[18] reported complete bony blockage of the sacral canal in 7.7% of cadaver specimens. They also noted other variations, such as a complete midline bony septum dividing the sacral canal into two small compartments or the presence of an extremely small sacral hiatus the size of pencil lead in a small percentage of subjects. An occasional extreme anteroposterior angulation in the sacrum was also reported. All of these variations would make a caudal epidural injection either more difficult or impossible. Moore[132] reported at least some anatomic abnormality in the bony structure of the sacrum in 20% of patients examined. Despite the presence of such bony abnormalities, Cousins and Bromage[50] reported successful caudal epidural anesthesia in 94% of their patients, which closely agrees with several more recent studies.

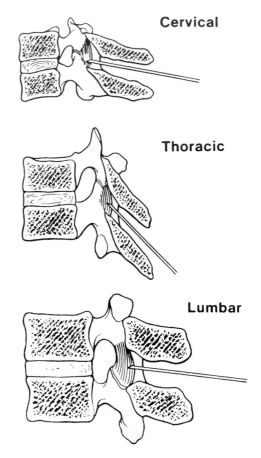

FIGURE 30-1. Spinous process and needle entry angle for cervical, thoracic, and lumbar spine midline epidural injection approaches. (From Cousins MJ, Bromage PR: Epidural neural blockade. In Cousins MJ, Bridenbaugh PO (eds): Neural Blockade in Clinical Anesthesia and Management of Pain. Philadelphia, J.B. Lippincott, 1988, with permission.)

Neuroaxial Compartment

The neuroaxial compartment includes all structures within the osseous and ligamentous boundaries of the spinal canal, including the posterior longitudinal ligament, the ligamentum flavum, and the epidural and epiradicular membranes (Fig. 30-2). Adequate knowledge of the cervicothoracic and lumbosacral epidural space is essential for proper epidural needle placement. The epidural space extends from the foramen magnum to the sacral hiatus and is located between the dura mater and the overlying ligamentum flavum and periosteum of the surrounding vertebral arches. No epidural space exists within the cranium due to the close adherence of the meningeal and endosteal dura, except where venous sinuses are present. At the foramen magnum, these two dural layers separate with the inner meningeal dura forming the spinal dura and the outer endosteal

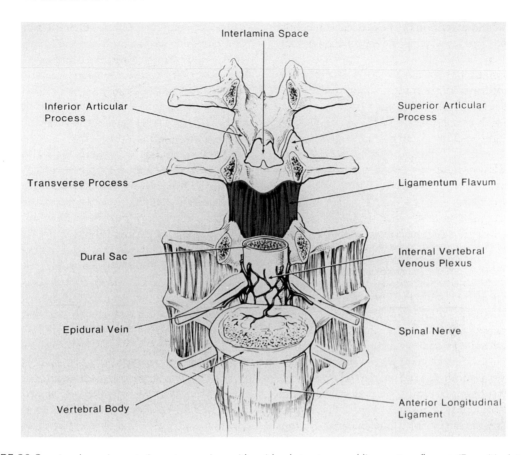

FIGURE 30-2. Lumbar spine anterior cutaway view with epidural structures and ligamentum flavum. (From Macintosh RR: Lumbar Puncture and Spinal Analgesia. Edinburgh, E & S Livingstone, 1957, with permission.)

dura forming the periosteum of the bony spinal canal. Within the dural covering resides the spinal cord and exiting nerve roots bathed in cerebrospinal fluid (CSF). In adults, the spinal cord generally extends inferiorly to the L1 or L2 level. The surrounding dural sac extends inferiorly in the sacrum to approximately the S2 level within the bony sacral canal and then terminates at the sacral hiatus at the S4 or S5 level. A sleeve of dura surrounds each nerve root as it exits through the neural foramen with a gradual thinning of the dural sleeve distally. Just distal to the dorsal root ganglion where the dorsal and ventral nerve roots join to form the spinal nerve, the dura adheres directly to the nerve, becoming continuous with the epineurium.

The width of the posterior epidural space beneath the neural arch at the midline varies throughout the length of the human spine. In the upper cervical region, the posterior epidural space is 1.5–2 mm wide and increases to 3–4 mm at the C7–T1 interspace, especially with spine flexion, but can become more narrow with neck extension. Cervical epidural injections in the midline at the C7–T1

interspace maximize the available epidural space and safety margin of the injection.[52] In the midthoracic region, the posterior epidural space is 3–5 mm wide and gradually expands to 5–6 mm at its greatest width in the midlumbar spine and then gradually decreases to about 2 mm at the S1 level.[45] At all levels, the triangular epidural space is widest in the midline underneath the junction of the lamina and narrows laterally beneath the zygapophyseal joints. The distance from the surface of the skin to the lumbar epidural space varies widely—from less than 3 cm to greater than 8 cm depending on the size and obesity of the patient.[51] The structures encountered during a midline epidural injection are skin, subcutaneous tissue, the supraspinous ligament, interspinous ligament, ligamentum flavum, and epidural space. The ligamentum flavum is a thick elastic fibrous band (3–5 mm in the midthoracic spine and 5–6 mm in the lumbar spine) running from the anteroinferior surface of the superior lamina to the posterosuperior edge of the lamina below (Fig. 30-3). The ligamenta flava on each side of the vertebral arch usually join in the midline and

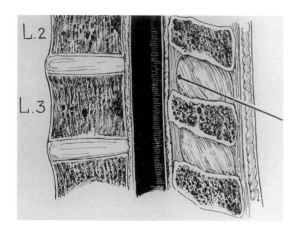

FIGURE 30-3. Lumbar spine sagittal view illustrating the ligamentum flavum and epidural space. (From Macintosh RR: Lumbar Puncture and Spinal Analgesia. Edinburgh, E & S Livingstone, 1957, with permission.)

taper in thickness laterally until connecting with the joint capsule of the adjacent zygapophyseal joint. The increased resistance to both needle advancement and injection afforded by the ligamenta flava is an important indicator of needle depth, as is the subsequent loss of resistance with needle penetration into the epidural space. Due to the vertical overlapping pattern of the ligamenta flava, the epidural space at any interspace is wider just above the edge of the inferior lamina, and placement of the epidural needle in this location is recommended for the paramedian approach.

The intervertebral foramen are bordered superiorly and inferiorly by the pedicles of adjacent vertebrae, anteriorly by the vertebral body and disc, and posteriorly by the zygapophyseal joint capsule (Fig. 30-4). The course of the spinal nerve roots exiting through the neuroforamen varies considerably as the nerve roots leave the spinal canal depending on the level of the spine. In the cervical spine, the nerve roots travel anteriorly and exit almost perpendicular to the long axis of the spine. In the thoracic and lumbar spine, the nerve roots travel more inferiorly and exit in a lateral plane without the anterior orientation seen in the cervical spine. The lumbar roots exit just under the pedicle with a downward course of 40–50° from horizontal and occupy the superior portion of each foramen. In order to safely inject medication as close to a lumbar nerve root as possible, the needle should be placed in the upper portion of the foramen just beneath the adjacent pedicle.

The sinuvertebral nerve is a branch of the somatic ventral nerve root and the sympathetic gray ramus communicans.[25] The sinuvertebral nerve originates just lateral to the neuroforamen and

enters the spinal canal just anterior to the dorsal root ganglion. Within the vertebral canal, the sinuvertebral nerve innervates the outer annulus of the disc, posterior longitudinal ligament, epidural membranes, and dura at the same segmental level and adjacent levels. Branches of the sinuvertebral nerve form a dense plexus throughout the anterior and lateral dura and extend within the dural sheaths covering the spinal roots and dorsal root ganglion.[59] Neuroaxial compartment pain is caused by irritation of the tissues innervated by the sinuvertebral nerve or direct stimulation of adjacent nociceptive fibers. The complex multisegmental innervation pattern of the sinuvertebral nerve probably is responsible, at least in part, for the diffuse pain referral patterns characteristic of neuroaxial pain. Once an injury involves local nerve root tissue, extremity pain in a radicular pattern occurs.

In addition to neural structures, the epidural space also contains veins, arteries, and adipose and loose aerolar tissues (Fig. 30-5). Epidural fat runs continuously throughout the epidural space and is most abundant in the dorsomedial region and less abundant in the ventromedial and lateral regions. Pads of loosely adherent epidural fat lie between the dural sac and the lamina or ligamenta flava and are apparently pushed aside by fluid injected into the epidural space. The presence of epidural fat can be important in the absorption and subsequent slow release of various medications (most importantly,

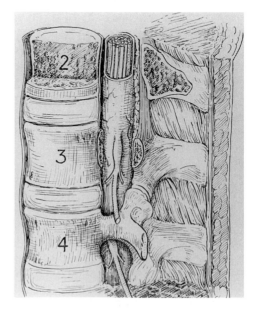

FIGURE 30-4. Lumbar spine sagittal view with exiting nerve roots. (From Macintosh RR: Lumbar Puncture and Spinal Analgesia. Edinburgh, E & S Livingstone, 1957, with permission.

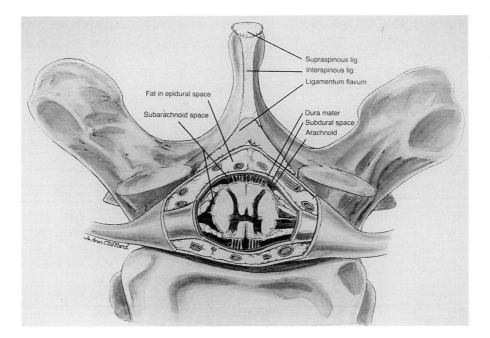

FIGURE 30-5.   Lumbar spine axial view with epidural structures. (From Brown DL: Atlas of Regional Anesthesia. Philadelphia, W.B. Saunders, 1992, with permission.)

local anesthetics such as bupivacaine). Also, epidural fat is thought to decrease in compliance with aging and may contribute to the increased resistance to epidural injection often reported in elderly patients.[51] Within the epidural loose areolar tissue reside small invaginations in the dura known as arachnoid villi, which are most plentiful in the lateral recesses of the epidural space. Due to the profuse vascularity of these villi, a portion of any medication injected into the epidural space may diffuse or be transported into the subarachnoid space and directly bathe the spinal cord and nerve roots.

Several other real or potential spaces within the dural sac are important when performing epidural injections. Just beneath the dura is the subdural space, which is a potential space between the dura and arachnoid mater containing only a small amount of serous fluid (Fig. 30-6). The subarachnoid space is between the arachnoid and pia mater and contains cerebrospinal fluid and blood vessels. The pia mater is a very thin, highly vascularized membrane adhering closely to the spinal cord and nerve roots. Advancing a needle into the subarachnoid space will lead to a "wet tap" often with return of CSF through the needle. The injection of medications unknowingly into the subarachnoid space, especially local anesthetics and possibly corticosteroids, can lead to serious complications as described later. Inadvertent needle placement into the potential subdural space will not be associated with CSF return, but also may be associated with significant complications similar to a subarachnoid injection.

Vascular Anatomy

Venous drainage of the epidural space occurs through the relatively large and valveless epidural veins, which are most abundant in the anterolateral portions of the spinal canal.[29] The epidural veins are part of the vertebral venous plexus, which communicates directly with the basivertebral veins located within the vertebral bodies. Superiorly, the vertebral venous plexus communicates with the occipital, sigmoid, and basilar venous sinuses within the cranium. Inferiorly, the vertebral venous plexus drains through many segmental epidural veins that exit the spinal canal through the intervertebral foramen and allow venous return to the inferior vena cava and azygos vein via thoracic and abdominal veins. Maintaining epidural needle placement as medially as possible will decrease the risk of puncturing the large lateral epidural veins through which medications can be inadvertently delivered directly to intracranial veins, potentially causing CNS side effects.

The arterial blood supply to the epidural and subarachnoid space, including the spinal cord, is delivered through segmental radicular arteries entering the intervertebral foramen from the aorta, subclavian and iliac arteries and from arterial vessels

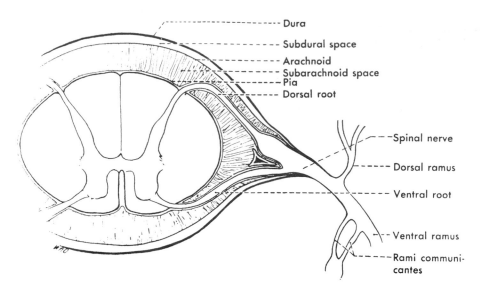

FIGURE 30-6. Schematic axial view of meningeal tissue layers. (From Hollingshead WH, Jenkins DB: Functional Anatomy of the Limbs and Back, 5th ed. Philadelphia, W.B. Saunders, 1981, with permission.)

descending from the posterior inferior cerebellar arteries. The radicular arteries entering the spinal canal pass through the dura in the neuroforamen at the region of the thin dural cuff. The anterior spinal artery, which primarily supplies the ventral motor spinal cord, receives most of its blood via these segmental radicular arteries. Most of the radicular arteries are quite small and supply only a minimal portion of the total spinal cord arterial blood flow. In fact, most of the arterial blood reaching the anterior spinal artery does so primarily through only six or seven major radicular arteries. Damage to one of the larger radicular arteries from a needle in the neural foramen at or above L2 could cause significant arterial compromise of the cord at that level. The largest of these major radicular arteries enters in the lumbar region to supply the enlarged lumbar cord and is called the radicularis magna (artery of Adamkiewicz). The radicularis magna enters the spinal canal through a single intervertebral foramen between T8 and L3 and is located on the left side 78% of the time. Obviously, needle damage to this important arterial feeder could result in significant ischemic damage to the lumbosacral cord with primarily motor deficits.[32] A common variant of spinal arterial circulation as described above involves a smaller than usual radicularis magna and multiple large lumbar radicular arteries from the iliac artery traversing the lower lumbar neuroforamen, any of which could incur needle damage from a transforaminal approach.

CLINICAL KNOWLEDGE

Cervicothoracic Spine: Clinical Trials

Cervical epidural steroid injections (CESIs) have been used in the treatment of both acute and chronic neck, shoulder, and arm pain.[46,47,148,161,190] CESIs also have been reported in the treatment of reflex sympathetic dystrophy, postherpetic neuralgia, postlaminectomy cervical pain, acute viral brachial plexitis, and muscle contraction headaches, with at least some good responses reported anecdotally for each of these conditions.[46,125,148,161,169,190,193] Rowlingson and Kirschenbaum[161] studied 25 patients with neck and at least some radicular pain, but not necessarily with neurologic deficits, with each patient receiving 50 mg of triamcinolone diacetate epidurally and at least 6 months of follow-up. Six patients (24%) achieved excellent pain relief with full return to activities; all six had radicular pain and at least mild sensory deficits prior to the injection. Of the remaining patients, ten (40%) reported good relief (≥ 75% pain relief), six (24%) reported fair relief, and three (12%) reported little or no relief. Purkis[148] administered 113 CESIs to 58 patients with at least 6 months of neck pain; each injection contained 130 mg of methylprednisolone. A total of 38 (65%) of the patients reported at least 50% pain relief 3 weeks after the injection; 9 of these had no pain at all. In prolonged follow-up, three patients noted significant relief 12 months after corticosteroid injection. Shulman[169] studied 96 patients receiving

80–160 mg of methylprednisolone; 41% reported at least 50% pain relief several weeks after the injection; 35% fair pain relief after several weeks; and 24%, poor or no relief.

More recently, Cicala et al.[46] treated 58 patients with CESIs using 1 mg/kg of methylprednisolone acetate; 24 (41%) had excellent relief (at least 90% pain relief for 6 months), 17 (~ 29%) noted good relief (50–90% pain relief for at least 6 months), and 17 (~ 29%) noted poor relief (no more than 50% or 6 weeks of pain relief). Cicala stated that excellent results were more likely in patients with cervical spondylosis, although some patients with subacute cervical strain also had excellent results; mostly poor results occurred with chronic cervical strains. Half of patients with pending litigation reported absolutely no pain relief. Mangar and Thomas[125] treated 40 patients with CESIs using 80 mg of methylprednisolone acetate; 15 (38%) of patients had excellent pain relief (greater than 70% relief); three (7%) had good relief (50–70%); nine (23%) had poor relief (1–50%); and 13 (32%) had no relief. Patients with cervical disc herniation had overall better responses with 75% noting at least 50% pain relief.

Castagnera et al.[41] compared patients injected with steroid versus steroid with 2.5 mg morphine during CESIs at the C7–T1 interspace. The morphine group had significantly better pain relief one day after injection, but pain relief was similar for the two groups at longer-term follow-ups. They did report at least a 78% positive response rate for both groups. Stav and associates[177] studied patients with cervicobrachalgia receiving either cervical intramuscular steroid injection or CESI. One week after the final injection, the CESI group reported good to very good pain relief in 76% of patients and similar relief in only 35% of intramuscular injection patients. At one year follow-up, 68% CESI patients still had at least good pain relief compared to only 12% in the intramuscular group. Finally, Ferrante[76] treated 100 patients with 235 CESIs, each containing 80 mg of methylprednisolone acetate; 40% of patients had at least 50% pain relief and at least partial return to activities. Patients with a true radiculopathy and associated neurologic deficits had a 62% probability of obtaining at least 50% pain relief. Also, 67% of all patients obtained at least some pain relief. The best results with CESIs occurred in patients with either a true radiculopathy (having symptoms and sensory and/or motor deficits at a specific root level) regardless of abnormalities on imaging studies or radicular pain only with structural abnormalities on imaging studies at the level corresponding to the symptoms. Better outcomes occurred in patients with cervical spondylosis or stenosis, without myofascial symptoms and with the presence of motor weakness.

According to the above studies, CESIs seem to work better in patients with cervical spondylosis, acute disc herniation, limited myofascial pain complaints, and significant radicular pain in a specific dermatomal distribution. No controlled, blinded studies of CESIs including a placebo group or an accounting of associated treatments or therapies have been reported. For these reasons, further scientific study is needed to fully quantify the efficacy of CESIs.

Regarding thoracic epidural steroid injections (TESIs), due to the relatively low incidence of thoracic spine disease, few studies documented their efficacy for either thoracic spine or radicular pain. As in the cervical and lumbar spine, TESIs have been recommended for the treatment of thoracic disc disease. Thoracic disc herniations, however, account for less than 1% of all symptomatic disc herniations.[69,207] At least 11–13% of thoracic disc herniations are asymptomatic based on diagnosis by CT-myelography[9] and MRI.[202,204] Thoracic disc herniations that do not cause significant pain or neurologic deficits are thought to remain relatively asymptomatic in most cases and, therefore, require no preventive treatments.[9] The treatment of symptomatic thoracic disc herniations remains somewhat controversial. Brown[35] has stated "the thoracic herniated disc appears to follow a course similar to cervical or lumbar disc disease in that these herniations frequently respond to a nonoperative therapy program." TESIs are known anecdotally to often provide pain relief in the treatment of painful thoracic disc herniations in patients without associated myelopathy.

TESIs also have been shown to provide pain relief from thoracic radiculopathies not only from disc disease, but also due to herpes zoster, trauma, or associated diabetes.[79,80] Degenerative scoliosis, generally seen in women, is the other condition most commonly associated with thoracic radiculopathies.[89] Reporting on the use of TESI in four cases of idiopathic thoracic neuralgia, Forrest[80] demonstrated a nearly 50% pain relief lasting 12 months in one case and a similar level of relief lasting about three months in two other cases. One of the authors (REW) has also found TESIs to be helpful in the management of painful thoracic spondylosis and chronic inflammatory thoracic pain unresponsive to more conservative measures.

Lumbosacral Spine: Clinical Trials

According to Kepes and Duncalf,[111] about 100 reports on the use of subarachnoid and epidural spinal injections for low back pain were published worldwide from 1960–1985. Recent review articles on the efficacy of lumbosacral epidural steroid injections (LESIs) by Kepes and Duncalf,[111] Benzon,[13] Haddox,[89] and Bogduk et al.[24] are recommended. All of these articles mention the lack of well-controlled studies on LESIs and the variability between studies in the type and dosage of corticosteroid used, injection technique, patient diagnosis, length of follow-up, and quantitation of pain relief. The response rate obtained with LESIs in past studies has varied from 20–100%,[89,111] with an average response rate calculated from many studies at 60% by Kepes and Duncalf[111] and 75% by White.[200] A summary of the results from studies on LESIs including at least 100 patients is presented in Table 30-1. The majority of these studies involve no attempt to randomize treatments or provide a control group of patients, and, although the studies do provide anecdotal information, no scientific conclusions regarding the efficacy of LESIs can be made from their data. The results of studies containing at least some control group of patients are presented in Table 30-2.

According to Bogduk,[24] more than 40 papers have been published on lumbar and caudal epidural corticosteroid injections involving a total of more than 4,000 patients. Only four of these papers have recommended against the use of lumbosacral

TABLE 30-1. Uncontrolled Epidural Steroid Studies Including at Least 100 Patients

Study	Number of Patients	Percentage of Patients Reporting Pain Relief	Volume Injected (ml)
Arnhoff, 1977	140	39	10
Burn & Langdon, 1979	138	78	40
Goebert et al., 1961	113	73	30
Heppner et al.	478	100	
Heyse-Moore, 1978	120	62	20
Ito, 1971	296	73	5–10
Jennings et al.	134	66	10–20
Mount	287	88	20
Sayle-Creer and Swerdlow, 1969	320	53	100
Swerdlow and Sayle-Creer, 1970	177	65	5
Warr et al., 1972	500	63	40

Adapted from Kepes ER, Duncalf D: Treatment of backache with spinal injections for local anesthetics, spinal and systemic steroids. A review. Pain 23:33–47, 1985.

TABLE 30-2. Controlled Epidural Corticosteroid Studies

Study	Number of Patients	Approach	Follow-up	Steroid Benefit
Beliveau, 1971	48	caudal	1–3 mo	yes
Dilke, 1973	100	lumbar	2 wk & 3 mo	yes
Breivik, 1976	35	lumbar	3 wk	yes
Snoek, 1977	51	lumbar	48 hr	no
Yates, 1978	20	caudal	1 mo	yes
Klenerman, 1984	63	lumbar	2 wk & 20 mo	no
Helliwell, 1985	39	lumbar	1 mo & 3 mo	yes
Ridley, 1988	39	lumbar	2 wk	yes
Bush & Hillier, 1991	23	caudal	1 mo & 1 yr	yes

epidural corticosteroids. Previous research has indicated that an epidural injection of saline or local anesthetic alone can be effective in relieving back and leg pain in some patients.[49,62,63,76] The occasional positive response to epidural saline or anesthetic questions the validity of these agents as experimental controls versus epidural corticosteroids. Numerous studies have, however, compared the efficacy of epidural injections using local anesthetic or saline compared to mixing these agents with corticosteroids. Beliveau[12] published one of the first such studies comparing patients with radicular pain injected by a caudal approach with procaine versus procaine plus 80 mg of methylprednisolone. He reported no significant difference in pain relief between these two groups. Snoek et al.[174] treated patients having unilateral radicular pain with lumbar epidural injections and used either 2 ml of saline or 80 mg of methylprednisolone (2 ml) and found no significant differences in pain relief between the two groups. Patients in both groups responded and reported pain relief ranging from 25–70%. Bush and Hillier[39] injected patients with either 25 ml of saline or 80 mg of triamcinolone plus 0.5% procaine up to a total of 25 ml. At 1 month of follow-up, patients treated with corticosteroid showed significant pain relief and increased mobility and quality of life. At 1 year follow-up, this treatment group continued to have a tendency (although not statistically significant) of less pain and more mobility and significantly fewer patients with a positive straight leg raise test.

Cuckler et al.[60] also reported no significant difference in pain relief between an epidural injection of procaine versus corticosteroid; this 1985 study has been quoted frequently as evidence against the efficacy of epidural corticosteroids. However, because the authors examined the patients for pain relief only once 24 hours after epidural corticosteroid injection, a period of time considered too brief for epidural steroids to work effectively, the results are generally not considered valid. In addition, Cuckler's patients all received epidural corticosteroids at the L3–L4 level regardless of the level causing pain, and fluoroscopic guidance was not used. Several other well-known studies[31,39,180,210] compared various combinations of epidural saline and/or local anesthetic solutions against epidural corticosteroids and concluded that the steroid did provide better pain relief for back and radicular pain. However, according to Bogduk et al.,[24] no statistically valid conclusions can be drawn from the results of these studies due to small sample sizes or a poorly controlled study design.

Several controlled studies have compared the pain relief resulting from an epidural corticosteroid injection to a placebo injection involving needle placement into the interspinous ligament. In 1973, Dilke et al.[70] performed a randomized, prospective, double-blind study involving patients with radicular pain and comparing the efficacy of lumbar epidural injection using lidocaine and 80 mg of methylprednisolone versus a 1-ml saline interspinous ligament injection. Compared with control patients, a significantly greater number of treated patients that reported pain being "clearly relieved," more treatment patients were pain-free at 3 months, and more had resumed work after 3 months. Ridley[157] evaluated epidural corticosteroid mixed with saline versus a control interspinous ligament injection of 2 ml saline and also reported a definite benefit from the epidural corticosteroid injection after 2 weeks. Klenerman et al.[113] studied patients who had radicular pain for less than 6 months and received an epidural injection of either 20 ml of saline, 80 mg of methylprednisolone in 20 ml of saline, or 20 ml of 0.25% bupivacaine or interspinous needling with a Touhy needle. These authors found no added benefit from the corticosteroid but did note a 75% response rate to epidural injection versus control patients. Finally, Helliwell et al.[95] injected patients having unilateral radicular pain with either 80 mg of methylprednisolone plus 10 ml of saline into the epidural space, or 5 ml of saline into the interspinous ligament. Follow-up was performed at 1 and 3 months, and a significantly greater number of patients receiving the epidural corticosteroid had "definite improvement," loss of a positive straight-leg raise test, and decreased pain with spine motion.

Two recent meta-analysis studies of prior LESI research results both have found at least some degree of benefit from epidural steroid procedures. First, Rapp et al.[153] reviewed 300 articles from 1966 to 1993 and identified 6 studies with sufficient experimental controls to include in the analysis. The meta-analysis revealed a small but statistically significant benefit for pain relief following LESI. In 1995 Watts and Silagy[196] combined the results of eleven Australian LESI trials for their meta-analysis study. Their report indicated that patients having significant radicular pain were 2.6–3 times more likely to have at least 75% back and leg pain relief up to 60 days following the injection as compared to placebo treatment. Study patients also were two times more likely to have significantly decreased back and leg pain 12 months following epidural steroid injection versus placebo treatment. These authors indicated that their study provided quantitative evidence supporting the efficacy of epidural steroids, particularly for the treatment of radicular pain.

According to Derby, Bogduk, and Kine,[67] the transforaminal approach may more reliably place corticosteroid in the anterior epidural space where the most pain-sensitive structures are located. Many studies report the usefulness of selective nerve root blocks to identify or confirm a specific nerve root as a pain generator when such a diagnosis is not clear based on other clinical evidence.[72,94,97,116,176] A recent study noted "considerable and sustained" relief in 22 of 28 patients with selective transforaminal epidural steroid injections with an average follow-up period of 3.4 years.[197] All treatment patients had either a lateral disc herniation within the foramen or a far-lateral herniation lateral to the foramen. Lutz et al.[124] also studied the efficacy of selective transforaminal epidural injections done under fluoroscopy. In their study, 52 of 69 (75%) patients treated had 50% pain relief or greater and a return to most preinjury physical activities at an average of 80 weeks after injections. Patients received an average of about two selective epidurals given an average of four months after onset of pain. Overall, less favorable results were obtained in patients having either more than 6 months pain since onset or severe lateral bony stenosis.

Previous studies have indicated that the majority of patients with substantial leg pain relief from a selective nerve root block, even if the relief is temporary, will benefit from surgery for the radicular pain when that nerve root injury is associated with a disc herniation or lateral bony stenosis.[72,97,116] It is thought that a single nerve root is almost always responsible for acute radicular symptoms. Kikuchi[112] treated patients diagnosed with acute radicular leg pain associated with intermittent claudication and was able to relieve the pain in 90% of the patients by blocking only one nerve root. Derby et al.[67] showed the significant negative predictive value of transforaminal corticosteroid injections in relation to the surgical outcome for the treatment of chronic radiculopathy. Of 38 patients with radicular pain for at least 12 months and less than 80% pain relief 1 week after a selective nerve root block with corticosteroid, only 2 had significant relief following surgery for radicular pain. In addition, 11 of 13 patients with a positive response to the corticosteroid nerve root block had a positive surgical outcome. Therapeutically, one or two corticosteroid nerve root blocks have been shown to occasionally provide relief from radicular pain for more than 6 months, allowing adequate time for recovery and avoiding the need for surgery.[112]

Several important factors may have been addressed incompletely in studies regarding lumbosacral epidural corticosteroids. Most of these studies did not use fluoroscopy, and a significant incidence of improper needle placement without fluoroscopy has been documented, especially for a caudal approach, which has been used frequently in past studies.[12,31,39,200,210] In general, study participants receiving improper (not epidural) placement of corticosteroid due to the lack of fluoroscopic guidance and not responding because of this technical error are routinely grouped with patients in the same study receiving properly placed epidural corticosteroids, thereby lowering the apparent response rate. Also, the specific approach used for an epidural corticosteroid injection has often been uncontrolled in previous studies and sometimes appeared poorly matched to the patient's condition, especially for the many studies using a caudal approach. If localizing the corticosteroid in the epidural space as close to the pain generators as possible does strongly affect the response, then prior estimates of the efficacy of lumbosacral epidural corticosteroids may remain underestimated. For example, the response from a caudal epidural injection for an L4 radiculopathy, especially if a relatively small volume of injectate is used, is probably not as effective as a well-placed selective transforaminal approach.

Various trends with epidural corticosteroid injections do seem apparent from previous research. First, patients with a more acute episode of back or leg pain generally respond better to epidural corticosteroids, particularly if the duration of pain is less than 3 months.[36,86,91] Unilateral radicular pain, especially

when due to active nerve root inflammation from acute disc pathology rather than bony stenosis, tends to respond more favorably than strictly low back pain.[89,200] Patients also tend to have poor responses to epidural corticosteroids postoperatively unless a significant reinjury causing an acute disc or nerve root injury has occurred. The temporary nature of pain relief generally afforded by epidural corticosteroids has been well documented by White et al.,[200] who reported 82% of patients with pain relief one day after an LESI, 24% after 1 month, 16% after 2 months, and 7% for at least 6 months. However, because back or leg pain occurring from an acute disc injury often improves dramatically without surgery,[164] temporary pain relief from epidural injections can provide time during which disc or nerve recovery may occur. Also, a small but undetermined percentage of patients receiving epidural corticosteroids for back or leg pain obtain persisting pain relief and avoid potential surgery, thereby saving substantial medical costs and avoiding the iatrogenic risks of surgery. The benefits gained from epidural corticosteroids regarding patients' long-term functional status, not simply pain relief, also remain unclear, although one study has shown decreased return to work time in patients treated with epidural corticosteroids.[70]

Mechanism of Pain Relief

Before the use of corticosteroids, epidural injections were performed with large volumes of saline solution, and relief of back and leg pain was thought to be due to the disruption of scar tissue in the epidural space.[76] Such a mechanism is now disputed since large volumes of radiographic dye injected in the lumbar epidural space flow along a path of least resistance out of the epidural space through the neuroforamen.[199] More likely, mechanisms for pain relief seen after a saline epidural injection are an osmotic effect decreasing local epidural and nerve root tissue edema or dilution of inflammatory mediators.[89] Response to an epidural injection of local anesthetic may be due in part to the physical effects of the fluid itself, but also to the interruption of afferent nerve impulses, which is known to decrease the associated level of pain.[40]

Soon after Lindahl and Rexed[121] attributed sciatica to the persistent inflammation of lumbosacral nerve roots, the widespread use of corticosteroids in epidural and intrathecal injections began. Since that time, the key role that inflammatory mediators originating from the disc play in the production of local inflammation and resulting discogenic and neurogenic pain is well documented.[57,115,128,164,183] It has followed that the proposed primary mechanism of action of epidural corticosteroid injections is the potent anti-inflammatory properties of the corticosteroids.[78,180,184,193,200] Winnie[208] provided further evidence for an anti-inflammatory mechanism as compared to injectate volume alone by achieving significant long-term responses from LESI after injecting only 2 ml of corticosteroid. The marked pain relief often noted with epidural corticosteroid injection for an acute radiculopathy may also be due to the stabilization of nerve root membranes by the corticosteroid suppressing the ectopic neuronal discharges, which can cause pain and paresthesias.[68,183,197] Corticosteroids also may exert an "anesthetic" action to block nociceptive C-fiber conduction independent of their anti-inflammatory properties.[171]

Siddall and Cousins[171] have recently reviewed the complex interacting mechanisms believed to contribute to spine pain, including radiculopathy. The intracellular chemicals released from both injured tissues and inflammatory cells at the site of acute spine injury can generate pain signals from local nerves and non-neural tissues such as the outer annulus and posterior longitudinal ligament. Phospholipase A2 is one such chemical mediator identified within spine tissue thought to play a role in spinal pain after injury. Lee et al.[118] performed animal studies documenting increasing phospholipase A2 levels early after rat nerve root injury from ligation and decreased levels following steroid infiltration associated with decreased pain behaviors by the animals as well. Prolonged exposure of spine neural tissue to these inflammatory mediators potentially may cause permanent alteration in nerve function and nociception unrelated to active inflammation.[171] The risk of permanent nerve abnormal function seems to encourage aggressive use of corticosteroids early after spine injury and may help to explain the relatively poor responses reported with epidural steroid injection for chronic radicular pain.

POTENTIAL COMPLICATIONS

Medications and Associated Risks

Local Anesthetics

Lidocaine and bupivacaine are the most common anesthetics used for epidural injection. The general characteristics and toxic effects of these two amide anesthetics have been presented earlier in this book.

All local anesthetics injected into the epidural space must be preservative-free because the effect of preservatives in the epidural and subarachnoid spaces has not been evaluated satisfactorily. A major concern when administering anesthetics into the epidural space is systemic toxicity. The two most common systemic effects from epidural local anesthetics involve the central nervous system (CNS) and the cardiovascular system. A rough estimate of the threshold plasma concentration in humans causing onset of CNS toxicity for lidocaine is 5–10 µg/ml (probably closer to 10 µg/ml), and for bupivacaine is 2–4 µg/ml (bupivacaine is about four times more toxic than lidocaine).[52] Braid and Scott[30] injected 400 mg of lidocaine epidurally in test subjects and recorded an average peak plasma concentration of about 4 µg/ml, slightly below the neurotoxic concentration given above. In order to give a total dose of 400 mg of lidocaine, 40 ml of 1% or 20 ml of 2% lidocaine would be required. Both of these doses are significantly above the usual dose of lidocaine used for epidural corticosteroid injections (generally 5–15 ml of 0.5 or 1% lidocaine for LESIs and less volume for selective nerve root blocks and CESIs). The maximum epidural dose recommended for a single injection is 500 mg for lidocaine and 225 mg for bupivacaine (90 ml of 0.25% bupivacaine).[52] These ranges for CNS toxicity are only estimates, however, and neurologic side effects have been reported at much lower doses. Higher concentrations of lidocaine (4 or 5%) can cause serious side effects at lower total dosages than cited above, requiring more cautious administration, but these concentrations are generally not used undiluted for standard epidural corticosteroid injections.[51] Peak plasma concentration of epidural anesthetics occurs 10–20 minutes after injection, so it is recommended that patients be monitored for at least 30 minutes following an epidural injection. Significant CNS toxicity caused by intravascular lidocaine is usually manifested by complaints of circumoral numbness, disorientation, light-headedness, nystagmus, tinnitus, and muscle twitching in the face or distal extremities.

Cardiovascular toxicity can occur from the direct effect of the anesthetic on the sympathetic nerves, which help to regulate cardiac function and peripheral blood flow. The onset of sympathetic blockade is known to be more rapid from subarachnoid versus epidural injections, but both can be associated with serious cardiac side effects.[168] Sympathetic blockade develops with local anesthetics placed in the thoracic region and does not occur with such agents in the lumbar region unless a volume large enough to cause an ascending epidural block to the thoracic level is injected or inadvertent subarachnoid injection occurs. Studies using healthy adult patients have shown that anesthetic blockade to the T5 level caused only minimal cardiac changes provided that bradycardia was avoided.[82,173] Complete sympathetic blockade to the T1 level is associated with potentially more serious complications, including decreased cardiac output, decreased mean arterial pressure, and decreased peripheral resistance requiring cardiovascular support measures.[51]

Acute cardiac complications can result from an intravascular injection of lidocaine or bupivacaine, the most significant of which is decreased cardiac contractility. Previous studies have shown, however, that excellent cardiovascular function is maintained in humans with plasma lidocaine concentrations of 4–8 μg/ml.[110] Also, serious cardiac complications from lidocaine toxicity are thought to occur at plasma lidocaine concentrations that are about seven times higher than the concentration causing CNS seizure activity.[133] Large doses of bupivacaine in particular have been shown to have the potential to cause depression of both myocardial contractility and cardiac conduction resulting in resistant bradycardia and ventricular arrhythmias.[154] In human volunteers though, slow IV injection of bupivacaine to achieve plasma concentrations equivalent to those occurring during epidural anesthesia failed to cause any significant cardiovascular changes.[126]

Other than the use of excessive dosages, the most serious complications occur when local anesthetics to be given epidurally are inadvertently injected into the subdural or subarachnoid space or given intravascularly. Although many factors determine the spread and effect of a subarachnoid anesthetic injection, the level of the injection and the total dosage of the anesthetic are most important. Obviously, cervical and thoracic level blocks pose a greater risk for possible cardiac, autonomic, or central nervous system complications. For most LESIs done at the L3–L4 level or below, a typical single dose of 10 ml of 1% lidocaine or 0.25% bupivacaine inadvertently injected in the subarachnoid space may cause a complete sensory or even motor block (less likely with bupivacaine), but would typically be limited to the sacral and lumbar levels.[32] More superior levels of spinal anesthesia are possible from a lumbosacral approach, however, and all the appropriate equipment should be immediately available to manage any cardiovascular, neurologic, or respiratory sequelae. In fact, the maximum single dose recommended for a

lidocaine subarachnoid injection is 100 mg, which is equivalent to 10 ml of 1% lidocaine, a dosage frequently used with epidural corticosteroid injections.

Improper subarachnoid needle placement during an epidural injection can be identified with the use of fluoroscopy. In addition, a 3–5 ml test dose of local anesthetic before the injection of the total volume of anesthetic and corticosteroid can help prevent complications. The onset of significant sensory changes within 3–5 minutes of the test dose strongly suggests subarachnoid rather than epidural placement and can be used to prevent possible serious side effects occurring with improper needle placement. Accidental intravascular administration of local anesthetics is relatively common in epidural injections but can be virtually eliminated with the use of fluoroscopy.[200]

Corticosteroids

The corticosteroids most commonly used for epidural injection of methylprednisolone acetate, triamcinolone diacetate, and betamethasone (Celestone Soluspan). Andrade[7] presented a study of epidural corticosteroid side effects in 301 patients and listed the following possible effects: insomnia, mood swings, euphoria, depression, postinjection pain flare, facial erythema, fluid retention, hypertension, congestive heart failure, hyperglycemia, headache, gastritis, and menstrual irregularities. The study examined side effects occurring 5–7 days after patients received 3–12 mg of betamethasone. The most common problems were insomnia (39%), facial erythema (29%), nausea (21%), rash and pruritus (8%), and "fever" (10%, although no patient was found to have an oral temperature higher than 100°F). About 14 days after LESI, no persistent complaints were reported, and Andrade concluded that the majority of side effects after LESIs were temporary. Most of these side effects are clearly associated with the systemic absorption of corticosteroid and subsequent transient hypercorticism. Burn and Langdon[38] documented depressed plasma cortisol levels occurring for about 2 weeks after epidural methylprednisolone injection with a return to normal levels within 3 weeks. Raff et al.[150] reported chronic suppression of adrenocorticotropic hormone (ACTH) secretion and decreased plasma cortisol levels for 3 months in patients receiving 80 mg of triamcinolone at weekly intervals for 3 weeks. These corticosteroid effects constitute a valid reason for avoiding an arbitrarily scheduled series of epidural injections.

The development of Cushing's syndrome from epidural corticosteroid injections with more prolonged abnormalities is rare, but also has been documented. Cushing's syndrome was noted in four patients receiving 300–600 mg of epidural methylprednisolone over 3 days, although this represents a higher total corticosteroid dose than most recommendations suggest.[114] Tuel[185] reported a case of Cushing's syndrome with cushingoid appearance and an undetectable plasma cortisol level after one CESI of 60 mg of methylprednisolone. The patient's signs and symptoms developed over 1 month and resolved after about 4 months. Patients suffering from severe symptomatic adrenal suppression and decreased plasma cortisol after an epidural corticosteroid injection should be diagnosed, if possible, before being subjected to additional significant stressors in order to avoid a possible adrenal crisis. One such stressor could be spinal surgery. Our review revealed no published cases of an adrenal crisis occurring with a spine surgery following epidural corticosteroids. In diabetic patients, complications from epidural corticosteroids due to transient hyperglycemia must be monitored closely and can usually be managed satisfactorily with frequent checks of blood sugar and adjustments in medication. Finally, congestive heart failure developing in cardiac patients after epidural corticosteroids due to fluid retention must be considered, although only one such case has been documented.[84]

Concerns regarding the use of methylprednisolone acetate for spinal injections arose in the 1970s after reports of associated chemical arachnoiditis were published.[138] At that time, subarachnoid corticosteroid injections were being done and the causative agent of the arachnoiditis was thought to be the polyethylene glycol contained in methylprednisolone, because years of similar injections with hydrocortisone did not seem to induce arachnoiditis. Animal studies have revealed no deleterious effect to neural tissue from repeated exposure to glucocorticosteroid alone.[65] Strict epidural without subarachnoid use of corticosteroid with polyethylene glycol has not been shown to cause arachnoiditis, but the potential always exists for accidental subarachnoid injection during an epidural procedure. No conclusive evidence has proven the cause and effect relationship between methylprednisolone with polyethylene glycol and arachnoiditis, so some authors continue to approve the use of this corticosteroid preparation,[14,33] whereas many physicians recommend using other corticosteroid preparations.[16,135,137,160] Soluble corticosteroid preparations, such as the betamethasone solution that we recommend, does not contain polyethylene glycol or other potentially damaging preservatives. Betamethasone should not be mixed with lidocaine or any other local anesthetic containing preservatives, such as methylparaben or propylparaben, because these additives tend to cause flocculation of the corticosteroid.

Allergic and Anaphylactic Reactions

The medications injected during epidural blocks can lead to allergic or anaphylactic reactions. Pruess[146] reported that most allergic reactions to corticosteroids are not caused by the carrier vehicle but by the corticosteroid alone. An allergic or pseudoallergic reaction in a previously nonsensitized individual may be delayed up to 1 week after depot corticosteroid injection due to the gradual systemic uptake of these medications. However, anaphylactoid reactions (without a histologic immune response) or actual anaphylaxis (with a histologic immune response) occur most often within 2 hours after the epidural injection but have been known to develop up to 6 hours later.[172] Regardless of the cause, fatalities from anaphylactoid reactions and anaphylaxis are generally caused by respiratory-related complications involving mechanical airway obstruction.[83] We found no cases of fatal anaphylaxis following an epidural corticosteroid injection in the literature. Close patient monitoring after epidural injection is recommended for approximately 30 minutes, as well as direct patient access to an informed on-call physician after an injection in case of delayed but emergent complications.

Medical Complications

Systemic Complications

Relatively few serious complications occur in patients receiving epidural corticosteroid injection from well-trained and experienced clinicians. For CESIs, Waldman[190] performed 790 injections and reported three episodes of vasovagal syncope (two of which required treatment with IV fluids and ephedrine), one superficial infection at the injection site, and two unintentional dural punctures. Cicala et al.[46] did 204 CESIs and noted one instance of intermittent nausea and vomiting lasting 12 hours, one episode of transient upper extremity weakness, and two dural punctures without sequelae.

For LESIs, Brown[36] reported no serious side effects in 500 patients, and White[198] quoted a rate for significant complications of about 0.4% after lumbar epidural injections in 300 patients. Minor medical complications from LESIs include headache, dizziness, transient hypotension, nausea, and transient aggravation of back pain or leg pain.[12,63] Some of these minor complications are apparently due to the injection of the corticosteroid into the epidural space.[17] Headache without dural puncture occurs occasionally, especially after injection of a large volume of epidural fluid. The incidence of such headaches has been estimated at 2%[91] and attributed to air injected into the epidural space, increased intrathecal pressure from the fluid injected around the dural sac, or possibly an undetected dural puncture.[4] A temporary increase in the patient's back or leg pain for 24–48 hours after epidural corticosteroid injection has been reported to occur 1–2% of the time either due to tissue irritation from the corticosteroid itself or from the rate or volume of the injectate and generally requires no treatment.[12,48,91]

Dural Puncture and Associated Headache

Unintentional dural punctures during epidural corticosteroid injections occur even in the hands of experienced physicians. The incidence of dural puncture during a cervical or lumbar epidural injection done by experienced physicians is estimated in the anesthesia literature as ranging from 0.5–1%,[58,148] 0–2%,[140] and up to 5%.[23] The incidence of dural punctures with caudal epidural injection is much lower, as expected and reported by White[199] as 2 dural punctures out of 2,000 caudal injections. If needle advancement is not carefully controlled during an injection, a dural puncture may be associated with direct spinal cord trauma for any block at or above the L2 level. All documented reports of needle injuries to the spinal cord occurring during spinal injections state that patients complained immediately of severe lancinating pain at or below the dermatomal level of needle placement at the time of the injury.[51] Following laminectomy, midline or paramedian epidural injection at the level of the surgery is not recommended because the epidural space may be obliterated due to scarring leading to a subarachnoid injection; performing the block at a level above or below the surgery site or with a transforaminal approach is recommended.[205]

After accidental penetration of the dura, injection of even small volumes of local anesthetics may cause complete and ascending spinal anesthesia. Subarachnoid placement of the needle can usually be detected with fluoroscopy and a 3–5 ml test dose of 1% lidocaine before more anesthetic or corticosteroid is injected. However, a negative test dose does not guarantee epidural needle placement, and continued close observation is necessary.[51] Following

an accidental dural puncture, White[199] suggests relocating the needle at a different interspace and injecting only corticosteroid with saline or sterile water to avoid possible complications from subarachnoid anesthetics.

The incidence of postdural puncture headaches in the anesthesia literature ranges from 7.5–75%[64] and depends significantly on needle size, with the highest estimates of 75% associated with 16- and 18-gauge epidural needles.[54,55] Lambert[117] reported postdural puncture headache requiring blood patch in 75% of patients with 17-gauge epidural needle use versus 13–39% of patients with 25- to 27-gauge spinal needles. Also, conical non-cutting needletip injections required significantly fewer blood patches than beveled cutting needle procedures. In addition to headache, dural punctures that remain patent also can be associated with early decreased hearing acuity and, less commonly, dysfunction of various cranial nerves presumably secondary to CSF leakage. As mentioned, not all headaches developing after an epidural corticosteroid injection are due to dural punctures. The clinical features of a postdural puncture headache include delayed onset of several to about 48 hours, most severe pain with an upright position, and often total resolution in the supine or prone position. The most likely mechanism of postdural puncture headaches is loss of CSF through the puncture site with resultant tension on cranial meningeal vessels and nerves, as well as reflex vasodilatation, thereby causing pain.[37] Early conservative care involves 24–48 hours of bed rest, intake of oral fluid increased to 3 liters per day, oral analgesics as needed, and occasionally an abdominal binder.[32] Another treatment option involves the use of oral or intravenous caffeine, which has been shown to be safe and often effective, although the recurrence rate following caffeine treatment is significant.[136] If resolution of the headache is not achieved in 1–2 weeks with more conservative management, then an epidural blood patch may be needed, which has a success rate of 90–95% and can be repeated once as necessary.[2,136] The procedure for the administration of a blood patch is presented in the Technical Considerations section of this chapter.

Durocutaneous fistulas after epidural corticosteroid injections are rare but have been reported and usually occur after multiple attempts are made to enter the epidural space at the same level using large-bore needles or a series of repeated injections at the same level.[11,89,108] Contributing factors are a blunt perforation of the skin with a large epidural needle or the deposition of substances along the needle tract such as corticosteroid or blood, which then interferes with proper healing of the tract. Recommendations to avoid dural fistula formation include flushing the corticosteroid solution out of the needle prior to withdrawal, cleaning the needle or using a new needle before attempting another injection, and puncturing the skin surface with a sharp introducer needle before pushing a blunt epidural needle through the skin.[108] Durocutaneous fistulas have been successfully treated with both blood patches and primary surgical closure of the dura and skin defect.[123]

With regard to cervical epidural injections, Hodges et al.[102] reported two cases of apparent permanent, intrinsic focal spinal cord injury with associated pain symptoms occurring in patients receiving these injections under fluoroscopic guidance. Both patients were apparently noncommunicative due to IV sedation during the actual spine injection. The authors stress the importance of maintaining verbal communication with the patient throughout the procedure to avoid unexpected spinal cord needle injury during cervical epidural procedures.

Epidural Abscess and Hematoma

Epidural abscess or hematoma formation following an epidural injection is the most serious potential complication of this procedure. Epidural abscess formation following an injection of corticosteroids is extremely rare and is almost always associated with the use of an epidural catheter. Baker[10] reviewed reported cases of epidural abscesses, and only one case in the 39 reviewed was from a single-shot epidural corticosteroid injection. Most of the other cases followed the use of an epidural catheter for spinal anesthesia in patients with preexisting systemic infections. No apparent increase in epidural abscess formation was associated with the use of corticosteroids during epidural procedures done on patients without systemic disease. An epidural abscess following an injection usually includes complaints of severe back pain, fever, and often chills with a leukocytosis developing about 3 days after the injection.[44] Prompt clinical evaluation and diagnosis is required for successful treatment of the infection, which is usually caused by *Staphylococcus aureus*. Immediate surgical laminectomy and debridement usually are required.[10] Patients with diabetes mellitus are possibly more susceptible to epidural abscess formation, as well as patients with a significant local or systemic infection before the epidural injection.

Epidural bleeding during injection is generally caused by damage to an epidural vein during the procedure and usually leads to minimal problems without any serious sequelae. Epidural hematoma formation with associated neurologic damage following an epidural injection is extremely rare in patients with normal blood clotting mechanisms; only one such case has been reported to date, and that case was associated with numerous epidural injections.[119] Any medications causing abnormalities in the clotting mechanism taken before the epidural injection could potentially increase the risk of an epidural hematoma. Such medications include heparin, Coumadin, aspirin, and all nonsteroidal antiinflammatory medications. Epidural injections also should be avoided in patients with a known platelet count of less than 100,000 platelets/ml.[1] Since epidural corticosteroid injection for pain management does not typically represent an emergency procedure, these procedures should be postponed until the clotting abnormalities can be corrected.

Serious concern regarding the presence of an epidural hematoma should be raised in patients complaining of severe neck or back pain associated with any significant neurologic complaints noted soon after receiving an epidural injection. Williams[202] reported a case of an epidural hematoma occurring after the seventh CESI performed in the same patient, all at the C7–T1 interspace; severe neck pain developed 20 minutes after the block and persistent sensory deficits within $2\frac{1}{2}$ hours. An immediate physical exam followed by a CT or MRI scan if necessary is essential for patients thought to have an epidural hematoma, because early surgical intervention can limit or even prevent permanent neurologic damage.[51]

The data and reports recently reviewed on the risk of dural puncture and epidural abscesses or hematoma are for posterior translaminar/transflaval epidural injections. The risk of these specific complications should be substantially lower for selective transforaminal epidural injections. However, selective epidurals have a significant risk of direct contact of the needletip to the nerve root and dorsal root ganglion if the needle traverses too deeply into the foramen.

TECHNICAL CONSIDERATIONS

Fluoroscopy

Most spine care specialists currently recommend fluoroscopy for diagnostic and therapeutic epidural injections for several reasons. Epidural injections performed without fluoroscopy are not always placed into the epidural space or at the desired interspace as intended.[74,178] Several studies have reported that experienced anesthesiologists misidentify the epidural space without the aid of fluoroscopy 25–30% of the time during lumbar epidurals and 30–40% of the time during caudal epidurals.[130,156,202] After performing many caudal procedures, El-Khoury[80] and Renfrew[155] recommended fluoroscopy due to the many variations of the sacrum and subsequent difficulty assessing proper needle location during caudal injections. Renfrew[155] used fluoroscopy after needle placement to evaluate anesthesiologists performing blind caudal injections to document how many needles were initially placed in the epidural space. He found that for experienced physicians caudal epidural needle placement was achieved 62% of the time, and, even when the sacral hiatus was easily palpated, initial epidural needle placement occurred in only 78% of patients. By definition, epidurals done strictly for anesthesia involve a sensory and motor blockade, which helps confirm proper needle placement, although such signs are not obtained during most midline or paramedian epidural corticosteroid injections. During diagnostic selective epidural nerve root injections when a sensory block is routinely produced, fluoroscopy is essential for exact needle placement so only a small amount of local anesthetic can be placed as close to that specific nerve root as possible.

Epidural corticosteroids are thought to provide prolonged pain relief because of the gradual absorption of the depot corticosteroid in the vicinity of the pain-generating tissues. It follows that using fluoroscopic guidance to ensure corticosteroid placement as close as possible to the pain generator probably will yield the best results. The presence of significant anatomic anomalies such as a midline epidural septum[19] or multiple separate epidural compartments[102] can restrict the desired flow of the epidural injectants to the suspected pain generator and will remain undetected without fluoroscopy. If an epidural corticosteroid injection fails and fluoroscopy was not employed, the failure may be due to either a genuine poor response and/or to improperly placed medications. Important diagnostic information may then be lost.

Fluoroscopy also prevents accidental intravascular injections, because the absence of blood return with needle aspiration before an injection is not a reliable indicator of intravascular needle placement. For caudal epidurals, White[198] reported a 6% incidence of

intravascular needle placement documented by fluoroscopy following no blood return with needle aspiration, and Renfrew[155] noted the same in about 9% of his caudal injections. Repeated injections of nonionic contrast into the epidural space causes no apparent histologic[69] or neurologic abnormalities.[100]

The various dye patterns seen with epidural injections must be recognized to avoid complications during these injections. The pattern typically seen with contrast injected into the epidural space is a fluffy spread of dye moving quickly away from the tip of the needle (Fig. 30-7). Other images indicating inappropriate needle placement include the rapid disappearance of dye in a vascular pattern (Fig. 30-8), the limited contained spread within a fascial plane, or the typical myelographic spread of a subarachnoid injection.

Needles and Equipment

Crawford and Tuohy needles are relatively blunt needles designed specifically for epidural injections. The blunt tip of these needles is ideal for less experienced physicians because it allows easier identification of the ligamentum flavum and less chance of puncturing the dura once the needle reaches the

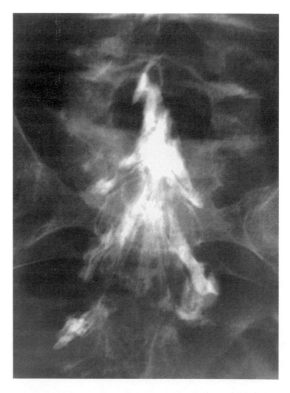

FIGURE 30-7. Caudal epidural injection contrast pattern or epidurogram.

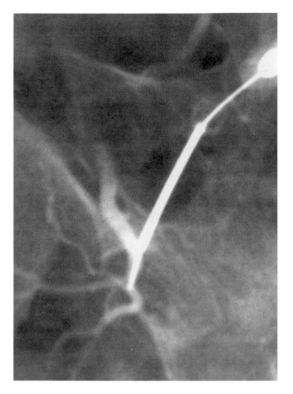

FIGURE 30-8. Vascular contrast pattern. (Courtesy of Ted Lennard, M.D.)

epidural space.[186] The curved tip of the Tuohy needle was initially designed to allow easier passage of a catheter through the needle into the epidural space. Winged needles or detachable wings for standard Tuohy needles are available for the hanging drop technique to allow the needle to be held with the fingers away from the fluid placed up to the needle hub during this technique.[51] Some experienced physicians prefer using needles designed for subarachnoid spinal procedures instead of an epidural needle for single-shot epidural injections. A 22-gauge standard spinal (Quincke-Babcock) needle is readily available and seems to be more comfortable for the patient than blunt epidural needles during an epidural injection. However, the risk of dural puncture is greater with a spinal needle because of the sharp point and medium-length cutting bevel. Most injectionists do choose the 22-gauge standard spinal needle for approaches that have less chance of a dural puncture, such as caudal approaches and single-needle selective nerve root blocks, and use epidural needles only for midline or paramedian approaches. For double-needle selective transforaminal injections, a standard 18- or 20-gauge spinal needle is inserted first, and a 23- or 25-gauge inner needle is placed through the larger

needle to complete the procedure. Other spinal needles have rounded, noncutting bevels (Green or Whitacre needles), which may decrease the risk of dural puncture and headache after accidental dural puncture as compared to standard spinal needles benefitting less experienced physicians.[32]

Whichever needle is used, the incidence of headaches after dural puncture is known to be significantly less with smaller gauge needles.[149,184,188] The incidence of dural puncture headaches also is decreased when the needle bevel is aligned parallel to the spinal axis and the longitudinal dural fibers.[131] The bevel of the needle always is placed on the same side of the needle as the notch on the hub to allow proper needle orientation during an injection, which can decrease the incidence of headaches should accidental dural puncture occur.

The supplies needed for epidural injections can be obtained in prepackaged trays (usually listed as myelogram trays), or the items can be opened separately as needed at the time of the injection. A list of essential equipment is presented in Table 30-3. One item not used for traditional anesthetic epidurals is a section of plastic IV tubing through which contrast can be injected under direct fluoroscopic view and significantly limit radiation exposure to the hands.

Identification of the Epidural Space

The standard technique used to identify needle-tip advancement into the epidural space relies on the loss of resistance to the injection of air or fluids when the needle enters the epidural space as compared to the marked resistance to injection within the tough overlying ligamentum flavum and other adjacent dense soft tissues (Fig. 30-9). Either the loss of resistance or the hanging drop technique can be

TABLE 30-3. Equipment Needed for Epidural Corticosteroid Injections

Betadine or other aseptic skin solution

Sterile drapes

Skin anesthetic: 1% lidocaine (for local anesthesia), 25- or 27-gauge, 1½-inch needles

Epidural anesthetic: 1%, 2%, 4% lidocaine or 0.25%, 0.5%, 0.75% bupivacaine as needed without preservative approved for epidural use

Epidural injection needle: 18- or 20-gauge Crawford or Tuohy needles (for midline or paramedian approach), 23- or 26-gauge Chiba needles (for double needle transforaminal approach), 22- or 25-gauge spinal needles as needed

Plastic IV tubing: 6–10 inches long

Glass syringes: 2 or 5 ml as needed

Fluoroscopy equipment

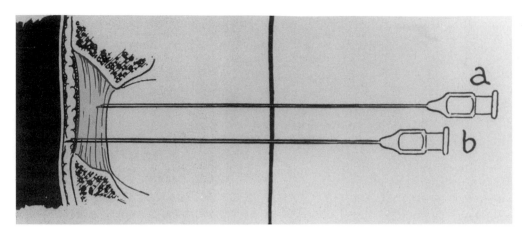

FIGURE 30-9.   Needle A entering the ligamentum flavum; needle B entering the epidural space, at which time a loss of resistance to injection would be noted. (From Macintosh RR: Lumbar Puncture and Spinal Analgesia. Edinburgh, E & S Livingstone, 1957, with permission.)

used. The loss of resistance technique traditionally uses a lubricated glass syringe partially filled with air or fluid (or both), and the substantial resistance to injection is noted while the needle is advanced through the muscle, spinous ligaments, and ligamentum flavum. For epidural injections performed on patients in the prone position under fluoroscopy, the heel of the hand being used to advance the needle is rested on the patient's back for support and control. Constant gentle pressure is placed on the syringe plunger, and significant resistance to both needle advancement and injection is noted when the needle has entered the ligamentum flavum. A noticeable loss of resistance to injection occurs as the needletip enters the epidural space. With fluoroscopy, the depth of the ligamentum flavum can be determined by first advancing the needle tip off the lamina and into the ligamentum flavum.

The hanging drop technique involves a similar process, except the needle is first filled with liquid to the top of the hub until the fluid meniscus is just visible. A winged-needle is used and advanced with a two-handed technique, and the epidural space is identified by the rapid disappearance of the fluid in the hub as it flows into the epidural space.[51] Two major disadvantages exist with the hanging drop technique. First, the increased resistance to injection characteristic of the ligamentum flavum is not experienced with the hanging drop technique, eliminating a useful landmark of needle depth. Also, a plug of epidermal or other tissues at the tip of the needle formed while advancing the needle through the skin will prevent the flow of fluid from the needle, signaling entrance into the epidural space.

Once the needle is thought to be in the epidural space, the hub should be observed for fluid dripping back from the needle, which could indicate a dural puncture with CSF drainage. Usubiaga[187] pointed out that a drip back of fluid (either dye or local anesthetic) just injected into the epidural space can occur possibly because of poor compliance of the epidural space and generally worsened by a rapid rate or increased volume of injection. Drip back of injected fluids, not CSF, usually ceases within 30 seconds as epidural pressure reequilibrates. In addition, a characteristic epidural dye flow pattern seen with fluoroscopy is most indicative of proper epidural needle position. The lack of fluid return with aspiration along with a negative test dose also indicates proper epidural needle placement.

Volume and Rate of Injection

Determining the most effective volume of injectate, especially for LESIs, has been considered since the onset of epidural injections. Large volumes of fluid, usually saline, have been recommended in the past for lumbar epidurals in the treatment of back and leg pain.[63] As the volume of injectate increases, however, gradually decreasing cephalad spread occurs as fluid spills out of the spinal canal through the paravertebral foramen. White[198] reported dye flow from the lumbar epidural space through the neural foramen often at volumes as low as 5–10 ml. According to Harley,[91] 10 ml of dye injected at the L4–5 interspace usually spreads from the L1 to the S5 level and is a sufficient volume to bathe the areas involved in most lumbar disc derangements. For caudal epidurals, however, reliable spread is thought to occur up to the L4–5 level only, and injection at a more cephalad interspace should be used for disc lesions above the L4–5 level.[81] From these considerations, the most appropriate volume for lumbar midline, paramedian, and caudal epidural injections is 10–15 ml. There is no conclusive evidence that epidural corticosteroid injections using a greater volume provide more reliable pain relief. Smaller volumes are generally used for cervical epidurals ranging from 3–7 ml, although Cicala[46] used 10–15 ml without a noticeable increase in complications. Smaller volumes are needed for selective nerve root blocks, especially with local anesthetics, to maintain the diagnostic quality of the block. Bogduk[24] and Derby[66] recommend injecting only 1–2 ml of contrast and a 1–2 ml mixture of anesthetic and corticosteroid to limit injectate spread to a single nerve root as much as possible.

The rate of epidural injection does not appreciably change the ultimate spread of injectate.[38] Faster rates of injection are, however, thought to be associated with more pain during and after the epidural block.[70] The rate of epidural lidocaine injection causes only minimal changes in the maximum resulting lidocaine plasma concentration. Scott[165] reported an increase in the maximum plasma lidocaine concentration of just 16% when the anesthetic was injected within 15 seconds versus 60 seconds. The two most important reasons for injecting epidural solutions slowly over a 3–5 minute period are to decrease pain and to allow the best chance to identify complications from local anesthetics such as vasovagal reactions or accidental subarachnoid placement.

Patient Selection and Monitoring

The initial evaluation needed before a patient is scheduled for an epidural corticosteroid injection should include a review of any pertinent medical conditions. Each patient should be asked about conditions such as diabetes, past and present infections or immunocompromising conditions, blood clotting abnormalities or treatments, previous allergic reactions, previous injections, and the possibility of pregnancy. For cervical injections, the lack of controlled data makes informed selection of patients for CESI with respect to diagnosis and duration of symptoms difficult. As mentioned previously, the literature seems to indicate better results in patients with spondylosis (cervical arthritis, disc degeneration), cervical radiculopathy and radiculitis, cervical disc herniation, and spinal stenosis. Patients with radiculopathy and associated sensory or motor

deficits generally respond well, at least temporarily, to CESIs.[77] According to Rowlingson and Kirschenbaum,[161] a negative EMG does not correlate with a poor response to CESI. Certainly, all patients receiving a CESI should receive conservative treatments (time for possible spontaneous recovery, oral medications, and therapy) and obtain only partial pain relief before being considered for a CESI due to the infrequent but potentially serious side effects of the injection.

No well-documented guidelines exist for the timing of an initial CESI, although much of the published outcome data for CESI involved patients having neck pain for 6 months (but some up to 60 months) before receiving their first CESI.[77,148,161] Ferrante noted no correlation between outcome and duration of symptoms in his patients with a median duration of symptoms of 10.5 months (range 1–60 months). No thorough prospective studies have evaluated the necessity or the optimal time interval for repeat CESIs. Although some physicians employ a series of two or three CESIs spaced days or weeks apart, we recommend a more conservative approach. Patients who do not achieve significant pain relief (more than 50%) lasting for at least 2 weeks rarely have a significant component of inflammatory pain. More often, patients who do not respond significantly to CESI have residual neck pain of a mechanical origin, and a repeat CESI does not result in further pain relief. Any repeat injections should not be done sooner than 2 weeks, because the anti-inflammatory effect of the first dose is still present at least up to 2 weeks after a CESI.[38] Another reason for not repeating CESIs on a scheduled 1- or 2-week interval is the significant number of patients with prolonged excellent pain relief from a single injection.[46] Probably no more than three CESIs are appropriate within 12 months due to possible cumulative side effects from the total dose of corticosteroids given.

Absolute contraindications for CESIs include significant local or systemic infection or any current anticoagulation treatments. Although no uniform guidelines exist, Cicala[46] discouraged CESI in patients with a "grossly" herniated disc or severe spinal canal stenosis. Obviously, extreme caution is needed for any CESI in a patient with a disc herniation or stenosis, especially in regard to the volume of injectate used.

Thoracic epidural corticosteroid injections can be used in patients with thoracic pain from intercostal neuralgia due to trauma or herpes,[79,80] thoracic disc herniation with or without radicular pain,[26] and chronic axial somatic pain.[130] It is imperative that viscerogenic sources of thoracic pain be excluded before performing a TESI. Timing of initial and repeat injections is performed as recommended in the previous section on CESIs.

For LESIs, no universally accepted guidelines exist regarding patient selection and timing of injections, although more informed choices are possible due to the larger base of clinical data versus cervicothoracic injections. According to Gamburd,[81] White et al.,[200] and Benzon,[13] LESIs are most effective in patients with pain of discogenic origin, especially if the condition is acute, involves a significant disc bulge or herniation, and is associated with significant radicular pain. Patients having internal disc disruption from an annular tear without significant disc degeneration or radicular pain respond less often to epidural corticosteroids.[81] Lumbar spinal stenosis is another diagnosis that will usually have a good, but often time-limited, response to LESI.[81,103,199] For any diagnosis, Jamison[107] listed the following factors associated with poor response to LESI: (1) numerous previous treatments for pain without any improvement, (2) current use of multiple medications, and (3) back pain that does not increase with activities.

Clinically, initial LESIs are often recommended and performed sooner than the first CESI, probably due to physicians having more experience with LESIs and the less severe potential iatrogenic sequelae. Approximately 85–90% of cases of acute low back pain resolve within 6–12 weeks, and allowing sufficient time for recovery without unnecessary treatments is important in patients showing gradual improvement.[6,7,201] However, several studies document better results for LESIs given within the first 3 months of low back or radicular pain.[91,145,199] Other factors must be considered when scheduling a patient's initial epidural injection, including (1) the failure of less invasive interventions, (2) the severity of the patient's pain and the need for pain control, (3) the use or misuse of oral analgesics, (4) the patient's ability to perform self-care activities, (5) the avoidance of hospitalization, (6) the facilitation of active rehabilitation, and (7) the allowance of an earlier return to work.[81] Routinely, the earliest an initial LESI is usually performed is about 6 weeks after the onset of back or radicular pain if other treatments are not effective. However, an LESI may be appropriate sooner if alternative pain management techniques are failing, especially in patients with severe radicular pain since there is a higher success rate from LESIs for this diagnosis. An experienced physician does not necessarily need a CT or MRI scan before giving an LESI, and the epidural injection can be done based on clinical judgment alone.[81] However, many physicians prefer to obtain a CT or MRI scan before performing a midline or paramedian epidural to assess the target epidural space.

No clear rationale exists for performing a series of LESIs at predetermined intervals since a positive response often lasts 4–8 weeks and sometimes longer. Also, a small percentage of patients with acute back with or without leg pain recover after one injection. It is generally accepted that if the initial epidural injection provides no relief, repeat injections are not recommended.[13,24,151,180,193] These authors also recommend a total of three LESIs per year due to possible cumulative side effects. Stambaugh[164] recommended the following absolute contraindications for LESIs: (1) cauda equina syndrome, (2) anticoagulation or bleeding disorder, and (3) suspected local or systemic infection.

Epidural corticosteroid injections at all levels of the spine are appropriate for an outpatient setting provided that all necessary resuscitative equipment is available, including oxygen, intubation equipment, and emergency drugs. For CESIs, Cicala[46] recommended always having IV access, monitoring pulse and blood pressure every 5 minutes during the injection, observing the patient for 45 minutes after the injection, and making a follow-up phone call 24 hours after the injection. Waldman[190] stated that IV access was not necessary for every patient receiving a CESI due to increased costs for the injection, risk of thrombophlebitis, and additional patient discomfort. He did suggest placing an IV in patients for whom IV access might be difficult during an emergency, such as obese patients or patients receiving previous chemotherapy or having peripheral vascular disease. Waldman also recommended premedicating overly anxious patients to prevent complications secondary to movement or hypertension during the injection. If patients are to receive any IV sedatives during an epidural injection, continuous monitoring of pulse, blood pressure, and respiratory status is advisable. Patients receiving IV sedatives should not be allowed to drive after the injection, and transportation should be arranged before the procedure. We strongly recommend IV access in all patients undergoing CESI along with equipment to monitor blood pressure, pulse, and oxygen saturation. We also advise postinjection monitoring of pulse and blood pressure every 15 minutes for about 45 minutes before releasing the patient after a CESI.

Epidural injections in the lumbosacral spine are typically associated with fewer and less serious side effects. Routine IV access is not needed for lumbar or caudal epidurals done under fluoroscopy and using limited volumes of local anesthetics. Obviously, adequate resuscitative equipment for any potential complication should be readily available. Close observation of the patient's condition, which may include blood pressure and pulse checks every 15–20 minutes, should be provided for about 30–45 minutes after any lumbosacral injection. Careful assistance with ambulation immediately following an epidural injection should be provided for every patient, especially if any sensory changes are noted after the block.

All medications used in the ACLS protocols for emergency resuscitation must be readily available. Ephedrine can often be used effectively for the treatment of mild to moderate hypotension in addition to any IV fluids that may be needed. Also, atropine alone often can be used to successfully treat transient bradycardia associated with vasovagal reactions occurring during an injection. Finally, flumazenil (Roazicon), which is a benzodiazepine antagonist, should be available if any patients are to receive IV sedation with a benzodiazepine.

Careful evaluation of the patient's response to both the diagnostic anesthetic portion of the block and the more prolonged therapeutic steroid anti-inflammatory portion can provide useful clinical information about that patient's spine condition. For midline or paramedian CESIs, Cicala[45] noted that transient upper extremity warming with tingling paresthesias following injection of epidural lidocaine was an indication of a well-placed injection. Similar symptoms in the legs following a midline or paramedian LESI with either partial or complete sensory block, including the painful dermatomes, suggests appropriate placement of the injectate. During sensory blockade, more detailed information regarding the pain response can be obtained with postinjection pain diagrams or diaries and provocative maneuvers including spine mobilization, straight-leg raising, and repetitive static or dynamic spine loading. An assessment of the patient's pain-coping abilities also can be gauged by the response to the pain and stress of the injection and the response to a common pain stimulus, such as local subcutaneous lidocaine infiltration.

For selective nerve root blocks, the onset of decreased sensation in an extremity restricted to a single dermatome corresponding to the level of the injection indicates a successful technique. The relief of radicular pain and negative responses to provocative maneuvers after the anesthetic block helps document the pain being generated from that specific nerve root. Complete pain relief of both spine (either neck or low back) and extremity pain after a selective epidural confirms the epiradicular tissues or dural sleeve as the source of both the somatic and radicular pain.[67] Complete relief of extremity pain without significant relief of spine pain suggests that the radicular pain is generated by the nerve root at the injected level, but the spine pain may be of a different origin. Selective epidural injections providing only partial relief may be followed by zygapophyseal joint and medial branch blocks and occasionally by discography to further define the pain generators as clinically indicated.

Choosing the Injection Approach

Many authors with vast experience performing epidural corticosteroid injections advocate injecting the anesthetic and corticosteroid as close as possible to the suspected pain generator. The choice of approach to the epidural space in any specific patient should be made with such localization in mind. Nonradicular cervical pain is one exception in which particular levels (C6–C7, C7–T1) are used almost exclusively for epidural injection due to technical and safety factors. A paramedian approach is appropriate for the treatment of corresponding paracentral disc herniation in the cervical, thoracic, or lumbar spine.

Lumbar nerve root blocks were first used to diagnose the source of radicular pain when imaging studies indicated more than one possible level of nerve root injury.[67] Localization of the needle near the nerve root relied on provocation of leg pain from physical irritation of the needletip just lateral to the foramen. A selective epidural injection is a variation of a selective nerve root injection and places anesthetic and steroid into the epiradicular membrane immediately surrounding the nerve root, dorsal root ganglion, spinal nerve, and ventral ramus.[142] Selective epidural injections are meant to infiltrate all the anatomic sites where pathology can affect the nerve from the paramedian annulus to the far-lateral extraforaminal region. Selective epidural injections also can be used to treat axial pain and may be a more reliable approach for delivering corticosteroid to the posterior annulus to treat midline and paracentral disc injuries.[24] Significant flow of injectate to the anterior epidural space adjacent to the posterior disc has been documented following

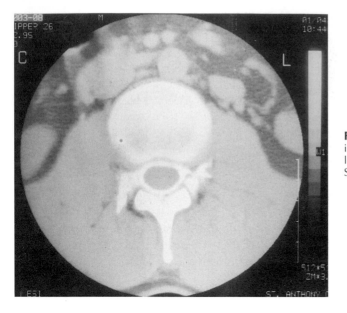

FIGURE 30-10. CT radiograph of contrast medium in the anterior and posterior lumbar epidural space following a translaminar epidural injection. (Courtesy of Stephen Andrade, M.D.)

posterior translaminar approach[6a] (Fig. 30-10), and similar studies are in progress for a transforaminal approach. It is important to understand that, based on the anatomy of a spinal nerve and its branches, a selective epidural injection at one level may anesthetize the dura and dural nerve root sleeves up to two segments caudally and one segment rostrally, the PLL and disc at the same level and one segment rostrally, and the Z-joints at the same level and one segment below. Therefore, in patients with predominantly axial pain, fully diagnosing the source of pain may require facet joint and/or disc injections.[142]

Occasionally, a transforaminal approach and a midline or paramedian approach is used in combination to ensure adequate spread of medication in the lateral foramen and central canal.[81] Midline or paramedian approaches should not be attempted routinely at postlaminectomy levels, and either an interspace just above or below the surgical scar should be chosen or a caudal or transforaminal approach should be used. The caudal epidural approach is used routinely for patients having suspected L5–S1 discogenic pain without unilateral radicular pain and is usually not recommended for patients thought to have a significant pain generator above the L4–5 level.

EPIDURAL INJECTION TECHNIQUE

Cervical Epidural Injections

Paramedian Approach

Cervical epidural injections should routinely be done at the C7–T1 interspace unless previous posterior cervical spine surgery has been performed

at this level, in which case the C6–C7 or T1–T2 level is substituted. The patient is placed in the prone position, and the skin at the appropriate level is prepared and draped aseptically. Under fluoroscopic view, the lamina forming the inferior border of the target interspace is identified and marked 2–3 cm lateral to the midline. Using a 1.5 inch, 25- or 27-gauge needle, a skin wheal is raised with 1% lidocaine, and the subcutaneous tissues are infiltrated down to the lamina under intermittent fluoroscopic control. A bicarbonate solution can be added to the lidocaine to reduce the burning sensation caused by the anesthetic. The skin needle is removed, and a nick is made in the skin with an 18-gauge needle before inserting the epidural needle down to the lamina under fluoroscopic control. The needle is then walked superiorly and medially off the edge of the lamina into the tough ligamentum flavum at or 1–2 mm lateral to the midline. The stylet is removed, and a syringe (often glass) filled with 2 ml of saline and 2 ml of air is attached to the epidural needle. Using a controlled grip with the hand holding the needle supported on the patient's back, the needle is slowly advanced while the other hand applies continuous pressure to the syringe. Loss of resistance should be felt within a few millimeters of needle advancement. Once loss of resistance is noted, aspiration to check for blood or CSF should be performed. If one is unsure if loss of resistance has been obtained, confirmation of position is critical by attempting aspiration followed by injection of a contrast agent. It is important to avoid the temptation to progress the needle deeper before documenting its location when a partial loss of

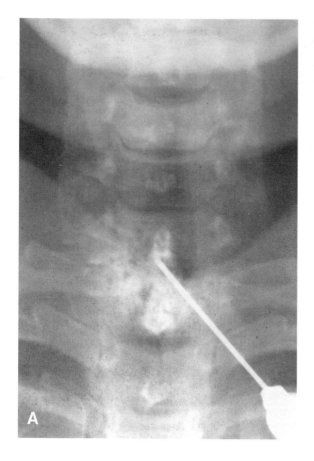

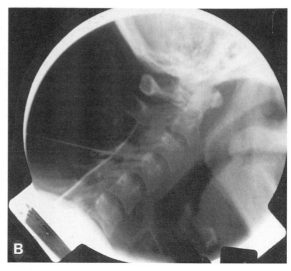

FIGURE 30-11. *A,* Anteroposterior view cervical epidurogram demonstrating a characteristic C7–T1 epidural contrast flow pattern. *B,* Lateral radiograph of a cervical epidurogram. (Courtesy of Paul H. Dreyfuss, M.D.)

resistance has been noted. Unless caution is exercised, inadvertent puncture of the dura and injury to the spinal cord may occur. After negative aspiration, a nonionic contrast agent may slowly be injected under direct fluoroscopic visualization looking for the spread of the contrast agent in the epidural space. Once the epidural space has been identified and confirmed radiographically (Fig. 30-11), a test dose of 1–2 ml of lidocaine is given. If there are no complaints of warmth, burning, significant paresthesias, or signs of apnea within 1–3 minutes, the corticosteroid preparation is slowly injected. After the injection, the needle is removed, the skin cleaned and a bandage is applied.

Some physicians perform cervical epidural injections with the patient in a sitting position with the head and chest supported and using C-arm fluoroscopy with a lateral view to document an epidural contrast pattern.[73a]

Transforaminal Approach

The cervical transforaminal approach or selective nerve root block is started by identifying the target neuroforamen with the patient in either the prone or oblique position. In the oblique position, the C2–3 foramen is both the most superior and the largest of all the cervical foramen. The foramen and associated nerve root levels can be counted down from the C2–3 level. The injection is performed with the patient in an oblique position with the side to be treated elevated and supported with pillows under the shoulder and back. Using C-arm fluoroscopy, the x-ray beam can be angled to more easily obtain an adequate oblique view. The skin over the target foramen is prepared and draped aseptically, and a local anesthetic is injected carefully down to the level of the bony posterior edge of the neuroforamen. A 25-gauge spinal needle is then advanced down to the posteroinferior edge of the neuroforamen until bone is contacted. The needle is slowly walked off the bone into the foramen and advanced only a few millimeters and no further medial than the midpoint of the adjacent pedicle, as seen in an anteroposterior (AP) projection. Care must be taken not to advance the needle too far medial where the nerve root and epidural veins are located. Needle position can be evaluated by rotating the C-arm to an AP view and slowly injecting 0.5 ml of contrast material under direct fluoroscopic view. An acceptable dye pattern includes filling of the round neuroforamen and

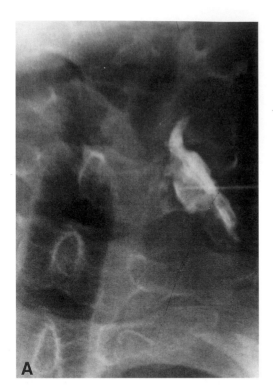
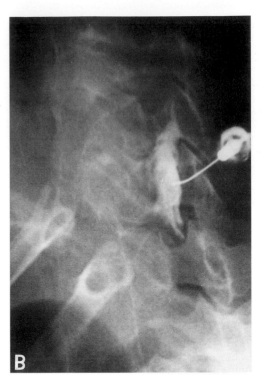

FIGURE 30-12.   *A*, Anteroposterior view cervical selective nerve root injection contrast pattern. *B*, Oblique view cervical selective nerve root injection. (Courtesy of Paul H. Dreyfuss, M.D.)

preferably contrast flow along the exiting nerve root (Fig. 30-12). The patient may often experience mild to moderate radiating arm pain during the injection of fluid into the foramen. Once an adequate dye pattern is achieved, about 2 ml of 1–2% lidocaine can be injected and the patient's response monitored

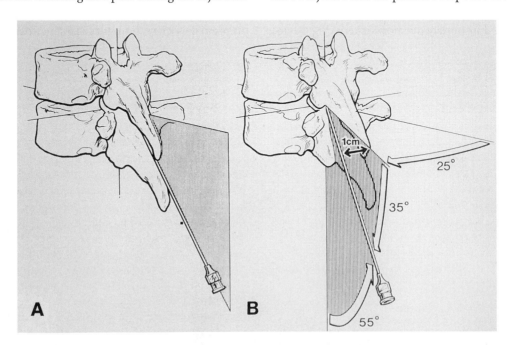

FIGURE 30-13.   Thoracic spine midline (A) and paramedian (B) epidural injection needle positions. (From Cousins MJ, Bromage PR: Epidural neural blockade. In Cousins MJ, Bridenbaugh PO (eds): Neural Blockade in Clinical Anesthesia and Management of Pain. Philadelphia, J.B. Lippincott, 1988, with permission.)

for diagnostic purposes. Celestone can be mixed with the lidocaine or injected separately; a volume of 1–2 ml is recommended.

Thoracic Epidural Injections

Paramedian Approach

The paramedian approach is usually used in the thoracic spine due to the bony anatomy of the thoracic lamina. Patient preparation and equipment are similar to that employed for CESIs. The skin over the lamina at the target interspace is injected with 1% lidocaine, and local anesthetic is slowly injected down to the lamina. A small nick is made in the skin with an 18-gauge needle, and the epidural needle is introduced through the skin. The bevel of the epidural needle is oriented cephalad, and the needle is introduced at a 50–60° angle to the axis of the spine and a 15–30° angle toward midline (Fig. 30-13). With C-arm fluoroscopy, the x-ray beam can be tilted parallel to the lamina, which helps visualize the thoracic interspace and indicates the appropriate entry angle of the needle. Under fluoroscopy, the epidural needle is advanced down to the superior edge of the lamina and then walked off the edge into the ligamentum flavum at or just lateral to the midline. The loss of resistance technique is used to locate the epidural space. After negative aspiration for blood and CSF, epidural placement is confirmed by injecting 0.5–2 ml of contrast material and visualizing the appropriate dye flow pattern (Fig. 30-14).

A test dose of 1–2 ml of 1% lidocaine without preservative is injected. If the test dose is negative, the corticosteroid preparation is slowly injected.

Transforaminal Approach

The thoracic transforaminal or selective nerve root block is performed with the patient in the prone position under fluoroscopy. The target neuroforamen and adjacent pedicle is marked, and the area is prepared and draped aseptically. Local anesthetic is applied to the skin and overlying soft tissues. A 22- or 25-gauge, 3½-inch spinal needle is placed into the skin 1–2 inches lateral to the target pedicle and centered between the ribs located above and below the target neuroforamen. The needle is advanced toward the inferior border of the rib above the neuroforamen until the rib is contacted. The needle is then redirected inferiorly and medially just under the pedicle, and a lateral view can be checked to verify an appropriate position in the neuroforamen. Care must be taken to redirect the needle as medial as possible after contacting the rib to avoid a possible pneumothorax. Once the needle is placed under the pedicle and into the neuroforamen, contrast can be injected and the needle readjusted until an acceptable dye pattern with some flow medially into the lateral epidural space and preferably some flow along the exiting nerve root is observed. Lidocaine and corticosteroid solutions can be injected as described in the cervical transforaminal block section. If the patient does not have

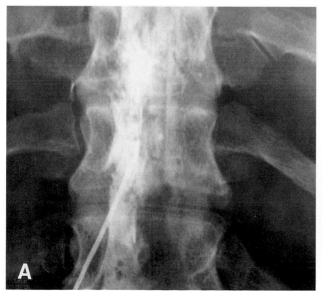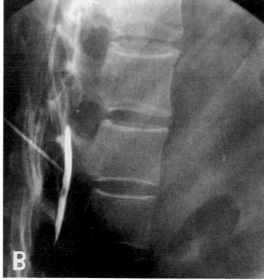

FIGURE 30-14. *A*, Anteroposterior thoracic epidurogram demonstrating a characteristic thoracic epidural contrast flow pattern. *B*, Lateral radiograph of a thoracic epidurogram. (Courtesy of Paul H. Dreyfuss, M.D.)

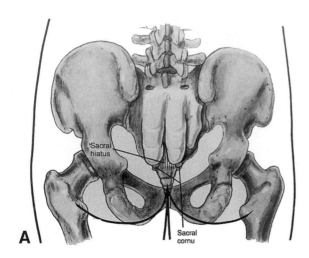
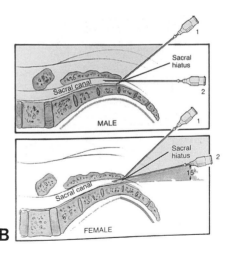

FIGURE 30-15. *A*, Schematic view of the sacrum and palpation of the sacral cornu. *B*, Needle 1 illustrates the initial angle of entry for a caudal epidural approach; needle 2 illustrates the redirected angle and advancement into the caudal epidural space. (From Brown DL: Atlas of Regional Anesthesia. Philadelphia, W.B. Saunders, 1992, with permission.)

significant immediate pain relief from the local anesthetic, repeating the injection at the level above or below should be considered because of the difficulty of localizing the exact painful level in the thoracic spine.

Lumbosacral Epidural Injections

Caudal Approach

A caudal epidural injection is started by placing the patient prone on the fluoroscopy table. The sacral region is prepared aseptically, and a fenestrated drape is placed over the midsacral region. Palpation of the sacrum with the fingers starting at the coccyx will provide a reliable bony landmark; the sacrum is then palpated superiorly until the two horns of the sacral cornu are identified (Fig. 30-15A). The sacral hiatus, which is the entry point into the caudal epidural space, lies between the cornu. While holding a finger (usually easiest with the nondominant hand) in place over the hiatus to maintain proper position, local anesthetic can be applied to the skin and then deeper to the sacral bone between the cornu. Using a 25- or 27-gauge, 1½-inch needle to slowly inject the local anesthetic is usually less painful to the patient than larger needles. A 22-gauge spinal needle is directed between the cornu at about a 45° angle with the bevel facing ventrally until the sacrum is contacted. The needle is carefully redirected more cephalad as the bony anatomy requires in the midline or slightly to the side of the patient's pain to allow entry into the caudal epidural space through the sacrococcygeal ligament (Fig. 30-15B). Once the needle is thought to be in the caudal

epidural space and a negative aspirate is achieved, nonionic contrast material is slowly injected under direct fluoroscopic view. Proper epidural placement is indicated by a typical epidural dye flow pattern (see Fig. 30-7). A dense, well-localized dye pattern indicates a subcutaneous position above the sacrum and is usually associated with increased resistance during injection. A lateral view of the sacrum with fluoroscopy can help determine both the initial and final needle placement using contrast to document adequate spread as needed. A vascular dye pattern necessitates careful withdrawal and repositioning of the needle. The volume of anesthetic and corticosteroid required to reach either the L4–5 or L5–S1 level can often be judged by the spread of dye, but at least 10 ml is generally required to reach the L5–S1 level and 15 ml to reach the L4–5 level.[22] The needle also can be carefully advanced more cephalad as superior as the S3 level to allow better flow of the injectate as desired. After appropriate needle placement is documented, the anesthetic and corticosteroid preparation may be slowly injected.

Lumbar Midline and Paramedian Approach

Lumbar epidural injections can be performed with either a midline or paramedian (also known as translaminar) approach (Fig. 30-16). Placing a pillow or cushion beneath the patient's abdomen to cause lumbar spine flexion often can facilitate lumbar epidural needle placement with the patient in a prone position. Some physicians prefer placing patients on their side and using a lateral view on fluoroscopy for a lumbar epidural injection. The midline approach is performed at the interspace

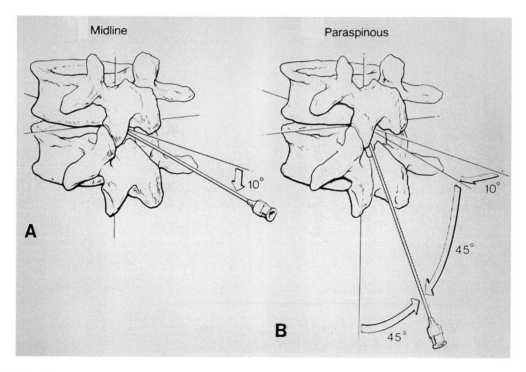

FIGURE 30-16.   Lumbar spine midline (*A*) and paramedian (*B*) epidural injection needle position. (From Cousins MJ, Bromage PR: Epidural neural blockade. In Cousins MJ, Bridenbaugh PO (eds): Neural Clinical Blockade in Clinical Anesthesia and Management of Pain. Philadelphia, J.B. Lippincott, 1988, with permission.)

most closely located to the level of the suspected source of pain, with the needle placed just below the target level due to the cephalad flow of most fluids injected into the epidural space. Fluoroscopy is used to accurately identify the appropriate interspace, and the skin is prepared aseptically. A 25- or 27-gauge needle is used to anesthetize the adjacent spinous processes. A 22- or 25-gauge, 1½-inch needle can be used to slowly anesthetize the interspinous ligament, being careful to constantly aspirate and check the resistance to injection because entry into the epidural space is possible. If an epidural needle is used, a nick in the skin is made with an 18-gauge needle and the 18- or 20-gauge epidural needle is placed through the skin. Alternatively, a 22-gauge spinal needle can be used for the injection. The needle is advanced at a slight upward angle (about 10° to horizontal) through the interspinous ligament. A 2-ml glass syringe can be used with the epidural needle to identify the epidural space by the loss of resistance technique. The hand used to advance the needle should be braced firmly against the patient's back at all times for controlled needle advancement. Proper midline needle placement during the injection can be assured by intermittent fluoroscopic imaging. Increased resistance to both needle advancement and injection with the glass syringe

can usually be detected once the needle enters the ligamentum flavum. The epidural space is then identified using the loss of resistance technique. The glass syringe is removed and the needle observed for CSF drip back. If no drip back occurs and aspiration is negative, contrast dye is slowly injected under fluoroscopy. When an appropriate epidural pattern is noted, a test dose of 3–5 ml of preservative-free 1% lidocaine is given, and the patient is monitored for several minutes. After a negative test dose, a solution of 0.5 or 1% lidocaine and corticosteroid can be slowly injected.

The technique used for a paramedian approach is identical to the midline technique except for the specific injection site. After skin preparation and marking, an epidural or spinal needle is placed 1–2 cm lateral to the caudal tip of the inferior spinous process of the target interspace on the side of the patient's pain. A more lateral needle placement is to be avoided, because such an approach increases the risk of encountering an epidural vein or adjacent nerve root. The needle is advanced under fluoroscopy until contacting the upper edge of the inferior lamina at the target interspace. The needle is walked superiorly into the ligamentum flavum, and the epidural space is identified by loss of resistance. After negative aspiration and no CSF drip back,

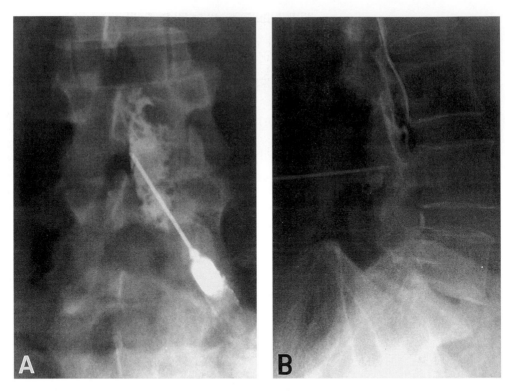

FIGURE 30-17. *A,* Anteroposterior view lumbar translaminar epidurogram demonstrating a characteristic contrast flow pattern. *B,* Lateral view lumbar translaminar epidurogram. (Courtesy of Paul H. Dreyfuss, M.D.)

contrast dye is slowly injected. If an acceptable epidural dye flow pattern is noted (Fig. 30-17) and a test dose is negative, the local anesthetic and corticosteroid solution may be injected.

Lumbar Transforaminal Approach

The patient is prepared in the prone position and fluoroscopy used to identify and mark the essential bony landmarks. Either an oblique or a posterior approach may be used with either a single- or double-needle technique. The most thorough presentation of transforaminal or selective nerve root blocks is by Derby, Bogduk, and Kine,[67] and many of the techniques described in this section were presented in their article. The bony landmark that is the target for transforaminal needle placement is just below the inferior aspect of the pedicle superior to the exiting nerve root of the "6 o'clock" position

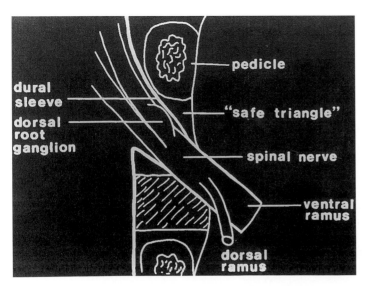

FIGURE 30-18. Schematic diagram of lumbar neuroforamen and safe triangle. (From Lutz GE, Vad VB, Wisneski RJ: Fluoroscopic transforaminal lumbar epidural steroids: An outcome study. Arch Phys Med Rehabil 79:1362–1366, 1998, with permission.)

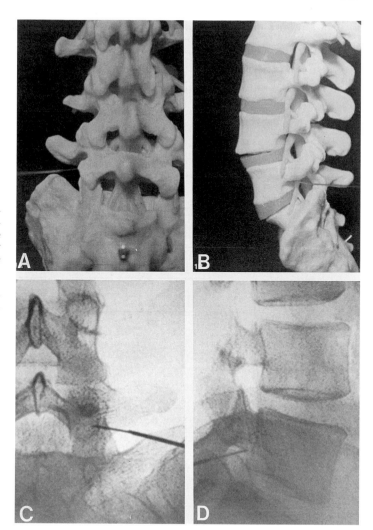

FIGURE 30-19. *A, B,* Spine model antero-posterior and lateral views, respectively, of appropriate needle position for left L5 selective nerve root injection. *C,* and *D,* Anteroposterior and lateral views, respectively, of appropriate needle position for right L5 selective epidural nerve root injection. (From Derby R, Bogduk N, Kine G: Precision percutaneous blocking procedures for localizing pain. Part 2. The lumbar neuroaxial compartment. Pain Dig 3:175–188, 1993, with permission.)

using the round pedicle as a clockface (Fig. 30-18). Derby et al.[67] describe a "safe triangle" at this location with the three sides corresponding to the horizontal base of the pedicle, the outer vertical border of the intervertebral foramen, and the connecting diagonal nerve root and dorsal ganglion. A needle placed into the safe triangle will lie above and lateral to the nerve root (Fig. 30-19).

For the oblique approach, the patient and the fluoroscopy unit are rotated as needed to provide an oblique projection of the pedicle on the side of the affected nerve root. The fluoroscopic image is adjusted until the superior articulating process is seen between the anterior and posterior edge of the vertebral body and the base of the articular process is in line with the pedicle above. After the skin and overlying tissues have been anesthetized, the needle is inserted just above the superior articulating process and directed toward the base of the pedicle. The needle is advanced slowly until bone is contacted

just below the pedicle. Nonionic contrast dye can be injected very slowly and the dye pattern assessed (Fig. 30-20). If leg paresthesias are noted as the needle approaches the neuroforamen, the needle should be withdrawn slightly (about 1 mm) and dye injected.

The posterior approach is done with the patient in the prone position and begins with the needle inserted into the skin over the lateral border of and about halfway between the two adjacent transverse processes at the target interspace. The needle is advanced slowly toward the lower edge of the superior transverse process, near its junction with the superior articular process. The needle is advanced until contacting the edge of the transverse process, at which time the needle is retracted slightly (2–3 mm) and redirected toward the base of the appropriate pedicle and advanced very slowly to the final position. The fluoroscopic dye pattern is assessed. Slightly curving the distal tip of the needle can

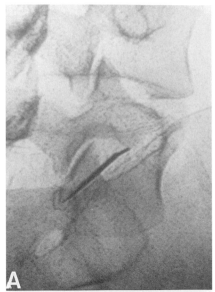

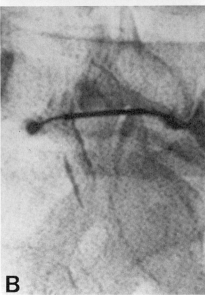

FIGURE 30-20. Lumbar spine oblique view of right L5 selective nerve root block using double-needle technique before (*A*) and after (*B*) contrast injection. (From Derby R, Bogduk N, Kine G: Precision percutaneous blocking procedures for localizing spine pain. Part 2. The lumbar neuroaxial compartment. Pain Dig 3:175–188, 1993, with permission.)

to the lower edge of the transverse process as described above. A 23- or 25-gauge, 6-inch Chiba needle is then placed through the introducer needle and redirected and advanced below the transverse process. The stiffness of the introducer needle enables easier redirection of the thinner and more flexible inner needle, which is potentially less damaging to the nerve root if contact with the nerve is made. The inner needle also can be curved at the tip and directed with the curve pointing toward the pedicle to allow easier advancement in the medial direction necessary to pass under the pedicle and into the neuroforamen.

After a needle has been placed at the 6 o'clock position of the pedicle, 0.5–1 ml of contrast dye is injected slowly at a rate of about 1.0 ml per 20 seconds.[24] If the needle has penetrated the epiradicular membrane surrounding the nerve root, a positive image of the nerve root will be seen on fluoroscopy, indicating an acceptable needle position (Fig. 30-21). Repositioning the needletip several millimeters more inferior to the pedicle sometimes will help localize the needle closer to the nerve and within the epiradicular membrane. A more negative image of the nerve with flow of contrast in the region of the epidural fat indicates the need to carefully readjust

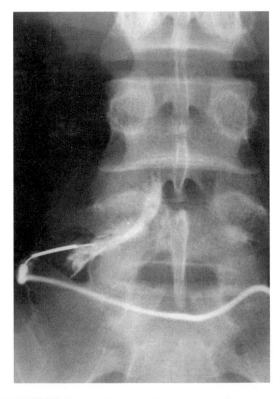

FIGURE 30-21. Left L5 selective nerve root injection contrast pattern. (Courtesy of Ted Lennard, M.D.)

facilitate precise localization of the needle into the lateral foramen. If the lateral border of the lamina can be visualized overlying the vertebral body on AP and oblique x-ray views, the needle can be inserted inferior to the transverse process and advanced slowly into the lateral foramen using the curved tip to proceed under the lamina and superior facet process.[123]

The double-needle technique is started by advancing an 18- or 20-gauge, 3½-inch spinal needle the needle to localize the tip closer to the nerve root if possible. A classic dye pattern or neurogram is not always achieved due to the patient's level of cooperation and type of local spine problem. The dye pattern may reveal pathology in the area of the exiting nerve root such as an abnormal position and course of the nerve secondary to a compressive vertebral osteophyte or lateral disc herniation. Derby et al.[67] describe other abnormal dye patterns and their possible clinical significance. After an adequate dye pattern is observed, an equal mixture of local anesthetic and corticosteroid is injected. A maximum volume of 2 ml of injectate is thought necessary to preserve the selectivity of the block to a single nerve root. Due to the small volume of local anesthetic injected, a higher concentration such as 4% lidocaine or 0.75% bupivacaine is recommended for this procedure.

The S1 nerve root also can be treated using a transforaminal approach, and a single-needle technique is usually adequate. The patient is placed in a prone position, and the S1 foramen is visualized under fluoroscopy. The S1 foramen appears as a small radiolucent circle just below the oval S1 pedicle. Using C-arm fluoroscopy, the S1 foramen is often seen best by directing the x-ray beam in a cephalocaudad direction so that the anterior and posterior foramina align. The needle is inserted slightly lateral and inferior to the S1 pedicle and advanced slowly through the posterior foramen to the medial edge of the pedicle. Care must be taken to avoid advancing the needle through both the posterior and anterior S1 foramen and into the pelvis. The appropriate depth can be gauged by first striking posterior sacral bone just above the posterior S1 foramen before directing the needle tip into the S1 neural canal. After the needle is properly located, the dye pattern is checked (Fig. 30-22) and the anesthetic and corticosteroid solution injected as with the lumbar selective nerve root blocks.

Blood Patch Procedure

The patient is first placed in the lateral or prone position depending on the physician's preference. Using strict aseptic technique, an epidural needle is placed into the epidural space using the loss of resistance technique. The needle is inserted at the same level of the spine as the previous epidural procedure at which time the dural puncture occurred. If that specific interspace is not available, the interspace one level inferior is chosen since most epidural injectates flow in a more cephalad than

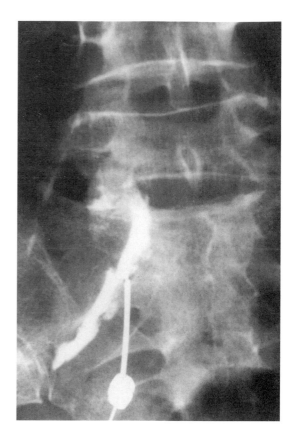

FIGURE 30-22. Left S1 selective nerve root injection contrast pattern.

caudad direction.[141] After the needle is properly placed in the epidural space, about 10–20 ml of intravenous blood is drawn into a plastic syringe also using strict aseptic technique (plastic instead of glass is used because the clotting process occurs more slowly in a plastic container). The blood is injected slowly into the epidural space, and the injection is stopped immediately if any significant pain is reported by the patient. The needle is removed and the patient is kept in the supine position for 30 minutes before being released, with no other precautions necessary. If the headache is not markedly improved or the pain returns after a brief period of relief, the procedure should be repeated once more.[141] The most effective volume of blood to inject for a blood patch has been thoroughly evaluated, and 12–15 ml seems to be both safe and effective.[55] Also, 15 ml of radioisotope-labeled blood injected into the epidural space has been shown to spread an average of nine spinal segments, providing more than adequate coverage.[181] Contraindications for an epidural blood patch are septicemia, local infection of the back, or active neurologic disease.[143]

REFERENCES

1. Abboud TK, David S, Nagappola S, et al: Maternal, fetal and neonatal effects of lidocaine with and without epinephrine epidural anesthesia in obstetrics. Anesth Analg 63:973–979, 1984.
2. Abouleish E, de la Vega S, Blendinger L: Long-term follow-up of epidural blood patch. Anesth Analg 54:459–463, 1975.
3. Abram SE: Subarachnoid corticosteroid injection following inadequate response to epidural steroid for sciatica. Anesth Analg 57:313–315, 1978.
4. Abram SF, Cherwenka RW: Transient headache immediately following epidural steroid injection. Anesthesiology 50:461–462, 1979.
5. Abram SE, Hopwood MB: What factors contribute to outcome with lumbar epidural steroids? In Bond MR, Charlton JE, Wolf DJ (eds): Proceedings of the 6th World Congress on Pain. Amsterdam, Elsevier, 1991, pp 491–496.
6. Anderson GB: Epidemiologic aspects of low back pain in industry. Spine 6:53–60, 1981.
6a. Andrade S: [Personal communication].
7. Andrade SA: Steroid side effects of epidurally administered celestone. International Spinal Injection Society 1(5), 1993.
8. Amadio JP: Peripherally acting analgesics. Am J Med 77:17–25, 1984.
9. Awwad EE, Martin DW, Smith KR Jr, et al: Asymptomatic versus symptomatic herniated thoracic discs: Their frequency and characteristics as detected by computed tomography after myelography. Neurosurgery 28:180–186, 1991.
10. Baker AS, Ojemann RG, Schwartz MN, et al: Spinal epidural abscess. N Engl J Med 293:463–468, 1975.
11. Ball CG, D'Alessandro FT, Rosenthal J, et al: Case history number 86: An unusual complication of lumbar puncture: A CSF cutaneous fistula. Anesth Analg 54:691–694, 1975.
12. Beliveau P: A comparison between epidural anesthesia with and without corticosteroid in the treatment of sciatica. Rheum Phys Med 11:40–43, 1971.
13. Benzon HT: Epidural steroid injections for low back pain and lumbosacral radiculopathy. Pain 24:277–295, 1986.
14. Benzon HT, Gissen AJ, Strichartz GR, et al: The effect of polyethylene glycol on mammalian nerve impulses. Anesth Analg 66:553–559, 1987.
15. Berman AT, Garbarino JL, Fisher S, et al: The effects of epidural injection of local anesthetics and corticosteroids on patients with lumbosciatic pain. Clin Orthop 188:144–150, 1984.
16. Bernat JL: Intraspinal steroid therapy. Neurology 31:168–171, 1981.
17. Bergquist-Ullman M, Larson U: Acute low back pain in industry. A controlled prospective study with special reference to therapy and confounding factors. Acta Orthop Scand 170(suppl):1–177, 1977.
18. Black MG, Holyoke MD: Anatomic reasons for caudal anesthesia failure. Anesth Analg 28:33–39, 1949.
19. Blomberg R: The dorsomedian connective tissue band in the lumbar epidural space in humans. Anesth Analg 65:747–752, 1986.
20. Boas RA, Cousins MJ: Diagnostic neural blockade. In Cousins MJ, Bridenbaugh PO (eds): Neural Blockade in Clinical Anesthesia and Management of Pain. Philadelphia, J.B. Lippincott, 1988, pp 885–898.
21. Bogduk N: The innervation of the lumbar spine. Spine 8:286–293, 1983.
22. Bogduk N, April C, Derby R: Precise localization of low back pain and sciatica. Presented at the International Spinal Injection Society Meeting, San Diego, 1993.
23. Bogduk N, Cherry D: Epidural corticosteroid agents for sciatica. Med J Aust 143:402–406, 1985.
24. Bogduk N, Christophidis N, Cherry D, et al: Epidural steroids in the management of back pain and sciatica of spinal origin. In Report of the Working Party on Epidural Use of Steroids in the Management of Back Pain. Canberra, Australia, National Health and Medical Research Council, 1993.
25. Bogduk N, Twomey LT: Clinical Anatomy of the Lumbar Spine, 2nd ed. New York, Churchill Livingstone, 1991.
26. Bonica JJ: Analgesic blocks for pain. In Bonica JJ, Procacci P, Pagin CA (eds): Recent Advances in Pain. Springfield, IL, Charles C Thomas, 1974, p 192.
27. Boudin G, Barbizet J, Guihard J: L'hydrocortisone intrarrachniclienne ses applications cliniques en particular dans le traitement de la méningite tuberculouse. Bull Soc Med Hop (Paris) 21:817–821, 1955.
28. Bowman SJ, Wedderburn L, Whaley A, et al: Outcome assessment after epidural corticosteroid injection for low back pain and sciatica. Spine 18:1345–1350, 1993.
29. Bowsher D: A comparative study of the azygous venous system in man, monkey, dog, cat, rat and rabbit. J Anat 88:400, 1954.
30. Braid DP, Scott DB: The systemic absorption of local analgesic drugs. Br J Anesth 37:394, 1965.
31. Breivik H, Hesla PE, Molnar I, et al: Treatment of chronic low back pain and sciatica: Comparison of caudal epidural steroid injections of bupivacaine and methylprednisolone with bupivacaine followed by saline. In Bonica JJ, Alba D, Fessard O (eds): Advances in Pain Research and Therapy. New York, Raven Press, 1976, pp 927–932.
32. Bridenbaugh PO, Greene NM: Spinal (subarachnoid) neural blockade. In Cousins MJ, Bridenbaugh PO (eds): Neural Blockade in Clinical Anesthesia and Management of Pain. Philadelphia, J.B. Lippincott, 1988, pp 213–251.
33. Bromage PR: Epidural Analgesia. Philadelphia, W.B. Saunders, 1978.
34. Bromage PR: Physiology and pharmacology of epidural analgesia. Anesthesiology 28:592–622, 1967.
35. Brown CW, Deffer PA Jr, Akmakjian J, et al: The natural history of thoracic disc herniations. Spine 17:S97–102, 1992.
36. Brown FW: Management of discogenic pain using epidural and intrathecal steroids. Clin Orthop 129:72–78, 1977.
37. Brownridge P: The management of headache following accidental dural puncture in obstetric patients. Anesth Intensive Care 11:4–15, 1983.
38. Burn JM, Langdon L: Duration of action of epidural methylprednisolone. Am J Phys Med 53:29–34, 1974.
39. Bush K, Hillier S: A controlled study of caudal epidural injections of triamcinolone plus procaine for the management of intractable sciatica. Spine 16:572–575, 1991.
40. Carr DB: Epidural steroids for radiculalgia. Journées de club anesthésie-douler 32:289–290, 1991.
41. Castagnera L, Maurette P, Pointillart V, et al: Long-term results of cervical epidural steroid injection with and without morphine in chronic cervical radicular pain. Pain 58:239–243, 1994.
42. Catchlove RF, Braha R: The use of cervical epidural nerve blocks in the management of chronic head and neck pain. Can Anesth Soc J 31:188–191, 1984.
43. Cathelin F: Mode d'action de la cocaine injecté dans l'espace epidural par le procédé de canal sacré. C R Soc Biol 53:478, 1901.
44. Chan S, Lueng S: Spinal epidural abscess following steroid injection for sciatica. Spine 14:106–108, 1984.
45. Cheng PA: The anatomical and clinical aspects of epidural anesthesia. Curr Res Anesth Analg 42:398, 1963.
46. Cicala RS, Westbrook L, Angel JJ: Side effects and complications of cervical epidural steroid injections. J Pain Symptom Manage 4:64–66, 1989.
47. Cichini MS: Epidural corticosteroid injections. J Post Anesth Nurs 7:163–166, 1992.

48. Cohn ML, Huntington CT, Byrd SE, et al: Epidural morphine and methylprednisolone: New therapy for recurrent low back pain. Spine 11:960–963, 1986.

49. Coomes EN: A comparison between epidural anesthesia and bedrest in sciatica. BMJ 1:20–24, 1961.

50. Cousins MG, Bromage PR: A comparison of the hydrochloride and carbonated salts of lignocaine for caudal analgesia in out-patients. Br J Anesth 43:1149–1154, 1971.

51. Cousins MJ, Bromage PR: Epidural neural blockade. In Cousins MJ, Bridenbaugh PO (eds): Neural Blockade in Clinical Anesthesia and Management of Pain. Philadelphia, J.B. Lippincott, 1988, pp 253–360.

52. Covino BG: Clinical pharmacology of local anesthetic agents. In Cousins MJ, Bridenbaugh PO (eds): Neural Blockade in Clinical Anesthesia and Management of Pain. Philadelphia, J.B. Lippincott, 1988, pp 111–144.

53. Covino BG, Scott DB: Handbook of Epidural Anesthesia and Analgesia. Orlando, Grune & Stratton, 1985.

54. Craft JB, Epstein BS, Coakley CS: Prophylaxis of dural-puncture headache with epidural saline. Anesth Analg 52:228–231, 1973.

55. Crawford JS: The prevention of headache consequent upon dural puncture. Br J Anesth 44:598–600, 1972.

56. Crawford JS: Epidural blood patch. Anaesthesia 40:381, 1985.

57. Crock HV: Internal disc disruption: A challenge to disc prolapse fifty years on. Spine 11:650–653, 1986.

58. Cronen MC, Waldman SD: Cervical steroid epidural nerve block in the palliation of pain secondary to intractable muscle contraction headache [abstract]. Headache 28:314–315, 1988.

59. Cuatico W, Parker JC Jr, Pappert E, et al: An anatomical and clinical investigation of spinal meningeal nerves. Acta Neurchir (Wien) 90:139–143, 1988.

60. Cuckler JM, Bernini PA, Wiesel SW, et al: The use of epidural steroids in the treatment of radicular pain. J Bone Joint Surg 67A:53–66, 1985.

61. Dallas TL, Lin RL, Wee W, et al: Epidural morphine and methylprednisolone for low back pain. Anesthesiology 67:408–411, 1987.

62. Daly P: Caudal epidural anesthesia in lumbosciatica pain. Anaesthesia 25:346–348, 1970.

63. Davidson JT, Robin GC: Epidural injections in the lumbosciatic syndrome. Br J Anesth 33:595–598, 1961.

64. Deisenhammer E: Clinical and experimental studies on headache after myelography. Neuroradiology 9:99–102, 1985.

65. Delaney T, Rowlingson RC, Carron H, et al: Epidural steroid effects on nerve and meninges. Anesth Analg 59:610–614, 1980.

66. Derby R, Bogduk N, Kine G: Precision percutaneous blocking procedures for localizing spinal pain. Part 2. The lumbar neuraxial compartment. Pain Digest 3:175–188, 1993.

67. Derby R, Kine G, Saal J, et al: Response to steroid and duration of radicular pain as predictors of surgical outcome. Spine 17:5176–5183, 1992.

68. Devor M, Gourin-Lippmann R, Raber P: Corticosteroids suppress ectopic neural discharge originating in experimental neuromas. Pain 22:127–137, 1985.

69. Dietze DD, Fessler RG: Thoracic disc herniations. Neurosurg Clin North Am 4:75–90, 1993.

70. Dilke TFW, Burry HC, Grahame R: Extradural corticosteroid injection in management of lumbar nerve root compression. BMJ 2:635–637, 1973.

71. Dirksen R, Rutgers MJ, Coolen JMW: Cervical epidural steroids in reflex sympathetic dystrophy. Anesthesiology 66:71–73, 1987.

72. Dooley JF, McBroom RJ, Taguchi T, et al: Nerve root infiltration in the diagnosis of radicular pain. Spine 13:79–83, 1988.

73. Dougherty JH, Fraser RAR: Complications following intraspinal injections of steroids; report of two cases. J Neurosurg 48:1023–1025, 1978.

73a. Dreyfuss P: [Personal communication].

74. Dreyfuss P: Epidural steroid injections: A procedure ideally performed with fluoroscopic control and contrast media. International Spinal Injection Society Newsletter 1(5), 1993.

75. El-Khoury GY, Ehara S, Weinstein JN, et al: Epidural steroid injection: A procedure ideally performed with fluoroscopic control. Radiology 168:554–557, 1988.

76. Evans W: Intrasacral epidural injection in the treatment of sciatica. Lancet 2:1225–1229, 1930.

77. Ferrante FM, Wilson SP, Iacobo C, et al: Clinical classification as a predictor of therapeutic outcome after cervical epidural steroid injection. Spine 18:730–736, 1993.

78. Flower RJ, Blackwell GJ: Anti-inflammatory steroids induce biosynthesis of a phospholipase A2 inhibitor which prevents prostaglandin generation. Nature 278:456–459, 1979.

79. Forrest JB: Management of chronic dorsal root pain with epidural steroid. Can Anaesth Soc J 25:218–225, 1978.

80. Forrest JB: The response to epidural steroid injections in chronic dorsal root pain. Can Anaesth Soc J 27:40–46, 1980.

81. Gaumburd RS: The use of selective injections in the lumbar spine. Phys Med Rehabil Clin North Am 2:79–96, 1991.

82. Germann PA, Roberts JG, Prys-Roberts C: The combination of general anesthesia and epidural block. I. The effects of sequence of induction on haemodynamic variables and blood gas measurements in healthy patients. Anaesth Intensive Care 7:229, 1979.

83. Giansiracers DF, Upchurch KS: Anaphylactic and anaphylactoid reactions. In Rippe JM, Irwin R, Alpert J, Dolen J (eds): Intensive Care Medicine. Boston, Little, Brown, 1985, pp 1102–1112.

84. Goebert HW, Jallow ST, Gardner WJ, et al: Painful radiculopathy treated with epidural injections of procaine and hydrocortisone acetate: Results in 113 patients. Anesth Analg 40:130–134, 1961.

85. Green LN: Dexamethasone in the management of symptoms due to herniated lumbar disc. J Neurol Neurosurg Psychiatry 38:1211–1217, 1975.

86. Green PW, Burke AJ, Weiss CA, et al: The role of epidural cortisone injection in the treatment of discogenic low back pain. Clin Orthop 153:121–125, 1980.

87. Gupta RC, Gupta SC, Dubey RK: An experimental study of different contrast media in the epidural space. Spine 9:778–781, 1984.

88. Gustafssan H, Rutberg H, Bengtsson M: Spinal haematoma following epidural analgesia. Anaesthesia 43:220–222, 1988.

89. Haddox JD: Lumbar and cervical epidural steroid therapy. Anesth Clin North Am 10:179–203, 1992.

90. Hakelius A: Prognosis in sciatica. Acta Orthop Scand Suppl 129:1–76, 1970.

91. Harley C: Epidural corticosteriod infiltration. A follow-up study of 50 cases. Am Phys Med 9:22–28, 1967.

92. Harrison GR, Parkin IG, Shah JL: Resin injection studies of the lumbar epidural space. Br J Anesth 57:333–336, 1985.

93. Hartman JT, Winnie AP, Ramamurthy S: Intradural and extradural corticosteroids for sciatic pain. Orthop Rev 3:21–24, 1974.

94. Hasueisen C, Smith BS, Myers SR, et al: The diagnostic accuracy of spinal nerve injection studies. Their role in the evaluation of recurrent sciatica. Clin Orthop 198:179–183, 1985.

95. Helliwell M, Robertson JC, Ellis RM: Outpatient treatment of low back pain and sciatica by a single epidural corticosteroid injection. Br J Clin Pract 39:228–231, 1985.

96. Herron LD: Selective nerve root block in patient selection for lumbar surgery. In North American Spine Society Meeting syllabus. Quebec, NASS, 1989, pp 28–29.

97. Herron LD: Selective nerve root block in patient selection for lumbar surgery—surgical results. J Spinal Disord 2:75–79, 1989.

98. Heyse-Moore G: A rational approach to the use of epidural medication in the treatment of sciatic pain. Acta Orthop Scand 49:366–370, 1978.

99. Hickey R: Outpatient epidural steroid injections for low back pain and lumbar sacral radiculopathy. N Z Med J 100:594–596, 1987.

100. Hindmarch T: Myelography with the non-ionic water-soluble contrast medium metrizamide. Acta Radiol 16:417–435, 1975.

101. Hodges SD, Castleberg RL, Miller T, et al: Cervical epidural steroid injection with intrinsic spinal cord damage. Two case reports. Spine 23:2137–2142, 1998.

102. Hogan GH: Lumbar epidural anatomy: A new look by cryomicrotome section. Anesthesiology 75:767–775, 1991.

103. Hoogmartens M, Morelle P: Epidural injection in the treatment of spinal stenosis. Acta Orthop Belg 53:409–411, 1987.

104. Hoppenstein R: A new approach to the foiled, failed back syndrome. Spine 5:371–379, 1980.

105. Howe JF, Loesser JD, Calvin WH: Mechanosensitivty of dorsal root ganglia and chronically injured axons—A physiological basis for the radicular pain of nerve root compression. Pain 3:25–41, 1977.

106. Irsigler FJ: Microscopic findings in spinal cord roots of patients with lumbar and lumbosacral disc prolapses. Acta Neurol 1:478–516, 1951.

107. Jamison RN, VadBoncouer T, Feriante FM: Low back pain patients unresponsive to an epidural steroid injection: Identifying predictive factors. Clin J Pain 7:311–317, 1991.

108. Jawalekar SR, Marx GF: Cutaneous cerebrospinal fluid leakage following attempted extradural block. Anesthesiology 54:328–349, 1981.

109. Johansson A, Hao J, Sjolund B: Local corticosteroid application blocks transmission in normal nociceptive C-fibres. Acta Anaesth Scand 34:335–338, 1990.

110. Jorfeldt L: The effect of local anesthetics on the central circulation and respiration in man and dog. Acta Anaesth Scand 12:153–169, 1968.

111. Kepes ER, Duncalf D: Treatment of backache with spinal injections for local anesthetics, spinal and systemic steroids. A review. Pain 22:33–47, 1985.

112. Kikuchi S, Hasue M, Nishiuama K, et al: Anatomic and clinical studies of radicular symptoms. Spine 9:23–30, 1984.

113. Klenerman L, Greenwood R, Davenport HT, et al: Lumbar epidural injections in the treatment of sciatica. Br J Rheumatol 23:35–38, 1984.

114. Knight CL, Burnell JC: Systemic side-effects of extradural steroids. Anesthesia 35:593–594, 1980.

115. Kornberg M: Discography and magnetic resonance imaging in the diagnosis of lumbar disc disruption. Spine 14:1368–1372, 1989.

116. Krempen JF, Smith BS: Nerve root injection: A method for evaluating the etiology of sciatica. J Bone Joint Surg 56A:1435–1444, 1974.

117. Lambert DH, Herley RJ, Hertwig L, et al: Role of needle gauge and tip configuration in the production of lumbar puncture headache. Reg Anesth 22:66–72, 1997.

118. Lee H, Weinstein JN, Meller ST, et al: The role of steroids and their effects on phospholipase A2, an animal model of radiculopathy. Spine 23:1191–1196, 1998.

119. Lerner SM, Gutterman P, Jenkins F: Epidural hematoma and paraplegia after numerous lumbar punctures. Anesthesia 39:550–553, 1973.

120. Lievre JA, Bloch-Michel H, Pean G, et al: L'hydrocortisone en injection locale. Rheumatism 20:310–311, 1953.

121. Lindahl O, Rexed B: Histologic changes in spinal nerve roots of operated cases of sciatica. Acta Orthop Scand 20:215–225, 1951.

122. Link S, El-Khoury G, Guilford B: Percutaneous epidural and nerve root block and percutaneous lumbar sympatholysis. Radiol Clin North Am 36:509–521, 1998.

123. Longmire S, Joyce TH: Treatment of a duro-cutaneous fistula secondary to attempted epidural anesthesia with an epidural autologous blood patch. Anesthesiology 60:63–64, 1984.

124. Lutz GE, Vad VB, Wisneski RJ: Fluoroscopic transforaminal lumbar epidural steroids: An outcome study. Arch Phys Med Rehabil 79:1362–1366, 1998.

125. Mangar D, Thomas PB: Epidural steroid injections in the treatment of cervical and lumbar pain syndromes. Reg Anesth 16:246, 1991.

126. Mather LE: Cardiovascular and subjective central nervous system effects of long-acting local anesthetics in man. Anaesth Intensive Care 7:215–221, 1979.

127. Matthews JA, Mills SB, Jenkins VM, et al: Back pain and sciatica: Controlled trials of manipulation, traction, sclerosant and epidural injections. Br J Rheumatol 26:416–423, 1987.

128. McCarron RF, Wimpee MW, Hudkins PG, et al: The inflammatory effect of nucleus pulposus: A possible element in the pathogenesis of low back pain. Spine 12:760–764, 1987.

129. Mehta M, Salmon N: Extradural block. Confirmation of the injection site by x-ray monitoring. Anaesthesia 40:1009–1012, 1985.

130. Merwin JD: Chronic thoracic pain. In Ramamurthy S, Rogers JN (eds): Decision Making in Pain Management. St. Louis, B.C. Decker, 1993, p 112.

131. Mihic DN: Postspinal headache and relationship of the needle bevel to longitudinal dural fibers. Reg Anesth 10:76, 1985.

132. Moore DC: A surface marking for caudal block. Br J Anesth 40:916, 1968.

133. Morishima HO, Peterson H, Finster M, et al: Is bupivacaine more cardiotoxic than lidocaine? Anesthesiology 59:A409, 1983.

134. Murphy RW: Nerve roots and spinal nerves in degenerative disc disease. Clin Orthop 129:46–60, 1977.

135. Murphy TM: Chronic pain. In Miller RD (ed): Anesthesia, 3rd ed. New York, Churchill Livingstone, 1990, p 360.

136. Neal JM: Management of postdural puncture headache. Clin Dialogues Reg Anesth 3:1–5, 1992.

137. Nelson DA: Dangers from methylprednisolone acetate therapy by intraspinal injection. Arch Neurol 45:804–806, 1988.

138. Nelson DA, Vates TS, Thomas RB: Complications from intrathecal steroid therapy in patients with multiple sclerosis. Acta Neurol Scand 49:176–188, 1973.

139. North RB, Kidd DH, Zahurak M, et al: Specificity of diagnostic nerve blocks: A prospective, randomized study of sciatica due to lumbosacral spine disease. Pain 65:77–85, 1996.

140. Okell RW, Sprigge JS: Unintentional dural puncture. A survey of recognition and management. Anaesthesia 42:1110–1113, 1987.

141. Olsen KS: Epidural blood patch in the treatment of post-lumbar puncture headache. Pain 30:293–301, 1987.

142. O'Neill C, Derby R, Ryan DP: Precision injection techniques for diagnosis and treatment of lumbar disc disease. International Spinal Injection Society Newsletter 3(2):34–58, 1999.

143. Ostheimer GW, Paluhniuk RJ, Schnider SM: Epidural blood patch for post-lumbar puncture headache. Anesthesiology 41:307–308, 1974.

144. Pasquier MM, Leri J: Injections intra et extra-durals de co- caine a dose minime dans le traitement de la sciatique. Bull Gen Therap 142:196, 1901.

145. Pearce J, Moll JMH: Conservative treatment and natural history of acute lumbar disc disease lesions. J Neurol Neurosurg Psychiatry 30:13–17, 1967.

146. Preuss L: Allergic reactions to systemic glucocorticoids: A review. Am Allergy 55:772–775, 1985.

147. Purcell-Jones G, Pitcher CE, Justins DM: Paravertebral so- matic nerve block: A clinical radiographic and computed tomographic study in chronic pain patients. Anesth Analg 68:32–39, 1989.

148. Purkis IE: Cervical epidural steroids. Pain Clin 1:3–7, 1986.

149. Quaynor H, Corbey M, Berg P: Spinal anesthesia in day-care surgery with a 26-gauge needle. Br J Anaesth 65:766–769, 1990.

150. Raff H, Nelson DK, Finding JW, et al: Acute and chronic suppression of ACTH and cortisol after epidural steroid administration in humans [abstract]. Program of the 73rd annual meeting of The Endocrine Society. Washington, D.C., 1991.

151. Raj PP: Prognostic and therapeutic local anesthetic block- ade. In Cousins MJ, Bridenbaugh PO (eds): Neural Blockade in Clinical Anesthesia and Management of Pain. Philadelphia, J.B. Lippincott, 1988, pp 899–934.

152. Ramsey HJ: Fat in the epidural space of young and adult cats. Am J Anat 104:345, 1959.

153. Rapp SE, Haselkorn JK, Elam K, et al: Epidural steroid in- jection in the treatment of low back pain: A meta-analysis. Anesthesiology 78A:923, 1994.

154. Reiz S, Nath S: Cardiotoxicity of local anesthetic agents. Br J Anaesth 58:736–746, 1986.

155. Renfrew DL, Moore TE, Kathol MH, et al: Correct place- ment of epidural steroid injections: Fluoroscopic guidance and contrast administration. AJNR 12:1003–1007, 1991.

156. Reynolds AF, Roberts PA, Pollay M, et al: Quantitative anatomy of the thoracolumbar epidural space. Neurosurgery 17:905–907, 1985.

157. Ridley MG, Kingsley GH, Gibson T, et al: Outpatient lumbar epidural corticosteroid injection in the management of sciatica. Br J Rheumatol 27:295–299, 1988.

158. Roberts M, Shepard GL, McCormick RC: Tuberculous meningitis after intrathecally administered methylpred- nisolone acetate. JAMA 200:894–896, 1967.

159. Rocco AG, Frank E, Kaul AF, et al: Epidural steroid, epidural morphine and epidural steroids combined with morphine in the treatment of post laminectomy syndrome. Pain 36:297–303, 1989.

160. Roche J: Steroid-induced arachnoiditis. Med J Aust 140:281–284, 1984.

161. Rowlingson JC, Kirschenbaum LP: Epidural analgesic techniques in the management of cervical pain. Anesth Analg 65:938–942, 1986.

162. Ryan MD, Taylor TKF: Management of lumbar nerve root pain. Med J Aust 2:532–534, 1981.

163. Saal JA, Saal JS: Nonoperative treatment of herniated lumbar intervertebral disc with radiculopathy. An outcome study. Spine 14:431–437, 1989.

164. Saal JS, Transon RC, Dobrow R, et al: High levels of in- flammatory phospholipase A2 activity in the lumbar disc herniations. Spine 15:674–678, 1990.

165. Scott DB, Jebson PJ, Braid DP, et al: Factors affecting plasma levels of lignocaine and prilocaine. Br J Anesth 44:1040–1049, 1972.

166. Shantha TR, Evans JA: The relationship of epidural anesthe- sia to neural membranes and arachnoid villi. Anesthesiology 37:543–557, 1972.

167. Shealy CN: Dangers of spinal injections without proper di- agnosis. JAMA 197:1104–1106, 1966.

168. Shimasoto S, Etsten BE: The role of the venous system in cardiocirculatory dynamics during spinal and epidural anesthesia in man. Anesthesiology 30:619, 1969.

169. Shulman M: Treatment of neck pain with cervical epidural injection. Reg Anesth 11:92–94, 1986.

170. Sicard JA: Sur les injections epidurales sacrococcygienes. C R Soc Biol 53:479, 1901.

171. Siddall PJ, Cousins MJ: Spine update: Spinal pain mecha- nisms. Spine 22:98–104, 1997.

172. Simon DL, Kung RD, German JD, et al: Allergic or pseudoallergic reaction following epidural steroid deposi- tion and skin testing. Reg Anesth 14:253–255, 1989.

173. Sjogren S, Wright B: Circulation, respiration and lidocaine concentration during continuous epidural blockage. Acta Anaesth Scand Suppl 46:5, 1972.

174. Snoek W, Weber H, Jorgenson B: Double blind evaluation of extradural methylprednisolone for herniated lumbar discs. Acta Orthop Scand 48:635–641, 1977.

175. Stambough JL, Booth RE Jr, Rothman RH: Transient hy- percorticism after epidural steroid injection. A case report. J Bone Joint Surg 66A:1115–1116, 1984.

176. Stanley D, McLoren MI, Evinton HA, et al: A prospective study of nerve root infiltration in the diagnosis of sciatica. A comparison with radiculopathy, computed tomography and operative findings. Spine 15:540–543, 1990.

177. Stav A, Ovadra L, Sternbert G, et al: Cervical epidural steroid injection for cervicobrachialgia. Acta Anaesth Scand 37:562–566, 1993.

178. Stewart HD, Quinnel RC, Dann N: Epidurography in the management of sciatica. Br J Rheumatol 26:424–429, 1987.

179. Strong WE, Wesley R, Winnie AP: Epidural steroids are safe and effective when given appropriately [letter]. Arch Neurol 48:1012, 1991.

180. Swerdlow M, Sayle-Creer W: A study of extradural med- ication in the relief of the lumbosciatic syndrome. Anesth- esiology 25:341–345, 1970.

181. Szeinfeld M, Ihmeidan IH, Moser MM, et al: Epidural blood patch: Evaluation of the volume and spread of blood in- jected into the epidural space. Anesthesiology 64:820–822, 1986.

182. Tajima T, Furukawa K, Kuramachi E: Selective lumbosacral radiculopathy and block. Spine 5:68–77, 1980.

183. Takata T, Inoue S, Takahashi K, et al: Swelling of the cauda equina in patients who have herniation of a lumbar disc: A possible pathogenesis of sciatica. J Bone Joint Surg 70A:361–368, 1988.

184. Tourtellotte WW, Henderson WG, Tucker RP, et al: A ran- domized, double-blind clinical trial comparing the 22- versus 26-gauge needle in the production of the post-lumbar puncture syndrome in normal individuals. Headache 12:73–78, 1972.

185. Tuel SM, Meythaler JM, Cross LL: Cushing's syndrome from epidural methylprednisolone. Pain 40:81–84, 1990.

186. Tuohy ER: Continuous spinal anesthesia: A new method of utilizing a ureteral catheter. Surg Clin North Am 25:834, 1945.

187. Usubiaga JE, Wikinski JA, Usubiaga LE: Epidural pressure and its relation to spread of anesthetic solutions in epidural space. Anesth Analg 46:440–446, 1967.

188. Vandam LD, Dfipps RD: Long-term follow-up of patients who received 10,098 spinal anesthetics. JAMA 161:586–591, 1956.

189. Viner N: Intractable sciatica—the sacral epidural injec- tion—An effective method of giving relief. Can Med Assoc J 15:630–634, 1925.

190. Waldman SD: Complications of cervical epidural nerve blocks with steroids: A prospective study of 790 consecu- tive blocks. Reg Anesth 14:149–151, 1989.

191. Wang LP, Schmidt JF: Central nervous side-effects after lumbar puncture. A review of the possible pathogenesis of the syndrome of post-dural puncture headache and associated symptoms. Dan Med Bull 44:79–81, 1997.

192. Warfield CA: Steroids and low-back pain. Hosp Pract (Off Ed) 20:32J–32R, 1985.

193. Warfield CA, Biber MO, Crews IA, et al: Epidural steroid injection as a treatment for cervical radiculitis. Clin J Pain 4:201, 1988.

194. Warr AC, Wilkinson JA, Burn JMB, et al: Chronic lumbosciatica syndrome treated by epidural injection and manipulation. Practitioner 209:53–59, 1972.

195. Watts RW, Silagy CA: A meta-analysis on the efficacy of epidural corticosteroids in the treatment of sciatica. Anaesth Intensive Care 23:564–569, 1995.

196. Weiner BK, Fraser RD: Foraminal injection for lateral lumbar disc herniation. J Bone Joint Surg 79B:804–807, 1997.

197. Weinstein J: Mechanisms of spinal pain: The dorsal root ganglion and its role as a mediator of low-back pain. Spine 11:999–1001, 1986.

198. White AH: Injection techniques for the diagnosis and treatment of low back pain. Orthop Clin North Am 14:553–569, 1983.

199. White AH: Injections, where do they fit? In Aggressive Non-Surgical Rehabilitation of Lumbar Spine and Sports Injuries. San Francisco, 1989.

200. White AH, Derby R, Wynne G: Epidural injections for the diagnosis and treatment of low back pain. Spine 5:78–82, 1980.

201. White AWM: Low back pain in men receiving worker's compensation. Can Med Assoc J 95:50–56, 1966.

202. Williams KN, Jackowski A, Evans PJD: Epidural hematoma requiring surgical decompression following repeated cervical epidural steroid injections for chronic pain. Pain 42:197–199, 1990.

203. Williams MP, Cherryman GR: Thoracic disc herniation: MR imaging. Radiology 167:874–875, 1988.

204. Williams MP, Cherryman GR, Husband JE: Significance of thoracic disc herniation demonstrated by MR imaging. J Comput Assist Tomogr 13:211–214, 1989.

205. Williamson JA: Inadvertent spinal subdural injection during attempted spinal epidural steroid therapy. Anesth Intensive Care 18:406–408, 1990.

206. Willis RJ: Caudal epidural blockade. In Cousins MJ, Bridenbaugh PO (eds): Neural Blockade in Clinical Anesthesia and Management of Pain. Philadelphia, J.B. Lippincott, 1988, pp 361–386.

207. Wilson TA, Branch CL Jr: Thoracic disc herniation. Am Fam Physician 45:2162–2168, 1992.

208. Winnie AP, Hartmen JT, Meyers HL, et al: Pain clinic II. Intradural and extradural corticosteroids for sciatica. Anesth Analg 51:990–1003, 1972.

209. Yamazaka N: Interspinal injection of hydrocortisone or prednisolone in the treatment of intervertebral disc herniation. Nippon Seikeigeka Gakkai Zasshi 33:689, 1959.

210. Yates DW: A comparison of the types of epidural injection commonly used in the treatment of low back pain and sciatica. Rheumatol Rehab 17:181–186, 1978.

211. Zimmerman M: Peripheral and central nervous mechanisms of nociception, pain and pain therapy: Facts and hypotheses. In Bonica JJ, Liebeskind JC, Alber-Fessard T (eds): Advance in Pain Therapy. New York, Raven Press, 1979, pp 3–32.

31

Spinal Cord Stimulation in Chronic Pain

Robert E. Windsor, M.D., Frank J. E. Falco, M.D.,
and Elmer G. Pinzon, M.D., M.P.H.

Since the first published paper on spinal cord stimulation (SCS) by Shealy in 1967, there have been over 2000 articles, presentations, symposia, and abstracts on the topic of neuroaugmentation.[72,76] The long-term results of SCS published in the 1970s were disappointing yet promising.[22,24,26,77] Most of the studies published in the 1970s and early 1980s demonstrated success rates of approximately 40%.[7] As with many new devices, problems included poorly designed hardware, inadequate patient selection criteria, and suboptimal surgical technique. The hardware typically consisted of an epidurally implanted single or dual electrode system. They provided a small electrical field and thus were unable to consistently stimulate the spinal cord. In addition, these systems were implanted via laminectomy or laminotomy with the patient under general anesthesia, thereby eliminating the possibility of surgeon-patient interaction. The electrodes commonly were implanted in the high thoracic or lower cervical region for lumbar pain syndromes. Patients were not consistently screened for psychological dysfunction, drug habituation, secondary gain issues, pain topography, and quality of pain. All of these factors have considerable impact on the overall efficacy of SCS.

Significant advances in SCS have been made in recent years. The hardware is more durable and more effective, and devices can be implanted percutaneously under fluoroscopic guidance, which allows operator-patient interaction and more accurate positioning of SCS leads. Two decades of experience have provided improved patient selection criteria. The net result is an improved capacity to control chronic pain.[7] This chapter discusses the clinical application of SCS, implantation technique, follow-up care, and the authors' clinical experience.

PAIN ANATOMY AND PHYSIOLOGY

Pain is an uncomfortable sensation associated with an emotional response.[28,87] The International Association for the Study of Pain (IASP) defined pain as "an unpleasant sensory and emotional experience associated with actual and potential tissue damage, or described in terms of such damage" (IASP, 1986).[28] It may originate from stimulation of chemical, mechanical, or thermal receptors found in free nerve endings within injured tissue. This is known as afferent pain and can occur in ligamentous or muscular injuries of the spine.[6,38,44,74] Pain also can occur from direct injury to the peripheral nerve that results in burning or shooting pain in the distribution of the affected nerve. Peripheral deafferentation (neuropathic) pain is demonstrated in conditions such as complex regional pain syndrome, peripheral neuropathy, or radiculopathy.[24,53,54] Central deafferent pain appears after injury to the central nervous system structures that are responsible for the transmission of pain, such as the thalamus.

Peripheral pain signals are transmitted by either thinly myelinated A-delta fibers or unmyelinated C fibers. The A-delta fibers convey discrete, sharp, fast pain at approximately 15 m/sec, whereas the C fibers transmit vague, chronic, burning, slow pain at less than 1 m/sec.[19,89]

Pain fibers typically enter the spinal cord through the dorsal root and then ascend or descend 2–6 segments within the dorsolateral fasciculus (Lissauer's tract). The A-delta fibers synapse with the dorsal gray horn neurons located in laminae 1, 2, 5, and 10, whereas the C fibers synapse with dorsal gray horn neurons located in laminae 1, 2, and 5. The majority of fibers then cross to the opposite ventrolateral portion of the spinal cord before ascending in the

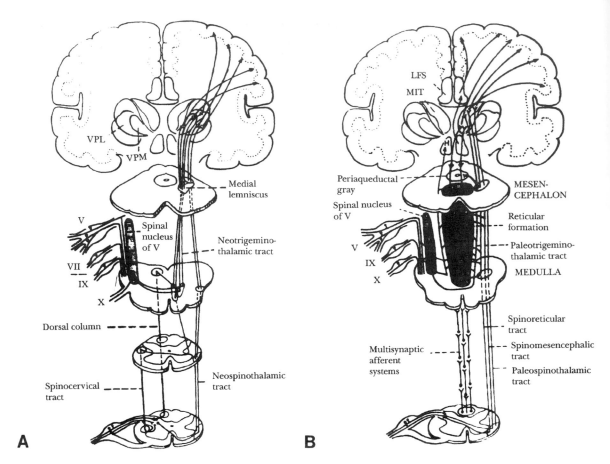

FIGURE 31-1. Neuroanatomic pathway for nociceptive pain transmission in the lateral (*A*) and medial (*B*) tracts. (From Bonica JJ: Anatomic and physiologic basis of nociception and pain. In Bonica JJ (ed): The Management of Pain, Vol. 1, 2nd ed. Philadelphia, Lea & Febiger, 1990, p 89, with permission.)

spinothalamic, spinoreticulothalamic, and spino-mesencephalic tracts. The lateral spinothalamic fibers terminate in the thalamic ventralis posterolateralis and posteromedialis nuclei, from which fibers are projected into other areas of the thalamus and to the somatic sensory cortex. The medial spinothalamic, spinoreticulothalamic, and spinomesencephalic tracts end in the reticular activating system within the medulla, pons, midbrain, periaqueductal gray, hypothalamus, and thalamic medial and intralaminar nuclei (Fig. 31-1).

The thalamus primarily is involved in conscious pain perception, and the cortex is involved in interpreting pain quality and locality. The A-delta fibers convey a distinctive, sharp pain, and C fibers conduct a characteristic diffuse, burning, or aching pain. This is likely a reflection of the A-delta fibers terminating at the cortical level versus C fibers that end diffusely in the brain stem and diencephalon.

In 1965 Melzack and Wall published their "gate control" theory in which they hypothesized that a "gate" system located in the dorsal gray horn within the substantia gelatinosa modulated pain (laminae 2 and 3).[51] They proposed that excess tactile signals traveling along the large myelinated A-delta fibers closed the gate, which then inhibit the propagation of pain impulses along the poorly myelinated C fibers (Fig. 31-2).

Although the pain pathway is still not completely understood, researchers have uncovered important parts of the neuronal system, including descending inhibitory influences from the brain that have been shown to suppress transmission of pain.[5,55,65,70] Evidence of an endogenous system of opioids that modulate sensory input also exists.[33,73,79]

Currently the prevailing belief in medicine is that the experience of pain is not merely physiologic but also is influenced by culture, religion, and psychological makeup.[23,30,49,50] In order to provide appropriate treatment, such factors must be considered when evaluating patients.

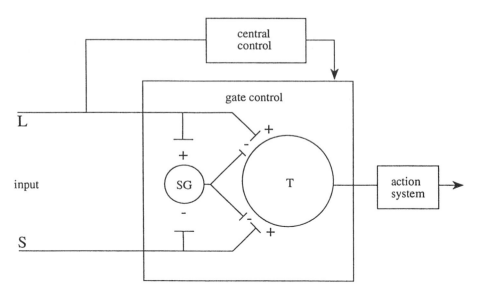

FIGURE 31-2.   Melzack and Wall gate-control theory of pain: large-diameter fibers (L), small-diameter fibers (S), substantia gelatinosa (SG), first central transmission cells (T), excitation (+), inhibition (–). (From Melzack R, Wall PD: Pain mechanisms: A new theory. Science 150:975, 1965, with permission.)

MECHANISM OF ACTION

Although the exact mechanism for pain control from SCS is not entirely understood, it is believed to result from direct or facilitated inhibition of pain transmission[22,24,26,32,51,76] (Fig. 31-3). The notable five mechanistic theories for SCS are:

1. **Gate control theory:** segmental, antidromic activation of A-beta efferents

2. SCS blocks transmission in the **spinothalamic tract**

3. SCS produces **supraspinal** pain inhibition

4. SCS produces activation of central inhibitory mechanisms influencing **sympathetic** efferent neurons

5. SCS activates putative **neurotransmitters** or **neuromodulators.**[32]

In 1967 the gate control theory motivated Shealy et al. to apply SCS as a means to antidromically activate the tactile A-beta fibers through dorsal column stimulation.[76] Shealy reasoned that sustained stimulation of the dorsal columns would keep the gate closed and provide continuous pain relief. Although the theoretical model put forth by Melzack and Wall has not been shown to be precisely correct, pain gating or pain control has been shown to exist.[22,24,26,51]

Other researchers believe that pain relief from SCS results from direct inhibition of pain pathways in the spinothalamic tracts and not secondary to selective large fiber stimulation.[16] This theory has been supported by Hoppenstein, who showed that the posterolateral stimulation of the spinal cord provided effective contralateral pain relief with substantially less current than posterior stimulation.[11]

Some investigators assert that the changes in blood flow and skin temperature from spinal cord stimulation may affect nociception at the peripheral level.[6,12,21,44,45] This postulate is further supported in

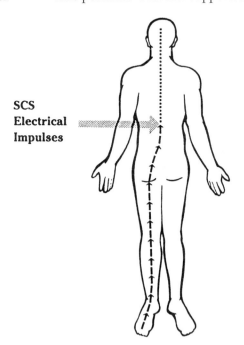

SCS Electrical Impulses

FIGURE 31-3.   Spinal cord stimulation blockage. The electrical impulses of spinal cord stimulation are directed at blocking pain signals to the brain. (Courtesy of Medtronic Neurological, Minneapolis, MN.)

Optimal steerability to target site due to:
- Coiled wire design
- Removable center stylet

PISCES-QUAD® LEAD
- Lead electrodes 3mm long, 6mm spacing
- Electrode span 30mm

PISCES-QUAD PLUS® LEAD
- Largest stim area available with a totally implantable device
- Lead electrodes 6mm long, 12mm spacing
- Electrode span 60mm

PISCES-QUAD® COMPACT LEAD
- For a more focused field
- Lead electrodes 3mm long, 4mm spacing
- Electrode span 24mm

SURGICAL LEADS

RESUME II® LEAD
- Lead paddle 8mm wide, 2mm thick

RESUME TL® LEAD
- Thinner and narrower than Resume II
- Fits more easily into small epidural spaces
- Lead paddle 6.6mm wide, 1.4mm thick

SYMMIX® LEAD
- Broader coverage option
- Lead paddle 10mm wide, 1.7mm thick

ON-POINT® PNS LEAD
- For single-nerve-distribution pain
- Anchorable mesh skirt surrounding paddle
- Lead paddle 6.6mm wide, 1.4mm thick

SPECIFY® LEAD
- More coverage where you want it, less coverage where you don't
- Ability to increase specificity of bilateral paresthesia patterns
- Lead paddle 8mm wide, 1.7mm thick
- For use especially with Mattrix System in DualStim Mode

TWIST-LOCK ANCHOR
- Helps prevent lead migration
- Reliably grasps the lead body of all Medtronic coiled wire, in-line SCS leads
- Designed to save OR time at initial implant and reduce need to surgically reposition the lead

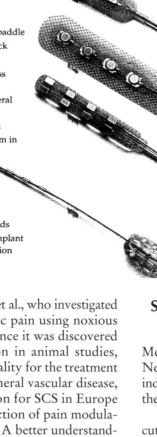

FIGURE 31-4. Medtronic SCS implantable leads. Percutaneous and surgically implantable SCS leads. (Courtesy of Medtronic Neurological, Minneapolis, MN.)

part by data from Marchand et al., who investigated the effects of SCS on chronic pain using noxious thermal stimuli.[17,25,29,47,59,71] Since it was discovered that SCS causes vasodilation in animal studies, clinicians have used this modality for the treatment of chronic pain due to peripheral vascular disease, and it is the leading indication for SCS in Europe today.[25,29,32,71,83] The precise action of pain modulation by SCS is still in debate. A better understanding of the pain system may lead to more effective stimulators and allow for even greater success.

SPINAL CORD STIMULATION LEADS

Two companies manufacture SCS systems: Medtronic, Inc. (Minneapolis, MN) and Advanced Neuromodulation Systems (Allen, TX) (refer to the individual company promotional brochures for further details).

Medtronic manufactures leads designed for percutaneous or laminotomy implantation (Fig. 31-4). The percutaneously implanted leads have either 4 or 8 electrodes. They have a tough, polyurethane outer covering and a helicoil substrate, which makes the leads very resilient with columnar strength and flexibility. The three different 4-electrode leads and one 8-electrode lead each have variable electrode lengths and interelectrode distances. The Pisces Quad Plus has four 6-mm electrodes with an interelectrode distance of 12 mm; the Pisces Quad lead has four 3-mm electrodes with an interelectrode distance of 6 mm; the Pisces Quad Compact lead has four 3-mm electrodes with an interelectrode distance of 6 mm; and the Octad has eight 3-mm electrodes with an interelectrode distance of 6 mm. In addition to these lead configurations, Medtronic is capable of individually producing a wide variety of 4- or 8-electrode leads to accommodate an individual physician's specifications or to treat complex or difficult pain patterns. In general, the smaller the interelectrode distance, the less risk for rootlet stimulation.

Medtronic also produces 5 electrodes for implantation via laminotomy: the Symmix, the dual paddle Symmix, the Resume TL, the Resume, and the Specify. The Symmix, Resume TL, and Resume leads have 4 electrodes each, the Specify has 8, and the dual paddle Symmix has two paddles with two electrodes each. The Symmix has 4 electrodes arranged in a diamond pattern, and the Specify has a total of 8 electrodes with 4 electrodes arranged side by side. Both of these electrode arrangements facilitate bilateral extremity stimulation. The dual paddle Symmix has two separate paddles designed to allow implantation over two contact sites on the spinal cord to cover a more complex pain pattern. The Resume lead is still the most commonly implanted paddle electrode.

Advanced Neuromodulation Systems (ANS) produces 3 leads for percutaneous placement with 4, 7, or 8 electrodes. The 4-electrode lead has an interelectrode distance of 10 mm, and the 8- and 7-electrode leads have an interelectrode distance of 7 mm. The 7-electrode lead is designed to treat upper extremity complex regional pain syndrome and has variable length electrodes spanning a much larger distance (144 mm) than the other leads to provide plasticity in the system for changing pain patterns. The notion of spanning a larger distance is to help thwart the effects of possible migratory pain patterns, which are thought to be a quality of complex regional pain syndrome type 1. Seven millimeters has been determined to be the optimal interelectrode distance for providing the greatest stimulation intensity with the least discomfort.[40]

ANS also produces 4 different surgically implanted paddle electrodes. They have a 4-electrode Lamitrode Four, an 8-electrode Lamitrode 44 that has 4 electrodes side by side, an 8-electrode Lamitrode 8, and a 16-electrode Lamitrode 88 with 8 electrodes side by side.

One of the clinical concerns with past ANS (previously Neuromed Inc., Davie, FL) leads was that they tended to break down in the body after 1–2 years, causing the system to malfunction. This was due to the bisthmus that was placed in the lead's insulation, which made it radioopaque. This concern was addressed by removing the bisthmus from the lead insulation and making the insulation out of polyurethane. ANS indicates that this has dramatically increased the life expectancy of their leads.

ANS makes its lead in 30- or 60-cm lengths with stylets for easier spinal placement. They also have extension leads to be used as needed when shorter spinal leads are clinically indicated.

PULSE GENERATORS AND RECEIVERS

Currently, only Medtronic makes a pulse generator allowing for a totally implantable system (Figs. 31-5 and 31-6). A pulse generator (Itrel-3) is powered by a pacemaker battery and lasts 3–5 years depending on use. The pulse generator is programmed transcutaneously by an external antenna attached to the physician's Medtronic Patient Programmer that gives off a radiofrequency signal that allows the physician to set the parameters of the electrical stimulation. In addition, two patient devices that control the pulse generator (although to a smaller extent than is possible with the physician's programmer) are available: a hand-held programmer and a powerful magnet. The hand-held programmer is about the size of an old-fashioned transistor radio and allows the patient to turn the system on and off and adjust the amplitude, pulse width, and rate within the parameters programmed by the physician. The powerful magnet is about the size of a refrigerator magnet and only will turn the device on or off. Both the hand-held programmer and the magnet are small enough to be easily carried by the patient all day. If the patient is a long-term user of a SCS system, he or she can turn the system on in the morning and leave the magnet at home, not turning it off until the evening or whenever he or she next returns home.

Both Medtronic and ANS manufacture externally powered radiofrequency systems that use implanted receivers (Figs. 31-6 and 31-7). Receivers are conductors that receive radiofrequency signals transcutaneously from a flat antenna placed on the skin over the receiver. The antenna is attached by a cable

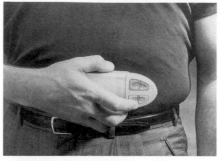

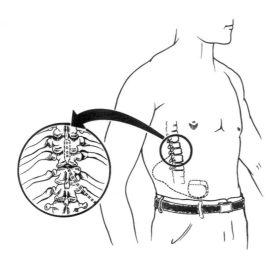

THE MEDTRONIC ITREL® 3 NEUROSTIMULATION SYSTEM

Diagram above shows typical implantation for control of chronic pain. Inset shows posterior view of the spine indicating lead placement. The photo at top right shows the EZ™ patient programmer used by the patient to adjust therapy between parameters set by the clinician. In photo at lower right, the EZ programmer is shown with the implantable Itrel 3 neurostimulation device.

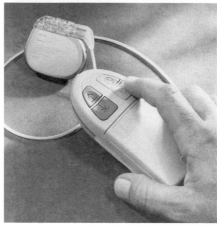

FIGURE 31-5. Medtronic Itrel 3 Neurostimulation System. The implantable Itrel 3 neurostimulation device is shown here with the EZ™ patient programmer. (Courtesy of Medtronic Neurological, Minneapolis, MN.)

to a programmable externally worn device known as a transmitter. The transmitter, which outwardly resembles a transcutaneous electrical nerve stimulation (TENS) unit, is powered by a 9-volt battery. The battery is changed every couple of days depending on use. Rechargeable 9-volt batteries also may be used.

Medtronic makes three different receivers, one for the 4-electrode leads (X-trel), one for the 8-electrode leads (Mattrix Octed), and one for two 4-electrode leads (Mattrix Dual Quad). The Mattrix Octed and the Mattrix Dual Quad systems both have 8 electrical contact points on the spinal cord and are used to treat more complex pain. ANS makes 6 different receivers to accommodate a variety of different lead combinations including one 4-electrode lead, two 4-electrode leads, two 4-electrode and one 8-electrode leads, 4-electrode leads, one 8-electrode lead, and two 8-electrode leads. In addition, the multichannel ANS receivers are able to program the leads in stereo fashion, which may provide some benefit in covering complex pain patterns that include axial pain. Stereo programming indicates that when the specified electrodes of one lead are activated, the specified electrodes on the other lead are silent and

vice versa. This occurs in an alternating pattern so rapidly that the brain perceives the stimulation pattern as continual and not intermittent. In addition, ANS has eliminated plastic boots and set screws from their system to make implantation easier.

PATIENT SELECTION CRITERIA

Proper patient selection is essential to the long-term success of an SCS system. Improper selection criteria were the principal reasons for suboptimal results reported in the 1970s. During the 1970s and early 1980s, most studies evaluating the long-term efficacy of dorsal column stimulation quoted success rates of approximately 40%. Technical advances leading to improved hardware coupled with improved patient selection have improved the rate of long-term efficacy to about 70%[7,76,77] (Tables 31-1 and 31-2).

An SCS system should be considered for patients who have not responded to reasonable measures of conservative care, including appropriate diagnostic, therapeutic, and rehabilitative techniques and have been given a reasonable period of time to recover from the condition.[7] The ideal patient should be

MEDTRONIC MATTRIX® NEUROSTIMULATION SYSTEM

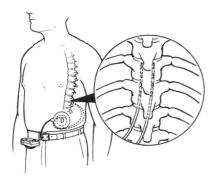

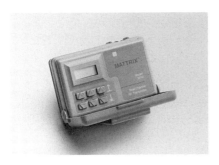

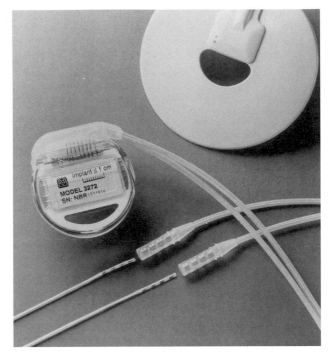

In the photo above, the two stimulation leads of the Mattrix system are shown with the receiver (left center) which is implanted under the skin. The external antenna (upper right) is affixed to the skin over the receiver. The belt-mounted transmitter, shown in the photograph at left, is easily adjusted by the patient with parameters set by the clinician to deliver stimulation impulses via the antenna to the receiver and then through the leads to the spinal column (inset in diagram). Dashed lines in diagram indicate implanted receiver and leads.

FIGURE 31-6. Medtronic Mattrix neurostimulation system. This diagram shows the two stimulation leads of the Mattrix system with the implantable receiver, the external antenna affixed to the skin over the receiver, and the belt-mounted transmitter. (Courtesy of Medtronic Neurological, Minneapolis, MN).

motivated, compliant, and free of drug dependence.[46] Psychological screening is recommended (but not mandatory) to exclude conditions that predispose to failure of the procedure. Diagnoses that are typical indications for this procedure include chronic radiculopathy, perineural fibrosis, neuropathic pain, and complex regional pain

TABLE 31-1. Medical Problems for Which Spinal Cord Stimulation Has Been Used

Angina pectoris	Paraplegia
Arachnoiditis	Peripheral neuropathy
Brachial plexopathy	Phantom pain
Cancer pain	Polyneuropathy
Causalgia	Postcordotomy dysesthesia
Cerebral palsy	Postherpetic neuralgia
Dysautonomia	Raynaud's disease
Dystonia	Reflex sympathetic dystrophy
Failed back surgery	Spinal cord infarction
Multiple sclerosis	Spinal cord neoplasia
Myelopathy	Thalamic syndrome
Pancreatitis	Vascular disease

From Robb LG, et al: Spinal cord stimulation: Neuroaugmentation of the dorsal columns for pain relief. In Weiner RS (ed): Pain Management, 5th ed. Boca Raton, St. Lucie Press, 1998, p 273.

TABLE 31-2. Etiologic Criteria

  I. Peripheral nerve lesion
   A. Postoperative hip pain
   B. Total hip replacement, persistent pain
   C. Intercostal neuralgia
   D. Thoracic disc disease, spondylosis, etc.
   E. Lumbar neuroradiculopathy
   F. Peripheral neuropathy—diabetic, toxic, idiopathic
   G. Cervical spondylosis with radiculopathy
 II. Deafferentation
   A. Postherpetic neuralgia
   B. Sympathetically maintained pain
   C. Phantom limb pain
   D. Thalamic syndrome
III. Vascular disease
   A. Thromboangiitis obliterans
   B. Arteriosclerosis obliterans with or without revascularization
   C. Retroperitoneal fibrosis
IV. Spinal cord lesions
   A. Posttraumatic
   B. Infarction
 V. Epidural fibrosis and arachnoiditis
   A. Postlumbar surgery pain syndrome
   B. Battered root syndrome
VI. Mixed lesions including combinations of the previous groups

From Robb LG, et al: Spinal cord stimulation: Neuroaugmentation of the dorsal columns for pain relief. In Weiner RS (ed): Pain Management, 5th ed. Boca Raton, St. Lucie Press, 1998, p 273.

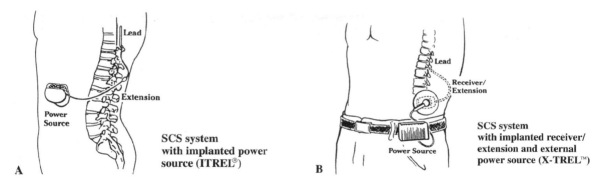

FIGURE 31-7. Medtronic SCS internal and external power sources. *A*, SCS system with implanted (internal) power source (Itrel®). *B*, SCS system with implanted receiver/extension and external power source (X-trel™).

syndrome.[4,11,19,35,48] In Europe, SCS also is used for peripheral vascular disease that is not amenable to medical therapy—excellent results have been reported.[2,25,29,71,81,83] In the United States, peripheral vascular disease is not an FDA-approved indication.

When considering pain topography, extremity pain responds better than axial pain, and the more distal the extremity pain the greater the clinical response (Fig. 31-8).[62,86] Middle and upper lumbar pain as well as thoracic, cervical, and chest pain are difficult to adequately control and maintain on a long-term basis. Pain due to severe nerve damage that is superimposed on cutaneous numbness (i.e., anesthesia dolorosa) also is difficult to treat with SCS. Central pain syndromes do not respond to SCS and are best treated by other modalities.

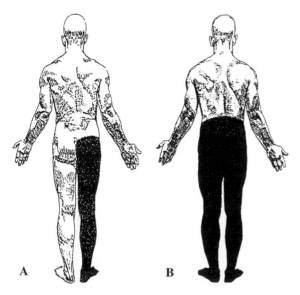

FIGURE 31-8. Ideal topographic pain pattern for treatment with spinal cord stimulation in patients with failed back syndrome and radiculopathy. *A*, Unilateral, multidermatomal pain pattern. *B*, Bilateral, with lower back pain pattern. (Courtesy of Advanced Neuromodulation Systems, Allen, TX.)

The use of 3–7 day outpatient trials with an SCS system has proved helpful in determining which patients will respond well enough to warrant a permanent implantation.[13,14,62,86] Absolute criteria that must be present for a patient to have a positive trial include tolerance of paresthesia, greater than 50% pain relief, and overall patient satisfaction. Relative requirements for a positive trial include improved functional level, reduced usage of pain medication, and reduced reliance on the health care system.

IMPLANTATION TECHNIQUE

Spinal cord stimulation may be performed by either percutaneous or open approaches. Only the percutaneous technique is described here. The SCS lead may be temporarily placed (Fig. 31-9) or permanently implanted in the cervical spine (Fig. 31-10).

Patients lie prone on the procedure table in a surgery suite. Placing a bolster under the bottom of the rib cage is optional. The entire posterior aspect of the torso is cleaned with an antiseptic solution such as Hibiclens or Betadine. Intravenous sedation is optional, although it does make patients more comfortable and does not compromise the reliability of patient-physician communication. The procedure must be interactive, because proper placement of the electrode is paramount to its success. Preprocedure antibiotics also are optional, but the authors use them consistently and have never had one surgical wound infection out of 400 lead implants in the last 8 years.

The T12–L1 interlaminar space is localized under fluoroscopic visualization as the point of entry to the epidural space. The L1–L2 interlaminar space may be used if the T12–L1 space is determined to be too small for maneuvering the epidural needle (Fig. 31-11). After choosing which space to enter, the physician must determine the optimal

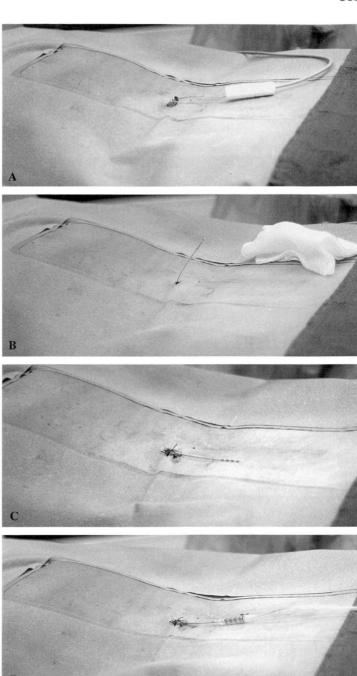

FIGURE 31-9. Series of photographs demonstrating a temporary spinal cord stimulator lead placement (*A–E*). (Courtesy of Robert E. Windsor, M.D., Georgia Pain Physicians, P.C.)

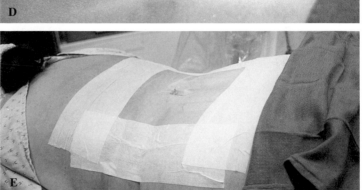

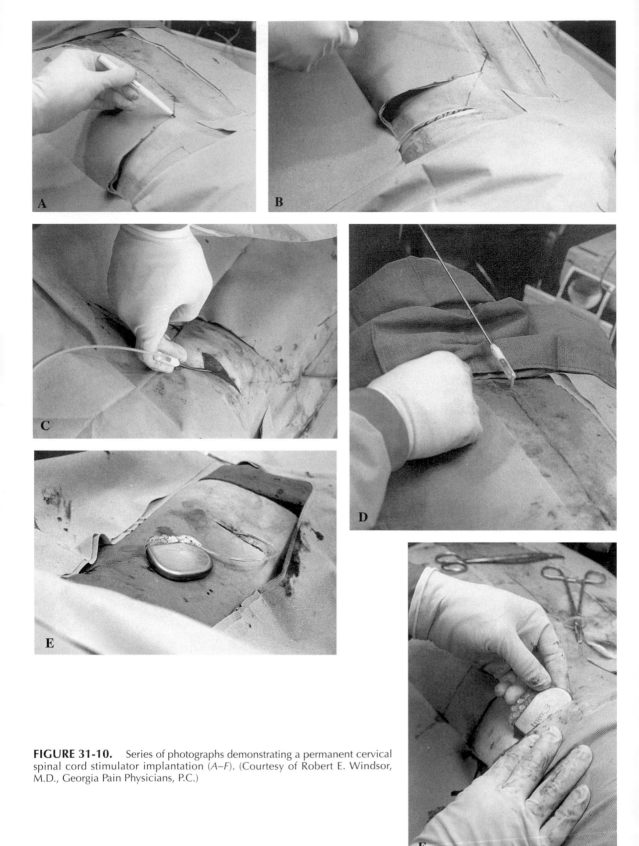

FIGURE 31-10. Series of photographs demonstrating a permanent cervical spinal cord stimulator implantation (*A–F*). (Courtesy of Robert E. Windsor, M.D., Georgia Pain Physicians, P.C.)

skin entrance site. Site selection is important because the final resting position of the epidural needle should be no more than 30° off the midline and 45° from the surface of the patient's back.

The skin entrance can be determined by using the following vector method. Under fluoroscopic visualization, a spinal needle is placed flat on the skin of the patient's back so that it intersects the midline of the cephalad portion of the chosen interlaminar space. The needle position is then adjusted on the patient's skin so that the tip contacts a point at the cephalad portion of the interlaminar space and the shaft contacts the ipsilateral side of the cephalad portion of the spinous process immediately caudal to the interlaminar space. The approximate skin entrance site for a large, medium, or small patient is 2½, 2, and 1½ vertebral bodies, respectively, caudal to the space chosen along the line of the needle. At this point, the physician should provide adequate local anesthesia along the trajectory the needle ultimately will take to reach the ipsilateral lamina of the interlaminar space to be entered.

After the patient is properly anesthetized, the epidural needle is advanced through the anesthetized soft tissues to the lamina and walked off the lamina in a cephalad and medial direction. The needle should penetrate the ligamentum flavum in the midline or 2–3 mm ipsilateral to the true midline. The epidural space is localized using loss of resistance. The lead is then advanced through the needle and up the posterior epidural space to the point of stimulation. The initial goal for stimulation of the cord for low back pain and lower extremity pain is the top of T9 (for lumbar coverage) or middle of C3–C7 (for cervical coverage) (Figs. 31-12 and 31-13). The lead should be placed in the midline if a bilateral stimulation pattern is desired, slightly to the right if a right-sided stimulation pattern is desired, and slightly to the left if a left-sided stimulation pattern is desired. If initial lead placement is difficult because of needle position, the needle may need to be repositioned. If adhesions prevent initial advancement, they may be slowly and cautiously lysed with either a lead blank or the lead itself. The lead may be steered by alternately rotating the bent stylet from its proximal end and advancing or retracting the lead. The needle also may be gently torqued to help place the lead.

After the lead has been positioned as outlined, the spinal lead is attached to an extension lead and the extension lead is attached to a screening device. The patient is then stimulated and the paresthesia pattern observed. If the paresthesia pattern covers

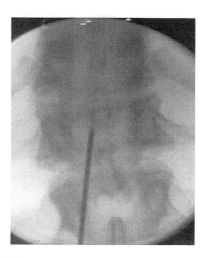

FIGURE 31-11. Proper epidural needle placement in preparation for percutaneous placement of a stimulating electrode. The epidural needle is placed into the L1–L2 interlaminar space on a line ipsilateral to the caudal end of the spinous process and directed toward the cephalad portion of the mid-interlaminar space. (Courtesy of Robert E. Windsor, M.D., Georgia Pain Physicians, P.C.)

the pain pattern with at least two different electrode settings, the needle is removed using a push-pull technique taking care not to move the lead, which is anchored to the skin. A sterile surgical dressing is placed over the entrance site. If abdominal stimulation occurs and adjusting the electrode montage does not rectify the pattern, the lead may be positioned above the sweet spot of the spinal cord that would yield an optimal stimulation pattern, the pulse width may be too wide, the lead's interelectrode distance may be too great, or the lead may be

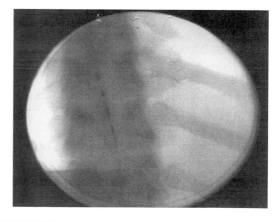

FIGURE 31-12. Spinal cord stimulator lead placement (lumbar stimulation). A Pisces Quad lead has been advanced up the posterior epidural space to the mid-body of T10 in preparation to initiate a stimulation trial. The zero (top) electrode is ~3 mm to the left of midline and the three electrode is ~5 mm to the right of midline. (Courtesy of Robert E. Windsor, M.D., Georgia Pain Physicians, P.C.)

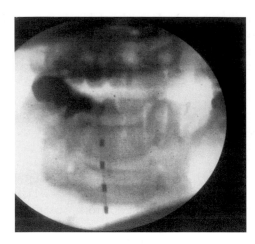

FIGURE 31-13. Spinal cord stimulator lead placement (cervical stimulation). A Pisces Quad lead is advanced up the posterior epidural space to the middle of the C3 vertebral body. The zero (top) electrode is ~2 mm to the left of midline. This lead position provided excellent neck, left shoulder girdle, and left upper extremity stimulation and pain relief from a chronic radiculopathy. (Courtesy of Robert E. Windsor, M.D., Georgia Pain Physicians, P.C.)

too laterally placed in the canal. In the first instance, the lead should be pulled down slightly and the patient restimulated. In the latter three conditions, a rootlet pattern of stimulation occurs in addition to or occasionally instead of a posterior column stimulation pattern. If the lead is too laterally placed, simply reposition the lead more medially. If the pulse width is too large, narrowing the pulse width and increasing the amplitude may be sufficient to solve the stimulation issue. If the interelectrode distance is too great, the lead must be removed and a lead with a smaller interelectrode distance inserted.

After the stimulation pattern has been optimally positioned over the patient's pain pattern, the patient is deeply sedated, and the soft tissues around the epidural needle are appropriately infiltrated with local anesthetic in preparation for surgery. The surgeon makes a longitudinal incision down to the supraspinous ligament. The incision should incorporate the epidural needle that should still be in place to protect the lead. The epidural needle is then removed using a push-pull technique under fluoroscopic visualization to ensure that the lead does not move. The lead is then anchored to the supraspinous ligament with a nondissolvable suture such as 2-0 silk, using the anchor supplied for the lead by the company. After the lead is adequately anchored, the incision should be packed with gauze infiltrated with 0.5% bupivacaine with epinephrine, and attention should be turned to creation of the subcutaneous pocket.

The position of the pocket should be determined and agreed upon with the patient before the procedure begins. It usually is created in the hip region beneath the belt line and slightly lateral to the longitudinal mid-gluteal line, although many implanters prefer the lower abdomen for implantation. The pocket should be no deeper than 1–2 cm deep to the skin and should be approximately 8 × 8 cm in area. The pocket should be created by primarily blunt dissection, and all bleeders must be controlled. The pocket then is packed off with gauze infiltrated with 0.5% bupivacaine with epinephrine to augment analgesia and bleeding control.

After the pocket has been made, the tract of tissue extending from the caudal end of the paramedian incision to the superomedial corner of the pocket should be infiltrated with 0.5% bupivacaine with epinephrine. After appropriate local anesthesia, a tunneling device with a tunneling tip should be advanced subcutaneously following the anesthetized tract, taking care to remain in the subcutaneous space and not violate the peritoneal cavity or get too near the under surface of the skin. After the tunneling tip has advanced through the subcutaneous tissues, it should be removed and replaced with a carrying tip. The female end of the extension lead is then placed in the carrying tip, and the extension lead is pulled back through the soft tissue tunnel until it comes out of the paramedian incision. A plastic boot is placed over the caudal end of the SCS lead, and then the extension lead is attached to the spinal lead. The plastic boot is then ligated over the junction of the SCS lead and the extension lead.

At this point in the procedure, the SCS lead is in place and is anchored to the supraspinal ligament; the SCS lead is attached to the extension lead; and the extension lead has been tunneled from the pocket to the paramedian incision. Both ends of the extension lead should be visible. The pocket and the paramedian incision may be irrigated with antibiotic solution and checked for bleeders. After determining that both paramedian incisions are dry, the caudal end of the extension lead is attached to the pulse generator (internally powered system—Itrel-3) or receiver (externally powered system—X-trel or ANS system), and the pulse generator or receiver is placed in the pocket with the writing visible to the operator (posteriorly directed). The pulse generator or receiver should fit within the pocket comfortably with 2–3 cm of pocket flap above the device. Any redundant extension lead should be placed anterior (deep) to the device in the pocket, and a small loop may be left at the caudal end of the paramedian incision. The pocket and the paramedian incision should be closed with deep absorbable sutures such as 2-0 Vicryl, and the skin may be closed with a subcuticular stitch or staples. After closing, there should be absolutely no stress on either suture line. A sterile pressure dressing should be applied to the surgical sites, and the patient should be discharged to the recovery area when appropriate.

TRANSMITTER PROGRAMMING PARAMETERS

When the patient is awake and alert in the recovery area, the patient's SCS settings should be optimized. The adjustable parameters of electrical stimulation in SCS are frequency (Hz), pulse width (stimulus duration), and amplitude (volts). A typical frequency is 50–80 Hz, although higher frequency may be used as a stronger counterstimulus. Increasing the pulse width increases the density of the stimulus, thereby providing deeper penetration into the spinal cord. Clinically, this usually results in a broader disbursement of paresthesia, which may be beneficial when, for example, the stimulation pattern needs to cover the back but only covers the hip. The pulse width can be increased, and the paresthesia pattern may then incorporate the low back. The amplitude represents the electrical force of the stimulus. Clinically, the patient usually experiences a more dense stimulation pattern, thus making it harder for the pain to "break through" the stimulation pattern. When the amplitude is adjusted too high, the patient may experience it as noxious sensation.

Initial stimulation settings are arbitrary and reflect programming experience. The amount of electrical output depends on the amount of epidural fat, anatomic variations, and the presence or absence of nerve injury in the posterior cord or afferent fibers in peripheral nerves. Typical transmitter settings begin with a frequency of 60 Hz, a pulse width of 250 msec, and the zero (top) electrode negative and the 3 electrode (bottom) positive. The amplitude slowly is increased until paresthesias are felt by the patient, typically between 2.5 and 4.5 volts. The intensity can be increased or decreased by changing any of the three parameters.

In order to generate current from the implanted lead, at least one electrode is made a cathode (negative) and another the anode (positive), which allows for current to flow from the anode to the cathode and results in nerve fiber depolarization. The density and flow of current from the implanted lead can be adjusted depending on which electrodes are selected to represent cathodes and anodes. A cathode and anode that are close together will generate a small, dense (higher intensity) electrical field, whereas two electrodes spaced far apart will provide a larger but less dense (lower intensity) electrical field. A larger and denser electrical field can be created with a cathode and anode spaced far apart by adding additional anodes or cathodes to the stimulation scheme and increasing the density of ion flow to the cathode. The "shape" of the stimulation pattern usually may be predicted by remembering that the cathode tends to "pull" electricity. That is, if the highest electrode is an anode and the lowest electrode is a cathode and the patient is not experiencing low back paresthesia, the lower back may be incorporated by switching the polarity of the electrodes. By switching the polarity of the electrodes, the highest electrode is made a cathode and the lowest electrode an anode. If a three-dimensional figure-of-eight pattern is desired, the highest and lowest electrode should be made cathodes, and the middle electrode should be made an anode (reverse bracketing, reverse guard banding). If a diamond field is desired, the highest and lowest electrodes should be anodes, and the middle electrode should be a cathode. The more cathodes involved in the montage, the higher the energy requirement and the sooner the batter will be discharged.

POSTPROCEDURE CARE AND FOLLOW-UP PROTOCOL

The patient undergoing a trial SCS is routinely recovered for one hour. As long as the recovery period is uneventful, the patient is discharged home. During the recovery period, the SCS programming is fine-tuned, the patient and/or patient's family is educated on how to use the device, and any questions are answered. The patient is told to keep the SCS area clean and dry and to take sponge baths only during the trial period instead of regular baths or showers. Prophylactic oral antibiotics are provided. Patients are instructed to avoid excessive bending or twisting because this may dislodge the SCS lead. In addition, they are told not to alter medication consumption and to maintain their routine activity level. They should alert the physician in case of any alteration in stimulation pattern, signs of infection, or any other unusual occurrences. Follow-up is usually within 7–10 days following implantation, when the lead is removed. The efficacy of the SCS is assessed, and the physician should then determine whether to proceed with a permanent SCS. Pain relief of greater than 50% is usually considered a positive response.

The patient undergoing a permanent implantation is brought into the ambulatory surgery center or hospital the morning of the procedure. A urinalysis, complete blood count with differential, and sedimentation rate should be obtained within 72 hours before the implantation. A chest x-ray and electrocardiogram should be obtained in all patients > age 45 years and those with a history of cardiac or pulmonary disease or ongoing signs or symptoms of cardiac or pulmonary difficulty. Preoperative and postoperative intravenous antibiotics are administered, and the patient is discharged following recovery with 7 days of oral antibiotics.

Upon discharge, the patient is given verbal and written instructions to avoid excessive lifting, twisting, or bending and to sponge bathe only for 2 weeks. The first postoperative visit is one week following the permanent insertion. The surgical site is checked, and any skin staples or sutures are removed. Slight swelling may be noted in the pocket. This probably is a normal finding representing a seroma, although suspicion of infection also is appropriate. A seroma may last for 3–4 weeks and may interfere with transmission with the radiofrequency-controlled devices (Medtronic X-trel or any of the ANS SCSs). The SCS is reprogrammed as needed during this visit. The patient should be seen in follow-up 2 weeks later and then again in one month. The patient then is seen as indicated. If a goal of returning the patient to work exists, aggressive rehabilitation is needed.

COMPLICATIONS

Serious complications from the percutaneous temporary or permanent procedure of SCS implantation are rare.[3] In one study, one nonfatal pulmonary embolism and one case of paraplegia lasting 3 months occurred.[39] The latter resulted from a laminectomy that was used to place the stimulating lead. Other rare reported complications include sphincter disturbance and gait abnormality.[66]

Most complications from the temporary or permanent devices include formation of scar tissue, poor localization of paresthesias, lead migration, lead fracture, pain at the pocket site or connection site, infection, nerve injury, and epidural hematoma.[2,3,19,20,34,56,59,80,82,90] In a comprehensive summary of different publications, lead migration or displacement varied from 3.7–69%, although most studies reported migration between 16% and 25%.[3] Rates of lead fractures were reported in various series from less than 1% to more than 20%, and superficial

infections occurred in 2–12% of cases. Serious surgical infections and clinically apparent epidural hematomas were rare. Cerebrospinal fluid leakage was found in one series in 2% of patients. Avoiding complications in spinal cord stimulation should follow an analytical, step-wise approach (Fig. 31-14).

In over 300 lead implants, the authors have experienced three in situ infections with permanent devices. One infection resulted from an occult bone stimulator infection from a previous fusion and presented more than 6 months following implantation; the second infection occurred 2½ months after implantation from an unknown source; and the third infection occurred 18 months following implantation and appeared to result from hematogenous seeding when the patient broke an abscessed tooth when he bit down on an apple the week before the infection presented. In the first two cases the SCSs were removed, and the patients were placed on intravenous antibiotics without further sequelae. In the third case the SCS was not removed, and the patient was adequately treated with oral antibiotics and dental care. We have had no complications with any of the trial lead placements.

CLINICAL RESULTS

Original long-term results of pain control from spinal cord stimulation in the late 1960s and 1970s were disappointing[22,24,26,77,80] and led to general widespread disappointment in SCS. Poor patient selection, inadequate equipment, and failure to perform implantations with the patient awake accounted for the dismal results. The advent of new technology, careful patient selection, trial implantation, percutaneous placement, and active physician-patient interaction during the procedure have contributed to the success of spinal cord stimulation over the past 15 years.

The most common SCS application in North America today is in the treatment of chronic low back and lower extremity pain due to chronic radiculopathy despite surgery.[14,37,64,75,80,86] This population represents the primary indication for SCS in our practice. The largest SCS study incorporates 320 consecutive patients who underwent either temporary or permanent implants at the Johns Hopkins Hospital between 1971 and 1990.[32] This series includes follow-up of 205 patients, the majority of whom were diagnosed with failed back surgery syndrome (FBSS). Permanent SCS implants were placed in 171 of these patients. At follow-up (mean interval 7.1 ± 4.5 yrs), 52% of patients had at least

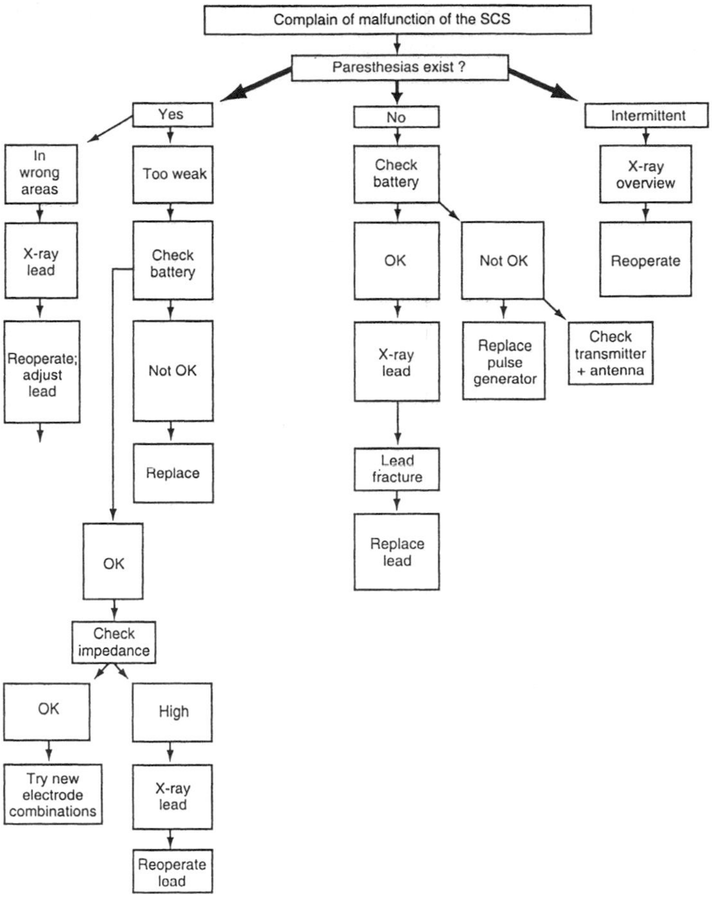

FIGURE 31-14. Avoiding difficulties in spinal cord stimulation (algorithm). Flow diagram for troubleshooting a malfunctioning spinal cord stimulation system. (From Augustinsson LE: Avoiding difficulties in spinal cord stimulation. In Waldman SD, Winnie AP (eds): Interventional Pain Management. Philadelphia, W.B. Saunders, 1996, p 429, with permission.)

50% continued pain relief, and 58% had a reduction or elimination of analgesic intake. About 54% of patients < 65 years were working at the time of follow-up; 41% had been working preoperatively.

The percentage of patients having long-term pain relief is similar in the majority of large published SCS series of implants for FBSS. The success rate in most of these studies, which is generally reported as 50% or more pain relief, is approximately 50–60%.[15,35,43,57,67,69] Some studies report success rates as high as 88% and others as low as 37%.[31,78] Although the latter studies differ in implantation technique and screening protocols, the success rate for pain reduction generally remains the same.

More recently published reviews have specifically looked at the efficacy of SCS in FBSS for pain control, reduction in narcotic consumption, function, and work status[18,41,58,59,68] and reveal that long-term pain reduction (at least 2 years after implantation) can be expected to range from 50–70% in approximately 60% of SCS patients. In 50–90% of individuals, opioid use is eliminated or reduced. The return to full employment rate after SCS reported by two studies is 25–59%, which is highly significant compared with the usual return-to-work rate (1–5%) in this population.[41,59] Reasons for the disparity between pain reduction and return-to-work rates appear to reflect the high percentage of unskilled laborers among this population, the prolonged periods of disability, and the attendant sociobehavioral changes that occur. Despite this disparity, level of function and activities of daily living increase overall.

The authors have implanted SCSs for the treatment of chronic pain in their practice for 7 years. The majority of patients have had FBSS, and the second leading indication has been complex regional pain syndrome (CRPS). Approximately 80% of the patients we have implanted report 50–80% pain relief and are satisfied with their device. The majority of patients who experienced < 50% pain relief still feel positively about their device and perceive it as having a positive impact on their pain. The vast majority of our patients who have been permanently implanted would have it done again. In general, we see a reduction in narcotic consumption and an improvement in function.

Most of our injured patients have a low educational level and were injured at work while doing relatively strenuous jobs. Although function generally improves with appropriate SCS implantation, few patients return to work. This is consistent with the observations of other researchers and appears to relate more to the chronicity of their disability, attendant psychosocial changes, and a relatively low job sophistication level. Such characteristics make it unrealistic to expect a high return-to-work rate regardless of the intervention. In the future, earlier intervention with stringent patient selection may help to improve return-to-work rates.

THE FUTURE

With the planned technological advances in implanted devices, the future of SCS looks promising.[8,35,36,62,63] Medtronic has an implanted pulse generator that is reported to adequately power a dual-lead system for several years in the final phase of Food and Drug Administration (FDA) approval at the time of this writing. In addition, a pulse generator that uses a capacitor instead of a battery that is rechargeable by an external radiofrequency-controlled device is in development and also in the final phase of FDA approval. ANS is developing an internalized pulse generator that will power its devices similarly to Medtronic's; however, it is not known when this device will be available. The reader is directed to outside sources for a more comprehensive analysis of subjects covered in this chapter.[1,9,10,17,52,85,88,89]

REFERENCES

1. Abram SE: Pain pathways and mechanisms. Semin Anesth 4:267–274, 1985.
2. Augustinsson LE, Carlsson CA, Holm J, et al: Epidural electrical stimulation in severe limb ischemia. Pain relief, increased blood flow, and possible limb-saving effect. Ann Surg 202:104–110, 1985.
3. Augustinsson LE: Avoiding difficulties in spinal cord stimulation. In Waldman SD, Winnie AP (eds): Interventional Pain Management. Philadelphia, W.B. Saunders, 1996, pp 427–430.
4. Barolat G, Schwartzman R, Woo R: Epidural spinal cord stimulation in the management of reflex sympathetic dystrophy. Stereotact Funct Neurosurg 53:29–39, 1989.
5. Basbaum AL, Fields HL: Endogenous pain control systems: Brain-stem spinal pathways and endorphin circuitry. Ann Rev Neurosci 7:309–315, 1984.
6. Bayliss WM: On the origin from the spinal cord of the vasodilator fibers of the hind-limb and on the nature of these fibers. J Physiol 382:173–209, 1987.
7. Bedder MD: Spinal cord stimulation and intractable pain: Patient selection. In Waldman SD, Winnie AP (eds): Interventional Pain Management. Philadelphia, W.B. Saunders, 1996, pp 412–418.
8. Bell GK, Kidd D, North RB: Cost-effectiveness analysis of spinal cord stimulation in treatment of failed back surgery syndrome. J Pain Symptom Manage 13:286–295, 1997.
9. Bonica JJ: Anatomic and physiologic basis of nociception and pain. In Bonica JJ (ed): The Management of Pain, Vol. 1, 2nd ed. Philadelphia, Lea & Febiger, 1990, pp 28–94.
10. Bowsher D: Pain mechanisms in man. Resident and Staff Physician 29:26–34, 1983.
11. Broseta J, Roldan P, Gonzalez-Darder V, et al: Chronic epidural dorsal column stimulation in the treatment of causalgic pain. Appl Neurophysiol 45:190–194, 1982.
12. Broseta J, Barbera J, de Vera JA, et al: Spinal cord stimulation in peripheral arterial disease. J Neurosurg 64:71–80, 1986.
13. Burchiel KJ, et al: Prognostic factors of spinal cord stimulation for chronic back and leg pain. Neurosurgery 36:1101–1111, 1995.
14. Burchiel KJ, Anderson VC, Brown FD, et al: Prospective, multicenter study of spinal cord stimulation for relief of chronic back and extremity pain. Spine 21:2786–2794, 1996.
15. Burton CV: Session on spinal cord stimulation: Safety and clinical efficacy. Neurosurgery 1:164–165, 1977.
16. Campbell JN: Examination of possible mechanisms by which stimulation of the spinal cord in man relieves pain. Appl Neurophysiol 44:181–186, 1981.
17. Crue BL: The neurophysiology and taxonomy of pain. In Brena SF, Chapman SL (eds): Management of Patients with Chronic Pain. Jamaica, NY, Spectrum Publications, 1983, pp 21–31.
18. De La Porte C, Van de Kelft E: Spinal cord stimulation in failed back surgery syndrome. Pain 52:55–61, 1993.
19. Devulder J, De Colvenaer L, Rolly G: Spinal cord stimulation in chronic pain therapy. Clin J Pain 6:51–56, 1990.
20. Erickson DL, Long DM: Ten-year follow-up of dorsal column stimulation. Adv Pain Res Ther 6:583–589, 1983.
21. Fedorcsak I, et al: Peripheral vasodilation due to sympathetic inhibition induced by spinal cord stimulation. In Proceedings of the IBRO World Congress of Neurosciences. Paris, France, IBRO, 1991, p 126.
22. Feldman RA: Patterned response of lamina V cells: Cutaneous and dorsal funicular stimulation. Physiol Behav 15:79–84, 1975.
23. Fields H: Depression and pain: A neurobiological model. Neuropsychiatry Neuropsychol Behav Neurol 4:83–92, 1991.
24. Foreman RD, Beall JE, Coulter JD, Willis WD: Effects of dorsal column stimulation on primate spinothalamic tract neurons. J Neurophysiol 39:534–546, 1976.
25. Groth DE: Spinal cord stimulation for the treatment of peripheral vascular disease. Adv Pain Res Ther 9:861–870, 1985.
26. Handwerker HO, Iggo A, Zimmerman M: Segmental and supraspinal actions on dorsal horn neurons responding to noxious and non-noxious skin stimuli. Pain 1:147–165, 1975.
27. Hoppenstein R: Percutaneous implantation of chronic spinal cord electrodes for control of intractable pain. Surg Neurol 4:195–198, 1975.
28. International Association for the Study of Pain: Classification of chronic pain: Descriptions of chronic pain syndromes and definitions of pain terms. Pain 28(Suppl 3):S1–S225, 1986.
29. Jacobs MJ, Jorning PH, Joshi SR, et al: Epidural spinal cord electrical stimulation improves microvascular blood flow in severe limb ischemia. Ann Surg 207:179–183, 1988.
30. Jensen MP, Turner JA, Romano JM, et al: Coping with chronic pain: A critical review of the literature. Pain 47:249–283, 1991.
31. Kalin MT, Winkelmuller W: Chronic pain after multiple lumbar discectomies—significance of intermittent spinal cord stimulation. Pain 40:S241, 1990.

32. Krames ES: Mechanisms of action of spinal cord stimulation. In Waldman SD, Winnie AP (eds): Interventional Pain Management. Philadelphia, W.B. Saunders, 1996, pp 407–411.

33. Krieger DT, Martin JB: Brain peptides. N Engl J Med 304:876–885, 1981.

34. Kumar K, Toth C, Nath RK, Laing P: Epidural spinal cord stimulation for relief of chronic pain. Pain Clin 1:91–99, 1986.

35. Kumar K, Nath R, Wyant GM: Treatment of chronic pain by epidural spinal cord stimulation: 10-year experience. J Neurosurg 75:402–407, 1991.

36. Kumar K, Toth C, Nath RK, Laing P: Epidural spinal cord stimulation for treatment of chronic pain—some predictors of success: A 15-year experience. Surg Neurol 50:110–121, 1998.

37. Kupers RC, Van den Dever R, Van Houdenhove B, et al: Spinal cord stimulation in Belgium: A nation-wide survey on the incidence, indications and therapeutic efficacy by the health insurer. Pain 56:211–216, 1994.

38. Larson SJ, Sances AJ Jr, Riegel DH, et al: Neurophysiological effects of dorsal column stimulation in man and monkey. J Neurosurg 41:217–223, 1974.

39. Law JD: Percutaneous spinal cord stimulation for the "failed back surgery syndrome." Pain Management Update 1:12, 1990.

40. Law JD: Spinal stimulation: Statistical superiority of monophasic stimulation of narrowly separated, longitudinal bipoles having rostral cathodes. Appl Neurophysiol 46:129–137, 1983.

41. Law JD, Kirkpatrick AF: Update: Spinal cord stimulation. Am J Pain Manage 2:34–42, 1992.

42. LeDoux MS, Langford KH: Spinal cord stimulation for the failed back syndrome. Spine 18:191–194, 1993.

43. LeRoy PL: Stimulation of the spinal cord biocompatible electrical current in the human. Appl Neurophysiol 44:187–193, 1981.

44. Linderoth B, Fedorcsak I, Myerson BA: Is vasodilation following dorsal column stimulation mediated by antidromic activation of small diameter fibers? Acta Neurochir Suppl (Wein) 46:99–101, 1989.

45. Linderoth B: Dorsal column stimulation and pain: Experimental studies of putative neurochemical and neurophysiological mechanisms [thesis]. Karolinska Institute, Stockholm, 1992.

46. Loeser JD, Parker G: Assessment and investigation of the patient with chronic pain at the University of Washington Multidisciplinary Pain Center. In Loeser JD, Egan KJ (eds): Pain Management. New York, Raven Press, 1989, pp 21–34.

47. Marchand S, Bushnell MC, Molina-Negro P, et al: The effects of dorsal column stimulation on measures of clinical and experimental pain in man. Pain 45:249–257, 1991.

48. Meglio M, Cioni B, Rossi GF: Spinal cord stimulation in management of chronic pain: A 9-year experience. J Neurosurg 70:519–524, 1989.

49. Melzack R: Psychological aspects of pain: Implications for neural blockade. In Cousins MJ, Bridenbaugh PO (eds): Neural Blockade in Clinical Anesthesia and Management of Pain, 2nd ed. Philadelphia, J.B. Lippincott, 1989, pp 845–860.

50. Melzack R, Casey KL: Sensory, motivational and central control determinate of pain. In Kenshalo DR (ed): The Skin Senses. Springfield, IL, Charles C Thomas, 1968, pp 423–443.

51. Melzack R, Wall PD: Pain mechanisms: A new theory. Science 150:971–979, 1965.

52. Melzack R: Anatomy and physiology of pain: Clinical correlates. In Waldman SD, Winnie AP (eds): Interventional Pain Management. Philadelphia, W.B. Saunders, 1996, pp 1–9.

53. Meyerson BA: Electric stimulation of the spinal cord and brain. In Bonica JJ (ed): The Management of Pain, 2nd ed. Philadelphia, Lea & Febiger, 1990, pp 1862–1877.

54. Meyerson BA, et al: Spinal cord stimulation in chronic neuropathic pain. Lakartidningen 88:727–732, 1991.

55. Miletic V, Hoffert MJ, Ruda MA, et al: Serotonergic axonal contacts on identified cat dorsal horn neurons and their correlation with nucleus raphe magnus stimulation. J Comp Neurol 228:129–134, 1984.

56. Mullet KR, et al: Design and function of spinal cord stimulators—theoretical and developmental considerations. Pain Digest 1:281–287, 1992.

57. Nielson KD, Adams JE, Hosobuchi Y: Experience with dorsal column stimulation for relief of chronic intractable pain. Surg Neurol 4:148–152, 1975.

58. North RB, Ewend MG, Lawton MT, et al: Failed back surgery syndrome: 5-year follow-up after spinal cord stimulator implantation. Neurosurgery 28:692–699, 1991.

59. North RB, Ewend MG, Lawton MT, et al: Spinal cord stimulation for chronic, intractable pain: Superiority of "multichannel" devices. Pain 44:119–130, 1991.

60. North RB, Fowler K, Nigrin D, et al: Patient-interactive, computer-controlled neurological stimulation system: Clinical efficacy in spinal cord stimulator adjustment. J Neurosurg 76:967–972, 1992.

61. North RB, Kidd D, Zahurak M: Spinal cord stimulation for chronic intractable pain: Experience over two decades. Neurosurgery 32:384–394, 1993.

62. North RB, Kidd DH, Lee MS, Piantodosi S: A prospective, randomized study of spinal cord stimulation vs. reoperation for failed back surgery syndrome: Initial results. Stereotact Funct Neurosurg 62:267–272, 1994.

63. North RB, Kidd DH, Wimberly RL, Edwin D: Prognostic value of psychological testing in patients undergoing spinal cord stimulation: A prospective study. Neurosurgery 39:301–311, 1996.

64. Ohnmeiss D, Rashbaum RF, Bogdanffy GM: Prospective outcome evaluation of spinal cord stimulation in patients with intractable leg pain. Spine 21:1344–1350, 1996.

65. Oliveras JL, Redjemi G, Besson J: Analgesia induced by electrical stimulation of the inferior centralis of the raphe in the cat. Pain 1:139–143, 1975.

66. Pineda A: Complications of dorsal column stimulation. J Neurosurg 48:64–68, 1978.

67. Pineda A: Dorsal column stimulation and its prospects. Surg Neurol 4:157–163, 1975.

68. Racz GB, McCarron R, Talboys P: Percutaneous dorsal column stimulator for chronic pain control. Spine 14:1–4, 1989.

69. Ray CD, Burton C, Lifson A: Neurostimulation as used in a large clinical practice. Appl Neurophysiol 45:160–206, 1982.

70. Reynolds DV: Surgery in the rat during electrical analgesia induced by focal brain stimulation. Science 164:444–449, 1969.

71. Robaina FJ: Spinal cord stimulation for relief of chronic pain in vasospastic disorders of the upper limbs. Neurosurgery 24:179–183, 1989.

72. Robb LG, Spector G, Robb MP: Spinal cord stimulation: Neuroaugmentation of the dorsal columns for pain relief. In Weiner RS (ed): Pain Management: A Practical Guide for Clinicians, 5th ed. Boca Raton, FL, St. Lucie Press, 1998, pp 271–293.

73. Ruda MA: Opiates and pain pathways: Demonstration of enkephalin synapses on dorsal horn projection neurons. Science 215:1523–1524, 1982.

74. Saade NE, Tabet MS, Soueidan SA, et al: Supraspinal modulation of nociception in awake rats by stimulation of the dorsal column nuclei. Brain Res 369:307–310, 1986.

75. Segal R, Stacey BR, Rudy TE, et al: Spinal cord stimulation revisited. Neurol Research 20:391–396, 1998.

76. Shealy CN, Mortimer JT, Reswick JB: Electrical inhibition of pain by dorsal column stimulation. Anesth Analg 46:489–491, 1967.

77. Shealy CN, Mortimer JT, Hagfors NR: Dorsal column electroanalgesia. J Neurosurg 32:560–564, 1970.

78. Siegfried J, Lazorthes Y: Long-term follow-up of dorsal column stimulation for chronic pain syndrome after multiple lumbar operations. Appl Neurophysiol 45:201–204, 1982.

79. Snyder SH: Opiate receptors in the brain. N Engl J Med 296:266–271, 1977.

80. Spiegelmann R, Friedman WA: Spinal cord stimulation: A contemporary series. Neurosurgery 28:65–71, 1991.

81. Steude U, Abendroth D, Sunder-Plassamann L: Epidural spinal electrical stimulation in the treatment of severe arterial occlusive disease. Acta Neurochir Suppl (Wien) 52:118–120, 1991.

82. Sweet W, Wepsic J: Stimulation of the posterior column of the spinal cord for pain control: Indications, technique and results. Clin Neurosurg 21:278–310, 1974.

83. Tallis RC, Illis LS, Sedgwick EM, et al: Spinal cord stimulation in peripheral vascular disease. J Neurol Neurosurg Psychiatry 6:478–484, 1983.

84. Tasker RR: Deafferentation in central pain. In Wall PZ, Melzack R (eds): Textbook of Pain, 2nd ed. Edinburgh, Churchill Livingstone, 1989, pp 154–180.

85. Thienhaus O, Cole BE: The classification of pain. In Weiner RS (ed): Pain Management: A Practical Guide for Clinicians, 5th ed. Boca Raton, St. Lucie Press, 1998, pp 19–26.

86. Turner J, Loeser JD, Bell KG: Spinal cord stimulation for chronic low back pain: A systematic literature synthesis. Neurosurgery 37:1088–1096, 1995.

87. Wall PD, Melzack R: Introduction. In Wall PD, Melzack R (eds): Textbook of Pain, 2nd ed. Edinburgh, Churchill Livingstone, 1989, pp 1–18.

88. Yaksh TL: Neurological mechanisms of pain. In Cousins MJ, Bridenbaugh PO (eds): Neural Blockade in Clinical Anesthesia and Management of Pain, 2nd ed. Philadelphia, J.B. Lippincott, 1988, pp 791–844.

89. Yaksh TL: Anatomy of the pain processing system. In Waldman SD, Winnie AP (eds): Interventional Pain Management. Philadelphia, W.B. Saunders, 1996, pp 10–18.

90. Young RF: Evaluation of dorsal column stimulation in the treatment of chronic pain. Neurosurgery 3:373–379, 1978.

32

Radiofrequency Neurotomy of the Zygapophyseal and Sacroiliac Joints

Paul Dreyfuss, M.D., and Christopher J. Rogers, M.D.

Effective treatment of chronic spine pain demands accurate identification of the primary source of pain. The spine has many potential pain generators, including the annulus fibrosus of the disc, zygapophyseal (facet) joint (z-joint), sacroiliac joint (SIJ) and supporting ligaments, dura, spinal nerves, dorsal root ganglia, paraspinal muscles, and spinal ligaments (including the posterior longitudinal ligament).[13,19,64,73,110,111,114,139] The zygapophyseal joints are a potent source of spinal and extremity pain. Not only are they well innervated,[10,19,21,22,26,77,138] but studies in healthy volunteers have shown that stimulating these joints or the nerves that innervate them produces cervical, thoracic, lumbar, and referred pain in the head, shoulder, scapula, buttock, thigh, and leg.[42,45,53–55,87,92] The sacroiliac joint also has been shown to be a potent pain source as it is innervated,[58,66,132,147] and experimental stimulation of this joint has been shown to produce primarily buttock pain.[50]

Spinal axis joint-mediated pain states cannot be ignored because the literature documents that they can be a source of chronic pain and impairment. Anesthetizing these joints with fluoroscopically guided, contrast-enhanced injection techniques relieves symptoms in patients with joint-mediated pain.[6,12,15,33,34,40,43,74,77,85,110,114,128,134] Controlled blocks in the cervical spine (C3–4 to C6–7) confirm that the prevalence of z-joint pain after whiplash is approximately 50%.[7,82] A similar study in patients with whiplash in whom headache was the main complaint revealed the C2–3 joint as the primary pain generator in 53% of cases.[81] No data exist on the prevalence of thoracic z-joint pain. Studies using controlled blocks confirm that the prevalence of chronic zygapophyseal joint pain in low back pain is 15% in younger patients[111,114] and as high as 40% in older patients.[116] The prevalence of sacroiliac joint pain in those with lower back and buttock pain

using controlled blocks is approximately 15%.[85,110]

Radiofrequency (RF) lesioning of nerves supplying painful tissues can provide an effective treatment after the pain source is established. Used appropriately, such procedures have the potential to offer relief of chronic pain when less invasive treatments and natural history have failed. Neurotomy of the medial branch nerves was devised on the premise that pain from a zygapophyseal joint could be relieved by coagulation of its afferent nerve supply. By blocking conduction in these nerves, coagulation simply reproduces the effect of a diagnostic medial branch block but for a longer time. Injection of phenol onto the target nerves has been reported as one method of joint denervation,[62,129] as has cryoneurolysis.[104,109] However, the greatest volume of literature on denervation of the zygapophyseal joints has described the use of percutaneous RF needle electrodes. This chapter will review the role of RF lesioning for cervical, thoracic, lumbar zygapophyseal and sacroiliac joint pain.

PRINCIPLES OF RADIOFREQUENCY LESIONING

Cushing and Bovie were the first to use RF energy for the cutting and coagulation of tissue in the 1920s.[25] Modifications have improved the control of current, power level, temperature, and consistency of lesion size. The basic RF circuit includes a voltage generator and both active and reference electrodes. The active electrode is placed near the target tissue. The electrodes typically used for spinal axis joint neurotomies are disposable 50- or 100-mm, insulated, 20- or 22-gauge RF needles with a 5–10-mm, noninsulated active tip. An adhesive surface dispersive (reference) electrode completes the electrical circuit. The RF lesion generator consists of a voltage source and stimulator with the ability to

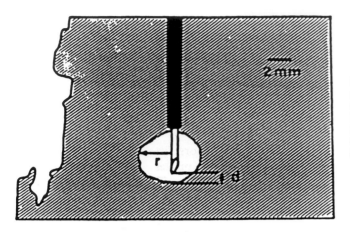

FIGURE 32-1. A tracing of a lesion produced in meat with a 22-gauge RF needle. The maximal circumferential radius (r) and distal radius (d) of the lesion is shown. (From Bogduk N, Macintosh J, Marsland A: Technical limitations to the efficacy of radiofrequency neurotomy for spinal pain. Neurosurgery 20:529–535, 1987, with permission.)

monitor impedance, temperature, power, voltage, current, and time. When a high-frequency alternating current (about 500,000 Hz) is applied, ionic currents are created in the tissue adjacent to the active electrode. Heat is generated as a result of friction. Tissues with an impedance greater than the current will generate higher temperatures that subsequently are recorded at the needle tip.

Temporary cessation of neural function occurs between 42.5 and 44°C.[70] Denervation of painful tissues is believed to occur by the application of heat energy at or exceeding the early cytotoxic range for nervous tissue (45–50°C).[23,137] Clinically, temperatures of at least 70–80°C are recommended for irreversible lesions.[93] As the lesion size increases with higher temperatures, the risk of boiling (100°C) or carbonization of tissues also increases.[145] The electrical and magnetic field energies generated are within normal physiologic levels.

Monitoring current, power, voltage, and impedance are less important clinically, but such measurements ensure that the generator functions appropriately. The size of the lesion created depends on the electrode diameter, electrode configuration (monopolar or bipolar), lesion time, and temperature utilized.[18,145] Monopolar electrodes of 1 mm in diameter (approximately equivalent to an 18-gauge needle) with a 5-mm exposed tip generated lesions with a mean diameter of 3.18 mm ± 0.41 in fresh egg white at 60 seconds at 85°C.[145] This equates to a radius lesion of 1.09 mm (after subtraction of the 1 mm diameter electrode). Increasing the temperature to 90°C for 60 seconds increased the lesion diameter to 3.39 mm ± 0.56, whereas increasing the time alone to 100 seconds only increased the lesion diameter to 3.25 mm (radius 1.13 mm) ± 0.50. In vivo measurements were then performed in subcortical white matter of adult New Zealand white rabbits.

Monopolar 1-mm needles with a 4-mm exposed tip produced lesion diameters of 4.91 mm ± 0.41 when lesioned at 80°C for 60 seconds. This equates to a radius lesion of 1.96 mm.[145] Others report a radius of 3.5 mm for lesions made in monkey brains using an electrode with a 1.05-mm tip diameter.[1,146]

The size and shape of lesions in both egg white and fresh meat using 18-gauge and 22-gauge needles have been evaluated.[18] The lesion radius made by the 18-gauge needle (2.2 mm ± 0.47) was twice that made by the 22-gauge needle (1.1 mm ± 0.25) in egg white at 80–85°C for 80 seconds. Equilibrium was obtained at 80 seconds once target temperature was established (80–85°C), and lesion times up to 145 seconds did not increase the lesion size. The mean radius was slightly (0.5 mm) but significantly (p < 0.01) larger at 90°C than at 80°C. The lesion was shaped like an oblate spheroid (elliptical), which concurs with prior research (Fig. 32-1).[18,145] The cardinal finding was that the lesion did not extend distal to the tip of the electrode. Thus, if RF electrodes are placed perpendicular to the nerve, the target nerve may not be incorporated within the lesion. Parallel needle placement to the target nerve is essential (Fig. 32-2).[18]

Temperature equilibrium depends on the rate at which heat is conducted away from and generated in the tissues. Total heating will be affected by heat sinks such as blood vessels and bone. Accurate temperature measurement ensures consistency of lesion size and safety. The objective of RF lesioning is to maintain the desired temperature for no less than 30 seconds and no more than 60 seconds, at which time lesion equilibrium is obtained.[70,145]

Combining the data from the above studies yields the following clinical conclusions and recommendations: (1) larger RF needles improve the lesion radius; (2) lesion times of at least 60 seconds and not greater than 80 seconds are ideal to improve

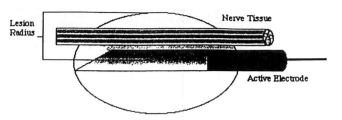

FIGURE 32-2. Lesion radius generated around the exposed tip of an active electrode positioned parallel to the medial branch nerve.

the lesion radius without using longer, nonproductive lesion times; (3) higher temperatures yield larger lesions, but temperatures greater than 90° involve excessive risks; and (4) the lesion shape is elliptical. The RF needles should be placed as parallel as possible to the target nerves.

The authors use 20-gauge RF needles for all cervical, thoracic, lumbar, and sacral neurotomies because they produce larger lesions than the 22-gauge needles but are more easily tolerated than the next available size (16-gauge, 1.6 mm Ray electrode). In the cervical and thoracic regions, 20-gauge needles are ideal, whereas 18-gauge needles are tolerated in the lumbar spine, if available. Temperatures are maintained at 85–90°C for 80–90 seconds in all spinal regions. Longer exposed tip needles (10 mm) are preferred for medial branch neurotomy to obtain a longer lesion parallel to the nerve without the need for a second burn along the course of the nerve when 4–5-mm exposed tips are used. A variable curved tip is useful in aligning the needle with the natural osseous course of the nerves.[47] For these reasons our needle of choice is a 20-gauge (0.9 mm), 10-mm exposed tip, precurved needle. The curve can be lessened manually, if desired.

REGIONAL NEUROANATOMY PERTINENT TO ZYGAPOPHYSEAL AND SACROILIAC JOINT NEUROTOMY TECHNIQUES

Cervical Joint Innervation

Each cervical z-joint from C3–4 to C7–T1 is innervated from the medial branches of the dorsal rami with each joint supplied from the branch above and below that joint. C2–3 is largely innervated from the third occipital nerve (TON), which is the superficial medial branch of the C3 dorsal ramus. The deep medial branch of the C3 dorsal ramus is referred to as the C3 medial branch proper. Articular branches may also arise from a communicating loop that crosses the back of the joint between the third occipital nerve and the C2 dorsal ramus.[10,11,77]

Each C3–C7 dorsal ramus crosses the same segment's transverse process and divides into lateral and medial branches. The medial branch curves consistently around the "waist" of the articular pillar of the same numbered vertebrae. The medial branch nerves are bound by fascia, held against the articular pillar, and covered by the tendinous slips of the origin of the semispinalis capitis.[77] Articular branches arise as the nerve approaches the posterior aspect of the articular pillar (Fig. 32-3). An ascending branch innervates the joint above and a descending branch innervates the joint below. At C7 the base of the transverse process occupies most of the lateral aspect of the articular pillar and pushes the medial branch higher than typical cervical medial branch nerves.[12,79] The TON continues around the lower lateral and dorsal surface of the C2–C3 joint embedded in the connective tissue

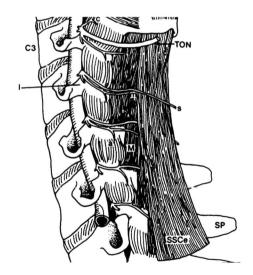

FIGURE 32-3. Cervical medial branch (m) and third occipital nerve (TON) anatomy from a lateral view. The lateral branches (l) of the dorsal rami have been cut. The articular branches (a) are seen to arise from the posterior portion of the medial branch nerve. The medial branch nerve is seen to ramify into the multifidus (M). The superficial medial branches (s) pass deep or dorsal to the semispinalis cervicis (SSCe) to become cutaneous. C3 = vertebral body of C3; SP = spinous process of C7. (From Lord S, Barnsley L, Bogduk N: Percutaneous radiofrequency neurotomy in the treatment of cervical zygapophyseal joint pain: A caution. Neurosurgery 36:732–739, 1995, with permission.)

that invests the joint capsule.[10,11] The TON provides muscle branches to the semispinalis capitis and becomes cutaneous over the suboccipital region. C4–C7 medial branch nerves typically lack any cutaneous branches.[10,11]

Radiographic anatomy has been evaluated using lateral and anteroposterior (AP) views of the TON and the C3–C7 medial branch nerves of 10 dissected cadavers. The courses of the C4 and C5 medial branch nerves were relatively constant following the waist of their respective articular pillars. C3, C6, and C7 showed more variation. Although in each cadaver the TON was rostral to the C3 medial branch, at times the C3 medial branch nerve adopts a more superior location at the upper third of the C3 articular pillar and often overlapped the TON. The C6 medial branch nerves coursed around the waist of the articular pillar or just above it, between the waist and the superior articular process. Most of the C7 medial branches (7 of 10) were located high on the C7 articular pillar and crossed the lateral image of the C6–C7 z-joint. A few were lower on the C7 transverse process and thus were lower on the lateral image of the C7 articular pillar. The distance between the bony articular pillar and the medial branches was greater than expected. Whereas some were adjacent to the bone, others were separated by 2–3 mm.[76] The third occipital nerve was large (approximately 1.5–2.0 mm) compared to typical medial branch nerves (approximately 1.0 mm).[79]

Thoracic Zygapophyseal Joint Innervation

Dissections of 84 thoracic medial branch nerves from 7 sides of four adult cadavers were performed (Figs. 32-4 and 32-5).[26,27] The nerves were found upon leaving the intertransverse space typically to cross the superolateral corner of transverse process. They then passed medially and inferiorly across the transverse process before ramifying into the multifidus muscle at the T1–T4 and T9–T10 levels. Exceptions to this occurred at mid-thoracic levels (T5–T8), where the nerve did not always assume contact with the transverse process. Although at times the nerve curved in a similar fashion, the inflection occurred at a point superior to the superolateral corner of the transverse process. Thus, the nerve did not run upon the transverse process but was suspended in the intertransverse space separated from the transverse process by the fascicles of the multifidus. The T11 medial branch course

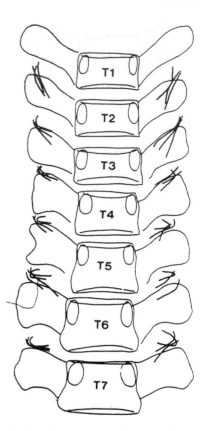

FIGURE 32-4. Diagram of the T1–6 medial branch nerves in relation to the transverse processes. (From Chua WH: Clinical Anatomy of the Thoracic Dorsal Rami [thesis]. Newcastle, Australia, University of Newcastle, 1994, with permission.)

varied due to the much shorter transverse process at T12. The T11 medial branch ran across the lateral surface of the root of the superior articular process of T12. Lastly, the T12 medial branch assumed a course analogous to lumbar medial branch nerves. Each medial branch nerve gave off a short ascending branch that entered the inferior aspect of the zygapophyseal joint as it passed caudal to the joint. A slender descending branch arose from the medial branch at the superolateral aspect of the transverse process. It has a sinuous course through the multifidus to enter the superior aspect of zygapophyseal below. The T1–T7 medial branches are musculocutaneous, whereas the lower thoracic medial branches have a muscular distribution only.[20]

Lumbar Zygapophyseal Joint Innervation

The lumbar zygapophyseal joints are innervated by the medial branches of the dorsal rami of L1–L5.[16,17,21,138] Each zygapophyseal joint is supplied by the two medial branches of the same levels

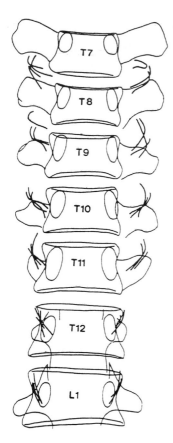

FIGURE 32-5. Diagram of the T7–12 medial branch nerves in relation to the transverse processes. (From Chua WH: Clinical Anatomy of the Thoracic Dorsal Rami [thesis]. Newcastle, Australia, University of Newcastle, 1994, with permission.)

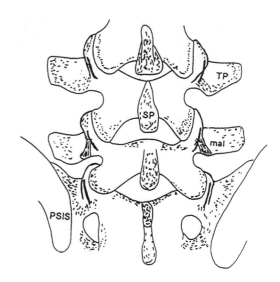

FIGURE 32-6. AP diagram of the lumbar spine depicting the medial branch nerves (short dark black lines) in the groove between the superior articular process and the transverse process. TP denotes the transverse process, SP the spinous process, PSIS the posterior superior iliac spine, and mal the mamilloaccessory ligament.

seal joint below. The L5 dorsal ramus crosses the ala of the sacrum rather than that of the transverse process. It then runs in a groove formed by the junction of the sacral ala and the root of the superior articular process of S1. The L5 dorsal ramus divides into medial and intermediate branches at the base of the L5–S1 zygapophyseal joint. The medial branch

comprising it. Therefore, the L4–L5 zygapophyseal joint is innervated by the L3 and L4 medial branches that cross the L4 and L5 transverse processes. The L5–S1 zygapophyseal joint is innervated by the L4 medial branch and dorsal ramus of L5. The L1–L4 dorsal rami divide off the spinal nerves and then divide into lateral, intermediate, and medial branches. The fifth dorsal ramus divides into medial and intermediate branches only. The intermediate and lateral branches of the L1–L5 dorsal rami enter the erector spinae muscles of the back. Each L1–L4 medial branch nerve crosses the base of the superior articular process at its junction with the transverse process. Within 1 cm, the medial branch enters the mamilloaccessory notch under the mamilloaccessory ligament (Figs. 32-6 and 32-7).[31] After exiting this notch, the medial branch supplies articular branches to the zygapophyseal joint above. It then courses inferiorly across the lamina to supply the interspinous ligament, the multifidus muscle, and the superior aspect of the zygapophy-

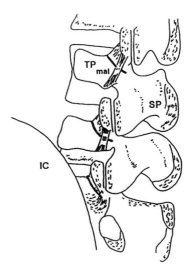

FIGURE 32-7. Oblique diagram of the lumbar spine depicting the medial branch nerves (short dark black lines) in the groove between the superior articular process and the transverse process. TP denotes the transverse process, SP the spinous process, IC the iliac crest, and mal the mamilloaccessory ligament.

wraps around the base of this joint before supplying it and then enters the segmental multifidus fascicles.[84] Each L1–L4 lumbar medial branch nerve lies across the transverse process of the vertebra below. Thus, the L3 medial branch is located at the junction of the superior articular process and transverse process of L4.[16,17,21]

Sacroiliac Joint Innervation

Free nerve endings that convey pain, thermal, pressure, and position sense are seen in the SIJ capsule and posterior ligaments.[58,66,132] Regional sacroiliac ligaments, including the sacrospinous and sacrotuberous ligaments, are innervated.[58,66] The sacrotuberous and sacrospinous ligaments are specifically innervated by the lateral branches of the S3 and S4 dorsal rami.[58]

In 1957, innervation to the SIJ was evaluated in 9 cadavers using macro- and microscopic techniques. Innervation was determined to be from the roots of L3–S2 and also from the superior gluteal nerve. Dorsally, innervation was from the dorsal rami of S1 and S2 in all cases.[132]

Eighteen Japanese cadavers were investigated with macroscopic and histologic evaluation to determine the innervation to the sacroiliac joint.[66] The upper ventral SIJ was innervated by the ventral ramus of L5, whereas the lower ventral aspect of the SIJ was innervated by the ventral ramus of S2 or branches from the sacral plexus. The upper dorsal aspect of the SIJ was innervated by the lateral branches of the dorsal ramus of L5, while the lower dorsal aspect was innervated by lateral branches from the dorsal rami of S1–S4.

Using gross, histologic, and immunocytochemical analysis the innervation to the SIJ was investigated in 8 cadavers.[58] Innervation was exclusively from the lateral branches of the S1–S4 dorsal rami. There were no branches to the SIJ from the obturator or sacral plexus. Nerves were distributed laterally between the superficial and deep portion of the sacroiliac ligaments. Laterally the S1–S4 nerves were seen at various layers to travel under the superficial and deep layers of the long posterior sacral ligament before passing through the gluteus maximus and emerging as cutaneous cluneal nerves. Furthermore, histologic and immunocytochemical studies on 2 fetal SIJs showed neurofilaments only in the dorsal portions.[58]

Recently, 10 cadavers were examined bilaterally to analyze the S1–S3 dorsal rami. Although the distribution of the dorsal sacral plexus was highly variable, several consistent features were appreciated. Each of the dorsal rami (S1–S3) had a medial and lateral division. The medial division penetrated the multifidus muscle and had fibers that extended to the midline. The lateral divisions anastomosed with each other within the multifidus compartment on the floor of the sacral gutter and sent branches into and through the capsule of the SIJ. The lateral division of S1 frequently passes through an isolated tunnel between the long posterior sacral ligament and the SIJ. As the lateral branches pass deep to the long posterior sacral ligaments, they flatten into thin ribbons. Once the S1–S3 nerves are through or over the long posterior sacral ligament, they turn inferiorly along the sacrotuberous ligament and pass through the gluteus maximus to become cutaneous in the perianal region.[147]

SELECTION CRITERIA FOR RADIOFREQUENCY NEUROTOMY

Patients most likely to benefit from radiofrequency lesioning have been diagnosed with functionally limited spinal zygapophyseal joint or SIJ pain that is resistant to at least 3 months of conservative treatments and natural history. Conservative treatment includes exercise-based physical therapy, modality- and passive treatment–based physical interventions, manual therapy (mobilization/manipulation), psychological interventions, anti-inflammatory agents, adjunctive nonopioid medications, fluoroscopically guided intra-articular and possibly extra-articular corticosteroid injections, and activity modification.

These conditions, however, cannot be diagnosed clinically. No clinical symptom or sign has been shown to be both sensitive and specific for zygapophyseal joint or SIJ pain.[36,37,40,85,113,114,128] Plain films, computed tomography, and bone or single photon emission computed tomography (SPECT) scans are not absolutely diagnostic.[15,32,86,102,117,127] The current mainstays for diagnosis are local anesthetic blocks of the putatively painful joint. These may be intra-articular blocks or blocks of the nerves that innervate the joint.[5,12,15,28,34,43,77,85,110,111]

The zygapophyseal joints (cervical, thoracic, and lumbar) may be anesthetized by direct intra-articular injections of local anesthetic or by anesthetizing the sensory innervation to the joint: the medial branches of the dorsal rami and also the L5 dorsal ramus for the L5–S1 zygapophyseal joint.[5,6,12,15,36,41,43,67,77] The SIJ can be anesthetized by direct intra-articular blocks or potentially by anesthetization of the L5 dorsal ramus and lateral branches of S1–S3 (4) dorsal rami if in fact the joint's innervation is only dorsal.[28,34]

Cervical and lumbar medial branch blocks have been shown to be target-specific if solutions are injected carefully at prescribed, osseous target points with additional attention to the needle's trajectory and direction of the bevel opening.[5,41] Contrast is necessary to ensure that inadvertent venous uptake does not occur.[12,41,67] By injecting prescribed osseous target points with 0.5 ml of 2% lidocaine, authors of a recent randomized, controlled, single-blind study found that medial branch blocks anesthetize the lumbar zygapophyseal joint at a rate of 89% provided that inadvertent venous uptake does not occur.[67] No literature exists on the target specificity or physiologic effectiveness of thoracic medial branch or S1–S4 lateral branch nerve blocks.

Because of a false-positive rate of single zygapophyseal joint injection procedures in the lumbar and cervical spine of 38% and 27%, respectively,[8,112] dual blocks of the joints or their nerve supply is recommended to obtain a secure diagnosis of zygapophyseal joint pain. Recently, subjects with chronic neck pain underwent dual medial branch blocks (lidocaine and bupivacaine [Marcaine]) and a placebo block with saline in a double-blind, controlled fashion.[80] The false-negative rate of time-contingent relief (longer relief with bupivacaine than lidocaine) with dual medial branch blocks was high (46%) against placebo, but the false-negative rate of non–time contingent relief (not having longer relief with bupivacaine than lidocaine but complete relief with both) with dual medial branch blocks was 0% (100% sensitivity). Eighty-eight percent (12% false-positive rate) of those with and 65% of those without time contingent relief after dual medial branch blocks withstood (no pain relief) a placebo challenge. Comparative medial branch blocks (lidocaine vs. bupivacaine [Marcaine]) substantially reduce the likelihood of a false-positive response; however, only a placebo injection can absolutely exclude a placebo response. Non–time contingent relief following dual medial branch blocks is a reasonable diagnostic compromise between single medial branch blocks that have an unacceptably high false-positive rate (27–38%) and triple blocks (comparative blocks and a placebo block) that incur additional time and expense. With this approach, sensitivity remains high (near 100%) and specificity greatly improves compared to single intra-articular or medial branch blocks.

We prefer to start with an intra-articular block with anesthetic and corticosteroid followed by medial branch blocks of the dorsal rami for zygapophyseal joint pain and L5 dorsal ramus and lateral branch blocks of the sacral dorsal rami for persistent sacroiliac joint pain. The first block set allows the patient the chance of a response to intra-articular corticosteroids, usually in combination with postinjection rehabilitation or joint mobilization/manipulation.[28,37,39] If this fails, the medial or lateral branch blocks test pain relief after temporary blockade of the nerves destined for coagulation and should theoretically be more prognostic than intra-articular blocks. Each block set should provide substantial pain reduction. Most clinicians consider substantial pain reduction as reduction of $\geq 80\%$ of the patients' pain in those with isolated spinal joint-mediated pain. Pain reduction of $\geq 80\%$ on two occasions using controlled (dual) medial branch blocks carries the highest likelihood of strongly positive RF results as is apparent in available prospective outcome studies that have used such strict criteria.[38,38a,83]

This argument is supported when these studies are compared to other reports using less stringent selection criteria. In studies using single medial branch blocks with less strict relief (e.g., $\geq 50\%$ relief) the percentage of subjects having high degrees of sustained pain relief is less.[63,95,98] Studies selecting patients on single intra-articular blocks of variable relief[3,96,100,106,130] or on clinical grounds alone[65,71,143,144] without diagnostic blocks generally reported even lower percentages of patients with high degrees (> 90% pain relief compared to pretreatment) of sustained pain relief.

OUTCOME STUDIES

Cervical Neurotomy

Early reports on cervical RF neurotomy were fraught with problems. Effectiveness was unconvincing. Major problems existed with selection criteria, including lack of reliable diagnostic block techniques, questionable accuracy of the RF technique, and lack of contemporary and objective outcome instruments. All reports were uncontrolled and practice audits rather than following a detailed, prospective design.[63,106–108,130,131,144] Selection criteria were often local tenderness and response to a single zygapophyseal joint block rather than controlled blocks (to limit false-positive blocks) including prognostic blocks of the target structures (medial branch nerves).[63,106–108,130] One report relied only on localized neck pain and tenderness over the zygapophyseal joints.[144] Many prior reports used a lateral approach so that their RF electrodes would not be parallel to the target nerves.[130,131,144]

Due to the limitations and less than optimal results of such studies, an audit of 19 patients was performed to determine if performance of a randomized, double-blind, controlled trial was justified.[79] This study used comparative local blocks of the medial branch nerves with complete pain relief required and longer relief from bupivacaine than lidocaine to satisfy entrance into the treatment phase. The RF neurotomy technique was altered from earlier reports so that parallel lesioning was performed using a posterolateral approach. A matrix of lesions was performed with two lesions per pass with three passes for the C3–C7 medial branch nerves. With each pass a lesion was made at the anterior and middle third of the articular pillar. One parasagittal pass was at the waist of the articular pillar and the others just above and below the waist of the articular pillar. Near completion of the study, the lesion at the anterior third of the articular pillar was made with a 30° oblique pass. For the third occipital nerve, the passes were at the level of the maximum convexity of the C2–C3 zygapophyseal joint at a point just above the waist of the C3 articular pillar and at one location between these points. A 22-gauge, 4-mm exposed tip was used for all lesions, but near completion of the study a Ray RRE™ electrode (1.6 mm diameter, 6-mm exposed tip) (Radionics, Burlington, MA) was substituted for lesions of the third occipital nerve. Seven of 10 patients who underwent lower medial branch neurotomy obtained complete pain relief for clinically useful periods. Pain relief was seen for 1 year or longer in many subjects. Only 4 of 10 patients undergoing third occipital nerve neurotomy obtained long-lasting relief. Ataxia and numbness were common but self-limited after third occipital nerve neurotomy. It was concluded that third occipital nerve neurotomy "should be abandoned" until the technical problems could be overcome but that lower cervical neurotomy should be formally evaluated with a randomized, controlled trial.[79]

The third occipital nerve neurotomy procedure was later modified using exclusively a larger diameter electrode and more lesions.[90] Eight patients (10 nerves) with C2–C3 joint pain established by controlled blocks were identified. Success was defined as a Visual Analogue Scale (VAS) of less than 5 out of 100, a McGill word count of 4 or less, and restoration of four of the most desired activities of daily living with pain relief lasting at least 3 months. Duration of relief was defined until 50% of pre-

treatment pain returned. Radiofrequency neurotomy was performed with a Ray RRE thermistor electrode, as previously described,[79] but with a larger number of lesions, especially over the C3 articular pillar just distal to the foramen.

Of the 10 procedures, 8 were successful. In contrast with earlier reports,[79] no early failures occurred. The median relief at the time of the audit was 202.5 days. Seven of the 8 patients experienced cutaneous hypersensitivity beginning around day 7 and lasting a median of 30.3 days. All patients had numbness in the cutaneous distribution of the TON, which usually remained as pain relief continued and subsequently reduced as pain returned, transforming into transient dysesthesia in 4 patients. It was concluded that this technique improves the success rate over previous reports but that "a significantly larger series of patients is needed before firm conclusions can be established."[90]

The only prospective, double-blind, controlled trial on the treatment of chronic cervical zygapophyseal joint pain was reported in 1996.[83] Twenty-four subjects with cervical zygapophyseal joint (C3–C4 to C6–C7) pain confirmed with triple double-blind, placebo-controlled medial branch blocks (lidocaine, bupivacaine [Marcaine], and placebo) were evaluated. Subjects were required to have complete pain relief with the anesthetic blocks and no relief with the placebo injection. Patients had a median of 34 months of pain prior to study entrance. They were randomized to RF or sham RF treatment. Outcome tools included the VAS, McGill Pain Questionnaire, and Symptoms Checklist 90R (SCL-90R) score. Radiofrequency treatments were conducted at 80°C for 90 seconds for the active group and at 37°C (machine off) for the control group. There was no difference between the groups except the machine being off or on when lesioning began. A 10-cm, 22-gauge electrode with a 4-mm exposed tip was used. Each electrode was inserted twice, once with a parasagittal pass (to reach the middle third of the articular pillar) and once with a 30° oblique pass (to reach the anterior third of the articular pillar). With each type of pass, 2–3 lesions were made to accommodate variations in the course of the nerve as previously described.[79] The median time that elapsed before pain returned to 50% of the pretreatment level was 263 days for the treatment group versus 8 days for the sham treatment group (p = 0.04) Although these results were strongly assertive, the authors caution that the results "cannot be generalized to apply to patients whose pain is confirmed by less stringent criteria or who are treated with less exacting variants of the technique."

The most recent study on cervical medial branch RF neurotomy[143] challenged the strict inclusion criteria used by Lord et al.[83] in a randomized controlled trial. In this prospective study, 15 subjects were chosen on the clinical grounds of having only cervicogenic headache without the use of any diagnostic blocks. Entrance criteria were based on clinical, diagnostic criteria for cervicogenic headache.[126] The authors did not use diagnostic blocks to select subjects because they question the specificity of all diagnostic blocks (especially zygapophyseal joint blocks) based on data from other investigators.[94,133]

Radiofrequency lesioning of the C3–C6 medial branch nerves was carried out with an oblique approach in the supine position on the symptomatic side(s). Outcomes were assessed at baseline, 8 weeks after treatment (short term), 4–14 months after treatment (intermediate term) (mean = 8.8), and 12–22 months after treatment (long term) (mean = 16.8). VAS, 7-point verbal rating scale (range: complete relief to excruciating pain), days per week with a headache, and analgesic intake per week were assessed. The mean VAS was 90.4 at baseline, 59 at short-term, 36.1 at intermediate, and 36.9 at long-term follow-up. This decrement was "statistically significant." According to the verbal rating scale, 1 of the 15 subjects (6.6%) had complete relief and 11 of the 15 experienced good relief (73%) at 8-week follow-up; 4 of the 15 (26%) had complete relief and 8 of the 15 (53%) had good relief at the intermediate follow-up; and 1 of the 15 (6.6%) had complete pain relief and 8 of the 15 (53%) had good relief at long-term follow-up. Using comparative blocks, a 70% complete pain relief success rate was obtained[79] versus only a 6.6% long-term complete pain relief success rate in this study.[143] Both studies were noncontrolled practice audits. Apparently, diagnostic blocks select those with the condition (zygapophyseal joint pain) amenable to RF neurotomy better than clinical grounds alone. The authors justify RF neurotomy without diagnostic blocks because they consider RF neurotomy to be a benign procedure and the likelihood of the success to be acceptable when considering the incidence of zygapophyseal joint pain as a causative factor in cervicogenic headache. The authors are currently conducting a randomized, double-blind, controlled trial using similar selection criteria without diagnostic blocks to formally compare their methodology to the results of Lord et al.[83]

Thoracic Neurotomy

The first attempts at thoracic medial branch neurotomy yielded poor results in a total of 19 combined patients, due primarily to an inaccurate understanding of the medial branch nerve anatomy.[75,120] The first publication dedicated to thoracic zygapophyseal joint RF neurotomy asserted that the nerves maintained an analogous course to the lumbar medial branch nerves.[135] Using two cadavers, the same investigators determined with cryomicrotome analysis that 44 RF needles fluoroscopically placed at the junction of the superior articular process and transverse process (as used clinically) never hit the "stem" of the medial branch.[136] Nervous tissue presumed to be smaller filaments of the medial branch nerves was hit in 61% of cases. Thus, the target nerve (the medial branch division of the dorsal ramus prior to its ramifications) was never targeted. When the true thoracic medial branch nerve anatomy is appreciated, it is obvious why such a technique would fail. The stem of the medial branch nerve is far more lateral on the superomedial border of the transverse process than the location where lesions were attempted.[135]

No peer-reviewed reports using known anatomic considerations exist on thoracic medial branch neurotomy. A final target position for RF neurotomy of the medial branch nerves at the superolateral aspect of the transverse process has been recommended, as has a medial and inferior starting position at the midline to obtain parallel needle placement to the target nerves.[26,35]

Lumbar Neurotomy

The first report of success with medial branch denervation was in 1971.[103] A 99.8% success rate after percutaneous medial branch destruction was claimed with the use of a knife in 1000 patients. However, it was later confirmed that this technique was inadequate because the knife was too short to reach the target medial branches.[69]

Shealy was the first to use radiofrequency methods for denervation of the zygapophyseal joints,[118,119,121] but these successful reports became suspect when it was determined that the technique used did not appropriately target the medial branches.[16,17] All studies that have used this technique are therefore invalid.[4,46,49,52,56,75,88,89,97,100,106,141]

Even studies that subsequently employed anatomically correct target points must now undergo scrutiny.[91,96,101] Studies have demonstrated that RF needles coagulate circumferentially and inadequately at the tip.[18] Consequently, electrodes introduced perpendicularly onto a nerve (the trajectory used for medial branch blocks) are unlikely to adequately coagulate the nerve.

In spite of these limitations, clinical medial branch RF neurotomy studies have demonstrated variable success.[4,24,30,38,38a,49,51,56,57,62,65,68,69,71,75,88,89,91,95–99,101,105,106,119,122,140] Success rates ranged from 17%[3] to 90%.[118,121] The measures of a successful outcome were varied and often arbitrary in these studies. Not one report used a comprehensive battery of outcome tools. The majority of the reports were retrospective practice audits with only three reporting a prospective design.[65,98,141]

Two randomized trials using the RF method of Shealy have been reported.[56,69] King and Lagger used physical examination alone to locate discrete areas of maximal tenderness in patients with chronic low back pain. This was the main inclusion criteria to identify 60 subjects that were randomized to one of three treatment groups; no diagnostic blocks were used. At 6 months, it was found that radiofrequency coagulation at a depth of 1.25 inches (RF myotomy) and RF neurotomy of the medial branches provided greater than 50% pain relief in 53% and 27% of subjects, respectively. These results were better than the control group, in which a stimulating rather than a coagulating current was used just cephalad to the point of maximal tenderness in the paravertebral gutter. No pain relief occurred in any control patient.[69]

In another study, 0.5 cc of 0.5% bupivacaine was injected "into and around the appropriate joints" as a single screening block to identify subjects for RF neurotomy who had experienced low back pain for more than 3 months.[56] Thirty patients with a "good" response to this injection were randomized to active or placebo RF neurotomy with all parameters the same "except for the radiofrequency heat lesion." Subjects underwent active (n = 18) and placebo (n = 12) lesions under double-blind conditions. Denervation was carried out in the manner described by Shealy, a technically flawed approach.[16,17] At 1 and 6 months, the active radiofrequency denervation group had a 42% and 24% VAS decrease in pain, respectively, versus a 17% and 3% VAS decrease of pain in the placebo group. The difference was statistically significant despite marginal results in the active group.[56]

Van Kleef et al. conducted the first prospective, randomized, double blind study of the effects of RF medial branch neurotomy in a selected group of patients with chronic low back pain.[142] It was clearly demonstrated that patients treated with placebo lesions did not obtain pain relief.[142] Thirty-one subjects were randomized into a group treated with a single 80°C lesion for 60 seconds at the L3, L4, medial branches, and L5 dorsal ramus unilaterally or bilaterally; electrodes were placed in the placebo group of patients, but no lesion was generated. A 22-gauge cannula with a 5-mm active tip was placed at the superior aspect of the junction of the transverse process and the superior articular process. The needle was positioned so that a 2-Hz stimulation produced a multifidus contraction, if possible, at < 1 volt (V).

Outcome measures included physical impairment according to Waddell, VAS, Oswestry disability scale, Dartmouth COOP/WONCA chart, and global perceived effect. Assessments were made at 8 weeks and 3, 6, and 12 months. A significant (p < 0.05) difference appeared at 8 weeks between the VAS and Oswestry scores of the active and placebo group. "Successes" were defined as at least 50% pain relief and a 2-point reduction in the VAS. Significantly more "successes" (p = 0.02) were found in the RF group at 3 (60%), 6 (47%), and 12 (47%) months follow-up.

However, for patients treated with active neurotomy, only modest results were obtained.[142] The mean average intensity pain scores of the actively treated patients dropped from 5.2 on a 10-point scale to 2.83 at 8 weeks after RF. Only a minority of patients obtained ≥ 90% pain relief.

The rationale of lumbar medial neurotomy predicts that patients with isolated zygapophyseal joint pain should obtain complete relief of their pain if the nerves that innervate their painful joint are coagulated. The failure of Van Kleef et al.[142] to secure this outcome consistently can be attributed to either of two factors. First, they selected their patients on the basis of single, diagnostic blocks (which carry a false-positive rate of 38%[112]) with at least 50% relief. Therefore, patients without true, isolated zygapophyseal joint pain may have been treated. Second, electrodes were placed less than optimally parallel (at an angle) to the target nerve.[142] Consequently, in some patients the target nerves may have failed to coagulate adequately. In their study, adequate coagulation of the target nerves was not assessed with segmental electromyography (EMG) of the multifidus.[59,60]

In a prospective audit, 15 subjects with chronic low back pain for > 1 year who met strict inclusion criteria were studied.[38] Multiple inclusion criteria were met, including primary low back pain, and ≥ 80% pain relief following two separate sets of medial branch blocks (maximum 6 nerves) without IV sedation at the painful levels. The first set of medial branch blocks was performed with 2% lidocaine and the second set, 1 week later, with 0.5% bupivacaine. A modified comparative block protocol was used; more than 1 hour of relief was required following lidocaine medial branch blocks and more than 2 hours of relief were required following bupivacaine medial branch blocks. Exclusion criteria included neurologic or dural tension findings, known disc pain or spinal stenosis, 75% disc space collapse on plain films, prior spinal surgery, depression as evidenced by a score of 20 or more on the Beck Depression Inventory (BDI), an abnormal multifidus EMG at any lumbar level, those involved in litigation, and those seeking or on disability or workers' compensation. There were 460 responses to public announcements for which 138 were examined and 41 were eligible for medial branch blocks. Of these, 15 completed the dual medial branch block paradigm. Eighty-seven percent of subjects had pain for more than 2 years while 54% had pain for more than 5 years.

A 16-gauge (1.6 mm) radiofrequency Ray needle was used incorporating parallel lesioning techniques with two 5-mm contiguous lesions at each targeted nerve. Prior to lesioning, both the impedance and the minimum voltage necessary to obtain a visual multifidus twitch was noted. Standard outcome tools administered at baseline included the BDI, VAS for that day and a weekly average, the Roland-Morris disability scale, 36-item Short Form health survey (SF-36), McGill Pain Questionnaire, expectation with treatment North American Spine Society (NASS) scale, medication and cointervention treatment inventory, isometric push, pull and above shoulder lift tasks, a dynamic floor to waist lift, and an L1–L5 multifidus EMG. All written outcome tools were administered at 6 weeks and 3, 6, and 12 months postneurotomy. The lift tasks and multifidi EMG were repeated only at 6 weeks after neurotomy.

Either no change or a slight increase in mean lift task scores occurred after versus before neurotomy. Cointerventions were absent in 93% of the subjects for the duration of the study. Treatment was successful with statistically significant improvements ($p = < 0.0001$ to 0.004) in the VAS, Roland-Morris disability scale, physical function and bodily pain subscales of the SF-36 questionnaire, and the McGill Pain Questionnaire when baseline was compared to 6 week and 3, 6, and 12 months postneurotomy. Sixty percent of subjects at 1-year follow-up had ≥ 90% pain relief, and an additional 27% had at least 60% pain relief.

Of the targeted nerves, 90.5% were lesioned as determined by a normal pre- and abnormal postsegmental multifidi EMG. No correlation was found between impedance values or the minimum voltage necessary to obtain a palpable multifidi twitch just before neurotomy and the presence or absence of denervation postneurotomy.

These results dispel some of the myths and conventions concerning the performance of medial branch neurotomy.[38,38a] The use of preliminary motor electrical stimulation to verify electrode placement appears to be superfluous and an unnecessary waste of operative time. Adjusting the electrode position to minimize the threshold for evoked activity in the multifidus also does not improve outcome. The essential requirement is that the electrode is placed in an anatomically sensible and accurate position, which may be judged radiologically and by the operator's sense of the needle in the target osseous groove.[38,38a] This study differs in several respects from previous studies of lumbar medial branch neurotomy:

1. It is the first prospective study to have treated only patients with zygapophyseal joint pain proven with controlled (dual) diagnostic medial branch blocks.

2. It is the only lumbar study to have used an anatomically and technically accurate operative technique using careful parallel needle placements.

3. It is the only study to have shown accurate and adequate coagulation of the target nerve by objective means.

4. It is the only study to have recorded multiple subjective and objective outcome measures over a prolonged period.

Under these conditions the present study shows that, in properly selected patients, lumbar medial branch neurotomy offers profound and lasting relief of chronic low back pain. In this regard, the results of the present study complement and extend those obtained by Van Kleef et al. in their controlled trial.[142] If patients are rigorously selected and if accurate surgical techniques are used, approximately 60% of patients can expect 90% improvement of their pain, and 87% can expect 60% improvement, lasting at least 12 months without the need for potentially costly and time-consuming cointerventions such as exercise-based physical therapy or manipulative care.

ASSESSING THE TECHNICAL SUCCESS OF LUMBAR MEDIAL BRANCH RADIOFREQUENCY NEUROTOMY

The theory of lumbar branch neurotomy maintains that if the target nerve is adequately coagulated, not only should pain-relief ensue, but also the appropriate bands of multifidus should be denervated. In addition to supplying the zygapophyseal joints, the medial branches of the lumbar dorsal rami also innervate specific bands of the multifidus muscle.[21,123] The pattern is such that each medial branch innervates only those fibers of multifidus that arise from the spinous process with the same segmental number as the nerve.[21,123] These fibers lie in constant, definable regions and are selectively accessible to EMG needles.[59-61] Thus, post- versus preoperative EMG is a means of testing the face validity of lumbar medial branch neurotomy and serves as an objective control for genuine relief. Patients who report relief in the absence of denervation of their multifidus cannot be claimed to have pain relief because of the neurotomy; nonspecific factors must apply. On the other hand, complete pain relief correlated with objective signs of denervation would support the credibility of an accurate and thorough neurotomy. Furthermore, persistence of pain after neurotomy in the presence of denervation of the multifidus indicates that the initial diagnosis was incorrect.

Using parallel needle placement techniques, three-view imaging, and operator feel of adequate placement of the electrode in the target osseous groove where the medial branch resides, a 90.5% denervation rate was appreciated by Dreyfuss.[38,38a] This was the first study that specifically incorporated baseline multifidi EMG to ensure lack of denervation prior to neurotomy from concomitant or alternative pathology. Baseline testing may be critical because dorsal rami neuropathy with multifidi denervation (e.g., from diabetic dorsal rami neuropathy),[9] a disc herniation,[72] or entrapment of medial branch nerve under the mamilloaccessory ligament can occur.[48,124] Additionally, multifidi denervation can be seen early in myopathies.[29] Thus, comparison of individual segmental multifidi muscles pre- and postneurotomy with EMG remains the most accurate method to document technical success (denervation) after neurotomy.

No segmental specific EMG techniques are available for examining the cervical or thoracic spine.[61] The multifidus muscles, however, can still be evaluated for the presence or absence of denervation at large, which can provide clinically helpful information. This is especially true when all examined multifidi levels where the RF lesions were made lack denervation potentials and pain persists.

Sacroiliac Joint Neurotomy

No formal peer-reviewed outcome studies exist on RF neurotomy for intra- or extra-articular SIJ-mediated pain. Radiofrequency lesioning has been used in an attempt to denervate the sacroiliac joint.[70] This method generates linear lesions between two bipolar electrodes. This occurs as long as the distance between the two cannulas does not exceed five times the diameter of an individual cannula. Fifteen to 20 continuous lesions are made along the posterior joint line in an attempt to incorporate all nerve filaments that are descending into and through the posterior SIJ capsule. Alternating, slightly overlapping bipolar lesions are made from S1 to the most inferior aspect of the SIJ.[70]

There are no reports on lesioning the stem of the nerves (L5 dorsal ramus and the lateral branches of S1–S3 dorsal rami) that innervate either the joint complex as a whole[58] or its dorsally innervated aspect including the joint capsule and overlying ligaments.[66] If the SIJ complex pain generator is innervated by these nerves that can be approached via RF lesioning, neurotomy should serve as a valuable treatment technique. This is provided, of course, that these nerves can be adequately lesioned. This has yet to be determined anatomically or validated via appropriate outcome studies. Additionally, as the L5 dorsal ramus and lateral branches of the S1–S3 dorsal rami provide sensory innervation to the skin of the superior to inferior buttock,[147] there is the additional theoretical risk of dysesthesias with lesioning these particular nerves as exists with third occipital nerve neurotomy.[90]

JOINT DENERVATION TECHNIQUES

General Principles and Practice

Similar precautions used for any spinal-related injection procedure should be addressed. For example, patients with an ongoing infection or those maintained on therapeutic doses of anticoagulants should not be treated.

In all RF neurotomy techniques strict aseptic technique is used. The patient is in a prone position. IV access is obtained, and continuous pulse oximetry, pulse, respiration, and electrocardiogram (ECG) measurements are monitored. The patient's blood pressure is checked every 5 minutes during the procedure. Conscious sedation with midazolam (Versed) and occasionally fentanyl (Sublimaze) is provided as necessary to prevent patient motion while aiding pain and anxiety reduction.

With all RF procedures it is recommended that three views (AP, lateral, and oblique) document safe and precise needle placement before lesioning. A C-arm is essential. Motor stimulation at 5 Hz, 1 millisecond duration using 1.0–1.5 V ensures that stimulation of the ventral ramus or nerve root does not occur after radiographic and operator sense of appropriate final needle position is obtained. Nerve root stimulation would be evident by myotomal activation of that nerve root with extremity movement. This maneuver further prevents inadvertent spinal nerve root injury that may easily be avoided through three-view imaging and an appreciation of spinal neuroanatomy. Searching for a segmental multifidi twitch at the needle position associated with the least voltage needed to produce such a twitch has not been correlated with a higher degree of segmental denervation. In fact, a segmental twitch may not be obtainable (especially at the L5 dorsal ramus), yet the lesion yields pain relief and segmental denervation as judged by pre- versus postsegmental multifidi EMG.[38,38a]

The authors do not routinely use sensory stimulation (50 Hz) in an attempt to evoke usual pain that many clinicians empirically trust to ensure placement adjacent to the target nerve. No literature addresses the prognostic value of sensory stimulation, and the prospective studies with the best clinical outcomes did not use this technique.[38,38a,83]

The authors prefer to use a moldable, precurved, 20-gauge (0.9 mm), 10-mm exposed tip needle. An example of such an RF electrode is the Racz-Finch Kit Disposable Cannula needles (RFK-C) (Radionics). The need may arise to use a larger electrode for repeat RF procedures or with TON neurotomies for which the larger Ray needle electrode has yielded better results with multiple lesions.[90] The curve is essentially removed for thoracic neurotomies and lessened approximately 50% for cervical and sacral neurotomies. The original molded curve is adequate for most L1–L4 medial branch neurotomies or, per the authors' preference, is slightly lessened (approximately 20%) for both L1–L4 medial branch and L5 dorsal ramus lesions.

Prior to lesioning, the target nerves are anesthetized with 0.5–0.75 ml of 2% lidocaine. If this fails to render the lesioning painless, an additional 0.25–0.5 ml of lidocaine is injected before formal lesioning. Lesioning parameters for all zygapophyseal and sacroiliac joint RF techniques include active tip temperatures of 85–90°C for 80–90 seconds for reasons previously cited.

RF Needle Placement Techniques

Cervical Zygapophyseal Joint

C3–7 Medial Branch Nerves

Although some clinicians use a supine, oblique approach to the cervical medial branch nerves,[70,131] the authors prefer a prone approach with the head positioned in a head-holding device. We believe this maximizes parallel needle placement to the target nerves as do other investigators.[79,83]

AP imaging is obtained with no rotation of the head or the C-arm. The C-arm is then declined (intensifier more caudal) to obtain a pillar view at the targeted segment. This allows imaging through the zygapophyseal joints. In this manner, the zygapophyseal joints are imaged similar to a posterior approach to zygapophyseal joint injections. The beam is then parallel to the target nerves and the segmental articular pillar and its waist is maximally visualized (Fig. 32-8). If a parasagittal approach is taken to reach the mid-third of the articular pillar,[79,83] the needle is placed directly down the beam into the target waist of the articular pillar that corresponds to the same numbered target nerve. If an oblique approach also is used to reach the anterior third of the articular pillar,[79,83] a 30° oblique from an AP view is used. The needle is then advanced down the beam. With these techniques, a 22-gauge, 4-mm exposed tip, noncurved RF needle is used.[83]

Many clinicians prefer to avoid using two needle passes because of increased patient discomfort. Instead, a modified 15° postero-oblique approach is used with the larger 20-gauge, 10-mm active exposed tip needle and the addition of an approximately 10° curved tip (Fig. 32-9). The C-arm is rotated 15° and the needle is advanced directly down the beam. With this approach, only one pass is needed as long as the targeted osseous plane is contacted with the exposed needle tip from the mid to anterior third of the articular pillar. The curved tip usually allows one to reach the more medial position of the articular pillar at its anterior third. With this modified oblique approach, it is assumed that the needle will lie close enough to the targeted nerve to lesion it along its length from the middle to anterior

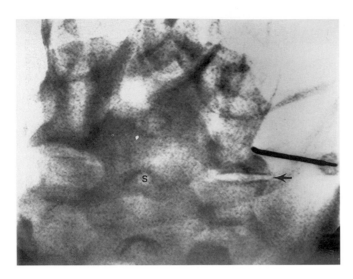

FIGURE 32-8. AP pillar view of the C3 segment. The C3–4 z-joint space is optimally imaged as denoted by the black arrow. The RF needle has been directly placed down the beam into the waist of the C3 articular pillar where the nerve resides. S denotes the spinous process.

third of the articular pillar. This approach, however, unlike Lord's,[79,83] has never been formally evaluated in any outcome study.

Regardless of the approach (postero-oblique with a precurved tip) or approaches (parasagittal and 30° oblique)[79,83] of the needle under pillar, declined view imaging of it should be directed just medial to the waist of the articular pillar until bone is contacted. This ensures avoidance of overzealous anterior placement. At this point the needle is then slowly redirected just off the articular pillar laterally; the C-arm is then repositioned so that pure lateral imaging (with the bilateral zygapophyseal joints overlapped) is obtained. The needle should be seen to rest just off the posterior edge of the articular pillar in parallel alignment with the course of the target nerve. It is then slowly advanced anteriorly and slightly medially until bone is gently contacted and the active tip

rests at the middle third of the articular pillar if one is using the parasagittal approach, at the anterior third of the articular pillar if one is using the 30° oblique approach, or at both if using the modified postero-oblique approach with a 10-mm exposed tip.

It has been recommended with each approach (parasagittal and oblique) and placement at the mid and anterior third of the articular pillar, respectively, that 2–3 lesions are made to account for superior to inferior nerve position variability.[79,83] With this, the needle is placed at the middle of the articular pillar in a cephalad-to-caudad plane and then additional lesions can occur. One lesion is one RF needle diameter superior and the other is one RF needle diameter inferior. Using validated techniques,[83] there may be up to six lesions per nerve.

Using the theoretically attractive modified 15–20° postero-oblique approach, a maximum of three

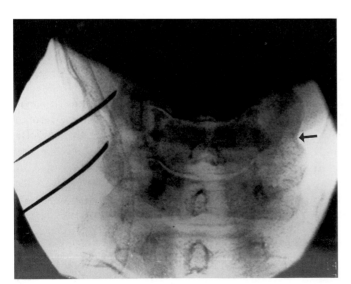

FIGURE 32-9. AP radiograph of the cervical spine showing RF needles in place at the waist of the articular pillar. A 15° oblique approach was utilized. The black arrow denotes the waist of the articular pillar on the contralateral side.

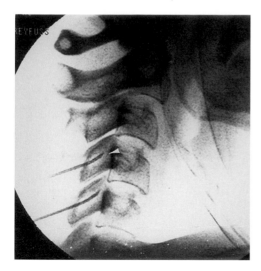

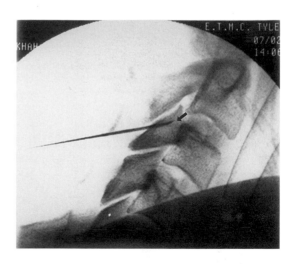

FIGURE 32-10. Lateral radiograph of the cervical spine. RF needles are in place for a C4 and C5 medial branch neurotomy. The C4 RF needle could be advanced anteriorly 2–3 mm to the tip of the white arrow and still be in a safe position.

FIGURE 32-12. Lateral radiograph of a C3 medial branch nerve neurotomy at the superior lesioning position, which accounts for nerve location variability. The needle could be safely advanced 2 mm to the tip of the black arrow before lesioning.

lesions are necessary to cover the same territory because of the longer exposed active tip. This approach, however, has not been scientifically validated. Furthermore, using the wider diameter needle renders the lesion radius larger. In theory, this makes lesioning of the target nerve more likely if this approach with a precurved needle indeed allows the needle to be placed consistently parallel to the target nerve with the same accuracy as using

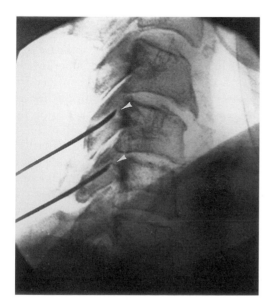

FIGURE 32-11. Lateral radiograph of the cervical spine. RF needles are in place for a C4 and C5 medial branch neurotomy. Both RF needles could be advanced anteriorly 2–3 mm to the tip of the white arrows and still be safe.

two separate approaches with an uncurved needle as previously recommended.[79,83]

Regardless of the approach or approaches used, after final needle placement is obtained on lateral imaging, the C-arm should be repositioned in an AP projection to ensure that the needle has not strayed too far lateral from the articular pillar. Finally, upon lateral imaging the needle tip should never rest more anterior than the anterior edge of the articular pillar. In an attempt to maximize safety, the authors prefer to be just (2 mm) posterior to this point for lesioning the anterior third of the articular pillar regardless of which approach is used (Figs. 32-10 and 32-11).

For the C4–C6 medial branch nerves the above technique suffices, but at C3 and C7 more superior lesions are necessary to account for this variability because of the possibility of a greater degree of superior nerve displacement (Fig. 32-12).[76]

Third Occipital Nerve

Similar prone positioning is used with the previously described needle approaches. The difference is that the target is not the waist of the articular pillar but the convexity of the C2–C3 joint on declined, pillar-view imaging. On lateral imaging, at least three and preferably four to five lesions are made superior to inferior on lateral imaging to account for the cephalad-to-caudad variation of the nerve position using at least a 20-gauge RF needle (Fig. 32-13). The target is at and up 2 needle diameters superior and inferior to the C2–C3 joint line at the anterior and middle third of the articular pillar.

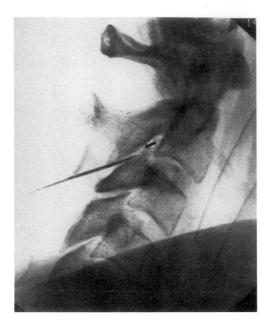

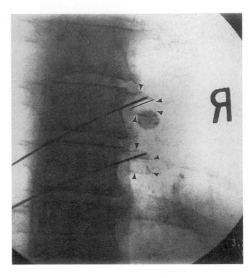

FIGURE 32-13. Lateral radiograph of a third occipital nerve neurotomy at one of the inferior lesioning positions. The needle could be safely advanced to the tip of the black arrow before lesioning.

FIGURE 32-14. AP radiograph of the mid-thoracic spine. Two RF needles have been placed for a thoracic medial branch neurotomy. The black arrowheads denote the lateral margin of the two targeted transverse processes. The inferior needle is appropriately placed to the superolateral aspect of the transverse process. The superior RF needle has been additionally placed one needle diameter medial and parallel to the first lesion location. The RF needle was first placed at the location of the thin black line.

Using primarily a 22-gauge RF needle, technical failure occurred with TON lesioning in 60% of cases.[79] For this reason, it is recommended that at least a 20-gauge RF needle is used, if not a Ray (16-gauge) needle[90] for this particularly larger and more variably located nerve.

Thoracic Zygapophyseal Joint

The following technique is used by the authors and has not been formally evaluated with either a retrospective or prospective outcome study design. Anatomically invalid techniques[135,136] will not be presented.

One begins with AP imaging with cephalad-to-caudad angulation so that the disc space margins are well defined at the level of the target transverse processes. The target transverse processes are marked. A midline skin mark is made from this mark so that a 20-gauge, 10-mm exposed tip RF needle (with the curve removed) can be advanced superiorly and laterally to lie parallel to the target nerve. After the needle is advanced through the skin, the transverse process should be contacted at the junction of its medial one-third and lateral two-thirds. From this location the needle is walked off laterally so that the tip rests just over the superolateral edge (inflection point) of the transverse process as previously endorsed.[26] If the transverse process cannot easily be appreciated, 5–10° of contralateral oblique imaging

usually enhances visualization. At this location, one lesion is made. The operator may elect to make one to two more parallel lesions medial to the first to account for variability in nerve location (Fig. 32-14).

The authors prefer to augment the above technique with phenol neurolysis for the T5–T8 levels rather than attempt RF lesioning in free soft tissue space. At these levels the target nerves may never reside on the superolateral aspect of the transverse process, but instead exist more superiorly displaced.[26,27] The authors have elected to use a mixture of 8–10% phenol, 80–85% glycerin, 2% lidocaine, and saline for an additional attempt at neurolysis. In theory, this viscous injectant will be limited in its diffusion away from the target nerve. After RF lesioning, contrast is injected with needle tip redirectioning as necessary through the 20-gauge needle until superior and medial flow is appreciated (Fig. 32-15). Then 0.5 ml of the phenol mixture is injected after appropriate, nonvascular flow is confirmed. Contrast dispersal at the appropriate location also should be subsequently appreciated.

Lumbar Zygapophyseal Joint

Declined ("Groove") View Starting Position

The starting position in the declined view approach allows the operator to directly image the

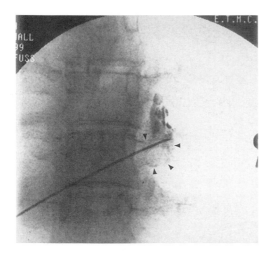

FIGURE 32-15. AP radiograph of the mid-thoracic spine. An RF needle is appropriately placed for a medial branch neurotomy. Additionally, contrast has been injected with appropriate flow prior to the injection of a phenol solution, which accounts for neurotomy of a superiorly displaced medial branch nerve. The black arrowheads denote the margin of the transverse process.

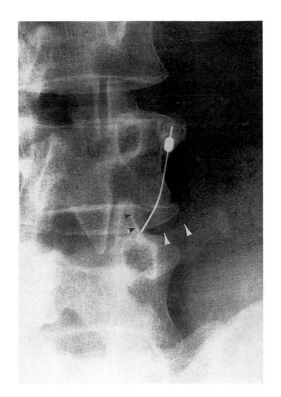

FIGURE 32-16. Groove view for the L3 medial branch nerve at the L4 transverse process. A needle has been placed on the nerve as in an L3 medial branch block directly in the groove between the transverse process (*white arrows*) and superior articular process (*black arrows*).

osseous groove where the nerve resides analogous to the cervical technique. If the needle is then advanced "down the beam," the needle will be placed parallel to the target nerve.

The C-arm is positioned with approximately 10–15° of ipsilateral rotation and 20° of cephalad tilt so that the osseous groove where the target nerves reside (between the superior articular process and transverse process) is maximally defined.[23] When angulation is appropriate, the cortical edges of convexity between the superior articular process and transverse process are crisp and maximally defined. This view is noted as the "groove view" (Fig. 32-16). For the L5 dorsal ramus, the groove between the superior articular process of S1 and the sacral ala is maximally imaged with avoidance of excessive oblique imaging that images the posterior superior iliac spine "over" the osseous groove where the L5 dorsal rami reside. Usually at L5, slightly more inferior angulation is needed than at the more superior levels.

The RF needle is then advanced down the fluoroscopy beam (using the groove view) (Fig. 32-17). Bone is contacted just proximal to the mamilloaccessory ligament, and the RF needle is then advanced slightly in this osseous groove while continuously feeling bone on two sides of the needle shaft. AP imaging is obtained to ensure that needle placement is medial enough and the needle is not advancing laterally along a defect in the transverse process. The needle should be medial to the

lateral silhouette of the superior articular process, if possible. After AP imaging confirms adequate medial position, an oblique "Scottie dog" view is

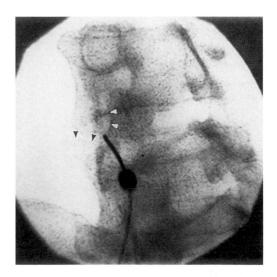

FIGURE 32-17. Groove view of the L4 medial branch nerve with an RF needle appropriately placed down the targeted groove. The white arrows denote the superior articular process, and the black arrows denote the transverse process.

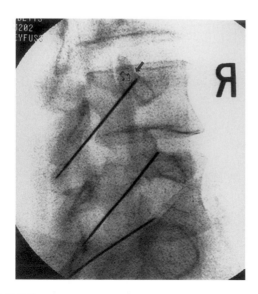

FIGURE 32-18. Oblique radiograph of an L3 and L4 medial branch and L5 dorsal ramus neurotomy. The L3 neurotomy needle is not yet in the ideal location because it is slightly lateral to its target. The needle should be at the tip of the open black arrow and in line with the superior junction of the transverse process and superior articular process (solid black arrow).

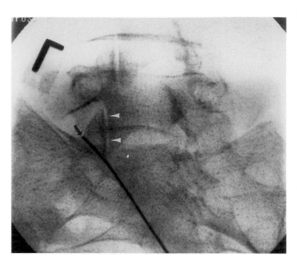

FIGURE 32-20. Oblique radiograph of an L5 dorsal ramus neurotomy. The white arrows denote the L5–S1 z-joint, and the black arrow indicates the most superior aspect of the junction between the sacral ala and the superior articular process of S1.

obtained. The needle should be seen to reside parallel to the target nerve in the osseous groove between the superior articular process and the transverse process just proximal to the mamilloaccessory ligament for the L1–L4 medial branch nerves. For the L5 dorsal ramus, the needle should be seen to reside just superior to the inferior aspect of the L5–S1 zygapophyseal joint in its osseous groove. The needle is then advanced to the superior-proximal osseous positions of the medial branch and L5 dorsal ramus nerves using this oblique view (Figs. 32-18, 32-19,

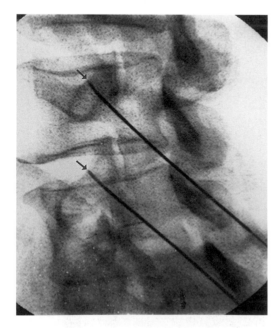

FIGURE 32-19. Oblique radiograph of an L3 and L4 medial branch neurotomy. The black arrows denote the superior junction of the transverse process and superior articular process where the nerve first rests in the targeted osseous groove.

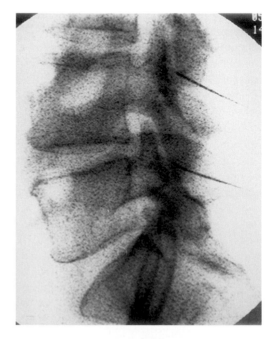

FIGURE 32-21. Lateral radiograph of the lumbar spine showing RF needles in place for an L3 and L4 medial branch neurotomy. Note that the needles are placed at the posterior margin of the foramen.

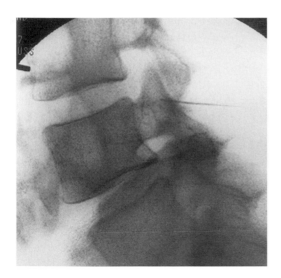

FIGURE 32-22. Lateral radiograph of the lumbar spine showing an RF needle in place for an L3 medial branch neurotomy. Note that the needle is placed at the posterior margin of the foramen.

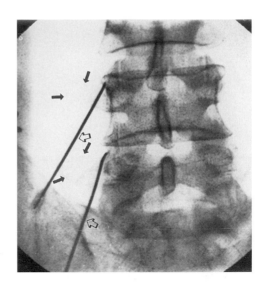

FIGURE 32-24. AP radiograph of an L3 and L4 medial branch neurotomy at the L4 and L5 transverse processes. The solid black arrows denote the superior and lateral margins of the transverse processes, and the open black arrows denote the skin starting positions.

and 32-20). The superior-proximal osseous position is at the proximal junction of the superior articular process and transverse process for the L1–L4 medial branch nerves, the proximal junction of the superior articular process of S1, and the sacral ala for the L5 dorsal ramus. A lateral view is then obtained to ensure the needles are placed no further anterior than the posterior aspect of the foramen (Figs. 32-21 and 32-22). The C-arm is then repositioned in an

AP projection to verify that the needles did not stray laterally while being advanced under oblique imaging (Figs. 32-23, 32-24, 32-25, and 32-26). If this occurred, the needles should be repositioned. With this technique, 10 mm of the target nerve is lesioned in a parallel fashion just proximal to the mamilloaccessory ligament.

Starting Position AP View

It is the experience of the authors that the groove view yields similar skin starting positions in relation to osseous landmarks on the AP image. In a majority of subsequent cases tested, starting at these common

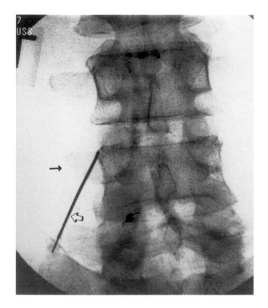

FIGURE 32-23. AP radiograph of an L3 medial branch neurotomy at the L4 transverse process. The solid black arrow denotes the lateral tip of the L4 transverse process, and the open black arrow denotes the skin starting position.

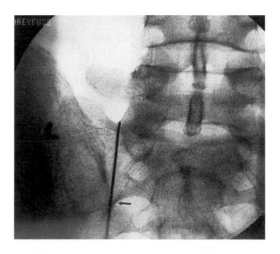

FIGURE 32-25. AP radiograph of an L5 dorsal ramus neurotomy. The black arrow denotes the skin starting position.

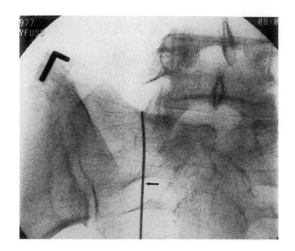

FIGURE 32-26. AP radiograph of an L5 dorsal ramus neurotomy. The black arrow denotes the skin starting position.

skin starting positions yielded appropriate parallel needle positioning without the need for the groove view. This was confirmed on AP, oblique, and lateral imaging. When effective, it reduces operator time and radiation exposure by removal of an additional view.

For L1–L4 medial branch nerve RF lesioning, the lateral skin starting position on AP imaging pertains to beginning "two-thirds" the distance of the lateral extension of the transverse process at the target level for long transverse processes and at the lateral extension of the transverse process for very short transverse processes. This difference is purely a judgment call by the operator. If the lateral silhouette of the superior articular process is large, it may impede medial and superior placement of the needle if the starting position is too far medial. In this scenario, one may need to start slightly more lateral regardless of the length of the transverse process, but almost never more lateral than the lateral aspect of the target transverse process. This decision also is best left to the experienced operator.

The inferior starting position pertains to just above the transverse process below the target level. For example, for an L3 medial branch nerve neurotomy, the needle is placed just above the L5 transverse process because this nerve resides at the L4 transverse process (see Figure 32-23). For the L4 medial branch nerve (at the L5 transverse process), the inferior starting position is just inside the posterior superior iliac crest and at the mid aspect of the S1 pedicle (see Figure 32-24).

For the L5 dorsal ramus the inferior needle position is just above the S2 pedicle and just lateral to a direct line that coincides with the lateral position of the target nerve. One must ensure advancing the

needle superiorly will not be impeded by the posterior superior articular process.

The needle is then advanced on AP imaging until it rests at the level of the mamilloaccessory ligament for the L1–L4 medial branch nerves or at the level of the inferior aspect of the L5–S1 zygapophyseal joint for the L5 dorsal ramus. After the needle is placed medial enough and it contacts bone, the C-arm is rotated to an oblique view. The needle should be seen to reside parallel to the target nerve in the osseous groove between the superior articular process and the transverse process just proximal to the mamilloaccessory ligament as occurs with use of the groove view. At the L5 dorsal ramus the needle should be seen to reside just superior to the inferior aspect of the L5–S1 zygapophyseal joint in its osseous groove. The needle is then advanced along the bone so that it remains medial enough to its final position as outlined in the declined view starting position section of this chapter.

Sacroiliac Joint

The following technique used by the authors has not been formally evaluated with either a retrospective or prospective study design. The authors believe that the following technique has theoretical advantages over the bipolar technique[70] to lesion the descending, multiple nerve twigs to the SIJ. The authors prefer to lesion not only the L5 dorsal ramus but also the stem of the lateral branches of the S1–S3 dorsal rami just lateral to the posterior sacral foramen. In this manner, the origin rather than the multiple distal twigs of the target nerves is lesioned. The L5 dorsal ramus and the lateral branches of S1 and S3 are chosen based on the consensus of recent anatomic findings of the dorsal innervation to the SIJ.[58,66,147]

The L5 dorsal ramus is lesioned as described earlier for lumbar zygapophyseal joint denervation (Fig. 32-27). The lateral branches of the S1–S3 dorsal rami are targeted within 5–10 mm of their exit from the posterior sacral foramen in an attempt to lesion the stem of the nerve. After this point, the S1–S3 lateral branches anastomose with each other within the multifidus compartment on the floor of the sacral gutter.[147] The lateral branches of the S1–S3 dorsal rami can exit at multiple angles from the posterior sacral foramen and are not consistent in their osseous relationship like the lumbar medial branch nerves.[147] The lateral branches leave the sacral posterior foramen at the 7–10 o'clock positions of the foramen as viewed as a clock face on the left side.[147] For this reason, the 7, half past 8, and 10 o'clock positions are used as the three target sites for lateral branch RF neurotomy at the left S1–S3 levels. In

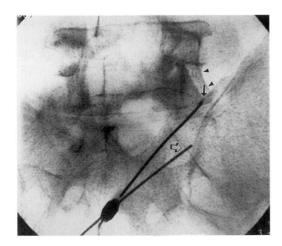

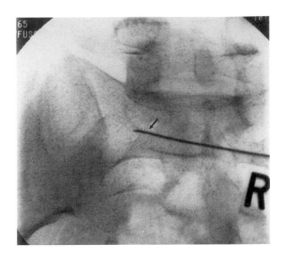

FIGURE 32-27. Oblique radiograph of an L5 dorsal ramus neurotomy and an S1 lateral branch neurotomy. The S1 RF needle is placed at the half past 8 o'clock position of the target nerve. The black arrowheads denote the lateral margin of the L5 vertebral body, which can at times be confused with the lateral edge of the L5–S1 z-joint. The longer, solid black arrow denotes the superior junction of the transverse process and superior articular process. The open, black arrow denotes the S1 posterior foramen.

FIGURE 32-28. AP radiograph of an S1 lateral branch neurotomy. The needle is placed at the 7 o'clock position. The black arrow denotes the S1 posterior foramen.

this way, the lateral branch stem should be lesioned within its variable exiting location.

AP imaging is obtained and the approximate target sites should be chosen. The posterior foramen should be viewed as one would image for cannulation of this foramen via a selective epidural or nerve root block technique. A 20-gauge, 10-mm exposed tip needle with a slight curve (10°) is placed from the midline in an angle that corresponds in parallel fashion to the 8:30 target location for the left side (See Figure 32-27). With this approach, the needle lies approximately

parallel to the target nerve and this angulation should prevent entry into and through the posterior foramen. The sacrum should be contacted at or just before the posterior foramen. The needle is then "walked" off laterally along the presumed nerve location at the 8:30 position while feeling the sacrum inferiorly until the distal end of the 10-mm exposed tip lies at the lateral aspect of the posterior foramen. Subsequent AP and lateral imaging confirms that the needle is placed on the dorsum of the sacrum and not in the sacral canal. Motor stimulation confirms the position before lesioning. Lesioning is performed and then the needle is placed to the remaining two target positions (7 and 10 o'clock) upon redirectioning from the same skin insertion site (Figs. 32-28, 32-29, and 32-30). Thus,

FIGURE 32-29. AP radiograph of an S1 lateral branch neurotomy. The needle is placed at the "10 o'clock" position. The black arrow denotes the S1 posterior foramen.

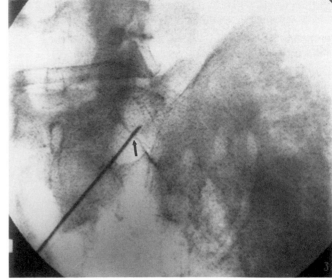

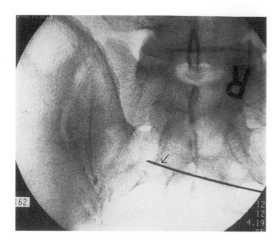

FIGURE 32-30. AP radiograph of an S2 lateral branch neurotomy. The needle is placed at the 7 o'clock position in relation to the posterior S2 foramen. The black arrow denotes the S2 posterior foramen.

three claw-like lesions are performed just lateral to each targeted posterior sacral foramen.

Postoperative Management

After the RF procedure is completed, the patient is not allowed to drive him- or herself home because of potential effects of lidocaine extravasation for medial branch anesthetization prior to neurotomy. Furthermore, many patients receive IV conscious sedation.

Following the procedure, patients may note increased soreness and local pain, which is especially prevalent in the first 3–5 days and usually abates within 10–14 days. Pain is easily managed with oral analgesics in the first 7–10 days. Patients may return to their usual daily activities the day after the procedure.

Generally, the authors endorse progression of patients' activities of daily living with inclusion of spinal strengthening and aerobics after the patient's pain is reduced to a manageable level that does not interfere with activity. No particular occupational or sport-related restrictions are placed on any patient after a successful RF neurotomy.

Complications

Rarely, patients may notice cutaneous related pain after the usual postoperative period, such as itching, burning, and hypersensitivity. This is more common in the cervical spine, especially with TON lesions.[79,90] When it occurs it is transient and usually subsides in approximately 4–6 weeks.[90] Tricyclic antidepressants can be very helpful for this condition,

as can gabapentin. Transient ataxia has been reported with TON neurotomy.[79] No long-term complications or serious adverse effects have been described with zygapophyseal or sacroiliac joint RF techniques, with the exception of one case report of presumed transection of the lateral branch(es) of the dorsal ramus at upper (L1–L3) levels from an RF neurotomy procedure, which resulted in a neuralgia-like pain syndrome.[14]

A recurrent concern at conferences on this topic is whether medial branch neurotomy causes Charcot's arthropathy.[44] This is not a valid concern. Notwithstanding the fact that Charcot's arthropathy involves vascular mechanisms rather than denervation,[2] it should be noted that Charcot's arthropathy classically affects the knee in the context of an entire lower limb without nociceptive innervation. Although medial branch neurotomy denervates a zygapophyseal joint, that segment is not totally denervated, nor is it rendered unstable. The disc of the segment remains intact and innervated, as do most of the muscles acting on the segment. Given that each lumbar medial branch is distributed to a single segmental band of multifidus,[21,84,123] medial branch neurotomy denervates not more than 20% of the multifidus per nerve coagulated. The erector spinae remains unaffected. Moreover, despite a 90.5% denervation rate of effected multifidi muscle fascicles, in one study no patient at 12-months follow-up exhibited any symptoms suggestive of "instability" or of disability that may be attributed to impaired function of the multifidus.[38] Furthermore, functional lift tasks remained the same or slightly improved (due to decreased pain) after RF neurotomy.

Patients frequently ask, "Will I be injured if I exert myself and I can't feel my spinal joints?" There is no report of injuries to insensate zygapophyseal joints with any technique, and the authors have never witnessed such an event. The spinal segment remains primarily innervated and possesses the necessary protective pain receptors and reflexes.

WHAT IF THE RF NEUROTOMY PROCEDURES FAILS?

The first question that should be asked is: Was the procedure a technical failure? The best way to determine this is with post-RF multifidi EMG. If no denervation potentials are appreciated, then technical failure occurred. The procedure should be repeated by alternative means, which usually implies the use of a larger needle electrode (e.g., a Ray electrode if a 20-gauge was previously used) and multiple lesions to account for anatomic variability in the course of the target nerve. If the above fails or the EMG was technically successful, then alternative pain generators should be pursued, such as intrinsic disc-mediated pain.

LONG-TERM MANAGEMENT

Although outcomes past the 12-month postprocedure period have not been formally performed, studies suggest that the therapeutic effect of RF neurotomy tends to diminish with time.[56,83,95,135,143] Only one study demonstrates the success of repeat RF neurotomies. An audit of 83 cervical medial branch neurotomy procedures found that if the first procedure provided complete relief for greater than 90 days, then repeat neurotomies had an 82% success rate.[78] No such data exist for the thoracic, lumbar, or sacral regions. The anecdotal experience of the authors is that pain relief following RF neurotomy for zygapophyseal joint pain continues for at least 12–14 months in the lumbar spine and 9–12 months in the cervical and thoracic spine. A large portion of patients, however, may not have recurrence of their pain even after 2–3 years. Anecdotally, the authors have repeated lumbar and thoracic RF neurotomies with equal success in most, but not all, cases.

CONCLUSION

Radiofrequency denervation of the medial branch nerves is a safe and effective treatment option for patients with persistent cervical and lumbar zygapophyseal joint pain after other noninvasive treatments and natural history have failed. Similar RF techniques hold promise for recalcitrant thoracic zygapophyseal and sacroiliac joint pain. Dual non–time contingent blocks with at least one block set representing medial branch blocks appear to best prognosticate relief with subsequent medial branch RF neurotomy. This treatment remains a viable option in the therapeutic armamentarium of the spine physician when used appropriately.

REFERENCES

1. Alberts WW, Wright EW, Feinstein B, von Bonin G: Experimental radiofrequency brain lesion size as a function of physical parameters. J Neurosurg 25:421–423, 1966.
2. Allman RM, Brower AC, Kotlyarov EB: Neuropathic bone and joint disease. Radiol Clin North Am 26:137–138, 1988.
3. Anderson K, Mosdal C, Vaernet K: Percutaneous radiofrequency facet denervation in low back and extremity pain. Acta Neurochir 87:48–51, 1987.
4. Banerjee T, Pittman H: Facet rhizotomy: Another armamentarium for treatment of low backache. N C Med J 37:354–360, 1976.
5. Barnsley L, Bogduk N: Medial branch blocks are specific for the diagnosis of cervical zygapophyseal joint pain. Reg Anesth 18:343–350, 1993.
6. Barnsley L, Lord S, Bogduk N: Comparative local anaesthetic blocks in the diagnosis of cervical zygapophyseal joint pain. Pain 55:99–106, 1993.
7. Barnsley L, Lord SM, Wallis BJ, et al: The prevalence of chronic cervical zygapophyseal joint pain after whiplash. Spine 20:20–26, 1995.
8. Barnsley L, Lord S, Wallis B, Bogduk N: False-positive rates of cervical zygapophyseal joint blocks. Clin J Pain 9:124–130, 1993.
9. Bastron JA, Thomas JE: Diabetic polyradiculopathy: Clinical and electromyographic findings in 105 patients. Mayo Clin Proc 56:725–732, 1981.
10. Bogduk N: The clinical anatomy of the cervical dorsal rami. Spine 7:319–330, 1982.
11. Bogduk N, Marsland A: On the concept of third occipital headache. J Neurol Neurosurg Psychiatry 49:775–780, 1986.
12. Bogduk N: International Spinal Injection Society Guidelines for the performance of spinal injection procedures. Part 1: Zygapophyseal joint blocks. Clin J Pain 13:285–302, 1997.
13. Bogduk N: Innervation of the lumbar spine. Spine 8:286–293, 1983.
14. Bogduk N: Lumbar lateral branch neuralgia: A complication of rhizolysis. Med J Aust 1:242–243, 1981.
15. Bogduk N, Aprill C, Derby R: Diagnostic blocks of spinal synovial joints. In White AH (ed): Spine Care Diagnosis and Conservative Treatment, Vol. 1. St. Louis, Mosby, 1995, pp 298–321.
16. Bogduk N, Long D: The anatomy of so-called articular nerves and their relationship to facet denervation in the treatment of low back pain. J Neurosurg 51:172–177, 1979.
17. Bogduk N, Long DM: Percutaneous lumbar medial branch neurotomy. A modification of facet denervation. Spine 5:193–200, 1980.
18. Bogduk N, Macintosh J, Marsland A: Technical limitations to the efficacy of radiofrequency neurotomy for spinal pain. Neurosurgery 20:529–535, 1987.
19 Bogduk N, Twomey LT: Clinical Anatomy of the Lumbar Spine, 2nd ed. London, Churchill Livingstone, 1991.
20. Bogduk N, Valencia F: Innervation and pain patterns of the thoracic spine. In Grant R (ed): Physical Therapy of the Cervical and Thoracic Spine. Edinburgh, Churchill Livingstone, 1988, pp 27–37.
21. Bogduk N, Wilson AS, Tynan W: The human lumbar dorsal rami. J Anat 134:383–397, 1982.
22. Bradley KC: The anatomy of backache. Aust N Z J Surg 44:227–232, 1974.
23. Brodkey J, Miyazaki I, Ervin F, Mark V: Reversible heat lesions: A method of stereotactic localization. J Neurosurg 21:49, 1964.
24. Burton C: Percutaneous radiofrequency facet denervation. Appl Neurophysiol 39:80–86, 1976–77.
25. Cosman B, Cosman E: RFG-3C Lesion Generator Operator's Manual, Version B, Appendix H. Burlington, MA, Radionics, 1995.
26. Chua W, Bogduk N: The surgical anatomy of thoracic facet denervation. Acta Neurochir 136:140–144, 1995.
27. Chua WH: Clinical Anatomy of the Thoracic Dorsal Rami [thesis]. Newcastle, Australia, University of Newcastle, 1994.
28. Cole A, Dreyfuss P, Stratton S: The sacroiliac joint: A functional approach. Crit Rev Phys Med Rehabil 8:125–152, 1996.

29. Czrny JJ, Lawrence J: Importance of paraspinal muscle electromyography in cervical and lumbosacral myopathies. Am J Phys Med Rehabil 74:458–459, 1995.

30. Demirel T: [Experience with percutaneous facet neurectomy]. [German]. Medizinische Welt 31:1096–1098, 1980.

31. Derby R, Bogduk N, Schwarzer A: Precision percutaneous blocking procedures for localizing spinal pain. Part 1: The posterior lumbar compartment. Pain Digest 3:89–100, 1993.

32. Dolan AL, Ryan PJ, Arden NK, et al: The value of SPECT scans in identifying back pain likely to benefit from facet joint injection. Br J Rheum 35:1269–1273, 1996.

33. Dreyer SJ, Dreyfuss P, Cole A: Zygapophyseal (facet) joint injections: Intra-articular and medial branch block techniques. Phys Med Rehabil Clin North Am 6:715–742, 1995.

34. Dreyer S, Dreyfuss P, Cole A: Posterior elements (facet and sacroiliac joints) and low back pain. Phys Med Rehabil State Art Rev 13:443–471, 1999.

35. Dreyfuss P: Differential diagnosis of thoracic pain and diagnostic/therapeutic injection options. Int Spinal Injection Soc Sci Newsl 2(6):10–29, 1997.

36. Dreyfuss PH, Dreyer SJ, Herring SA: Contemporary concepts in spine care: Lumbar zygapophyseal (facet) joint injections. Spine 20:2040–2047, 1995.

37. Dreyfuss P, Dreyer S: Lumbar facet injections. In Gonzalez EG, Materson RS (ed): The Nonsurgical Management of Acute Low Back Pain. New York, Demos Vermande, 1997, pp 123–136.

38. Dreyfuss P, Halbrook B, Pauza K, et al: Lumbar radiofrequency neurotomy for chronic zygapophyseal joint pain: A pilot study using dual medial branch blocks. Int Spinal Injection Soc Sci Newsl 3(2):13–31, 1999.

38a. Dreyfuss P, Halbrook B, Pauza K, et al: Efficacy and validity of radiofrequency neurotomy for chronic lumbar zygapophyseal joint pain. Spine [in press].

39. Dreyfuss P, Michaelsen M, Horne M: MUJA: Manipulation under joint anesthesia/analgesia: A treatment approach for recalcitrant low back pain of synovial joint origin. J Manipulative Physiol Ther 18:537–546, 1995.

40. Dreyfuss P, Michaelsen M, Pauza K, et al: The value of medical history and physical examination in diagnosing sacroiliac joint pain. Spine 21:2594–2602, 1996.

41. Dreyfuss P, Schwarzer A, Lau P, et al: The target specificity of lumbar medial branch and L5 dorsal ramus blocks. A computed tomography study. Spine 22:895–902, 1997.

42. Dreyfuss P, Tibiletti C, Dreyer S: Thoracic zygapophyseal joint pain patterns: A study in normal volunteers. Spine 19:807–811, 1994.

43. Dreyfuss P, Tibiletti C, Dreyer S, Sobel J: Thoracic zygapophyseal joint pain: A review and description of an intraarticular block technique. Pain Digest 4:44–52, 1994.

44. Drinka PJ, Jaschob K: Treatment of chronic cervical zygapophyseal joint pain. N Engl J Med 336:1530–1531, 1997.

45. Dwyer A, Aprill C, Bogduk N: Cervical zygapophyseal joint pain patterns 1: A study in normal volunteers. Spine 15:453–457, 1990.

46. Fassio B, Bouvier J, Ginestie J: Denervation articulaire posterieure per-cutanee et chirurgicale. Sa place dans le traitement des lombalgies. Rev Chir Orthop 67(suppl 11):131–136, 1980.

47. Finch PM, Racz GB, McDaniel KZ: A curved approach to nerve blocks and radiofrequency lesioning. Pain Digest 7:251–257, 1997.

48. Fisher MA, Kaur D, Houchins J: Electrodiagnostic examination, back pain, and entrapment of posterior rami. Electromyogr Clin Neurophysiol 25:183–189, 1985.

49. Florez G, Elias J, Ucar S: Percutaneous rhizotomy of the articular nerve of Luschka for low back and sciatic pain. Acta Neurochir Suppl 24:67–71, 1977.

50. Fortin JD, Dwyer AP, West S, Pier J: Sacroiliac joint: Pain referral maps upon applying a new injection/arthrography technique. Part I: Asymptomatic volunteers. Spine 19:1475–1482, 1994.

51. Fox J, Rizzoli H: Identification of radiologic co-ordinates for the posterior articular nerve of Luschka in the lumbar spine. Surg Neurol 1:343–346, 1976.

52. Fuentes E: La Neurotomia apofisaria transcutanea en el tratamento de la lumbalgia cronica. Rev Med Chile 106:440–443, 1978.

53. Fukui S, Ohseto K, Shiotani M: Patterns of pain induced by distending the thoracic zygapophyseal joints. Reg Anesth 22:332–336, 1997.

54. Fukui S, Ohseto K, Shiotani M, et al: Referred pain distribution of the cervical zygapophyseal joints and cervical dorsal rami. Pain 68:79–83, 1996.

55. Fukui S, Ohseto K, Shiotani M, et al: Distribution of referred pain from the lumbar zygapophyseal joints and dorsal rami. Clin J Pain 13:303–307, 1997.

56. Gallagher J, Petriccione di Vadi P, Wedley J, et al: Radiofrequency facet joint denervation in the treatment of low back pain: A prospective controlled double-blind study to assess its efficacy. Pain Clin 7:193–198, 1994.

57. Golcer A, Cetinalp E, Tuna M, et al: Percutaneous radiofrequency rhizotomy of lumbar spinal facets: The results of 46 cases. Neurosurg Rev 20:114–116, 1997.

58. Grob KR, Neuhuber WL, Kissling RO: Die innervation des sacroiliacalgelenkes beim Menschen. Zeitschr Rheumatol 27:117–122, 1995.

59. Haig AJ: Clinical experience with paraspinal mapping II: A simplified technique that eliminates three-fourths of needle insertions. Arch Phys Med Rehabil 78:1185–1190, 1997.

60. Haig AJ, Moffroid M, Henry S, et al: A technique for needle localization in paraspinal muscles with cadaveric confirmation. Muscle Nerve 14:521–526, 1991.

61. Haig AJ, Parks TJ: Paraspinal muscles: Anatomy and electrodiagnostic testing in the cervical and lumbar regions. Phys Med Rehabil Clin North Am 5:447–463, 1994.

62. Hickey RFJ, Tregonning GD: Denervation of spinal facets for treatment of chronic low back pain. N Z Med J 85:96–99, 1977.

63. Hildebrandt J, Argyrakis A: Percutaneous nerve block of the cervical facets: A relatively new method in the treatment of chronic headache and neck pain. Manual Med 2:48–52, 1986.

64. Hirsch D, Ingelmark B, Miller M: The anatomical basis for low back pain. Acta Orthop Scand 33:1–17, 1963.

65. Ignelzi RJ, Cummings TW: A statistical analysis of percutaneous radiofrequency lesions in the treatment of chronic low back pain and sciatica. Pain 8:181–187, 1980.

66. Ikeda R: Innervation of the sacroiliac joint. Macroscopic and histological studies. J Nippon Med School 58:587–596, 1991.

67. Kaplan M, Dreyfuss P, Halbrook B, Bogduk N: The ability of lumbar medial branch blocks to anesthetize the zygapophyseal rhizotomy of lumbar spinal joint: A physiologic challenge. Spine 23:1847– 1852, 1998.

68. Katz SS, Savitz MH: Percutaneous radiofrequency rhizotomy of the lumbar facets. Mt Sinai J Med 7:523–525, 1986.

69. King J, Lagger R: Sciatica viewed as a referred pain syndrome. Surg Neurol 5:46–50, 1976.

70. Kline MT: Radiofrequency techniques in clinical practice. In Waldman S, Winnie A (eds): Interventional Pain Management. Philadelphia, W.B. Saunders, 1996, pp 185–217.

71. Koning HM, Mackie DP: Percutaneous radiofrequency facet denervation in low back pain. Pain Clin 7:199–204, 1994.

72. Kuruoglu R, Oh SJ, Thompson B: Clinical and electromyographic correlations of lumbosacral radiculopathies. Muscle Nerve 17:250–251, 1994.

73. Kuslich S, Ulstrom C, Michael C: The tissue origin of low back pain and sciatica: A report of pain response to tissue stimulation during operations on the lumbar spine using local anesthesia. Orthop Clin North Am 22:181–187, 1991.

74. Lippet A: The facet joint and its role in spine pain. Spine 9:764, 1984.

75. Lora J, Long DM: So-called facet denervation in the management of intractable back pain. Spine 1:121–126, 1976.

76. Lord SM: Cervical Zygapophyseal Joint Pain after Whiplash Injury: Precision Diagnosis, Prevalence, and Evaluation of Treatment by Percutaneous Radiofrequency Neurotomy [doctoral thesis]. Newcastle, Australia, University of Newcastle, 1996.

77. Lord SM, Barnsley L, Bogduk N: Cervical zygapophyseal joint pain in whiplash injuries. Spine State Art Rev 12:301–322, 1998.

78. Lord SM, McDonald GJ, Bogduk N: The repeatability of percutaneous radiofrequency neurotomy for cervical zygapophyseal joint pain: An audit of 83 procedures [abstract]. In Proceedings of the Australians Anesthesia Society Congress. Hobart, Australia, AAS, 1997, p 67.

79. Lord S, Barnsley L, Bogduk N: Percutaneous radiofrequency neurotomy in the treatment of cervical zygapophyseal joint pain: A caution. Neurosurgy 36:732–739, 1995.

80. Lord S, Barnsley L, Bogduk N: The utility of comparative local anesthetic blocks versus placebo-controlled blocks for the diagnosis of cervical zygapophyseal joint pain. Clin J Pain 11:208–213, 1995.

81. Lord S, Barnsley L, Wallis B, et al: Third occipital nerve headache: A prevalence study. J Neurol Neurosurg Psychiatry 57:1187–1190, 1994.

82. Lord S, Barnsley L, Wallis BJ, et al: Chronic cervical zygapophyseal joint pain after whiplash: A placebo-controlled prevalence study. Spine 22:1737–1744, 1996.

83. Lord S, Barnsley L, Wallis B, et al: Percutaneous radiofrequency neurotomy for chronic cervical zygapophyseal joint pain. N Engl J Med 335:1721–1726, 1996.

84. Macintosh JE, Valencia F, Bogduk N, Munro RR: The morphology of the human lumbar multifidus. Clin Biomech 1:196–204, 1986.

85. Maigne JY, Aivalikilis A, Pfefer F: Results of sacroiliac joint double block and value of sacroiliac pain provocation tests in 54 patients with low back pain. Spine 21:1889–1892, 1996.

86. Maigne JY, Boulahdour H, Chatellier G: Value of quantitative radionuclide bone scanning in the diagnosis of sacroiliac joint syndrome in 32 patients with low back pain. Eur Spine J 7:328–331, 1998.

87. McCall IW: Induced pain referral from posterior lumbar elements in normal subjects. Spine 4:441–446, 1979.

88. McCulloch J, Organ L: Percutaneous radiofrequency lumbar rhizolysis (rhizotomy). Can Med Assoc J 116:30–32, 1977.

89. McCulloch JA: Percutaneous radiofrequency lumbar rhizolysis (rhizotomy). Appl Neurophysiol 39:87–96, 1976–77.

90. McDonald G, Govind J, Lord S, Bogduk N: Percutaneous radiofrequency neurotomy for C2–3 zygapophyseal joint pain. In Proceedings of the Combined Meeting of the International Spinal Injection Society and the Australasian Faculty of Musculoskeletal Medicine. Sydney, Australia, ISIS/AFMM, 1998, pp 14–15.

91. Mehta M, Sluijter M: The treatment of chronic low back pain. Anaesthesia 34:768–775, 1979.

92. Mooney V, Robertson J: The facet syndrome. Clin Orthop 115:149–156, 1976.

93. Moringlane JR, Koch R, Schafer H, Ostertag CHB: Experimental radiofrequency coagulation with computer-based on line monitoring of temperature and power. Acta Neurochir 96:126–131, 1989.

94. North R, Kidd D, Zahurak M, Piantadosi S: Specificity of diagnostic nerve blocks: A prospective, randomized study of sciatica due to lumbosacral spine disease. Pain 65:77–85, 1996.

95. North RB, Han M, Zahurak M, Kidd DH: Radiofrequency lumbar facet denervation: Analysis of prognostic factors. Pain 57:77–83, 1994.

96. Ogsbury JS, Simon RH, Lehman RAW: Facet denervation in the treatment of low back syndrome. Pain 3:257–263, 1977.

97. Oudenhoven R: Articular rhizotomy. Surg Neurol 2:275–278, 1974.

98. Oudenhoven R: Paraspinal electromyography following facet rhizotomy. Spine 2:299–304, 1977.

99. Oudenhoven R: The role laminectomy, facet rhizotomy and epidural steroids. Spine 4:145–147, 1979.

100. Pawl R: Results in the treatment of low back syndrome from sensory neurolysis of lumbar facets (facet rhizotomy) by thermal coagulation. Proc Inst Med Chicago 30:150–151, 1974.

101. Rashbaum R: Radiofrequency facet denervation. A treatment alternative in refractory low back pain with or without leg pain. Orthop Clin North Am 14:569–575, 1983.

102. Raymond J, Dumas JM, Lisbona R: Nuclear imaging as a screening test for patients referred for intra-articular facet block. J Can Assoc Radiol 35:291–292, 1984.

103. Rees W: Multiple bilateral subcutaneous rhizolysis of segmental nerves in the treatment of the intervertebral disc syndrome. Ann Gen Pract 26:126–127, 1971.

104. Saberski LR: Cryoneurolysis in clinical practice. In Waldman S, Winnie A (eds): Interventional Pain Management. Philadelphia, W.B. Saunders, 1996, pp 172–184.

105. Savitz M: Percutaneous radiofrequency rhizotomy of the lumbar facets: Ten years experience. Mt Sinai J Med 58:177–178, 1991.

106. Schaerer J: Radiofrequency facet rhizotomy in the treatment of chronic neck and low back pain. Int Surg 63:53–59, 1978.

107. Schaerer JP: Radiofrequency facet denervation in the treatment of persistent headache associated with chronic neck pain. J Neurol Orthop Surg 1:127–130, 1980.

108. Schaerer JP: Treatment of prolonged neck pain by radiofrequency facet rhizotomy. J Neurol Orthop Med Surg 9:74–76, 1988.

109. Schuster GD: The use of cryoanalgesia in the painful facet syndrome. J Neurol Orthop Surg 3:271–274, 1982.

110. Schwarzer AC, Aprill CN, Bogduk N: The sacroiliac joint in chronic low back pain. Spine 20:31–37, 1995.

111. Schwarzer AC, Aprill CN, Fortin J, et al: The relative contributions of the disc and zygapophyseal joint in chronic low back pain. Spine 19:801–806, 1994.

112. Schwarzer A, Aprill C, Derby R, et al: The false positive rate of uncontrolled diagnostic blocks of the lumbar zygapophyseal joints. Pain 58:195–200, 1994.

113. Schwarzer AC, Derby R, Aprill CN, et al: Pain from the lumbar zygapophyseal joints: A test of two models. J Spinal Disord 7:331–336, 1994.

114. Schwarzer AC, Aprill CN, Derby R, et al: Clinical features of patients with pain stemming from the lumbar zygapophyseal joints. Is the lumbar facet syndrome a clinical entity? Spine 19:1132–1137, 1994.

115. Schwarzer AC, Scott AM, Wang S, et al: The role of bone scintigraphy in chronic low back pain: Comparison of SPECT and planar images and zygapophyseal joint injection. Aust N Z J Med 22:185, 1992.

116. Schwarzer AC, Wang SC, Bogduk N, et al: Prevalence and clinical features of lumbar zygapophyseal joint pain: A study in an Australian population with chronic low back pain. Ann Rheum Dis 54:100–106, 1995.

117. Schwarzer AC, Wang S, O'Driscoll D, et al: The ability of computed tomography to identify a painful zygapophyseal joint in patients with chronic low back pain. Spine 20:907–912, 1995.

118. Shealy CN: Facets in back and sciatic pain. Minn Med 57:199–203, 1974.
119. Shealy C: Percutaneous radio frequency denervation of spinal facets. J Neurosurg 43:448–451, 1975.
120. Shealy C: Facet denervation in the management of back and sciatic pain. Clin Orthop 115:157–164, 1976.
121. Shealy C: The role of the spinal facets in back and sciatic pain. Headache 14:101–104, 1974.
122. Shearer J: Radiofrequency facet rhizotomy in the treatment of chronic neck and low back pain. Int Surg 63:53–59, 1978.
123. Shindo H: Anatomical study of the lumbar multifidus muscle and its innervation in human adults and fetuses. Nippon Ika Daigaku Zasshi 62:439–446, 1995.
124. Sihvonen T, Lindgren KA, Airaksinen O, et al: Dorsal ramus irritation associated with recurrent low back pain and its relief with local anesthetic or training therapy. J Spinal Disorders 8:8–14, 1995.
125. Silvers H: Lumbar percutaneous facet rhizotomy. Spine 15:36–40, 1990.
126. Sjaastad O, Fredriksen T, Pfaffenrath V: Cervicogenic headache: Diagnostic criteria. Headache 30:725–726, 1990.
127. Slipman CW, Sterenfeld EB, Chou LH, et al: The value of radionuclide imaging in the diagnosis of sacroiliac joint syndrome. Spine 21:2251–2254, 1996.
128. Slipman CW, Sterenfeld EB, Chou LH, et al: The predictive value of provocative sacroiliac stress maneuvers in the diagnosis of sacroiliac joint syndrome. Arch Phys Med Rehabil 79:288–292, 1998.
129. Silvers R: Lumbar percutaneous facet rhizotomy. Spine 15:36–40, 1990.
130. Sluijter ME, Koetsveld-Baart CC: Interruption of pain pathways in the treatment of the cervical syndrome. Anaesthesia 35:302–307, 1980.
131. Sluijter M, Mehta M: Treatment of chronic back and neck pain by percutaneous thermal lesions. In Lipton S, Miles J (eds): Persistent Pain: Modern Methods of Treatment, Vol 3. London, Academic Press, 1981, pp 141–179.
132. Solonen KA: The sacroiliac joint in light of anatomical, roentgenological, and clinical studies. Acta Orthop Scand Suppl 27:1–127, 1957.
133. Stolker R, Vervest A: Pain Management by Radiofrequency Procedures in the Cervical and Thoracic Spine: A Clinical and Anatomical Study. Utrecht, University of Utrecht Press, 1994, pp 1–187.
134. Stolker R, Vervest A, Groen G: The management of chronic spinal pain by blockades: A review. Pain 58:1–20, 1994.
135. Stolker RJ, Vervest A, Groen G: Percutaneous facet denervation in chronic thoracic spinal pain. Acta Neurochir (Wien) 122:82–90, 1993.
136. Stolker R, Vervest A, Groen G: Parameters in electrode positioning in thoracic percutaneous facet denervation: An anatomical study. Acta Neurochir 128:32–39, 1994.
137. Strohbehn J: Temperature distributions from interstitial RF electrode hyperthermia systems: Theoretical predictions. Int J Radiat Oncol Biol Phys 9:1655–1667, 1983.
138. Suseki K, Takahashi Y, Takahashi K, et al: Innervation of the lumbar facet joints. Origins and functions. Spine 22:477–485, 1997.
139. Travell J, Simons D: Myofascial Pain and Dysfunction. The Trigger Point Manual. Baltimore, Williams & Wilkins, 1983.
140. Uematsu S, Udvarhelyo G, Benson D: Percutaneous radiofrequency rhizotomy. Surg Neurol 2:319–325, 1974.
141. Uyttendaele D, Verhamme J, Vercauteren M: Local block of lumbar facet joints and percutaneous radiofrequency denervation. Preliminary results. Acta Orthop Belg 47:135–139, 1981.
142. Van Kleef M, Barendse G, Kessels A, et al: Randomised trial of radiofrequency lumbar facet denervation for chronic low back pain. Spine 24:1937–1942, 1999.
143. Van Suijlekom HA, Van Kleef M, Barendse G, et al: Radiofrequency cervical zygapophyseal joint neurotomy for cervicogenic headache: A prospective study of 15 patients. Funct Neurol 13:297–303, 1998.
144. Vervest A, Stolker R: The treatment of cervical pain syndromes with radiofrequency procedures. Pain Clin 4:103–112, 1991.
145. Vinas F, Zamorano L, Dujovny M, et al: In vivo and in vitro study of the lesions produced with a computerized radiofrequency system. Stereotact Funct Neurosurg 58:121–133, 1992.
146. Von Bonin G, Alberts WW, Wright EW, Feinstein B: Radiofrequency brain lesions. Arch Neurol 12:25–29, 1965.
147. Willard FH, Carreiro JE, Manko W: The long posterior interosseous ligament and the sacrococcygeal plexus. In Proceedings of the Third Interdisciplinary World Congress on Low Back and Pelvic Pain. Vienna, Austria, 1998.

Index

Entries in **boldface** type indicate complete chapters.